Confronting Alzheimer's Disease and Other Dementias

**OFFICE OF TECHNOLOGY
ASSESSMENT TASK FORCE**

Robert M. Cook-Deegan, Project Director
Nancy Mace, Consultant in Gerontology
Mary Ann Baily, George Washington University
David Chavkin, Maryland Disability Law Center
Catherine Hawes, Research Triangle Institute,
    North Carolina

 Science Information Resource Center

 **J.B. LIPPINCOTT COMPANY
PHILADELPHIA**

London   Mexico City   New York   St. Louis   São Paulo   Sydney

Authorized Hardbound Edition, 1988

Science Information Resource Center
East Washington Square
Philadelphia, Pennsylvania 19105

Publisher's Note:

This permanent edition contains the complete text of
the Office of Technology Assessment Special Report
entitled *Losing a Million Minds—Confronting the Tragedy of Alzheimer's Disease and Other Dementias.* Under
the direction of the OTA Dementia Project Staff and
with the help of a distinguished Advisory Panel more
than 10,000 pages of existing reports and 40 new
research papers were reviewed, distilled, and compiled
into this comprehensive volume.

Science Information Resource Center is a cooperative
venture of J.B. Lippincott Company and Hemisphere
Publishing Corporation, subsidiaries of Harper & Row,
Publishers, Inc., New York.

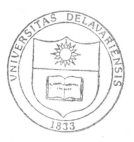

Library of Congress Cataloging-in-Publication Data
    Confronting Alzheimer's disease and other
dementias.
    Reprint. Originally published: Losing a million
minds. Washington, D.C. 1987.
    Includes bibliographies and index.
    1. Alzheimer's disease. 2. Dementia.
I. Cook-Deegan, Robert M. II. United States.
Congress. Office of Technology Assessment.
III. Title. [DNLM: 1. Alzheimer's Disease.
WM 220 L879 1987a]
RC523.L67   1988   618.97'683   87-26322
ISBN 0-397-53000-5

Foreword

Congressional concern about the plight of those suffering from Alzheimer's disease and other dementias has steadily mounted for the past five years. This report grew out of a previous OTA report on *Technology and Aging in America*; it was requested by the following seven committees:

- **U.S. Senate:**
  —Committee on Finance,
  —Committee on Labor and Human Resources,
  —Committee on Veterans' Affairs, and
  —Special Committee on Aging.
- **U.S. House of Representatives:**
  —Committee on Energy and Commerce,
  —Committee on Science and Technology, and
  —Select Committee on Aging.

In addition to the requesting committees, the House and Senate subcommittees that appropriate funds to the Department of Health and Human Services have frequently expressed interest, as have the Senate Committee on the Budget and the House Committee on Ways and Means. Members and staff of the requesting committees, other committees, and personal staff have been directly involved in identifying subjects that are covered in this report. The unusual length of this report is testimony to the diversity of issues associated with dementia that fall within the jurisdiction of various committees.

Writing this report involved collection of more than 10,000 pages of existing documents and preparation of more than 40 papers by outside experts under contract to OTA. Many of the OTA contract reports have been released to the National Technical Information Service or published elsewhere (see appendix C). OTA staff also gathered information through discussions with more than 130 congressional staff and hundreds of others—including government employees at the State and Federal levels and representatives of more than 100 nongovernment organizations in the United States and other countries. The resulting document has been reviewed by the project's advisory panel and more than 50 other experts in various relevant fields. More than one hundred other individuals have reviewed specific chapters or early drafts.

On behalf of OTA, I wish to express my thanks to the myriad of individuals who contributed either directly or indirectly to this study. It distills a mass of information into a form that I hope will be useful to policymakers. As with all OTA reports, however, the content is the sole responsibility of OTA and does not necessarily constitute consensus of or endorsement by the advisory panel or the congressional Technology Assessment Board.

JOHN H. GIBBONS
Director

Advisory Panel for OTA Assessment of Disorders Causing Dementia

Daniel Wikler, *Chairman*
Program in Medical Ethics, University of Wisconsin Medical School
Departments of Philosophy and History of Medicine

John Blass
Cornell University Medical College, and
  Director, Dementia Research Service
Burke Rehabilitation Center

Stanley Brody
University of Pennsylvania Medical School
Department of Physical Medicine and
  Rehabilitation, and
Wharton School of Finance

Donna Campbell
Veterans Administration
Geriatric Research and Education and Care
  Center
Bedford, MA

Gill Deford
National Senior Citizens Law Center
Los Angeles, CA

Karl Girshman
Hebrew Home of Greater Washington

Lisa Gwyther
Duke University Medical Center
Center for the Study of Aging and Human
  Development
Family Support Program

Thomas Jazwiecki
Office of Reimbursement and Financing
American Health Care Association

Purlaine Lieberman
Equitable Life Assurance Society of the United
  States

William Markesbery
Professor of Pathology and Neurology
University of Kentucky College of Medicine

Paul Nathanson
University of New Mexico
Institute of Public Law

Nancy Orr
Hillhaven Corporation Special Care Units

Diana Petty
Family Survival Project
San Francisco, CA

Dominick Purpura
Albert Einstein College of Medicine

Betty Ransom
National Institute on Adult Daycare, and
  National Center on Rural Aging
National Council on the Aging

Donald Schneider
Management Health Systems
Rensselaer Polytechnic Institute School of
  Management

Jerome Stone
President, Alzheimer's Disease and Related
  Disorders Association

Sallie Tisdale
Writer and Long-Term Care Nurse
Portland, OR

Ramon Valle
College of Human Services
San Diego State University

Philip Weiler
Department of Community Health, and
  Director, Center for Aging and Health,
  University of California, Davis, School of
  Medicine

Peter Whitehouse
Alzheimer's Neuroscience Center and
  Department of Neurology, Case Western
  Reserve School of Medicine; Division of
  Behavioral Neurology, University Hospitals
  of Cleveland

NOTE: OTA appreciates and is grateful for the valuable assistance and thoughtful critiques provided by the advisory panel
  members. The panel does not, however, necessarily approve, disapprove, or endorse this report. OTA assumes full
  responsibility for the report and the accuracy of its contents.

OTA Dementia Project Staff

Roger Herdman, *Assistant Director, OTA*
Health and Life Sciences Division

Gretchen S. Kolsrud, *Biological Applications Program Manager*

Robert M. Cook-Deegan, *Project Director*
Dana A. Gelb, *Research Analyst*
L. Val Giddings, *Analyst*
Katie Maslow, *Analyst*
Teresa S. Myers, *Research Analyst*

Authors Under Contract
Nancy Mace, Consultant in Gerontology, Towson, MD
Mary Ann Baily, George Washington University
David Chavkin, Maryland Disability Law Center
Catherine Hawes, Research Triangle Institute, North Carolina

Support Staff
Sharon Kay Oatman, *Administrative Assistant*
Linda Rayford, *Secretary*
Barbara Ketchum, *Secretary*
Bryan Harrison, *Office Automation Systems Analyst*

CONTENTS

Chapter 1
Dementia: Prospects and Policies

"It may be two or three decades before a favorable treatment is available. If this is so, developing increasingly efficient health care delivery grows in importance on a more immediate time scale."

—David Drachman
chairman of the Scientific Advisory Board,
Alzheimer's Disease and Related Disorders Association,
July 28, 1986.

" 'Old family values' do not need restoration simply because they have not diminished. The fact is that government and agency services supplement but do not supplant family services. . . . The evidence points unmistakably to the need for family-focused services to alleviate the burden of parent care. These are basic to all other efforts and can only be made available by social policy. . . . Alzheimer's patients are not eligible for "skilled" care [as defined by Medicare and Medicaid], though they need the most skilled care of all."

—Elaine Brody
before the Subcommittee on Health and Long-Term Care,
Select Committee on Aging, and
Subcommittee on Health and the Environment,
Committee on Energy and Commerce, U.S. House of Representatives,
Aug. 3, 1983.

"Most families are heroically fighting a devastating illness. Supporting them can be rewarding to professionals and, we believe, a legitimate goal for the Congress. We must be realistic and not oversell our abilities to dramatically cut costs or resolve problems, but cannot turn our backs on the families of 2 or 3 million people. Families can do so much for themselves; however, five things need the leadership of Congress:

1. ongoing support for research,
2. support for training of professionals,
3. provision of a variety of alternative respite services,
4. equitable funding for quality long-term care when it is necessary, and
5. equitable disability policies."

—Nancy Mace
before the Subcommittee on Health and Long-Term Care,
Select Committee on Aging, and
Subcommittee on Health and the Environment,
Committee on Energy and Commerce, U.S. House of Representatives,
Aug. 3, 1983.

CONTENTS

Tables

Figures

Dementia: Prospects and Policies

Disorders causing dementia—the loss of mental functions in an alert and awake individual—will constitute a large and growing public health problem until well into the next century. Today, an estimated 1.5 million Americans suffer from severe dementia—that is, they are so incapacitated that others must care for them continually. An additional 1 million to 5 million have mild or moderate dementia (27). Ten times as many people are affected now as were at the turn of the century (79). The number of people with severe dementia is expected to increase 60 percent by the year 2000. Unless cures or means of prevention are found for the common causes of dementia, 7.4 million Americans will be affected by the year 2040—five times as many as today (see figure 1-1). The middle line on figure 1-1 assumes no change over time in the probability of developing severe dementia at a given age, and it does not hinge on new births but rather projects cases of dementia based on those already born. Further increases in life expectancy would increase the number of cases expected, and finding means to prevent dementing disorders would lower it.

The public has only recently become aware of the problems posed by dementing illnesses. Dementia and Alzheimer's disease (AD) have become household words only in the last few years. Efforts of national organizations, such as the Alzheimer's Disease and Related Disorders Association (ADRDA), have emphasized the plight of families and publicized the problems faced by nationally famous individuals who have developed dementia (e.g., Rita Hayworth). The most prevalent disorder causing dementia, Alzheimer's disease, has risen from relative obscurity to the cover of *Newsweek* magazine, the pages of *Life*, and prime-time television ("Do You Remember Love?" a made-for-television movie aired by CBS in May 1985). One book on caring for patients with dementia, *The 36-Hour Day* (74), has sold over 500,000 copies, and several other books for the general public have found sizable audiences (21, 48,84).

Figure 1-1.—Current and Projected Cases of Severe Dementia in the United States, 1980-2040

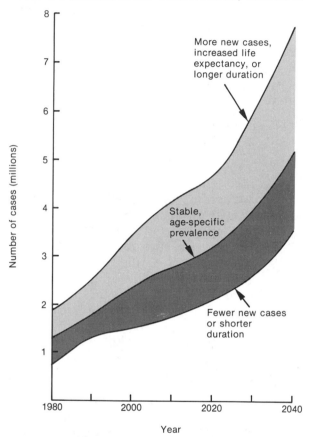

SOURCE: P.S. Cross and G.J. Gurland, "The Epidemiology of Dementing Disorders," contract report prepared for the Office of Technology Assessment, 1986.

Interest among health and social service professionals has risen in parallel with public awareness. Medical attention to Alzheimer's disease began to increase in the 1970s, catalyzed in 1976 by an editorial in a medical journal calling attention to the high prevalence and perniciousness of the disease (61) and by activities supported by various Federal research institutes (the National Institute on Aging, the National Institute on Neurological and Communicative Disorders and Stroke, and the National Institute of Mental Health). Dozens of professional books, special issues of professional journals, and symposia proceedings on problems related to dementia have appeared since then. Two new journals—the *American Journal of Alzheimer's Care*, for caregivers, and *Alzheimer's Disease and Associated Disorders: An International Journal*, for scientists and clinical investigators—deal specifically with this topic.

Professional recognition of the problems posed by dementia is also reflected in (and partly caused by) increased funding for biomedical research and training. Federally funded research on dementing conditions has increased from $3.9 million in 1976 to an estimated $67 million in 1987. Federal funding has been supplemented by support from nongovernment organizations and foundations such as ADRDA, the American Federation for Aging Research, and the John Douglas French Foundation on Alzheimer's Disease.

Most recently, policymakers have become concerned with problems related to dementia because of the substantial costs of dealing with the diseases, and the relatively poor financial coverage of long-term care services needed by individuals with dementia and their families (14).

GOALS OF PUBLIC POLICY RELATED TO DEMENTIA

Consensus on the goals of public policy related to dementia is necessary as a background for policy change. Policy goals presuppose a set of accepted premises. One such premise is that individuals with dementia should be accorded the same respect for their person that they could have expected if they had not lost mental abilities. This does not imply, however, that the same decisions will always be reached—decisions to forgo life-sustaining treatment, for example, may be more acceptable in the presence of irreversible dementia than without it.

Another common assumption is that the family has the best interests of a dependent person with dementia in mind, and the best available information about what the patient would have wished. This is not always the case, but it is a starting point for many medical, financial, and legal decisions, and puts the burden of proof on those who believe that the assumption is unwarranted in a particular case. A final assumption is that the government has some role in protecting the rights and health of an individual with dementia, although the proper degree of government involvement in financing, coordinating, and directly providing services is subject to debate.

The degree to which funds should be transferred from one generation to another is an underlying unresolved issue in many public policies. Transfers within families are generally left to the individuals involved, but many government programs either directly transfer funds from one group to another (e.g., Social Security and Medicare for older Americans, and education and recreation subsidies for the young) or attempt to enforce familial responsibilities in public programs (e.g., requiring spouses to pay expenses incurred under Medicaid). The care of dependent adults has been a traditional concern, but the aging of the population has brought out the uncertainties and lack of consensus much more forcefully in recent decades, and public policies reflect these tensions.

Overall policy goals can be roughly categorized into two groups: those intended to diminish the magnitude of the problem for future generations, and those directed at ameliorating problems already facing patients with dementia and those who care for them, which are relevant now and in the next few years. The long-term goals include searching for ways to eliminate the diseases causing dementia, or at least to diminish their severity and consequences. The ultimate solution for the problem of dementia would be a "technical fix"—a fully effective way to prevent all dementing diseases, or a drug or surgical procedure to reverse their symptoms. There is no assurance that such a solution is possible at all, and it is certainly not likely in the next several years. That does not detract from the long-term practical benefits of supporting research, but it does suggest that it would be unwise to rely exclusively on the hope of a cure for all the diseases. A balanced policy will ensure support for research combined with efforts to address existing problems—to deal with those who now have dementia or will develop it before there are technical means to prevent or eradicate it.

Near-term goals include training caregivers (family, volunteer, and professional), improving care practices in acute and long-term care, and devising means to pay for the catastrophic expenses brought on by dementing illness. Some policies can influence both immediate and long-term goals. Research on clinical care and service delivery, for example, can both improve current practice and assist future generations. Education raises general awareness and also improves the prospects for finding an ultimate solution.

Several general short-term goals are repeatedly stressed in the literature dealing with the care of persons with dementia, although they are rarely stated explicitly. Some of these objectives are:

- to preserve maximum independence of the affected individual;
- to provide a continuum of care—a full range of services available at different stages of ill-

ness and adaptable to changes in the individual's family, finances, and needs;
- to efficiently coordinate the provision of care to maximize the match between available services and the needs and preferences of the individual and the family;
- to preserve the dignity of the affected individual;
- to reduce the severity of symptoms;
- to treat medical problems that may worsen dementia or cause pain and suffering;
- to cultivate preserved abilities and reduce the adverse effects of lost abilities;
- to foster the integrity of the family and minimize family stress; and
- to distribute the catastrophic costs of caring for those with dementia across the population without encouraging overuse of publicly financed services.

Attaining these goals may not be possible in many cases, and consensus on how best to achieve them has proved elusive. The role of government in assuring quality and paying for long-term care, for example, is the subject of extensive debate, and current policies reflect this lack of consensus.

FEDERAL POLICY PRIORITIES

The Federal Government can influence the problems posed by disorders causing dementia in hundreds of ways, many of which are described in this report. Federal policy options range from direct intervention to indirect encouragement of others to act. The Federal Government can catalyze actions by State or local governments, citizens' groups, or private organizations (e.g., by disseminating information about dementia, services, or methods of caring for patients). In other areas, the Federal Government has a more direct or exclusive role (e.g., support for biomedical research). The ways in which the issues arising from dementing illness are addressed will be subject to political and technical debate, but the *objectives* of public policy are likely to revolve around these priorities:

- support for biomedical research,
- support for health services research,
- education,

- financing long-term care,
- patient assessment and coordination of services,
- increasing the range of services available, and
- assuring quality care.

Several of the priority areas overlap, and policies that affect one will necessarily have an impact on the others. Programs to educate consumers would, for example, depend on biomedical and health services for reliable information. Educated consumers would, in turn, be in a better position to assure quality care, obtain financing through existing mechanisms, plan their own finances prudently, and become knowledgeable about available services. Policies affecting financing would influence all other aspects of care because payment methods often determine the range of services made available; many observers believe, therefore, that policy change should focus first on financing. Yet no service system can work without all the pieces in place, including available trained personnel and mechanisms for coordinating services and assessing needs (whether formally or informally).

Policy changes on one front will thus need to be assessed for their overall impact. A balanced approach, with greatest efforts centering on those areas for which the Federal Government is most responsible, is most likely to lead to improved care.

ORGANIZATION OF THE REPORT

The issues relating to these policy priorities are covered briefly in this chapter. Other chapters cover issues in greater detail, and contain more specific policy options, with discussions about the advantages and disadvantages of the options.

Chapters 2 and 3 provide the technical background for the rest of the assessment: chapter 2 describes the symptoms and special problems related to dementing illnesses, while chapter 3 describes the diagnostic process and treatment methods for the various disorders, and briefly reviews what is known about the most prevalent disorders. Chapter 4 describes how families and other informal caregivers provide care for individuals with dementia.

Chapter 5 highlights some of the difficult issues that arise when people develop dementia and can no longer make legal, financial, or medical decisions for themselves. Difficulties in making decisions about medical care are covered in much greater depth in a series of papers commissioned by OTA and reviewed at an OTA workshop. (Those papers—covering philosophical, legal, ethical, and practical aspects of making medical decisions— will be published as a supplement to the *Milbank Quarterly* in 1987.)

Chapter 6 begins the section on long-term care. It describes the general system of long-term care—where it is provided and what it entails— and leads into chapters 7 through 12, which deal with more specific aspects of long-term care. Chapter 7 reviews the emerging movement in nursing homes, day care centers, and home care services to design programs specifically for those with dementia. Chapter 8 reviews how diagnosis of dementia itself is insufficient to predict care needs, and emphasizes the difficulties in doing so. Chapter 9 covers professional staffing and training. It includes a brief discussion of physician qualifications. It emphasizes long-term care, and especially the training of nurses and nurse's aides. Chapter 10 addresses the difficult issue of how to assure quality in the care provided in nursing homes and other long-term care settings.

Two chapters deal with how long-term care is structured and financed for those with dementia in the United States. Chapter 11 describes how the Medicare and Medicaid programs are organized, highlighting aspects that are particularly relevant for those with dementia. Chapter 12 builds on that description and discusses the merits of various methods of paying for long-term care. It contains options for changing the financing system, including charity, various private methods, incentives for private savings, private and public insurance, tax incentives, modifications of existing public health programs, and major reform of public financing. The final chapter discusses Federal policies on biomedical research.

Several other documents, based in part on activities connected with this OTA study, will be published elsewhere. These documents are listed in an appendix to this report.

REASONS FOR INCREASED INTEREST IN DEMENTIA

The new awareness of dementia can be traced to several sources, including the aging of the population, changing medical practices, and the activities of lay organizations.

Life expectancy at birth has risen from 47.3 years in 1900 to 74.5 years in 1982 (105). More than four of every five Americans born this year can expect to reach age 65, compared with two of every five in 1900. The oldest groups are expanding most rapidly. The prevalence of severe dementia rises from approximately 1 percent (ages 65 to 74), to 7 percent (ages 75 to 84), to 25 percent (over age 85) (27). The aging of the population, particularly the rising numbers of those over 85, thus results in many more cases of dementia. Longevity among those over age 65 has also increased dramatically in the last decade (105), adding further to the number of people at risk of developing dementia. These population trends partly explain the greater public awareness of dementia.

As physicians and other health professionals see more elderly patients, medical problems associated with aging receive more attention. The creation of the National Institute on Aging in 1974 (Public Law 96-296) resulted in part from greater awareness about aging. But diagnostic classifications have also changed radically. For example, the standard classification system used now for dementia—the *Diagnostic and Statistical Manual* of the American Psychiatric Association, 3rd edition (DSM-III)—was published in 1980. Diagnostic labeling has changed as well. In the past, neurologists and psychiatrists commonly labeled dementia beginning before age 65 as presenile dementia or Alzheimer's disease. Those whose symptoms appeared after age 65 were said to have senile dementia. This distinction has largely been eliminated, with both groups of patients categorized as having Alzheimer's disease or dementia of the Alzheimer type.

New terminology and shifting theories of causation have unified a large number of disorders under the term dementia. Until recently, many physicians believed that dementia was usually caused by atherosclerosis (a common disease of the blood vessels, often called "hardening of the arteries"). Many patients were said to have "cerebral arteriosclerosis" (a particular form of atherosclerosis) based on insufficient evidence. (This is still a common diagnosis in many nursing homes, reflecting outmoded diagnostic practices among referring physicians.) Work done in the United States and Europe from the late 1950s to the present, however, has found that the most common type of dementia is Alzheimer's disease (66 percent according to aggregate data from several studies) (64). Several forms of dementia *are* due to vascular disease, and as a group they constitute the second most common cause of dementia. Vascular diseases causing dementia also have been differentiated and more specifically classified.

Many public organizations have formed around issues related to dementing conditions. ADRDA, for example, was created in June 1979 by several family support groups that had sprung up independently throughout the country. It has since become the largest national organization focused on dementia and the needs of caregivers. ADRDA has also played an important role in attracting media attention to the problems faced by families. There are many other national foundations—the John Douglas French Foundation and national organizations concerned with Huntington's disease, Parkinson's disease, multiple sclerosis, head injury, stroke, and other brain impairments that cause dementia. Some organizations deal with specific diseases while others, such as the Family Survival Project in California (83), focus on issues common to brain impairment in adults caused by a multitude of diseases. Such nongovernment organizations have helped raise public awareness of the severe problems posed by dementia.

Policymakers have also become more interested in dementia, because their constituents express concern and because many problems stemming from dementia affect and are affected by government activities. Finally, the economic costs of dementing illness have caused concern to those who must pay for the care of a loved one and to government administrators and legislators concerned about spending, particularly for long-term care. Individuals with dementia constitute perhaps the largest definable population group of those who require long-term care for extended periods, and payments for long-term care under the Medicaid program account for up to 10 percent of some State budgets (14).

POLICY INTEREST IN DEMENTIA

Growing congressional interest in Alzheimer's disease is reflected in the number of bills that specifically mention the condition—three bills (having to do with designation of National Alzheimer's Week) in the 97th Congress (1981 to 1982), and 26 in the 98th Congress (1983 to 1984). Several called attention to the problem by designating November as Alzheimer's Disease Month, while others dealt with health care and biomedical research. During the 98th Congress, five Alzheimer's disease research centers were established by the National Institutes on Aging. In the 99th Congress (1985 to 1986), 38 bills were introduced. The major health care issues for patients with dementia have been more directly addressed than in previous Congresses. Another five research centers have been created, a prototype Alzheimer's disease registry will soon be started, and several demonstration projects to deliver respite care will be funded.

Federal executive agencies have also shown increased awareness of the problems caused by dementia. Most health and social service programs relating to this issue are administered by the U.S. Department of Health and Human Services (DHHS). In 1981, Margaret Heckler created a Task Force on Alzheimer's Disease as her first act upon confirmation as Secretary of DHHS. The Task Force issued a report in 1984 (110), and continues to function under the current Secretary, Otis Bowen. In one article, then-Secretary Heckler noted:

The cost of AD is very high. Many Alzheimer's patients are maintained in family homes. The total cost for nursing homes alone is estimated at over $13 billion per year; by 1990 that figure could exceed $41 billion. But the financial cost is in many ways secondary to the real toll that Alzheimer's exacts. This disease robs society of the contribution of productive individuals with a wealth of accumulated wisdom and life experience. It also pulls into its eddy friends and family members who give up their own pursuits to look after their afflicted loved ones (46).

The Veterans Administration (VA), military health services, and Indian Health Service are also concerned with dementia, because these agencies deliver health and social services to eligible populations, either directly or under contract to other providers. State governments have shown interest in the problems of dementia as well. At least 21 States have major legislative initiatives, including over 80 bills on Alzheimer's disease (at least 20 of which became State laws in 1985 and 1986) (3,36,55). Several others have made administrative changes in the absence of new legislation. Some States (e.g., California, Maryland, Kansas, Texas, Minnesota, Rhode Island, and Illinois) have developed carefully planned and widely publicized approaches to problems of dementia.

WHAT IS DEMENTIA?

Dementia is a complex of symptoms that can be caused by many different underlying diseases. The process of classifying dementia requires that symptoms be identified and carefully assessed before the underlying disease or condition causing the dementia is diagnosed.

Symptoms of Dementia

Although loss of recent memory is its hallmark, the term dementia implies global impairment of mental functions. The symptoms can include loss of language functions, inability to think abstractly,

inability to care for oneself, personality change, emotional instability, and loss of a sense of time or place.

Dementia is different from mental retardation because it indicates a *loss* of previous abilities. (Those with mental retardation have below average mental ability rather than a loss of previous capabilities; they can also develop dementia if their abilities decline further.)

Dementia differs from *delirium* because delirium is associated with diminished attention or temporary confusion. Delirium implies a tran-

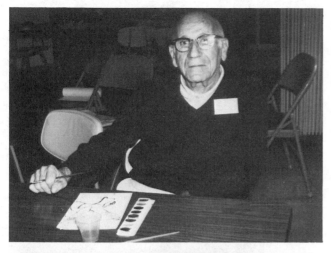
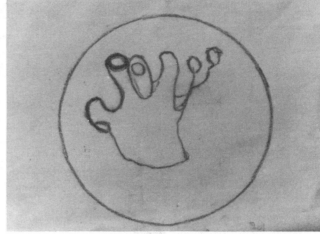
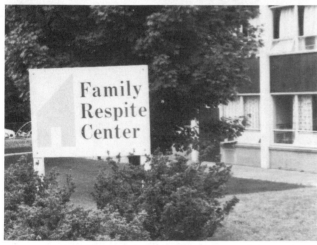
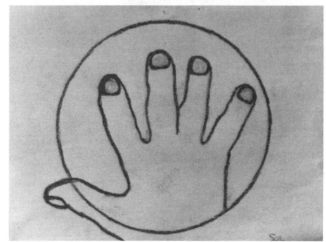

Photo credit: Office of Technology Assessment

S (upper left) goes to the Family Respite Center in northern Virginia for day care (lower left). He is a graphic artist who now has Alzheimer's disease. When asked to draw the hand pictured at bottom right, he draws the picture seen in the upper right. S's drawing is smaller than the model and shows distortion of spacial relationships, incorrect counting of fingers, and misplacement of fingernails. Such errors are typical of those due to damage to the brain caused by Alzheimer's disease.

sient loss of mental abilities, as during intoxication or following acute head injury. It is not always easy to distinguish dementia from retardation or delirium, particularly among the very old or those about whom there is little available medical information. But differences are usually clear, and diagnostic classification relies on maintaining the distinctions.

Disorders Causing Dementia

More than 70 conditions can cause dementia (63). Identifying the symptoms leads to a search for the cause—the process of diagnosis. The dis-

orders covered in this report (see table 1-1) can be classified into several groups. Degenerative disorders are diseases whose progression cannot be arrested. The ultimate cause of most such diseases is not known, and these disorders cause progressive deterioration of mental and neurological functions, often over years. Alzheimer's disease is by far the most prevalent degenerative dementia, found in 66 percent of all cases (64). The remaining disorders in table 1-1 are listed by cause. A few of them can be reversed following treatment, but truly reversible dementia occurs in only 2 to 3 percent of cases (64,80). In most cases, dementia is stable or progressive (although the severity

Table 1-1.—Disorders Causing or Simulating Dementia

Disorders causing dementia:

Degenerative diseases:
  Alzheimer's disease
  Pick's disease
  Huntington's disease
  Progressive supranuclear palsy
  Parkinson's disease (not all cases)
  Cerebellar degenerations
  Amyotrophic lateral sclerosis (ALS) (not all cases)
  Parkinson-ALS-dementia complex of Guam and other
    island areas
  Rare genetic and metabolic diseases (Hallervorden-
    Spatz, Kufs', Wilson's, late-onset metachromatic
    leukodystrophy, adrenoleukodystrophy)
Vascular dementia:
  Multi-infarct dementia
  Cortical micro-infarcts
  Lacunar dementia (larger infarcts)
  Binswanger disease
  Cerebral embolic disease (fat, air, thrombus fragments)
Anoxic dementia:
  Cardiac arrest
  Cardiac failure (severe)
  Carbon monoxide
Traumatic dementia:
  Dementia pugilistica (boxer's dementia)
  Head injuries (open or closed)
Infectious dementia:
  Acquired immune deficiency syndrome (AIDS)
    AIDS dementia
    Opportunistic infections
  Creutzfeldt-Jakob disease (subacute spongiforn
    encephalopathy)
  Progressive multifocal leukoencephalopathy
  Post-encephalitic dementia
  Behcet's syndrome
  Herpes encephalitis
  Fungal meningitis or encephalitis
  Bacterial meningitis or encephalitis
  Parasitic encephalitis
  Brain abscess
  Neurosyphilis (general paresis)
Normal pressure hydrocephalus (communicating
    hydrocephalus of adults)
Space-occupying lesions:
  Chronic or acute subdural hematoma
  Primary brain tumor
  Metastatic tumors (carcinoma, leukemia, lymphoma,
    sarcoma)
Multiple sclerosis (some cases)
Auto-immune disorders:
  Disseminated lupus erythematosis

  Vasculitis
Toxic dementia:
  Alcoholic dementia
  Metallic dementia (e.g., lead, mercury, arsenic,
    manganese)
  Organic poisons (e.g., solvents, some insecticides)
Other disorders:
  Epilepsy (some cases)
  Post-traumatic stress disorder (concentration camp
    syndrome—some cases)
  Whipple disease (some cases)
  Heat stroke

Disorders that can simulate dementia:

Psychiatric disorders:
  Depression
  Anxiety
  Psychosis
  Sensory deprivation
Drugs:
  Sedatives
  Hypnotics
  Anti-anxiety agents
  Anti-depressants
  Anti-arrhythmics
  Anti-hypertensives
  Anti-convulsants
  Anti-psychotics
  Digitalis and derivatives
  Drugs with anti-cholinergic side effects
  Others (mechanism unknown)
Nutritional disorders:
  Pellagra (B-6 deficiency)
  Thiamine deficiency (Wernicke-Korsakoff syndrome)
  Cobalamin deficiency (B-12) or pernicious anemia
  Folate deficiency
  Marchiafava-Bignami disease
Metabolic disorders (usually cause delirium, but can be
    difficult to differentiate from dementia):
  Hyper- and hypo-thyroidism (thyroid hormones)
  Hypercalcemia (calcium)
  Hyper- and hypo-natremia (sodium)
  Hypoglycemia (glucose)
  Hyperlipidemia (lipids)
  Hypercapnia (carbon dioxide)
  Kidney failure
  Liver failure
  Cushing syndrome
  Addison's disease
  Hypopituitarism
  Remote effect of carcinoma

SOURCE: Adapted from R. Katzman, B. Lasker, and N. Bernstein, ''Accuracy of Diagnosis and Consequences of Misdiagnosis of Disorders Causing Dementia,'' contract
report prepared for the Office of Technology Assessment, U.S. Congress, 1986.

can often be reduced by treating other medical problems that exacerbate the symptoms). Although the diseases causing dementia are generally not reversible, they are treatable. Treatment for most cases centers on minimizing the effects of the illness rather than attempting to return to normal mental function.

Alzheimer's disease is marked by distinctive changes and loss of nerve cells that can be detected microscopically in brain tissue. The term may actually refer to a *group* of diseases with possibly different causes and perhaps distinguished by their symptoms, rate of progression, inheritance patterns, and age at onset. These are grouped under one term because scientific understanding has not progressed sufficiently to distinguish them.

Dementia caused by disease of the blood vessels (vascular dementia) accounts for the second largest number of cases in most studies, although the interpretation of such studies is being reevaluated to ascertain the degree to which vascular disease itself can cause dementia. It is clear, however, that vascular disease may worsen the symptoms of dementia.

Some cases of dementia can be prevented: Toxic dementias and those caused by infections are clear examples. Once the brain is structurally damaged, however, dementia from these causes is usually permanent.

Disorders that can simulate dementia, in contrast, include conditions for which treatment may eliminate dementia. Treatment of these can be instituted *in order to* restore mental function. Dementia will not invariably disappear with treatment, but it is more likely to do so than for diseases in the other categories. The difference between these diseases and the first category of disorders is the rapidity of improvement and the higher likelihood of complete recovery of mental functions.

There is substantial overlap in the categories. Many older people suffering from depression, for example, show signs of dementia. Some reports have found that as many as 31 percent of those thought to have dementia have depression instead (94). Yet the rate of misdiagnosis is not as high today, because physicians have become more sophisticated in separating the various types of dementia and differentiating this condition from other mental symptom complexes. Those thought to be "misclassified" as depressed have been studied years later and found to be at much higher risk of eventually developing obvious dementia— suggesting they had an underlying dementia at the time of "misclassification" (64). One author notes the continuum from normal mental function to severe dementia including intermediate points such as "forgetfulness," "at risk of dementia," and various severities of clinical dementia (62). The overlap between disorders that cause dementia and those that simulate it cannot always be clearly defined with current medical knowledge,

and it is sometimes difficult to pinpoint where individuals are on the continuum of mental capacity. Scientific discoveries might shift any one of the degenerative disorders into another category if a cause were found or a treatment discovered that could halt the loss of brain cells. The categories suggested in table 1-1 are intended to clarify and highlight conceptual distinctions rather than to imply that diseases fall neatly into separate categories.

The distinctions among disease categories are nonetheless important for several reasons. Those with Alzheimer's disease (with or without other conditions) constitute a large portion of patients with dementia. At present there is no cure, and treatment focuses on changing the environment and adapting caregiver behavior to meet the needs of patients, rather than on curing the dementia through medication or surgery. Making the specific diagnosis of Alzheimer's disease precludes certain types of therapy, and also highlights the need to begin training caregivers about what to expect and how to deal with the expected worsening dementia. Diagnosis is therefore important in informing families about what to expect, but it is not sufficient to determine care needs without also assessing family support, severity of the disease, and the individual patient's symptoms. Decisions about medical care, social services, and family expectations all hinge on accurate diagnosis. The diagnosis of dementing illnesses will be the topic of a consensus development conference at the National Institutes of Health July 6-8, 1987.

Public policy priorities differ for those whose dementia can be eliminated. The paramount need of such patients is for accurate diagnosis and appropriate treatment, both of which are aspects of acute medical or mental health care. Public policies to identify these patients can reduce the number misdiagnosed with "irreversible" dementia and wrongly channeled into long-term care (64). The number of individuals with dementia whose symptoms can be treated and eliminated is estimated at 2 (80) to 3 percent (64), and the costs of unnecessarily providing long-term care for them are likely to offset the costs of diagnosis for all cases of dementia (64). Policy issues related to disorders causing progressive dementia, on the other hand, center on appropriate long-term care for those

Table 1-2.—ICD-9 Codes for Disorders Causing Dementia

094	**Neurosyphilis**
094.1	General paresis
290	**Senile and presenile organic psychotic conditions**
290.0	Senile dementia, simple type
290.1	Presenile dementia
290.2	Senile dementia, depressed or paranoid type
290.3	Senile dementia with acute confusional state
290.4	Arteriosclerotic dementia
291	**Alcoholic psychoses**
291.1	Korsakov's psychosis, alcoholic
291.2	Other alcoholic dementia
294	**Other organic psychotic conditions (chronic)**
294.0	Korsakov's psychosis, nonalcoholic
294.1	Dementia in conditions classified elsewhere
294.8	Other chronic organic psychotic conditions
294.9	Unspecified chronic organic psychotic conditions
310	**Specific nonpsychotic mental disorders following organic brain damage**
310.1	Nonpsychotic cognitive or personality change following organic brain damage
310.9	Unspecified nonpsychotic mental disorders following organic brain damage
331	**Other cerebral degenerations**
331.0	Alzheimer's disease
331.1	Pick's disease
331.2	Senile degeneration of the brain
331.3	Communicating hydrocephalus
331.5	Creutzfeldt-Jakob disease
331.6	Progressive multifocal leukoencephalopathy
331.7	Cerebral degeneration in other disease elsewhere classified
331.8	Other cerebral degeneration
331.9	Unspecified cerebral degeneration
333	**Other extrapyramidal disease and abnormal movement disorders**
333.4	Huntington's chorea
437	**Other and ill-defined cerebrovascular disease**
437.0	Cerebral atherosclerosis
437.1	Other generalized ischemic cerebrovascular disease
437.2	Hypertensive encephalopathy
797	**Senility without mention of psychosis**

Any patients have dementia, but category also includes some without dementia:

279	**Disorders involving the immune mechanism**
279.19	Acquired immune deficiency syndrome (AIDS dementia)
290	**Senile and presenile organic psychotic conditions**
290.8	Other senile/presenile organic psychotic conditions
290.9	Unspecified senile/presenile organic psychotic conditions
323	**Encephalitis, myelitis and encephalomyelitis**
323.0	Kuru
323.1	Subacute sclerosing panencephalitis
323.2	Poliomyelitis
323.3	Arthropod-borne viral encephalitis
323.4	Other encephalitis due to infection
323.5	Encephalitis following immunization procedures
323.6	Postinfectious encephalitis
323.7	Toxic encephalitis
323.8	Other
323.9	Unspecified cause
332	**Parkinson's disease**
333	**Other extrapyramidal disease and abnormal movement disorders**
333.0	Other degenerative disease of the basal ganglia
438	**Late effects of cerebrovascular disease**

SOURCE: *International Classification of Diseases,* 9th Revision Conference, 1975 (Geneva: World Health Organization), vol. 1, 1977 and vol. 2, 1978; modified by *Coding Clinics for ICD-9 CM,* American Hospital Association, various issues.

already affected, and on research to identify new treatments or means of prevention.

A different way to classify disorders causing dementia is found in the International Classification of Diseases (see table 1-2) (56). That system, called ICD-9, is used to code diagnoses in most hospitals and clinics, and is the starting point for diagnosis-related group reimbursement under Medicare. The classification is well adapted for many specific disorders. No specific code exists for several disorders, however, and a large number of diagnostic categories that include many persons with dementia (e.g., someone with Parkinson's disease) do not separate individuals with dementia from those without it. Many diseases listed in table 1-1 do not have ICD-9 codes, and individuals with them would be classified in nonspecific categories. These shortcomings limit the usefulness of ICD-9 in refining epidemiologic studies because it is impossible to specify only those persons who have dementia.

The State of California recently reviewed the various systems of nomenclature for dementing disorders (70). The analysts suggested grouping disorders under a new broad category "acquired cognitive impairment," according to the subcategories noted in table 1-3. The confusion over terminology may be reduced if revisions of the two most widely used diagnostic classifications are made compatible. Revision of the ICD-9, to be called ICD-10, is scheduled for 1989. DSM-III is a set of guidelines for making diagnosis of mental disorders (7). It is the most widely used classification for the symptoms of dementia, and its criteria have been used in most recent studies. The revision of DSM-III will be called DSM-IV and will likely be made available after release of ICD-10. The two classifications are promised to be more compatible than DSM-III and ICD-9 (70).

Table 1-3.—California State Listing of Acquired Cognitive Impairments

Primary (cortical) degenerative dementias—DSM-III:
  Alzheimer's disease
  Pick's disease
Degenerative dementias with involvement of motor systems:
  Amyotrophic lateral sclerosis
  Cerebellar degenerations
  Guam-Parkinson-dementia complex
  Huntington's disease
  Parkinson's disease
  Progressive supranuclear palsy
  Other rare disorders: including Hallervorden-Spatz disease,
    Kufs' disease, Wilson's disease, metachromatic leu-
    kodystrophy, adrenoleukodystrophy
Vascular:
  Binswanger disease
  Cerebrovascular accident: including hemorrhage,
    stroke, aneurysms (recent and past)
  Cortical microinfarcts
  Lacunar infarctions
  Multi-infarct dementia
Postanoxia or postischemia—due to:
  Carbon monoxide
  Cardiac arrest
  Strangulation, asphyxiation, or suffocation
Traumatic:
  Intracranial injury without skull fracture:
    open and closed
  Intracranial injury with skull fracture:
    open and closed
  Fat embolism
  Post-traumatic brain syndrome:
    nonpsychotic
    psychotic
Auto-immune:
  Disseminated lupus
  Multiple sclerosis
  Primary CNS vasculitis
Central nervous system infections:
  AIDS (primary or opportunistic infections)
  Behcet syndrome
  Creutzfeldt-Jakob disease
  Encephalitis, herpes simplex
  Fungal, parasitic, and chronic bacterial meningitis,
    abscesses, and granuloma
  Neurosyphilis
  Postencephalitic dementia

Progressive multifocal leukoencephalopathy
Hydrocephalus, adult onset (normal pressure)
Space-occupying lesions:
  Hematomas: including subdural, epidural, and in-
    tracerebral
  Metastatic carcinoma, lymphoma, leukemia
  Primary brain tumors
Toxic dementias:
  Alcoholic dementia
  Drugs: including neuroleptics, diazepam-related
    hypnotics, anticonvulsants, beta blockers, digitalis
  Korsakoff's syndrome
  Metallic poisons: including lead, mercury, arsenic,
    manganese
  Organic poisons: including solvents, organophosphates
Psychiatric illness presenting as dementia:
  Chronic schizophrenia
  Conversion disorder
  Depression
  Ganzer's syndrome
  Paranoia
Nutritional disorders:
  Marchiafava-Bignami disease
  Pellagra
  Thiamine deficiency (Wernicke-Korsakoff syndrome)
  Vitamin B-12 or folate deficiency
Metabolic disorders:
  Addison disease
  Cushing syndrome
  Hepatic failure
  Hypercalcemia
  Hypercapnia
  Hyperlipidemia
  Hypoglycemia
  Hypo- and hyper-thyroidism
  Hypopituitarism
  Hypo- and hyper-natremia
  Remote effects of carcinoma
  Uremia
Sensory deprivation (agnosia)
Other disorders
  Concentration camp syndrome
  Epilepsy
  Heat stroke
  Whipple disease

SOURCE: D.A. Lindeman, N.G. Bliwise, G. Berkowitz, et al., "Development of a Uniform Comprehensive Nomenclature and Data Collection Protocol for Brain Disorders," Institute for Health and Aging, University of California, San Francisco, June 1986.

COURSE OF THE ILLNESSES

The course of a dementing illness varies from one person to another as well as among the different disorders. A few generalizations can be made, however, about progressive dementing illnesses. Onset is usually noticed by the person with the disorder, family members, friends, or colleagues at work (rather than by a physician). Although some disorders appear suddenly, most—including Alzheimer's disease—are insidious. People lose some mental ability, usually memory, or begin to show poor judgment or incompetence at work. They often succeed in hiding their symptoms for months or even years (if symptoms are mild), but the disability eventually becomes serious enough to merit medical investigation.

A physician is typically consulted by the individual or family, initiating the diagnostic process. If the indvidual is seen early by a physician knowledgeable about dementia, the first visit will result in the scheduling of appropriate tests or referral to another specialist (usually a neurologist or psychiatrist) who will direct and monitor the use of diagnostic tests. An estimated 80 percent accuracy in diagnosis can be obtained through medical history and physical examination, while 90 percent accuracy can be achieved when these are supplemented by a battery of psychological and laboratory tests and by radiological examinations (63).

Once diagnosis is completed, treatment can be started for some dementing conditions (and any other medical conditions detected during diagnostic evaluation). Medications may assist in managing some symptoms (93), the progression of which can be slowed or arrested in a few cases. The focus of most medical management, however, is family education—training caregivers to adapt to the patient, simplifying the individual's living space, and referring relatives to family support services (121,122). Current medical management of dementia is based largely on anecdotal reports and clinical impressions rather than on solid data, since there have been relatively few clinical investigations (122). Drug treatment to improve intellectual function and memory has been a topic of intense investigation, but results have not yet shown clinically significant improvement. Drug management of behavioral disorders can benefit patients and ease the burden for caregivers, but it must be carefully planned and monitored (93,122).

Diagnosis and treatment can continue for several years. Repeated visits for evaluation may be necessary to establish a final diagnosis—particularly for cases of early dementia, unusual progression, or atypical symptoms. Treatment, including medication, may be changed from time to time in response to changing needs or adverse drug effects.

An individual with dementia also often requires intermittent medical care for other illnesses. Because dementia is most prevalent among the very old, and because the very old are at risk of multiple medical disabilities, it is common for those with dementia to require attention for diseases of the heart, lungs, kidneys, or other organs. Their mental incapacity also places them at increased risk of falls, mistakes in medication, and household accidents. Individuals with dementia frequently need dental care. Those with dentures often lose them or break them; those with other dental problems may not become aware of them until they have become serious or caused undue pain.

Most dementing conditions last years, often decades. One recent study found the average duration of illness, from first onset of symptoms to death, was 8.1 years for Alzheimer's disease and 6.7 years for multi-infarct dementia (9). The time from *diagnosis* to death averaged 3.4 years for Alzheimer's disease and 2.6 years for multi-infarct dementia, suggesting that patients typically show symptoms for over 4 years before a diagnosis is made. Recent improvements in professional education and increased public awareness may eventually shorten this period. The duration of a dementing illness is unpredictable, however—Alzheimer's disease can last up to 25 years.

Patients with dementia generally die of some other illness (17,18), and dementia is associated with increased overall mortality (64). Alzheimer's disease is often cited as the fourth leading cause of death in the United States (although not reflected on death certificates or in official statistics). Such statements assume that each year the number of new cases roughly equals the number of deaths of those with Alzheimer's disease (see discussion in ref. 79), and that shortened life expectancy is related to the presence of Alzheimer's disease—both untested assumptions. *Mortality* caused by dementing conditions is, in any case, not the only consideration; of equal or greater concern are deterioration of valued human mental capacities, loss of autonomy, and catastrophic expenses caused by the ensuing need for long-term care.

Long-term care refers to medical, mental health, and personal services rendered to those with diminished capacity for self-care due to illness. Brain damage caused by a disease process results in loss of mental functions and dependency on others. Long-term care is often needed from the beginning of the disease, and can precede diagnosis. Individuals' needs differ markedly. Some remain at home throughout the illness, while others benefit from day care or nursing home placement soon after symptoms are noted. Recent research has shown that the use of formal services is, in fact, more strongly correlated with characteristics affecting the person most responsible for taking care of someone with dementia than with severity of symptoms or other characteristics of the ill individual (23). Yet there would be no dependency on a caregiver if not for the illness.

Since all individuals with dementia eventually become dependent (if their disease runs full course), they all require long-term care. Individuals typically need long-term care from onset to death, although the degree to which *formal* services are used varies. Most families keep someone with dementia at home for as long as possible, often despite extreme cost, health risk, and stress to themselves (12,20,23,37,124).

Two general hypotheses about long-term care for persons with dementia are important to public policy, but their validity has not been confirmed. One posits that care needs intensify as the disease worsens until the afflicted person dies. The other suggests that most of the caregiving burden is due to changes in behavior and personality. As the dementia worsens, behavioral problems diminish as the individual becomes weaker, less mobile, and eventually mute. If the second hypothesis were correct, the need for care would be greatest at midcourse of the illness, and services to support families through the worst periods might forestall institutional placement.

The complex interactions between the affected person's symptoms and stresses affecting the caregiver and family are equally important in predicting a need for formal long-term care services, but the crucial factors are only now being studied. The concept of a smooth progression of illness and dependency caused by it is illusory, with large variations in types of symptoms, rapidity and severity of progression of disease, and strength and resilience of informal supports.

Those with dementia generally die after years of being dependent on others for their care. The cause of death is usually a disease of a different organ system—pneumonia, heart disease, or kidney failure, for example. These individuals are logical candidates for hospice care in their last months, with an emphasis on allaying pain and suffering rather than prolonging life. Autopsy following death is often the only means of confirming what disease the person had, but the rate of autopsy in the United States has fallen dramatically, and an accurate diagnosis may never be ascertained. Failure to confirm a diagnosis at autopsy can interfere with accurate genetic counseling and analysis of the efficacy of medical care.

MAGNITUDE OF THE PROBLEM

The problems posed by disorders causing dementia will increase as the population ages and more people either develop a dementing disorder themselves or must care for a relative or friend. The magnitude of the problem can be gauged by projecting the number of people likely to be affected (the prevalence of dementia), estimating the costs of caring for those who now have dementia, and assessing some of the indirect burdens.

Prevalence of Dementia

Dementia can be divided into several categories by severity and type. Studies over the past several decades have varied widely in reported prevalence rates. These variations can be attributed to the different age groups studied, the inclusion or exclusion of people in long-term care facilities, degree of severity involved, methods of assessing mental function, or other sample characteristics. Most studies conducted since 1980 have followed DSM-III criteria (7), dramatically reducing the degree of variation from study to study (64).

Recent studies show a relatively narrow range of prevalence of severe dementia, from 5 to 7 percent of those over 65, with a median of 6.5 percent (27). Although the criteria for "severe" dementia vary from study to study, the degree of variation for this category is much less than if "mild" and "moderate" cases are also included. The extreme variation of results on mild and moderate cases makes projections of future prevalence impossible. Further, those with mild and moderate dementia in community studies are those about whom there is the greatest possibility of diagnostic error. For these reasons, projections of cases have been done only for severe dementia (see table 1-4). The total number of all cases can be estimated from these studies by assuming that for each case of severe dementia, probably at least one person and possibly up to three people have milder dementia and will eventually develop severe dementia if they live long enough.

Prevalence is most often reported as a percentage of people age 65 or older affected at a particular time. Average prevalence figures mask significant differences among different age groups. As noted earlier, the prevalence of severe dementia among those 65 to 74 is roughly 1 percent, compared with 25 percent for those over 84 (27).

Some authors have used the terms "epidemic" and "rising pandemic" to describe the projected increase in prevalence of dementia. Use of such terms is subject to misinterpretation, however, because of their associations with uncontrolled infection. Although the number of people with dementia will rise substantially over the next several decades, it will not do so explosively. (One demen-

tia, associated with acquired immune deficiency syndrome, is epidemic, but uncertainties about its prevalence, reversibility, and mortality preclude accurate projections.) Vascular dementia may drop in prevalence, paralleling the decline of stroke and hypertension. The prevalence of Alzheimer's disease, because it accounts for the largest number of cases, will largely determine the overall prevalence of dementia. Alzheimer's disease is expected to rise slowly in prevalence, in tandem with aging of the population.

Studies show general agreement on the overall prevalence of severe dementia among the population 65 or older, but substantial uncertainty exists about mild and moderate dementia, the oldest age group, ethnic and racial subgroups, nursing home populations, and subtypes of dementia. Some data, for example, suggest that the risk of developing dementia after age 84 begins to decline (79); other data do not support that hypothesis (97). That could be due to real decline, inadequate reporting (since dementia is "expected" in the very old and therefore not recorded), or insufficient sampling of the very old cohort. Many of these groups about which there is little information are among those expanding most rapidly (see figure 1-2). Policy planning will thus require rigorous investigation of prevalence rates among the very old, minority groups, and nursing home residents.

Table 1-4.—Current and Projected Cases of Severe Dementia in the United States, 1980-2040
(thousand cases)[a]

Age group	1980	2000	2020	2040
Under 65	78	88	150	150
65-74	160	180	300	290
75-84	550	860	1,000	1,700
Over 85	570	1,300	1,800	5,200
Total cases	1,400	2,400	3,300	7,300

[a]These projections are based on prevalence of severe dementia of 1 percent ages 65 to 74, 7 percent 75 to 84, and 25 percent 85 and over (Cross and Gurland, 1986). Cases under 65 have been estimated as follows: the 75,000 current cases (Mortimer and Hutton, 1985) under age 60 correspond to 48 percent of cases in the next oldest cohort (ages 65 to 74) (Cross and Gurland, 1986). Projections of future cases under 65 have been conservatively calculated as 50 percent of cases in the 65 to 74 cohort, for simplicity and to account partially for those aged 61 to 64. Another method would be to use the estimated 13.5 per 100,000 prevalence estimate among those 30 to 59 (Kokman, 1984, as cited in Mortimer and Hutton, 1975), but this is more complicated and more subject to error due to the shifting age structure within this very large age group. The table yields estimates of cases under age 65 at the conservative end of the range reported (5 to 10 percent of all cases—Cross and Gurland, 1986).

SOURCES: P.S. Cross and B.J. Gurland, "The Epidemiology of Dementing Disorders," contract report prepared for the Office of Technology Assessment, U.S. Congress, 1986.

Costs of Dementia

Although the exact costs of dementing illness to the Nation cannot be calculated, all agree that they are already high and bound to rise at least in proportion to the expected increase in prevalence. The many studies of costs noted in this section do not provide estimates that are sufficiently accurate and reliable to permit refined policy planning, but they are a starting point for analysis of spending for different services. Policies that affect the largest spending categories (informal care and long-term care) are those accorded high priority by caregivers as well as those concerned about government spending.

Overall Costs

Two studies have attempted to estimate the overall costs to the Nation of caring for those with

Figure 1-2.—Contribution of Elderly Age Groups to Projected Increase in Cases of Severe Dementia

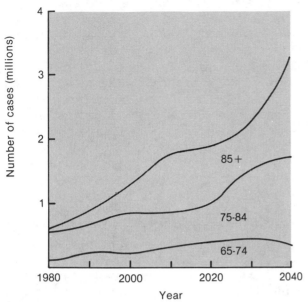

SOURCE: P.S. Cross and G.J. Gurland, "The Epidemiology of Demential Disorders," contract report prepared for the Office of Technology Assessment, 1986.

dementia. The National Institute on Aging (NIA) sponsored a study that estimated total costs of just over $38 billion in 1983 (51). That study attempted to estimate only those costs exclusively due to dementia, but the projections (particularly those for the largest cost components) were contingent on small pilot studies. A review of these cost estimates, prepared for the State of California, concluded that costs of dementia were large but could not be precisely defined (75). A Battelle Memorial Institute study commissioned by OTA estimated $24 billion to $48 billion total costs (projected to 1985) (10). That study, too, tried to estimate only the costs specifically due to dementia, but it used different projection methods for estimating community and nursing home costs for long-term care. The estimates from these studies are similar in range, but they can be misinterpreted. Both the NIA and Battelle studies estimate costs of diagnosis, treatment, nursing home care, informal care, lost wages, and other indirect costs. Each component is large but cannot rigorously be projected, due to the paucity of relevant information, not study design.

In addition to studies of overall costs, some researchers have estimated costs related to demen-

tia stemming from diagnosis, medical treatment, nursing home care, and informal long-term care; these are discussed below.

Costs of Diagnosis

The costs of diagnosis can be estimated by assuming that 200,000 new cases of severe dementia will occur each year, and that at least as many mild and moderate cases will come to the attention of physicians for diagnostic evaluation. The estimated incidence of 200,000 is calculated by assuming 1.5 million affected people (27) and 7.5 year average duration, based on the average from one recent survey (9). That estimate is conservative, because it is based on figures at the low end of prevalence estimates, assumes only one diagnostic evaluation per case, and neglects those persons who are evaluated for dementia but are not found to have a dementing illness.

The cost of diagnosis per case depends on the number of times a patient must be seen (the patient may need periodic reevaluation if dementia is mild or presents atypically), local medical costs, and whether the diagnostic testing is done on an outpatient or inpatient basis (i.e., during repeated clinic visits or in the hospital). Outpatient diagnosis entails an estimated $1,000 to $2,000 for physician charges, laboratory tests, neuropsychological testing, brain imaging studies, and ancillary services (64). Costs for the laboratory tests alone can range from about $154 to about $1,110 per patient (65). Those figures suggest that it costs at least $400 million to $800 million each year nationwide to diagnose disorders causing dementia.

The Medicare program's costs for inpatient diagnosis differ according to geographic location, type of hospital, and discharge diagnosis. A hospital discharging a patient with the diagnosis of Alzheimer's disease would be reimbursed from $6,800 to $7,200 in most areas (87). If all cases were diagnosed following a single hospitalization, the national cost of diagnosis would be approximately $2.8 billion. Although no data show whether inpatient or outpatient diagnosis is more common, a survey of caregivers commissioned by OTA for this assessment did find that 30 percent of patients had never been hospitalized (123). Diagnosis in a hospital could have been done on a maximum of 70 percent, although the number is likely much lower because most hospitalizations would be for purposes other than initial diagnosis of dementia.

Hospital admission for diagnosis is not the norm in most centers; physicians who see many patients with dementia report that inpatient diagnosis is performed only for a small minority of patients. In fact, diagnosis as the sole reason for hospital admission would likely be disallowed for reimbursement under Medicare except in rural areas or special circumstances. Diagnosis is thus largely done on an outpatient basis, with attendant costs in the outpatient range rather than the much higher estimate for inpatient diagnosis.

Given all the uncertainties, a firm figure for cost of diagnosis cannot be stated. A reasonable estimate for the national cost of diagnosis would be $500 million to $1 billion each year—high, but relatively small compared with long-term care costs. The diagnostic process is more likely to be covered by Medicare and private health insurance than long-term care is, and therefore requires smaller out-of-pocket payment by patients.

Costs of Drugs and Medical Services After Diagnosis

Once a diagnosis is made, medical management of patients with dementia requires continued visits to physicians, drug treatment of behavioral symptoms and ancillary medical problems, mental health services, and intermittent hospital care for concurrent illnesses. One study estimated these medical costs due to dementia at just over $10 billion in 1983 (51). Another study did not specify costs in dollars, but found that those with dementia were more likely to die during a hospital admission, had longer lengths of hospital stay, and were more likely to be discharged to a nursing home or require home assistance. The study also reported that:

> . . . . Cognitive impairment at the time of admission may be regarded as a marker for sicker, less stable, more clinically complex patients. Such patients can be expected to fare worse than their mentally intact counterparts and to require more intense social service support if they survive to discharge (31).

Costs of Nursing Home Care

In 1984, total national expenditures for nursing home care reached $32 billion; for 1986, the estimate is $38.9 billion (8). The 1986 estimate includes $19.5 billion from individuals (50 percent), $500 million from insurance (1.3 percent), $10.4 billion in Federal funds (27 percent), $8.2 billion in State and local payments (21 percent), and $300 million (0.8 percent) from other sources (8) (see figure 1-3). Medicaid was the single largest payer for nursing homes (29). In 1980, Medicaid accounted for more than three-quarters of the total spent on long-term care under the six largest Federal programs (the other five are Medicare, Older Americans Act programs, State supplements to income, Title XX funds, and VA programs) (22). Nursing home care is a small part of Medicare, and the services covered are restricted to short stays after hospitalization. Nursing home payments under Medicare were only $600 million of $64.6 billion total Medicare outlays in 1984 (8), and accounted for 1.9 percent of the total spent nationwide on nursing home care.

Nursing home payments surged from 1.7 percent of all health care expenditures in 1950 to 5.8 percent in 1965, and then to an estimated 9.7 percent in 1986 (8). Health care costs are significant,

Figure 1-3.—1986 Estimated Costs of Nursing Home Care (billions of dollars)

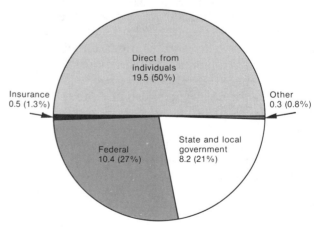

Total = $38.9 billion

SOURCES: R.H. Arnett, D.R. McKusick, S.T. Sonnefeld, et al., "Projections of Health Care Spending to 1990," *Health Care Financing Review* 7:1-36, spring 1986.

Figure 1-4.—Personal Payments for Health Care and Health Insurance

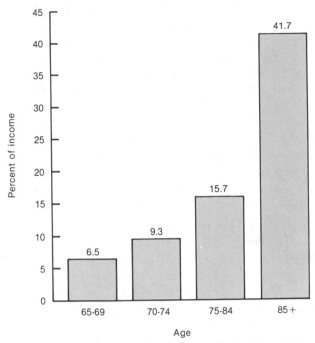

SOURCE: ICF, Inc., "The Role of Medicare in Financing the Health Care of Older Americans," submitted to American Association of Retired Persons, July 1985, table 21, adapted by the Office of Technology Assessment.

especially for older Americans (see figure 1-4). Among those over 64, fully 9.9 percent of their expenditures go for health care (compared with 2.6 percent for those under 25, and 5.4 percent for those 55 to 64) (11). The difference is even more dramatic within the older age group. One study estimated out-of-pocket expenditures for health care and health insurance at 6.5 percent of income for those 65 to 69, compared with 15.7 percent for those 75 to 84, and 41.7 percent for those over 85 (54, table 21).

The proportion of these expenditures directly caused by dementing illness is not known. The National Nursing Home Survey of 1977 found that 57 percent of nursing home residents had "chronic brain syndrome" or "senility" (112, table 8) as noted by nursing home staff. Most people in these categories likely had what would now be called dementia, although some older adults with mental retardation might also have been misclassified as "chronic brain syndrome."

A recent sample of people admitted to nursing homes in Texas showed that 40 to 60 percent had diagnoses indicating dementia (103). A sample of 3,427 residents of 52 New York State nursing homes found 41 percent had diagnoses indicating dementia or extensively overlapping with it (32). Both samples used the admitting diagnosis (the accuracy of which depends on the quality of prior medical evaluation and varies widely from site to site) and are likely low for two reasons. First, dementia is commonly missed, especially in the very old, because it is "expected," even by many physicians. Second, physicians wishing to facilitate nursing home placement are often willing to list other diagnoses rather than dementia because nursing homes may be less willing to admit dementia patients (58).

Researchers at Johns Hopkins Medical School recently undertook the most reliable study to date, but it is small and preliminary. A research team performed thorough diagnostic investigations of 50 residents of a proprietary nursing home in Baltimore. The study found 39 (78 percent) had a dementing condition (an additional 7 residents had other mental diagnoses) (95). More studies of nursing home populations that include rigorous diagnosis could shed light on these disturbingly high figures.

Several studies of dementing illness assume that costs can be calculated by taking the proportion of nursing home residents with dementia and multiplying by the overall costs of long-term care. That assumes that all long-term care for individuals with dementia is *caused by* their dementia, an assumption that creates many potential inconsistencies. One problem is best explained by analyzing an even larger disabled population—those with arthritis. Symptomatic arthritis is roughly three times more prevalent than severe dementia in the population over 64. Its prevalence in nursing homes approximates that of dementia (112). Cost estimates that assumed arthritis caused nursing home placement would thus yield figures as high as those for dementia. Yet each disorder cannot account for half of all costs. Similar analyses could be done for residents with partial deafness, visual impairment, or incontinence, each highly prevalent in nursing home populations. The difficulty in determining *why* an individual needs personal or nursing services limits the interpretation of simple cost projections.

Although it is more plausible that dementia directly causes institutional placement more than arthritis does, no study has confirmed this. The rigorous costs studies that can be performed (as in the case of incontinence, for example) (82) presume carefully constructed models of care that do not exist for individuals with dementia. As a result, the fraction of nursing home costs due to dementia have not been estimated reliably. Yet cost projections for such care are important in considering policy changes that would promote delivery of services to persons with dementia. Information about costs and use rates for services would thus be quite useful for determining long-term care policy.

One study attempted to estimate the costs of nursing home care due directly to dementia, and estimated that 3 percent of all elderly people in nursing homes were admitted because of such conditions, with subsequent costs of $1 billion (in 1983 dollars) (104). That figure is almost certainly a significant underestimate because of the strong incentives for underdiagnosis of dementia in nursing homes. That study also reported 36 percent higher labor costs for residents with dementia, in contrast to a 6 percent figure found in New York State (32). Which is the correct figure for the costs of caring for those with dementia is purely speculative; each may be accurate for its own sample. The New York figure, for example, included a large number of nursing home residents who did not have significant functional impairments, and who may have required less care. Given uncertainties in the accuracy of diagnosis, type of service provided, and sensitivity to uncontrolled economic factors, using current estimates to predict costs of public policies should be done only with great caution.

Costs of Informal Long-Term Care

Most studies report that the majority of long-term care is delivered outside nursing homes—in board and care homes, adult day care centers, and patients' homes. Costs are extremely difficult to estimate, and most overall projections necessarily underestimate this component. One recent study based on a national sample of long-term care recipients estimated that 1.2 million Americans were receiving informal care (100). That figure compares to the estimated 1.4 million people in nursing homes (26,54). Some authors have estimated that 70 to 90 percent of long-term care is informal care, but it is unclear whether these estimates refer to numbers of persons, proportion of services, or some other measurable factor. If it is true that only 1.2 million Americans now receive informal care, then the magnitude of the problem may be less than previously stated—and the cost implications proportionately less worrisome to Federal, State, and local governments.

Costs of informal care include the wages and salaries forgone by family members caring for patients, the lost productivity that results when experienced workers leave the work force to care for relatives, and the stresses borne by patients and their families (37,125; see also chs. 2 and 4). The stress induced by loss of mental functions and personality change is enormous for individuals with dementia and for their families, and can lead to illness among caregivers. Such stress can be exacerbated by difficulties in finding and coordinating services to relieve the caregiving burden.

The bulk of informal care is delivered first by spouses, then by children (especially daughters) (38,100). The burden falls disproportionately on women. The very late onset of most dementing illnesses often means that a woman in her fifties or even late sixties may be the primary caregiver (14). The efforts of spouses and children are not generally captured by economic surveys—the costs of caring are hidden because no one pays for them directly.

A few indirect indicators of cost have been identified. Of those responding to the national survey conducted for OTA—which, because the sample was drawn from the national mailing list of ADRDA, likely represents more well-to-do families than average—30 percent reported they had "cut back sharply" in spending in order to care for their affected relative, 10 percent reported some impact, 22 percent noted little or no impact, and 48 percent had not used their own funds at all (123). (These figures add up to over 100 percent because of multiple answers from some respondents.)

A survey of women in Philadelphia found that 28 percent of those taking care of dependent mothers had quit their jobs to give care at home, and a similar proportion were considering it or had reduced their hours of work (12). A study of a national sample of long-term care recipients found 9 percent of caregivers had quit their jobs (100). Researchers studying the social breakdown syndrome (a combined index of functional limitations and difficult behavior) concluded that "most of the functional limitation and troublesome behavior occurring in the community is unrelated to the presence of a mental disorder in the elderly person. Nonetheless, persons with dementing disorders contribute to the community burden of disability disproportionately" (88). These studies are further indications of the cost of informal long-term care for patients with dementia.

Finally, two recent studies have been combined to estimate the community costs of caring for those with dementia. A small pilot study of 19 community-dwelling older Americans estimated average costs at $11,700 (in 1983 dollars) to take care of someone with dementia at home, based on what the care would have cost if families hired outside caregivers at prevailing wage rates. This study yielded national estimates of $26.7 billion for such care (50,51).

Costs to Government

Costs borne by government are of special interest to policymakers. The amount is not known and has not been specifically analyzed in any major national survey. Several factors suggest the services needed by individuals with dementia may be more costly than for other long-term care populations. The duration of nursing home stay for those with chronic brain syndrome and senility in the 1977 National Nursing Home Survey was 5 percent longer than average (111, combining tables H and 8). That figure significantly understates the likely length of nursing home stay for residents who enter *because* of dementia, for it is averaged over a diverse group of residents who stay for shorter periods. Those with chronic brain syndrome who are still in a nursing home at 90

days are expected to remain approximately 3 years (1,104 days), much longer than for any other diagnostic group. The average expected stay at time of admission is 97 percent greater (72). (These data are not specific to dementia patients, however, because while those in the category of "chronic brain syndrome" are largely residents with dementia, other groups—including a fraction of adults with mental retardation—are also included.)

Residents staying longer in a nursing home are more likely to spend down to Medicaid eligibility as they run out of financial resources by paying for care, although that has not been confirmed specifically for those with dementia. The RUG-II long-term care demonstration project in New York State found that patients with diagnoses indicating dementia had levels of disability 6 percent higher than average (32). That higher level of disability would lead to a higher level of care—and thus cost—in turn causing increased State and Federal payments to nursing homes for such residents under the RUG-II payment system (98). Indirect analysis thus suggests that length of stay and level of disability are both higher for residents with diagnoses indicating dementia, and that **individuals with dementia are more likely to be publicly subsidized by the Medicaid program and their care is more expensive than average nursing home residents.**

A range of long-term care costs can be estimated. The maximum possible cost would assume nursing home care for all with severe dementia, with estimates in the range of $33 billion (1.5 million residents times $22,000 per year average cost of nursing homes). The $22,000 is calculated by dividing total estimated costs for nursing homes in 1986 ($32.8 billion) (54) by the estimated number of nursing home residents (1.493 million) (106). That calculation accords well with one estimate based on a direct survey of 25 nursing home residents with dementia, which found costs of $22,500 per resident per year (in 1983 dollars) (49). If the Federal Government paid 30 percent of this, then its costs would be roughly $10 billion.

The $10 billion figure has a misleading ceiling, however. A more realistic figure for government costs is based on the assumption that half of current nursing home residents have dementia and that Medicare nursing home payments are not for dementia. That hypothesis yields an estimate of $4.4 billion for the Federal Government and $4.1 billion for the States in 1986. That estimate implies that **the Federal and State Governments are each bearing roughly 10 to 15 percent of the overall costs of long-term care for those with dementia**, with the remainder coming from individuals. (Some individual payments, however, also come indirectly from government through social security, VA pensions, and Supplemental Security Income, which provide over 45 percent of income for those over 65.) These estimates are necessarily quite imprecise, and more refined service planning will require much better information and analysis.

The amount of long-term care covered by government programs depends on several factors: degree of subsidy of services, access to services, eligibility criteria for programs, range of services provided, and method of payment. Expanding eligibility, access, range of services, or degree of subsidy would increase government costs, while narrower eligibility or restricted access to facilities would either reduce overall costs or shift expenses to individuals and families.

COORDINATING SERVICES FOR THOSE WITH DEMENTIA

Although several chronic disorders of old age increasingly confront the American health care system and cause people to need long-term care, several features of dementia make it especially difficult to coordinate services for anyone with this condition. Medical, mental health, and social services are frequently adapted only poorly to the needs and abilities of those with dementia. Services are typically intended for targeted populations, and those with dementia can "fall through the cracks." Families are often referred from agency to agency, each of which may exclude individuals with dementia from their services for different—and legitimate—reasons (83).

That need not be the case. In some regions, referral networks and family support groups have been established to deal with this problem (30, 35,83). Services adapted to patients with dementia are increasingly common, but still serve only a small fraction of the total population. For now, many individuals are left in an administrative limbo between services intended for aged, mentally ill, and acutely ill Americans (13).

Some States, local governments, or organizations have developed innovative and effective methods for delivering and coordinating care. The ADRDA chapters in Portland, OR and Atlanta, GA, for example, have developed in-home respite programs (30,35). The Family Survival Project and On-Lok have both coordinated and managed financing of a wide range of services in the San Francisco Bay area (73,83). These programs demonstrate that services for patients with dementia can be provided and financed successfully.

Several States have commissioned studies, developed plans, or established special programs that cover individuals with dementia. Georgia, Illinois, Kansas, Maryland, Massachusetts, Rhode Island, and Texas have issued major reports (2,19,38,41, 42,61,92,101). Minnesota has produced a comprehensive plan to serve those with brain impairments (77). California has passed several bills to fund pilot projects and is preparing a Task Force report (90). These States have taken the lead in studying the needs and planning services for those with dementia.

The Care System

The system for taking care of individuals with dementia includes a wide range of services provided in many settings. The informal care system consists of family, friends, and communities. The formal system consists of government agencies and nongovernmental organizations whose primary purpose is to provide services. Most of the needs of those with dementia are met by the informal care network. Formal service providers are usually used when the informal care system breaks down (e.g., a caregiver moves, gets sick, or dies) or when informal supports are not available (e.g., those without families and living alone).

Surveying the history of formal services, two researchers observed that:

> . . . public policy, in the last 50 years, has responded to the demographic imperatives of an aging society unevenly. In the two areas of income maintenance and medical services there has been substantial, and for the most part effective, response. But public policy has faltered in the area of health/social services (14).

People 65 or older have become much more economically independent, largely as a result of greater general affluence and Federal income support programs—primarily Social Security, government pension plans, and Supplemental Security Income (14,40). Medicare, the main Federal health program for those over 64 or with a disability, has broadened access to acute medical and short-term transitional care. Medicaid, the health program jointly funded by States and the Federal Government, has increased access to acute medical care for the indigent and become a major funding source for long-term care of the elderly. Long-term care for those who are not indigent and social services in general have not been as heavily subsidized by the Federal Government.

The protracted course of most dementing illnesses often leads to years during which an affected individual needs constant supervision. Most of the caregiver's activity is directed not at relieving medical problems, but rather at preventing the patient from inflicting harm and at enhancing the quality of the individual's life by taking advantage of preserved mental and physical functions. Those with dementia, for example, often can sing after they lose the ability to speak in long sentences, and they typically retain emotional responsiveness long after their intellectual functions are severely impaired.

Long-term supervisory care of the sort needed for someone with dementia is a service not generally covered by government-supported programs (except for the indigent). In addition, government programs usually focus on the person needing care; yet the person and caregiver function as a unit in most cases of dementia. Hiring a trained supervisor occasionally to watch and take care of someone with dementia gives caregivers respite—time needed to perform routine errands, socialize, or reinstate a sense of their own lives. Such services are not widely available, and formal programs generally do not cover them.

The system of care for those with dementia has several components. Patients must be medically evaluated, their medical illnesses treated, the severity of their illness assessed, their care needs identified, various services coordinated, and use of services financed. Each of these functions must be performed for each person. The ideal situation is a "continuum of care" in which the individual's informal supports and formal resources are assessed, and services identified and provided according to varying needs at different times. The system rarely functions smoothly, however, and the long-term care part of the system is particularly noted for its gaps in services and the paucity of financing alternatives.

Inventory of Services

In the survey undertaken for OTA, those caring for individuals with dementia were asked about their assessment of the importance of various services (regardless of current cost and availability constraints) (see ch. 4). The following 10 services were listed as most important, starting with those most often rated "essential or most important":

1. a *paid companion* who can come *to the home* a few hours each week to give caregivers a rest;
2. assistance in *locating people or organizations* that provide patient care;
3. assistance in *applying for government programs*, such as Medicaid, disability insurance, and income support programs;
4. a *paid companion* who can come to the home for *overnight care* so caregivers can go away for one or more days;
5. *home care* to provide personal care for the individual with dementia, such as bathing, dressing, or feeding in the home;
6. *support groups* composed of others who are caring for individuals with dementia;
7. *special nursing home care* programs only for individuals with dementia;
8. short-term *respite care* in nursing homes or

hospitals to take care of individuals with dementia while the caregiver is away;

9. *adult day care* providing supervision and activities away from the home; and

10. *visiting nurse* services for care at home (123).

In-home care, information about availability of services and government programs, and various forms of respite care were all highly ranked in the survey. These services do not exactly match those now available. Many of the services could be provided in a variety of settings, or by more than one type of professional.

Services are generally provided by agencies that focus on particular target groups in the population. The Federal Government funds services through several programs, including:

- *Medicare*, providing acute medical services for those at least 65, disabled, or suffering from end-stage renal disease;
- *Medicaid*, a joint State and Federal program to provide acute and long-term care for those with low income;
- *Social Services Block Grants*, under title XX of the Social Security Act—the services are not specified by the Federal Government, and States may provide foster care, adult day care, home care, homemaker services, meal preparation and delivery, transportation, or other services;
- *Supplemental Security Income*, a Federal program that makes monthly payments to the aged, disabled, and blind with incomes and assets below a Federal standard—individual States may supplement the Federal benefit to cover specific groups, such as those in board and care facilities, and can also cover services such as home care and homemaker services;
- *Services for the Aged*, under title III of the Older Americans Act—the range of services and eligibility are determined by States and Area Agencies on Aging (which are affiliated with the Administration on Aging); services may include adult day care, home care, homemaker services, transportation, telephone reassurance, senior center activities, and others;
- *Mental Health Services*, under Mental Health Block Grants to the States—the services include family counseling, drug use counseling, and support groups, and may include diagnosis and treatment in some areas; and
- *Income Programs*, under Social Security and government pensions programs—Social Security accounts for 37.6 percent and government pensions for 8.5 percent of the income to couples over 64; for individuals, the figures are 44.5 percent from Social Security and 7.8 percent from government pensions (40).

Government programs thus can overlap extensively in providing services for persons with dementia, can leave gaps in available services, and can vary in coverage from region to region and from one person to another. In addition to variable coverage, there is also variability of how services are organized. Services are usually organized according to the agency providing them. One study observed:

Health services for the aged are multiple, parallel, overlapping, and noncontinuous and at the very least confusing to the elderly consumer. Rarely do they meet the collective criteria of availability, accessibility, affordability, or offer continuity of care in a holistically organized system. Planning for health services for the aged is similarly confused. Parallel systems of service have their own planning mechanisms. As a result, the various planning efforts overlap, contradict, and are unrelated one to the other. Virtually all the services are funded by differing public money streams and have varied administrative arrangements, widely ranging eligibility requirements, and different benefits for the same or similar services (15).

Government and nongovernment programs are similar in grouping services into acute medical services, long-term care services, mental health services, senior services, and social services. The specific services included under these groupings often cover similar services and leave gaps among others. Personal care service may be included as a social benefit, a long-term care benefit, or in some cases a medical benefit. In most areas, however, it would not be available under any agency programs. Some of the services are noted in table 1-5. The settings in which the services are provided can be either residential (where the client lives) or nonresidential (a place the client goes to obtain services). The settings most often used are

Table 1-5.—Care Services for Individuals With Dementia

Adult day care	Patient assessment
Case management	Personal care
Chore services	Personal emergency
Congregate meals	response systems
Dental services	Physical therapy
Home delivered meals	Physician services
Home health aide services	Protective services
Homemaker services	Recreational services
Hospice services	Respite care
Information and referral to	Skilled nursing
services	Speech therapy
Legal services	Supervision
Mental health services	Telephone reassurance
Occupational therapy	Transportation
Paid companion/sitter	

SOURCE: Office of Technology Assessment, 1986.

listed and briefly defined in table 1-6. Chapter 6 contains a more detailed discussion of the settings, and the way that services and settings are provided and allocated.

Senior Services

Although dementing conditions are increasingly prevalent with age, only a minority of those in any age group ever develops dementia. Services for older Americans are usually targeted at the needs of the greatest number, and include senior centers, transportation, counseling, and homemaker chores. These are important services, but many programs exclude mentally impaired individuals, and many services useful to most older Americans are not helpful to those with dementia. Departments of aging and Federal agencies have increasingly focused on "frail" elderly individuals in recent years, but this grouping includes a heterogeneous population with a large variety of medical conditions.

Dementing conditions are among the most prevalent and severe age-associated diseases. But recognition of this fact is relatively recent, and services have not fully adapted to the needs of those with dementia. Under the Administration on Aging, several Area Agencies on Aging and Long-Term Care Gerontology Centers have established programs on Alzheimer's disease (108,110), but these serve only a small fraction of those with de-

Table 1-6.—Care Settings for Individuals With Dementia

Residential settings:

In-home services may include home health care, personal care, chore services, and homemaker services to the client's house, apartment, or other residence. Some in-home health services are provided by home health care agencies, most of which are certified by Medicare and must meet Federal standards for staffing and range of services. Other services are provided by community agencies funded by Federal, State, and local governments or nongovernmental organizations. Such agencies are generally not licensed or regulated.

Nursing homes are health care facilities that provide 24-hour care, nursing, and personal services in an institutional setting. Most are certified to provide care under Medicare and Medicaid to eligible residents, and are regulated by States, subject to Federal and State standards.

Board and care facilities are nonmedical residential care facilities that provide room and board and variable degrees of protective supervision and personal care. These range in size from foster care units with a few residents to large domiciliary facilities that house several hundred people. Many board and care facilities are licensed by State governments, but regulations are generally limited to physical structure and fire safety rather than patient care.

State mental hospitals are generally large State-funded institutions that provide acute and long-term psychiatric care primarily for mentally ill people, but also for some patients with dementia—especially those with behavioral symptoms that are difficult to manage.

Hospitals are facilities for medical care of those temporarily residing in them. The primary services available are diagnosis and treatment, but hospitals also often serve as foci for rehabilitation, case management, counseling, family support. They may also be affiliated with nursing homes, day care centers, home health agencies, or other settings and services.

Hospices are facilities for the care of terminally ill people. The emphasis in hospices is on alleviating symptoms and providing personal support, rather than cure and rehabilitation. Hospice services can be delivered in other settings, if the intent is to diminish suffering rather than prolong life.

Nonresidential settings:

Adult day care centers are day treatment facilities, some of which provide intensive medical, physical, or occupational therapy. Others provide primarily social activities and personal services for several hours during the day. Adult day care centers are licensed by some States, and must meet fire and safety codes of local jurisdictions, but are not subject to Federal regulation unless they provide services reimbursed by Medicare or Medicaid.

Community mental health centers are psychiatric and psychological treatment facilities that provide a variety of mental health services for people with acute and chronic mental illnesses. Most services are provided on an outpatient basis. Most centers were originally developed in accordance with Federal regulations tied to Federal funding but are now regulated by States and funded by them, supplemented by Federal funding through Mental Health Block Grants.

Outpatient facilities and clinics are medical settings for diagnosis and treatment of diseases. They may also become involved in delivering other services such as case management and counseling.

Senior centers are facilities intended for use by older Americans. They are often funded by a combination of private charity and local, State, and Federal Government contributions. Day care, recreational activities, family support, case management, and mental health services are available at some but not all senior centers.

SOURCE: Office of Technology Assessment, 1986.

mentia. In most areas, services for the elderly population do not include those specifically intended for individuals with dementia, and are poorly adapted to their needs (59). Although many commentators question whether services should be made available to those with dementia that are not available to similarly disabled groups (108), the degree of mismatch between services and the needs of persons with dementia could clearly be reduced without creating special eligibility groups.

Acute Care Services

Acute medical care for dementia includes identifying symptoms, diagnosing their cause, and treating illnesses discovered in the diagnostic process. Diagnosis and medical treatment for dementia are generally covered by insurance and government programs to the same extent as other medical conditions. Patients are not excluded from eligibility for acute medical care because of the nature of their symptoms. One inequity, a limitation of outpatient psychiatric care, has been addressed in recommendations of the DHHS Task Force on Alzheimer's Disease (110), but that represents a relatively small component of the acute care needs of those with dementia.

Methods of prevention also need attention in the acute care system. While there is no known way to avoid the most common dementia—Alzheimer's disease—diet, personal habits, and medical care can prevent many of the other disorders (e.g., diet can influence the risk of vascular disease and thus vascular dementia, and cessation of smoking can reduce the likelihood of lung cancer with spread to the brain—one of the most common types of brain tumors in those over 64). Even if the disorders causing dementia cannot be prevented, however, excess disability related to them can be reduced—preventing unnecessary suffering and costs of medical attention—avoiding infections (through vaccination and prompt treatment), careful use of medications (to avoid side effects), and altering personal habits (e.g., stop smoking to enhance lung function and reduce fire hazard, or reduce drinking that intensifies disorientation).

Diagnosis and treatment presuppose trained doctors, nurses, and other health professionals.

Alzheimer's disease and dementia were once the province of specialists such as neurologists and psychiatrists, but the aging of the population and increased awareness of dementia are making these conditions also a problem for family practitioners, internists, and other primary care physicians. In addition, there is a movement in medicine to provide specialized training for those dealing with the medical problems of older people. That type of practice, called geriatrics, is not now a medical specialty, but existing medical boards are offering special recognition of geriatric training (see ch. 9). Medical aspects of dementia are important in such training because dementia is primarily, although not exclusively, a geriatric problem.

The main issues in acute medical care are: 1) accurate diagnosis; 2) adequate treatment of general medical problems and controllable symptoms; and 3) training physicians, nurses, nurse's aides, and other caregivers. The main mechanisms for improving care are to educate health professionals and to ensure that full diagnostic evaluation and treatments are fairly reimbursed.

Long-Term Care Services

Although no single definition of long-term care has been accepted, it is generally agreed that its goal is to maintain or improve an individual's ability to function as independently as possible, and that services will be needed over a prolonged period, even if only needed intermittently. Medical care is an essential component, but a variety of other services are also important (60). "Long-term care" in public policy contexts sometimes means primarily nursing home care, although recent definitions are careful not to so restrict themselves. The White House Conference on Aging, for example, noted:

> Long-term care represents a range of services that address the health, social, and personal care needs of individuals who, for one reason or another, have never developed or have lost the ability for self-care. Services may be continuous or intermittent, but it is generally presumed that they will be delivered in the "long-term," that is, indefinitely, to individuals who have demonstrated need usually measured by some index of functional incapacity (113).

In terms of spending, however, Federal long-term care policy is mainly concerned with nursing home care. Even within the nursing home population, there is an important division of types and duration of long-term care. Nursing home care covered by Medicare, for example, is intended for those who primarily need medical treatments and intensive nursing care, called "skilled care" (e.g., changing of catheters, postsurgical care, and physical therapy) for short periods (generally less than 2 months). Medicaid coverage includes "skilled" care and also less specifically medical components, called "intermediate" care, but the emphasis remains on medical, as opposed to supervisory, care. Medical care in nursing homes tends to be needed most by those who are there for fewer than 90 days. Those residing in nursing homes for longer periods differ from others in type of disease (72) and in the services needed (14,52).

One study found that those with severe dementia admitted to a VA hospital were much more likely than other patients to come from a nursing home and to still reside in a nursing home one year later (96). Another study found that impairments that include dementia have the longest expected duration of residency in nursing homes among groups studied (72). Some have called attention to the two different populations in nursing homes, calling them "short-term long-term care" versus "long-term long-term care" (16), or "skilled" versus "chronic" care (52).

Individuals with dementia are likely to be in the long-stay group, needing supervisory and personal care more than medical attention. One analysis estimates that those with dementia constitute 60 to 70 percent of the long-stay group (14), making dementia one of the major determinants of those staying longer than 90 days in nursing homes. The distinction between short- and long-stay patients is particularly relevant in considering the potentially catastrophic costs of nursing home care. Catastrophic costs would accrue primarily to the long-stay residents of nursing homes. Five percent of Americans 65 and over are in nursing homes at any one time, but only 3.5 percent are long-stay patients (16). That implies the risk of incurring catastrophic long-term care costs is restricted to a smaller fraction of the population than is often cited, and makes risk-sharing through insurance more practical.

Nursing home care is by far the largest cost component of long-term care. Costs vary from region to region, ranging from just over $750 per month to over $3,000.[1] A recent study estimates that out-of-pocket costs for hospital care will account for $3.3 billion of the $63 billion total (5.2 percent) spent on inpatient services, and $600 million of the $5.8 billion (10.3 percent) on outpatient services in 1986 (see figure 1-5). That estimate contrasts with $16 billion in out-of-pocket payments of the estimated $32.8 billion (49 percent) spent on nursing home care (54). (The projection of 1986 costs differs from the $38.9 billion used by the Health Care Financing Administration cited earlier (8)—as it is based on a different economic model.)

Direct comparisons between hospitals and nursing homes are somewhat misleading, however. Nursing home and hospital costs include several components such as room and board, laundry, meal preparation, and cleaning. Residents of nursing homes and hospitals would pay for such "basic" living costs even if they were healthy and not in either facility. Other services are needed because of disability, such as nursing care and access to diagnostic treatment facilities, and these costs can be attributed to illness. Yet nursing home and hospital charges do not separate basic from medical service components. Comparisons of nursing home and hospital costs should compare the costs due to illness, not overall costs. The proportion of basic living costs is higher for nursing homes than hospitals, accounting for some of the discrepancy in what is covered by insurance and health care programs. It is unlikely, however, that basic living costs account for all or even most of the differential coverage. There is even evidence to suggest that hospitals are more expensive than nursing homes in delivering the same services (102), and costs in hospitals would more likely be covered by insurance or government health programs.

The availability of nursing home beds varies dramatically. In Wisconsin there is a surfeit of beds, particularly in the summer. In other States, health

---

[1]These figures are taken from fiscal year 1982 costs for intermediate care facility reimbursement in Kansas under Medicaid ($25.11 per day) as the minimum, and for a proprietary nonprofit facility in New York (over $100 per day) as the maximum. The Kansas figure is taken from Health Care Financing Administration data organized by the American Health Care Association (57).

Figure 1-5.—Out-of-Pocket Expenditures by Type of Service and Care, Estimated for 1986

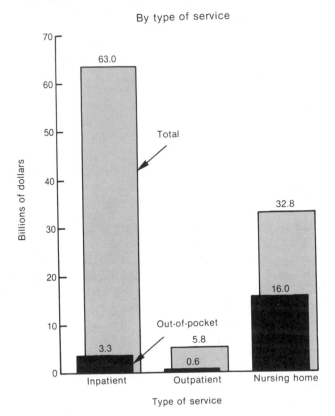

By type of service

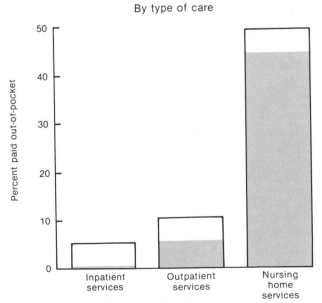

By type of care

SOURCE: ICF, Inc., "The Role of Medicare in Financing the Health Care of Older Americans," submitted to American Association of Retired Persons, July 1985, table 21, adapted by the Office of Technology Assessment.

systems agencies or other health planning boards have deliberately restricted the number of nursing home beds available in order to reduce costs under Medicaid. They have done so by using a process called certificate-of-need legislation, requiring a facility to receive State approval before adding beds. The constraint in number of beds has increased pressures for new beds by creating an unmet demand in many States.

The dearth of insurance and Medicare coverage of long-term care (particularly for stays of more than 90 days) is not widely recognized by most older Americans. A survey of elderly people performed by Gallup for the American Association of Retired Persons showed that 79 percent believed that Medicare would pay for all or part of their nursing home care (6). Another survey found that only 25 to 47 percent of those asked knew that Medicare does not cover a 6-month nursing home stay (76). Yet Medicare covers less than 2 percent of expenditures for nursing homes, and private insurance pays for less than 1 percent (54).

Medicaid is a program intended only for the indigent, and eligibility is contingent on nearly complete depletion of financial resources. Two recent surveys of older people in Massachusetts showed the high risk of families "spending down" to become financially eligible for Medicaid coverage soon after admission to a nursing home. Among those 75 and over, from 57 to 72 percent would become Medicaid-eligible by the end of one year in a nursing home; the figures for those over 65 were 57 to 83 percent (depending on marital status) (104). Figures for other areas will differ significantly because Medicaid varies in coverage and eligibility from State to State (see ch. 11) (19,67).

Social Services

Social services include housekeeping, transportation, and assistance in daily living (e.g., dressing, eating, shopping, meal preparation). Social services emphasize providing clients with what they need but cannot do for themselves, regardless of why they cannot do them. These services can be provided at the client's home or in community facilities, and not only at specialized medical or mental health centers. Many services, such as assistance with dressing or meal preparation, are needed by most individuals with dementia.

The home services needed by individuals with dementia are a particularly troublesome public policy issue. Medicare home health benefits are intended for use by those who would otherwise be accepting medical care in a hospital or nursing home. Although meal preparation, supervision, and personal care are the services most frequently needed by individuals with dementia at home, they are not covered by Medicare (or by Medicaid in most areas). Some social service agencies include those with dementia among their eligible population groups. The need for those delivering services to be trained to deal with the behavioral problems and mental confusion associated with dementia, however, may prevent some agencies from including persons with dementia in their client groups. In some regions, social services are coordinated with long-term care, health care, mental health care, or senior services (e.g., providing transportation to day care centers or delivering "meals on wheels"). In most areas, however, social services are only poorly coordinated with other services (19,58). Yet these services are among the ones most desired by caregivers and are significantly less expensive than home *health* care.

Medical and other health and social service administrators are reluctant to increase the range and availability of home services in some areas, however, because of anticipated escalating costs. They fear that such services would be abused by a variety of people who are not ill or needy. The potential for abuse would be reduced if recipients of the service were required to have an assessment of needs (based on diagnosis, functional disability, or some combination of factors), but it is not clear that there is a practical assessment method available that is cheap, accurate, reliable, and auditable.

Inexpensive home care for persons with dementia has been successful in some areas, often sponsored or coordinated by local ADRDA chapters or Area Agencies on Aging (30,35,89). A pilot project to train volunteer caregivers about dementia so they can provide social services in the home is beginning under the Senior Companion Program of ACTION. Such programs rely on funding through charity, volunteers, and nongovernment organizations, and the client's family is usually the source of payment. That is an economic way to control use. Another method is to set an upper limit on subsidized benefits by limiting the total days or budget, or through a voucher system (83).

Mental Health Services

Until the 1960s, institutional care for individuals with dementia was largely provided in State mental hospitals. Public policies to reduce the population in such facilities decreased the number of persons with dementia in mental institutions, and the availability of joint Federal and State coverage of nursing home care accelerated this trend (58,64). One careful investigation suggests that older persons who once would have been sent to mental hospitals are now referred to nursing homes (47 of 50 residents in one nursing home—94 percent—had a mental disorder) (95). The displacement has not been due to transferring residents directly from mental hospitals to nursing homes, however. (In the study just cited, only 1 resident out of 50 had been so transferred.) The data are most simply explained by older persons with behavioral and cognitive symptoms being preferentially admitted to nursing homes instead of mental institutions in recent years.

The behavioral aspects of dementia are among the most difficult symptoms to manage, and facilities using a mental health model (focusing on adapting to the individual's behavior) rather than a medical one (focusing on correcting a disability) appear in preliminary studies to benefit people more (25). A pattern of care is emerging that emphasizes careful medical evaluation and drug management, combined with a mental health model of care in nursing homes and day care centers that coordinate their services with available social and aging services.

Persons with dementia become dependent because of their inability to understand the intricacies of daily life. Although symptoms are caused by physical brain damage, dependency is induced by loss of *mental* function, rather than *physical* disability. That contrasts with arthritis or hip fractures, for example, where immobility is directly caused by joint and bone problems, and the disability is easier to observe and measure. There is less opportunity for confusing physical disabilities than mental ones, and concern for overutilization of health care services overall has engendered a conservative approach that puts the burden of proof on individuals with mental symptoms to show the legitimacy of their needs.

The behavioral symptoms of dementia often relegate individuals to categories for which coverage by health programs is ambiguous. They may be eligible for medical care, mental health services, both, or neither. In times of budget restraint, programs typically cut back on services not central to their mandate. Dementia is at the margin of both medical care and mental health services. Patients may be seen by a family physician, an internist, a neurologist, or a psychiatrist, and each specialty has its own orientation for diagnosis and treatment. Agencies delivering mental health services may exclude someone with dementia because their resources only cover drug rehabilitation, for example, or rape counseling, and yet health care programs typically focus on acute rather than long-term care. Those with dementia may thus be left with access to no services except family care at home or nursing home placement.

The Federal Government supports mental health research at the National Institute of Mental Health (NIMH) and pays for some mental health services through payments to States. Federal and State Governments jointly fund Community Mental Health Centers (CMHCs) throughout the Nation, but these must deliver a full range of services to all population groups. A recent survey found that at most 20 percent of CMHCs had programs for persons with dementia and their families; these programs were five times as common in CMHCs specialized in mental health for older individuals, and they were heavily used where available (68,69). NIMH has established three Clinical Research Centers on Psychopathology of the Elderly, two of which focus on Alzheimer's disease (108). These are important centers for investigating individual needs, treatment methods, and family support mechanisms. They also train many clinicians who can then care for patients in their practice. Yet because of the extent of the problem, the NIMH national centers and those CMHCs covering dementia miss large sections of the population. Findings from these centers must be applied nationwide before most Americans can benefit from them.

Mental health services for *caregivers* are also important. That applies to family caregivers as well as professionals and aides working in home care services, day care centers, and nursing homes. Services for caregivers include support groups, counseling, and treatment of stress-induced disorders. Much of the support for families has been provided by volunteer groups such as ADRDA and dozens of smaller local organizations at little cost to taxpayers. Such support cannot cover the full range of needs, however, and large geographic areas are still not served by such groups. Expanding the range of services and geographic coverage are both high priorities for ADRDA in its current organizational plan (4). Services for caregivers in long-term care facilities are not as well organized, and that issue deserves increased attention from home care, day care, board and care, and nursing home providers.

GROUPS OF SPECIAL CONCERN

Several groups are of special concern in policy discussions of care and services for persons with dementia:

- those without families,
- minority and ethnic groups,
- individuals experiencing disease onset in middle age,
- individuals residing in rural areas,
- veterans,
- low-income groups, and
- caregivers.

Each group has special needs and problems not shared by everyone with dementia that influence how providers must adapt services. The first four groups are at special risk of reduced access to services. They represent especially vulnerable populations, and those most likely to benefit from public services. The different risk factors can reinforce one another to identify those in particular jeopardy. A black woman with dementia living in a rural area on low income without a family, for example, would be unlikely to be receiving services but might especially need them.

Those Without Families

Much public interest has centered on problems faced by the families of those with dementia. Yet while many policies designed to improve the situation of someone with dementia rely on relatives or friends who can make decisions about care, finances, or the person's rights, many individuals with dementia do not have families or friends available. A 1975 General Accounting Office study of those age 65 or older in Cleveland, found 13 percent did not have a primary source of help in the event of disability (107). A recent national sample of long-term care recipients found that 10.7 percent lived alone (100).

The number without family may be higher for those with dementia because so many are quite old, and likely to be widowed. Extreme old age also increases the chance that someone's children are disabled or deceased. People who are not married are more likely than married individuals to reside for long periods in nursing homes (72). They are less likely to have access to alternative services such as day care because of difficulty finding the service and arranging for transportation. Informal care directly provided by families and coordination of care often managed by family members are likewise unavailable. Patients without families are thus disproportionately dependent on formal long-term care services such as nursing home care and case management by public agencies. Special methods of identifying and assisting patients without families are available only in a few areas, however, and there is little information about them.

Identifying those without families who may need services is especially difficult, but can be done by alerting police, ministers, grocers, and others in the community to look for older people who may be ill and to refer them to a lead agency. One program that does this is the "gatekeeper" program in Spokane, WA, which links a Community Mental Health Center, an Area Agency on Aging, and 13 other agencies together in a disseminated referral network with a single central process for screening candidates and determining eligibility for services (67,89).

Minority Groups

Minority groups have lower average incomes and use fewer public services than comparable groups in the general population. They frequently have different social support systems, religious affiliations, and cultural norms. Disparate minority groups cannot be analyzed as a homogeneous whole. Few studies have been done of older Americans in minority groups in general, and almost no information exists on dementia in particular (73). Although the prevalence of dementia appears similar across national boundaries and races, a few variations have been reported. The high rate of hypertension among blacks and Native Americans may make them more likely to develop vascular dementia (33,118). The ratio of vascular dementia to Alzheimer's disease also appears higher in Japan, and surveys of Chinese and Taiwanese populations report dramatically reduced prevalence of dementia (although such differences may be due to reporting rather than true prevalence) (78).

International studies of prevalence rates in different races can give clues about the expected prevalence among those minority groups in the United States, but rates in native countries can be affected by economic and cultural factors. Life expectancy among most minority groups is rising with more older individuals at risk of developing dementia. Minority groups also tend to be undercounted in the census, so projections of dementia among them would understate the true prevalence in the population. Each of these factors suggests that more minority elderly Americans will develop dementia, and that a higher proportion of persons with dementia will come from minority groups (73,118). Direct assessment of the prevalence and cause of dementia among minority groups in the United States is therefore important.

Disability among members of minority groups is higher (88), but statistics show lower use of many public services (73). That pattern might be altered, however, by programs designed for specific minority populations. The Keiko nursing homes in Los Angeles focus on the needs of Americans of Japanese descent, while the successful On-Lok program in San Francisco serves a population that is 70 percent of Chinese descent (73).

Social, medical, and long-term care services are usually structured for the majority population and frequently are only poorly adapted to the cultural norms of minority groups. Most minority groups, particularly those with sufficient concentrations of people in an area, have informal networks of family, religious, community, and service supports. These supports generally are also linked at the local level with service providers, but Federal and State Government policies frequently fail to permit local agencies sufficient latitude to take advantage of minority group social supports (118).

Service systems for minority groups work best when they take advantage of existing supports within the community. Black Americans tend to rely on churches for social and emotional support; Hispanics often have a network of *consejeras* (informal counselors) or *servidores* (people who informally take on the role of providing information and support); the Chinese have *Yau Sum* ("person of good heart"); American Japanese may have *Shinsetsu sua hito* ("kind person") networks; and Native Americans have tribal councils and designated spiritual leaders (73,118). The capacity of such informal supports, as in the majority culture, can be exceeded. Individuals with dementia typically go beyond the ability of the informal system to adapt at some point in the illness, but that point can be delayed by programs that foster informal networks, or that at least do not interfere with them (118).

Although family support groups have grown rapidly throughout the United States, the early growth has been concentrated in the majority Caucasian population. In the survey conducted for OTA, drawn from the ADRDA national mailing list, 94.8 percent of respondents were white, 1.6 percent black, and 0.7 percent other (2.9 percent did not respond to this question) (123). That compares with 88.5 percent white, 8.8 percent black, and 2.7 percent other minority in the U.S. census of those aged 55 to 64 (73). Family support groups

can, however, be successful among minority groups, as demonstrated by an Hispanic support group started in the Tampa area (47). Outreach to minority groups is high on the agenda of many of the support group organizations, including ADRDA.

Individuals Experiencing Onset of Dementia in Middle Age

The majority of dementing illnesses do not begin until after age 65. An estimated 5 to 10 percent of persons with dementia, however, develop the disease in middle age (27). The exact proportion of cases that begin before age 65 is uncertain, but an estimated 75,000 Americans under 65 have severe dementia (79).

The problems caused by onset in middle age add to those associated with later onset. Individuals who are working almost invariably lose their jobs and are usually unable to find other employment. They and their families not only suffer loss of income, but also incur substantial medical expenses for diagnosis and treatment, often complicated by loss of health insurance caused by unemployment (although this effect should be mitigated by recent changes in Federal law that require extension of health insurance for most categories of employees).

In addition, those in middle age are more likely to have young children with financial and emotional needs, who are less likely to understand declining mental function and personality change. Finally, many families discover that finances have been mismanaged for months or years before diagnosis. In many cases, the persons failed to maintain health, automobile, and life insurance payments, left important bills unpaid, or spent family funds frivolously.

These problems can be compounded by the difficulty in dealing with public programs. A person under 65 may encounter difficulty establishing eligibility for Social Security Disability Insurance (SSDI) (19). The survey done for OTA of those caring for someone with dementia found that 11 percent had applied for SSDI and 35 percent had been denied benefits (123). That finding is particularly important for those under age 65 because denial of disability benefits also generally precludes Medicare eligibility (19). Those declared ineligible for SSDI are also barred from Medicare coverage; those found eligible for SSDI must wait a minimum of 29 months until they are covered by Medicare (see ch. 11). The House and Senate Appropriations Committees requested that the Social Security Administration address disability policies regarding dementia, in consultation with the National Institutes of Health (conference report on Public Law 99-500).

The number of those developing dementia before age 65 could dramatically increase as a consequence of acquired immune deficiency syndrome (AIDS). The majority of those who develop AIDS also develop dementia due to brain infection by the virus that causes the disease (85). They thus become dependent on others for medical and daily care. Nine thousand cases of AIDS were reported in the United States in 1985, and 46,000 to 90,000 are expected in 1991; 20 to 30 percent of the estimated 1 to 1.5 million Americans infected by the AIDS virus as of June 1986 are projected to develop AIDS by 1991 (24). If 70 percent of those with AIDS develop dementia, then the proportion of those with dementia under 65 would almost double. There are several uncertainties in that estimate. The mortality of AIDS is quite high and so the duration of illness would be short. The proportion of those with virus infection who develop dementia but not AIDS is unknown, and the duration might be longer for such individuals. The AIDS pandemic is thus likely to dramatically increase care needs for those under age 65 with dementia, but the amount and duration of needed care are highly uncertain—both overall and for each patient.

Rural Residents

Rural residents have access to fewer specialized services, and hence a restricted range of long-term care options. Rural areas may be served by a single general physician unfamiliar with dementia, have only one local hospital, and only one nursing home. Few have adult day care or in-home services, and participation in family support groups, the few places they exist, may require substantial travel time. Reduced access to services may be exacerbated if there are no family members

in the area to help care for the individual with dementia, or if there are no neighbors nearby to provide intermittent help.

Veterans

The Veterans Administration is concerned about the rising prevalence of dementia among those eligible for its services (28,116,117). The rise in prevalence among veterans will peak 10 to 20 years before it does in the general population because of the special demographics of those who served during World War II, the Korean war, and in Vietnam (see figure 1-6).

The care received by veterans depends on why and when their illnesses began. The first priority for VA services goes to those whose disability or illness is service-connected. Dementia is only rarely service-connected (e.g., because of severe head trauma). Other services are provided on a space-available basis. Some VA facilities have developed special programs for those with dementia, but VA hospitals do not guarantee access to long-term care or to specialized services for those with dementia (see figure 1-7). Most VA facilities cover care for diagnosis and treatment of intercurrent illnesses. Veterans Administration hospitals and nursing homes treated over 20,000 veterans with a diagnosis of dementia in fiscal year 1983. Special care units for individuals with dementia have been developed at 12 VA medical centers. Yet the survey of caregivers done for OTA

Figure 1-6.—Number of Veterans Age 65 and Over

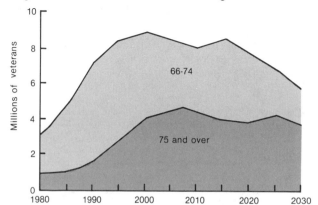

SOURCE: Veterans Administration, International Working Group, *The Veterans Administration and Dementia, Recommendations for Patient Care, Research, and Training,* October 1985.

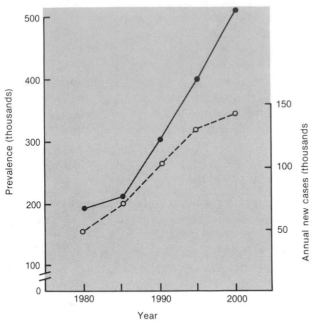

Figure 1-7.—Prevalence and Annual New Cases of Dementia, U.S. Veterans, 1980-2000

SOURCE: Veterans Administration, International Working Group, *The Veterans Administration and Dementia, Recommendations for Patient Care, Research, and Training*, October 1985.

found that 45 percent of those who had applied for extended care were refused VA services, most often because the disability was not service-connected (123).

For several reasons, the VA system is under increasing political pressure to provide care to those with dementia and other chronic illnesses. First, the number of veterans reaching advanced age is expanding rapidly (see figure 1-6). In 1980, only 3 million veterans were 65 and older, but this will increase to 9 million by the year 2000 (representing 63 percent of all men 65 and older) (115). Second, veterans and their families often expect the VA to cover all care. Explanations that particular illnesses or disabilities will not be covered often are not understood or are rejected, particularly if families know that the type of care they seek is available at VA facilities in other geographical areas.

Those With Low Incomes

Americans with low incomes are particularly dependent on government programs. Lack of income restricts them to those services that are free

through charity, subsidized, or inherently inexpensive. A substantial proportion of their low income is directly provided by the Federal Government. Among those 65 and over with less than $10,000 income, for example, social security provides on average 82.2 percent of income, compared with 17.8 percent for those with incomes over $30,100 (40). In addition, the Medicaid program to cover medical services is intended primarily for this group, yet both the lack of awareness and the complexity of the program hinder full use of the benefits. Ironically, those with higher incomes may benefit more from Medicaid, particularly the long-term care component, because they have easier access to the information needed to obtain eligibility and can afford to enter a nursing home as private pay clients, who later find they have "spent down" to Medicaid eligibility. People with lower incomes cannot pay initially, and nursing homes that have a choice prefer to admit private pay residents because Medicaid reimbursement rates are low.

Caregivers

Middle-aged caregivers are at high risk of becoming secondary victims of dementia. Volunteer groups and government services could productively target this group. The majority of those caring for dependent parents are middle-aged women (12,100), a fact that appears to be true not only for dependent older people in general, but also for those with dementia (37). These women may also be responsible for the care of children or adolescents, or may just be starting careers after their children have left home (12). Yet family support groups are the only services available to them in many areas.

A recent study of a national sample of long-term care recipients found that roughly three-fourths of caregivers lived with the dependent older person 7 days a week, and only 9.7 percent purchased formal services (100). Of those caring for dependent older people, 44 percent had done so for more than 1 year but less than 4 years, and over 20 percent had been caregivers for 5 years or more.

Caregivers who are themselves old face different stresses from those in middle age. Older caregivers are more likely to have an illness that in-

Box A.—A Case History

P was a bookish man with a robust sense of humor. He was an excellent student, had an easy time in college, and received his medical degree in 1947 from Louisiana State University. He did an internship, and several years of residency in pathology and medicine (doing work on kidney physiology with Homer Smith, an investigator of international reknown), and completed a residency in psychiatry. His interests over the years drifted towards Zoroastrianism, Tibetan Buddhism, psychoanalysis, and other widely divergent topics. He practiced as a psychiatrist and teacher for two decades, earning the intense loyalty of a large circle of patients and students.

In the fall of 1975, at age 50, he startled the guests at a dinner party by picking up the meat from his plate, rather than using his knife and fork. Although P had long been regarded as unusual, that was markedly eccentric, and far outside the range of his usual punctilious behavior. Soon after Christmas, his family found he did not remember that Christmas had passed. His humorous anecdotes became fragmented and impossible to follow. He became paranoid, and got lost returning home from work despite having had the same clinic and home addresses in New York City for many years. In January 1976, he was evaluated by a neurologist who said he had Alzheimer's disease.

The family adjusted to the simultaneous traumas of losing P's substantial income, dealing with his increasingly distressful disabilities, incurring large medical bills, and arranging his care. In March 1976, the informal care arrangement broke down under stress, and P was moved to Baton Rouge, Louisiana, to live at his childhood home with his mother. His wife moved to Canada, the country of her citizenship, his daughter found alternative financing for college, and his son left home for college. P's mental symptoms worsened. He could not remember where he was, what had happened to his patients, or why he could not return to New York. He had his first seizure in 1977, and his behavior became too difficult to manage so he was no longer taken to church. Where once he had never been found without a book in hand (he was the sort who would take a book to a picnic), he found it impossible to read. In 1978, he began to wander and get lost (to be picked up by the police), so the outside doors were locked. He began to hallucinate and talk to himself and show increasingly unstable emotional reactions.

In 1980, a day worker was hired to help at home because P could no longer get into and out of bed, and needed assistance eating and dressing. In 1981, his mother developed heart failure and had to be rushed to the hospital. That precipitated a crisis for the family. Nursing homes were regarded as either too expensive or unsafe, so home care was elected. Financial assistance was not available under disability or government programs because P did not require "skilled" care, but rather needed personal care and supervision. Home care services were not available in Baton Rouge in any event. The family, after several days on the phone, hired three "sitters" to cover 20 hours a day (one attendant during the day and two for evening and night). P's condition worsened over the next several years, with uncontrolled movements, inability to talk, and failure to recognize others.

In January 1985, P lapsed into a stuporous state of unknown cause. In early February, he was rushed to the hospital, where aggressive medical treatment was not pursued. Six days after admission, he died quietly at age 60, almost a decade after diagnosis.

creases the stress and health risk of caregiving. The finances of a person with dementia and the caregiver are closely commingled when the caregiver is a spouse, so the costs of care can have a catastrophic impact on two or more people, not just the ill person. Decisions about an individual's legal status (and control of family finances) likewise affect the person with dementia and the spouse alike.

POLICY ISSUES

The problems faced by persons with dementia and their families impinge on public policy in many ways. There is no cure, no means of prevention, and no fully effective treatment for most dementias. The government strategies for addressing this public health problem are: 1) to support research in hopes of discovering a cure or means of prevention, and 2) to deliver or facilitate delivery of services for those who develop dementia. The roles played by the Federal Government that are relevant to the problems of dementia include:

- supporting research, including basic science, clinical research, and the study of health care delivery;
- directly providing health care to special populations;
- paying for care through Medicaid, Medicare, Mental Health Block Grants, and tax subsidies;
- training and educating health professionals and caregivers;
- assuring the quality of acute and long-term care;
- planning health and social services; and
- disseminating information on care, research, and services.

Table 1-7 contains a brief list of some of the most important Federal programs that deliver or fund care for persons with dementia.

Should There Be Special Programs for Dementia?

Any discussion of the government's role in this field must consider whether there should be special programs for individuals with dementia. Furthermore, judgments about the fairness and effectiveness of different policies require a clear distinction between special services, entitlements, and research.

Specialized Services

Specialized services for those with dementia include support groups, day care centers, nursing home units, and in-home respite care programs designed specifically to aid those with mental impairment. Such specialized emphasis helps in the training of caregivers and focuses attention on the special problems of delivering services to those with dementia. The existence of specialized services for one group of diseases need not discourage developing specialized services for others. Patients with cancer, for example, do not receive the same treatment as those with heart disease, and yet may be covered under the same medical program (e.g., Medicare).

There is no consensus that persons with dementia should receive specialized services. Yet special care units at nursing homes, special day care centers, special board and care facilities, and even special hospitals for patients with Alzheimer's disease are proliferating. The rationales for such units are the opportunity to improve the care of persons with dementia by having better trained staff and adaptive environments, reduced interference with residents without dementing disorders, and the need for activities that specifically take account of diminished intellectual and communicative skills. Many worry, however, that such facilities will become the repository for neglected individuals. At present, no separate guidelines are available for special care units and programs, and philosophies and methods for administering them differ markedly. The ferment of activity in special care is generally improving care for those with dementia, however, and is generating innovative care techniques.

Special Entitlements

Special entitlements for individuals with dementia would make eligibility for services contingent on a particular diagnosis or type of disability. A special Medicare or Medicaid entitlement for dementia could be created, analogous to the special Medicare eligibility reserved for those with end-stage renal disease (although a special dementia entitlement would be primarily for long-term personal, rather than medical, care). Those favoring special entitlements contend that the problems of patients with dementia are so severe and different from those with other disorders that they deserve special eligibility. Others contend that those with dementia are merely one group among many vying for services in a fragmented health care market. They point to other groups with similar prob-

Table 1-7.—Federal Roles in Dementia Issues

Function	Primary agency or method	Agency delivering service
Research:		
Biomedical research	Public Health Service	National Institutes of Health (NIH)
		National Institute on Aging (NIA)
		National Institute of Neurological and Communicative
		Disorders and Stroke (NINCDS)
		Other NIH institutes
		National Institute of Mental Health (NIMH) (Alcohol, Drug
		Abuse, and Mental Health Administration)—the majority of
		research under the Public Health Service is conducted at
		universities or medical centers.
	Veterans Administration (VA)	VA investigators; geriatric research, education, and clinical
		care centers
	Department of Education	National Institute on Disability & Rehabilitation Research
Research on health services	National Center for Health Services Research and Health Care Technology	
	Assessment (NCHSR/HCTA)	
	NIMH	
	NIH	
	Health Resources and Services Administration (HRSA)	
	VA	
	Health Care Financing Administration (HCFA)	
	Administration on Aging (AOA)	Long-term care gerontology centers
	National Center for Health Statistics (NCHS)	
	Bureau of the Census	
Direct health care:		
	Department of Defense	Military hospitals and clinics
	VA	VA hospitals and facilities, contractors
	Indian Health Service	Indian Health Service facilities
Payment for care:		
Medicare (acute care)	HCFA	Hospitals, clinics, institutions, other providers
Medicaid (with States)	HCFA	Providers through State administrative offices
Mental Health Block Grants (with States)		Community Mental Health Centers
Tax policies	Department of Treasury	Internal Revenue Service
Contract care	DHHS	Indian Health Service
		VA
Training and education:		
	AOA	Long-term care gerontology centers
	HRSA	Bureau of Health Professions
	Veterans' Administration	Geriatric Research, Education, and Clinical Care Centers;
		Fellowships; Nurse Training; Interdisciplinary Teams
	Public Health Service	NIH Fellowships and Centers; NIMH Fellowships and Centers
	HCFA (Medicare)	Teaching hospitals
	Student Loan Programs	
Quality assurance:		
Acute care	HCFA	Professional review organizations
Nursing home care	HCFA and States (Medicaid)	State certification and inspection offices
Mental health advocacy— block grants to States		
Adult protective services		AOA, others
Planning:		
	Office of Assistant Secretary for Planning and Evaluation	
	Office of Assistant Secretary for Health (Alzheimer's Disease Task Force)	
	Public Health Service	HRSA
		NIMH
	HCFA (Medicare and Medicaid services)	
	AOA	Area agencies on aging
	VA (veterans)	
	Department of Defense (military personnel)	
	Indian Health Service (native Americans)	
Information dissemination:		
	Public Health Service	NIH
		NIMH
	Office of Assistant Secretary for Health (Task Force on Alzheimer's Disease)	
	AOA	Area agencies on aging
	HCFA (Medicare and Medicaid eligibility and coverage)	

SOURCE: Office of Technology Assessment, 1986.

lems in obtaining needed services, particularly long-term care. Other groups also have limited access to long-term care (e.g., adults with mental retardation or adults with spinal injury) and difficulty finding adequate mental health or social services (e.g., schizophrenics or the homeless). Still others may need health services from public programs with limited budgets (e.g., maternal and child health for the indigent under Medicaid).

Some of the consequences of developing special entitlements for dementia can be predicted. A special long-term care program for those with Alzheimer's disease would face several problems. If based on diagnosis, it would be unduly restrictive (eliminating services for those with multi-infarct or other dementias) or it would be vulnerable to inappropriate utilization because of vague definitions of the conditions covered. Making services contingent on diagnosis or a restricted list of conditions would put severe strain on the accuracy of diagnosis. While special diagnostic centers report 90 percent diagnostic accuracy (64), that proportion would likely drop if there were incentives favoring one diagnosis over another. Physicians wishing to aid their patients would likely list the diagnosis of Alzheimer's disease in preference to other dementing conditions if there were any room for doubt, thereby increasing the number of persons reported to have Alzheimer's disease even if the true prevalence did not change. If services were triggered by severity of disability, then a method to screen out those with lesser disability would have to be in place. That would likely entail mandatory assessment for eligibility, and would necessitate a measure of mental disability that is quick, accurate, reliable, and auditable.

A special entitlement for dementia, or specifically for Alzheimer's disease, also raises a question of fairness. An adult with spina bifida, Huntington's disease, or multiple sclerosis needs many of the same services as an individual with dementia. A special entitlement restricted to persons with Alzheimer's disease would likely promote conflict among interest groups for different diseases. A broader definition encompassing "related disorders" will be vague and difficult to implement. The prudent course appears to involve providing the services most needed but not restricting their use to *only* those with dementia.

Specialized Research

Although no consensus exists about the risks and benefits of special care or special entitlements, it is generally agreed that specialized *research* on relevant science, clinical care, and service use is essential. Serious study of the large group of people with severe functional disabilities due to dementia has only begun in the past few years, and much more information is necessary before public policies, medical practices, and service use can be rationally assessed. Such information can come only from research that focuses on individuals with dementia. Studies need not deal exclusively with persons with dementia to yield useful information. Those that survey long-term care or mental health in elderly people could shed light on the problems of someone with dementia if they include sufficient information to evaluate cognitive function (measured by a standard scale), service use, diagnosis, assessment of lost functions, efficacy of special care, and costs.

Diagnosis and Treatment

The main policy concern about diagnosis and treatment is rapid dissemination of knowledge to permit accurate diagnosis and appropriate treatment. The primary mechanisms for improving diagnosis and treatment are research and education (discussed in detail later in this section).

Also of concern is how to link medical evaluation to long-term care service planning, patient assessment, and social services. Creating new entitlements restricted to those with dementia would, for example, provide strong incentives to widen diagnostic criteria for those conditions, in order for more patients to qualify for public programs. The fragmented nature, complex organization, limited access, and uncertain eligibility criteria for long-term care services cause problems for individuals with dementia and their families. The physician is commonly responsible for coordinating medical services, but there is no analogous person to coordinate long-term care, mental health, social, and aging services. The concern here is for clients to have a person to turn to for information, and to begin planning service needs as soon as possible so that long-term care decisions are not made in a crisis atmosphere.

One mechanism to begin service planning would be to refer persons who receive the diagnosis of a disorder causing dementia to another professional or organization that can deal with the family and client in planning and coordinating services. This role is variously referred to by such terms as case management, case coordination, or linkage. Having such a professional available for referral from physicians would greatly improve the rational provision of services, but the costs are uncertain. Results from a national demonstration project to study case management and some alternatives (the Channelling project, supported by the Health Care Financing Administration will be available for analysis in late 1986, and information from that analysis will bear directly on policy regarding case management).

A third issue related to diagnosis and treatment concerns methods of diagnosis. The National Institute of Neurological and Communicative Disorders and Stroke (NINCDS), NIA, ADRDA, and the American Psychiatric Association each have published general criteria for diagnosis of dementing conditions, but none is specific as to which tests should be ordered and how they should be interpreted. Consensus may not be possible or advisable, but current criteria are not useful for the general practitioner trying to determine the diagnosis of a patient. An NIH consensus conference on diagnosis of dementia will be held in July 1987, and may help address this need.

One recent bill passed by Congress and signed by the President (Public Law 99-509) will establish up to 10 centers for diagnosis and treatment of dementing disorders. These would be distinct in function from the existing biomedical *research* centers, although they might be related geographically and administratively. The State of California has established six such centers, and reports that, even without publicity, the centers cannot meet demand for service (34). The centers are intended to diagnose and treat local cases of dementia, foster research, provide training for health professionals, aid families, and collect and analyze standardized information of use in planning services.

California reports that budget cutbacks at the State level have seriously impaired delivery of the expected services at the State-supported centers (34).

Diagnosis and treatment centers could be useful in training, setting standards for care, and focusing clinical research, but they should not be expected to make the diagnosis and treat all cases of dementia in the United States. The cutbacks California has reported could also occur at the national level.

Legal and Ethical Concerns

Decisions about medical care, family finances, and other important topics are often difficult enough even when all parties are mentally competent. They become even more difficult when someone has dementia. Eventually decisions must be made on behalf of the individuals—decisions about driving an automobile, working, controlling financial assets, or participating in research that may not be of direct benefit. Such decisions are particularly difficult when someone's employment involves professional work that is not closely supervised, such as medicine or law, yet these are jobs in which good judgment is essential.

State and Federal laws include several ways to appoint someone to make decisions for another person. Guardians and conservators can be appointed by a court following a procedure to decide that an individual is indeed incapable of autonomous choice. Durable powers of attorney allow a person to set certain constraints on finances or medical care and to appoint someone to make decisions *before* becoming mentally incompetent. Living wills can indicate what types of medical care an individual would wish to receive or refuse.

Each of these mechanisms for making decisions raises difficult questions. At what point is someone mentally incompetent? That is not a purely medical or purely legal question, and competence (legally defined) depends not only on the individual's mental ability, but also on the type of decision being made. Other questions include who is to oversee the decisions made by an appointed surrogate and how someone can be protected from conflicts of interest. Few of these questions can be directly addressed by Federal legislation.

Most are now being decided through the judicial system at both the State and Federal levels. Many States have also passed or considered laws about living wills, powers of attorney, guardianship, and conservatorship.

Legal issues related to Federal programs such as Medicare and Medicaid are also important. A family that receives legal advice soon after a diagnosis of progressive dementia is made may transfer the assets of the person with dementia more quickly, and thus establish patient eligibility for Medicaid sooner. Medicaid law stipulates that patient assets cannot be transferred for *purposes* of establishing Medicaid eligibility, and assets cannot have been transferred more recently than 2 years before becoming eligible. In most cases of dementia, assets would be transferred because of mental incompetence of the patient, but the burden of proof rests with the family. If transfer is completed early in someone's illness, the person is more likely to be eligible for Medicaid by the time nursing home care is needed.

These considerations make asset transfer a particularly difficult issue for families and State Medicaid administrators. Families benefit from early advice to legally transfer someone's assets, but individuals' rights to control their possessions must also be protected. And Medicaid is not intended to pay for the care of those who have impoverished themselves only on paper. Medicaid administrators would prefer to target their resources to those who need medical services and cannot afford them. The degree of responsibility of families in this context is unresolved. Idaho attempted to make children financially responsible for the care of their elderly parents in a 1983 law, but the legislation resulted in few recovered funds, was ruled in violation of Federal statutes, and was politically unpopular.

No clear legal method can resolve the dilemma, and those with different ideological views differ markedly about the form a remedy would take. The issue might become moot if the incentive to rely exclusively on Medicaid to cover long-term care were reduced significantly. The incentive is strong now because Medicaid is the only public program available, and lower incentives would require a substantially higher rate of private financing (e.g., long-term care insurance, life care communities, or private savings) or availability of alternative publicly financed long-term care services.

Another set of legal problems arises in government income support and health care programs. Those entitled to income and health benefits who are deemed mentally incompetent generally have a "representative payee" designated by the program disbursing funds. The representative payee becomes, in effect, the individual's guardian for social security payments. Yet the legal processes of establishing guardianship are not necessarily recognized by the Social Security Administration, the Veterans Administration, or other government agencies. Legal proceedings may be taken into account, but the agencies' own determinations carry more weight, despite being much less formal and providing less protection for the individual's rights.

Representative payees receive funds for an estimated 4 million to 5 million Americans. The Department of Health and Human Services has been sued on this issue, in *Jordan* v. *Heckler* (U.S. District Court, Western Oklahoma, CIV-79-944-W, Jan. 18, 1985) and the case is pending. Section 16 of the Social Security Disability Benefits Reform Act of 1984 (Public Law 98-460) mandated an annual accounting of representative payees, and sought a report on the proposed accounting system to be prepared for Congress in 1985. A six-page report was submitted in September 1985 (110), but it contained no data on rates of auditing or details about ascertaining mental competence for purposes of assigning representative payees. Nor did it describe procedures for identifying misuse of funds or special safeguards for those judged mentally incompetent who are cared for outside State mental institutions.

Education and Training

Providing high-quality services for those with dementia presumes the availability of trained people to deliver them. The sudden increase in awareness about dementia has meant that few centers are expert in care and research on this topic. Efforts to correct that deficiency have begun in the last 5 years, but most of those who care for individuals with dementia have never had special training.

Family members and other informal caregivers need information about the nature of the diseases and how their daily lives might change. That knowledge can improve their ability to plan and anticipate problems. They also need information about how to provide care. Persons with dementia are increasingly receiving special care, yet the results of innovations are not widely disseminated. When they are published, it is frequently in professional journals not readily available to family members. Health professionals can assist by preparing books, pamphlets, videotapes, and other educational materials intended for family caregivers. A few such materials are available: a guide to home care has been prepared (4), and several books have been published in recent years (21, 48,74,84).

The care of someone with dementia, as with other chronic illnesses, demands a range of skills and duration of service that no individual can fully supply. That realization has led to the development of interdisciplinary teams consisting of physicians, nurses, psychologists, social workers, and others. Multidisciplinary teams can better coordinate different services and bring their various areas of expertise to bear on the problems of someone with dementia.

Physicians now in general practice have had little formal training in geriatrics, although those who graduated from medical schools recently are likely to have had some courses. Attention to dementia has increased dramatically in some specialties, particularly neurology and psychiatry. Other specialties, such as family practice and internal medicine, are also publishing more articles, developing continuing education courses, and modifying medical school and residency curricula to include more material about dementing illness. Physician training in geriatrics should be improved by supportive provisions in the Omnibus Health Act of 1986 (Public Law 99-660). The results of such efforts should be felt over the next decade.

The physician's role in dementing illness extends well beyond making a diagnosis and rendering medical treatment. It also involves interacting with the care team and referring patients and their families to support groups, social services, and long-term care agencies.

Nurses are the backbone of long-term care, but long-term care is a low prestige and low paying specialty among these professionals. A shortfall of 75,000 nurses in long-term care is projected by 1990 (111). The medical training that nurses receive may not prepare them for the predominantly administrative and supervisory roles they perform in long-term care settings, and coverage of dementia varies among nursing schools even more than among medical schools.

Geriatric nurse practitioners, who receive special training in geriatrics, typically learn about the medical needs of older people, including coverage of dementia, and can perform many of the diagnostic, assessment, and treatment functions of physicians. They also generally learn about the service delivery system and how to coordinate services. They can form a bridge between the medical and social service systems, and are less costly to use than physicians.

Nurse's aides provide an estimated 80 to 90 percent of direct patient contact hours in long-term care (1,39). Yet they are poorly paid (usually minimum wage), have low educational levels, and have high turnover rates (45,49). Nurse's aides frequently have different socioeconomic and cultural backgrounds than those of their clients. The responsibility to train nurse's aides falls to long-term care facilities. Administrators are reluctant to invest heavily in training because aides are unlikely to remain long at the facility, but patient care depends on such training. Even those facilities that do wish to train aides have been hampered by lack of materials on dementia. Materials for training have recently become available through a cooperative effort of ADRDA and the American Health Care Association (44), and through the Hillhaven Corp. (91).

Other professionals are also involved in the care of those with dementia. Complete care frequently involves social workers, psychologists, physical and occupational therapists, speech therapists, and administrators who are familiar with the problems faced by individuals with dementia and knowledgeable about available services.

The Federal Government could play a critical role in ensuring that health and social service personnel working with persons with dementia receive the education and training necessary to deliver high-quality care. This role extends to educational institutions, programs that train professionals, and facilities that provide care.

Disseminating information about care to professional networks, family support groups, and the lay press can be an important function. The role of the Federal Government in providing information is most important in those areas in which it predominates (e.g., biomedical research, health services research, and how to use government programs). One example is the Alzheimer's Resource Center of New York City, which is preparing a book on nationwide resources about dementia available through the network of Area Agencies on Aging and State Units on Aging. The effort is the result of cooperation between a local chapter of ADRDA, the New York State Department for the Aging, and the Administration on Aging.

Accreditation of educational programs that train health and social service professionals is generally performed at the State level, but it is subject to Federal guidelines for those services reimbursed by Federal monies (e.g., Medicare and Medicaid). **Licensure** of professionals is also largely a State function, subject to Federal standards. **Training and staffing** requirements for acute, mental health, and long-term care facilities are written by States subject to Federal regulations. Requiring training about the care needs of those with dementia could be incorporated into certification guidelines. Although certification is a State function, the Federal Government could make receipt of Federal funds conditional on certain certification requirements.

Direct funding of training programs for physicians, nurses, and other health professionals is supported by the Department of Health and Human Services and the Veterans Administration. Continued support, with increased emphasis on geriatrics and particularly dementia, is likely to result in faculty whose talents are multiplied by teaching others to tackle the problems related to dementia.

Delivery of Long-Term Care

Formal long-term care services for persons with dementia are provided in nursing homes, board and care facilities, day care centers, mental health facilities, or individuals' homes (see table 1-6). Until recently, there has been little study of which services are used or needed by persons with dementia and by their caregivers. Equally little is known about which settings are best suited to deliver many of the needed services. Some studies suggest that 40 to 75 percent of those in nursing homes have dementia; data on prevalence of dementia in other settings are unavailable.

Individuals with dementia often need personal care, chore, and homemaker services in addition to—and often more than—medical care. Personal and social services are less widely available and less likely than medical care to be covered by government programs. Families may need temporary respite from continual supervision and care, but few agencies deliver care that is intended to relieve the burden of caregivers rather than patients (although most services do both).

Who Delivers Care?

Several factors determine who delivers long-term care for persons with dementia. For any one person, care may come from family at home, day care centers, home care providers, or a nursing home. Which provider is most appropriate depends on the extent of family and community informal supports, the quality and range of available services, the individual's symptoms, and the cost of the various options.

Families play a predominant role in providing long-term care for older Americans. A General Accounting Office study of the elderly population in Cleveland conducted in 1975 concluded that families were providing more than 50 percent of all long-term care services received, and that as the impairment of the patient increased, so did the proportion of services provided by the family. For the extremely impaired group, families provided 80 percent of needed services (107).

The degree of informal support may diminish in coming decades, however, for several reasons. Those most at risk of developing dementia are people in their eighties, and the children and spouses of such individuals are also likely to be older and themselves at risk of disability. At the same time, the declining birth rate in the United States has reduced the proportion of those who will be available to care for tomorrow's older people. The rapid influx of women into the work force also portends reduced availability of family caregivers; although women today report that work is important, one study found that they act as though they give caregiving priority over employment in most cases (12). Rising divorce rates and remarriage rates also complicate determining who will render care to an older relative; a person newly married into a family may feel less obliged to care for the new spouse's parent with dementia. Finally, the growing mobility of families increases geographic dispersion, and may make family caregiving less likely. Each of these trends weakens the informal care system, and may increase dependence on government services.

Caregiver Support

The primary needs of informal caregivers are respite care, information about the diseases and care methods, information about services, and a broadened range of services. **Family members' efforts can be aided by the Federal Government by giving them optimal information (especially that arising from federally supported research), assisting them in finding out about or obtaining services, and extending some benefits to caregivers and the person needing care as a unit, rather than restricting them to the individual with dementia.**

Range of Services

Caregivers believe that more services should be available to care for individuals with dementia. The caregiver survey conducted for OTA found that the majority of those who listed respite care, adult day care, board and care, and nursing home care as "essential" either knew these services were not available or did not know if they were available. That finding suggests that there is an unmet need both for services and for information about them.

Increasing the number of choices for care of persons with dementia will not necessarily diminish demand for nursing home care or reduce institutional care costs borne by government. Day and home care is much more widely available in the United Kingdom, for example, but rates of

nursing home residency are not significantly lower (43). Community-based care has not led to cost savings over nursing home care according to many recent studies (120). Some studies, however, report better patient outcomes with home care, and—of particular importance for persons with dementia who tend to reside for long periods in nursing homes once admitted—studies have not predicted what "the benefits of coordinated, expanded home care services might be for older, chronically impaired individuals who do not meet the skilled care requirement but, rather, need ongoing maintenance care" (52).

Patient Assessment and Eligibility for Services

Assessment is the process of identifying, describing, and evaluating patient characteristics associated with illness. While diagnosis of a dementing illness identifies the disease, assessment describes its impact on the individual, quantifies its severity, and is therefore essential in determining long-term care needs.

Eligibility for Medicare and Medicaid long-term care services and reimbursement levels for covered services are based primarily on the medical and nursing care needs of the individual. Some States are now using assessment instruments that measure cognitive and behavioral deficits and limitations in activities of daily living to determine Medicaid eligibility or reimbursement levels. These case mix assessments can reduce incentives to discriminate against heavy care patients, but have not been rigorously studied to ascertain their impact on persons with dementia. The RUG-II classification system in New York, for example, places 22 percent of those with diagnoses indicating dementia into the least reimbursed category (32). That placement could be either because these people indeed have only minimal disability (and might be better cared for outside a nursing home), because the diagnosis is incorrect, or because the RUG-II assessment process does not accurately capture the disabilities of such individuals.

Other case mix assessments may retain that uncertainty for those with dementia. It is important to determine whether the individuals do not need to be in a nursing home or whether their needs are not being identified by the assessment procedure, because low reimbursement will incline nursing homes against admitting individuals who fall in the minimal disability category. In New York, that has already occurred, with a marked drop in admissions of those showing minimal disability as measured by RUG-II assessment. It will be important to find out if those with dementia constitute a large fraction of that group and if there are alternative methods of care for those not admitted to nursing homes.

The assessment process is often the starting point for planning services, educating family members, and referring people to support groups and other community resources. Early engagement of a formal assessment process can thus serve as a focal point for bringing health professionals and families together to determine the prognosis for the individual with dementia, to learn about care options, and to find sources of relevant information.

Special Services for Individuals With Dementia

An increasing number of long-term care facilities and agencies are developing special services for persons with dementia, but these services are not yet widely available and most such individuals are treated elsewhere. Preliminary data suggest that **1 to 2 percent of nursing home residents with dementia are in special care units**. These facilities appear to be raising the standard of care, and are focusing attention on the large subpopulation of nursing home residents who suffer from dementia. Special care involves training of nurses and aides, redesign of rooms and common areas, and activities intended to take advantage of spared mental functions. Adapting the environment to altered needs of those with dementia appears to be useful, but the optimal way to do so is a topic of debate. The number of special care units has increased dramatically in recent years, yet no national body is responsible for identifying them, coordinating studies (to reduce duplication and disseminate results rapidly), or evaluating their efficacy.

Several policy issues are raised by special care units and programs. First, there is an apparent shortage of people highly knowledgeable about dementia available to staff such units or evaluate them. Second, evaluation and coordination of different units is currently haphazard. Third, standards for quality are unclear. Fourth, the type of individual eligible for care on special units is not uniform among different units, and optimal care methods may differ according to severity, type of symptoms, or disease. Finally, the costs and fair reimbursement rates for special units merit further inquiry. Do special care units cost more? Should they be paid more to care for those with dementia? Will special reimbursement lead to inequitable treatment of other types of patients, or will failure to pay more for those with dementia diminish their care?

Quality Assurance

Persons with dementia are at particular risk of receiving substandard care. They cannot communicate effectively, and their complaints may be discounted or ascribed to mental instability or misunderstanding. Reduced intellectual abilities interfere with rational consumer choice, an important component of quality assurance. Family members can act on behalf of individuals with dementia to assess and ensure the quality of care. If they are not available or the family is not cohesive, then ombudsmen, case managers, or designated surrogates must do so.

Quality of care in hospitals paid by Medicare is subject to the review of Professional Review Organizations. Outpatient and ambulatory acute care are less subject to direct inspection. The threat of malpractice is a strong incentive for providing adequate care in most acute care settings, but it has not been widely applied in long-term care settings.

The quality of care in nursing homes is regulated by States, subject to certification standards for Medicare and Medicaid. The system for assessing quality under Medicaid and Medicare is changing from a focus on inspection of facilities and physical plant to one that adds a client-centered assessment. Residents with dementia, however, are unlikely to be able to answer many of the questions about quality; inspection of their physical condition will yield clues as to their physical care, but will not assess overall quality of staff interactions or the resident's emotional satisfaction and staff regard for the person's dignity. These concerns are difficult to solve through purely regulatory means. Family assessment of a relative's health and happiness is another means of quality assurance. It is not available to residents without families, however, and its efficacy hinges on facilities' willingness to attend to suggestions or the availability of alternative care settings if they do not.

For Medicare and Medicaid administrators, only limited options exist to ensure compliance with care standards. In many areas, the scarcity of nursing home beds makes moving out of a poorly managed facility an unattractive option for the resident because an alternative one may not be available; that same scarcity makes State agencies reluctant to close down facilities. Less stringent enforcement actions have been successful in some States, and legislation permitting more use of them might be useful (see ch. 10). Professional organizations (e.g., American Health Care Association and the American Association of Homes for the Aging), proprietary and nonprofit nursing home chains, and new programs in teaching nursing homes can also promote higher standards and adherence to existing standards.

Day care, home care, board and care, and other community-based settings are licensed and regulated much less than nursing homes. Information about quality in such settings is sparse and much less thoroughly analyzed than information regarding quality of care in hospitals or nursing homes. Payment levels are generally lower and tend to be direct rather than through public subsidy, making any government regulation beyond licensing unlikely. Family or case manager assessment of quality is thus the main assurance of quality, perhaps supplemented by final resort to the legal system. Organizations (e.g., the National Association for Home Care and the National Council on the Aging) can help develop guidelines for care and suggest means of quality assurance. Federal and State Governments could also choose to have a direct role. If the range of services is expanded, examination of the quality of care in day care, home care, and board and care settings would be an important topic for health services research —to identify innovative ways to ensure that individuals have quality care that respects their rights and preserves their dignity.

Financing Long-Term Care

Financing long-term care for persons with dementia is one of the policy issues of greatest concern to caregivers and policymakers, and about which there is the least consensus. Policy options fall into several groups, according to the range of services reimbursed; the source of payment (individual, Medicaid, Medicare, insurance); and the relative responsibility of individuals and government.

These factors are woven together in a confusingly complex fabric of existing policies and priorities. Caregivers would prefer to see an expanded range of services available, whatever the source of payment. Government program administrators, legislators, and insurers also wish to fund the broadest number of options, but they do not want to leave commitments open-ended or to pay for services used by those who do not need them. The extremely complex set of laws, regulations, and contract arrangements for long-term care services reflects that concern for overutilization. Restricting payment to institutional settings has been one way to discourage illegitimate use and to attempt to concentrate resources on those who most obviously need them.

The source of payment determines not only who pays but also which services are covered and how those services are regulated and financed. Acute care under Medicare, for example, is paid under the diagnosis-related group payment system in most States, covers only some medically necessary services, and is relatively uniform—from the point of view of the individual—throughout the United States. Medicaid, in contrast, varies tremendously among the States in its eligibility criteria, funding levels, extent of coverage of nonmedical services, access to home services, method of payment, and enforcement of quality standards—for both acute and long-term care (19).

Options for financing long-term care also differ in degree of public subsidy, ranging from complete private financing to heavy public subsidy. At one end of the scale, private financing would include:

- direct individual or family payments not derived from government income programs,

- group cooperatives (for bargaining reduced rates with providers and insurers),
- charities, and
- conversion of home equity or other illiquid assets.

Numerous options that combine private financing with indirect public subsidy have been suggested:

- direct payments derived in part from government income programs;
- volunteer programs (generally by tax-subsidized nonprofit organizations, but also including government aid as in ACTION's Senior Companion programs);
- social/health maintenance organizations (S/HMOs);
- cooperatives (composed of groups of individuals with similar needs either directly providing care on a mutual help basis, directly financing services, or sharing information about services and financing options);
- private long-term care insurance (tax-subsidized);
- life care communities (tax-subsidized);
- dependent care tax deductions or tax credits; and
- individual medical or retirement accounts (tax-subsidized).

Finally, financing could involve increased direct public subsidy, with individuals contributing partial costs through expanded Medicaid eligibility, range of services, or level of payment, and through Medicare coverage of long-term care services.

Policy changes affecting Medicaid and Medicare could involve either small incremental changes in eligibility, scope of services, or reimbursement mechanisms or major long-term care reform. Major reform might entail private options dovetailed to public programs, publicly managed voluntary insurance options, or mandatory long-term care coverage. Options that extend complete public subsidy of all costs have not been discussed because proposals for such programs are not before the U.S. Congress.

The full range of policy options is more fully discussed in chapter 12, with brief discussions of some of the advantages and disadvantages of each.

They are also covered in the report of the OTA workshop held in May 1986, to be released by the Senate Committee on Labor and Human Resources and the House Select Committee on Aging. In addition, reports on long-term care financing are expected from the Brookings Institution and the Congressional Budget Office.

Secretary of Health and Human Services Otis Bowen transmitted a report on catastrophic illness to the President in November 1986. That report discussed acute medical care and also recommended several changes to improve long-term care financing, noting that "long-term care is the most likely catastrophic illness risk faced by individuals and families." Long-term care recommendations included: 1) Federal and private support for a broad educational effort regarding risks, costs, and options; 2) establishment of Individual Medical Accounts and withdrawal provisions for Individual Retirement Accounts (see ch. 12); and 3) support for private long-term insurance through tax provisions and removal of employer disincentives to cover long-term care in health insurance plans. Preparation of the report involved several public hearings in different regions, deliberations by three committees, and is based in part on a report to the Secretary by the Private/Public Sector Advisory Committee on Catastrophic Illness (86).

Financing of long-term care is one of the issues affecting individuals with dementia (and their families) that is most sensitive to public policies. Through Medicaid, Federal and State Governments are important payers of long-term care, covering the majority of those in nursing homes. The amounts paid by State and Federal Governments for nursing home care are roughly equal to total payments by individuals. The American Health Care Association estimates that 70 percent of nursing home residents are covered by Medicaid, and the figure is well over 80 percent for some States (58). The proportion of patients covered by Medicaid is higher than its fraction of payments for two reasons:

1. some patients on Medicaid also receive some income (from social security or other sources) that is paid to the facility to reduce Medicaid payments, and

2. levels of reimbursement per person are generally lower through Medicaid than other sources of payment.

The dominance of Medicaid means that decisions about the Medicaid program have a great effect on how nursing homes operate. Policies affecting nursing home coverage under Medicare affect a smaller, but still significant, fraction of nursing homes. Because of the absence of private insurers in long-term care, Federal and State Government decisions about financing are pivotal in determining access to and availability of day care, home care, respite care, and other services outside nursing homes.

Biomedical Research

Biomedical research includes basic biological, clinical, and public health research. It roughly corresponds to the type of research conducted under the auspices of the National Institutes of Health (either directly or through universities and medical centers). Basic research is conducted in the pursuit of scientific knowledge without primary regard for the applications of such knowledge. Clinical research applies basic knowledge in the search for preventive measures, treatments, and methods of diagnosis. Public health research builds on both basic and clinical research and applies it to population aggregates. The most common type of dementia, Alzheimer's disease, cannot be prevented or its symptoms reversed with current knowledge and techniques. The severity of future medical and social problems could be dramatically reduced if an effective drug or surgical treatment were found to significantly reduce symptoms or arrest the disease. Only a small proportion of those expected to develop dementia now have it, so finding a means of prevention could drastically reduce the projected number of people affected.

NIA, NIMH, and NINCDS are the three primary agencies supporting biomedical research (see table 1-8). Federal support for biomedical research (excluding funding for the Administration on Aging (AOA) and the Health Care Financing Administration (HCFA), whose research is primarily on health service delivery) has gone from less than $4 million in 1976 to over $65 million estimated for 1987. The number of publications on "Alzheimer's disease," "dementia," and "senility" leapt from 30 in 1972 to 87 in 1976, and then to 548 in 1985, reflecting the importance of increased Federal support. Nongovernment organizations such as ADRDA, the John Douglas French Foundation on Alzheimer's Disease, the American Federation for Aging Research, and the Howard Hughes Medical Institute are also contributing research funds, at levels corresponding to 5 to 10 percent of Federal funding. Private pharmaceutical and medical products companies are supporting applied research to find effective drugs and diagnostic devices, but their work builds on the basic research supported by the Federal Government.

Biomedical research on dementing conditions is likely to yield benefits in addition to its clinical

Table 1-8.—Federal Funding for Research on Dementia, 1976-87 (thousand dollars)

Agency[a]	1976	1977	1978	1979	1980	1981	1982	1983	1984	1985	1986[b]	1986[c]	1987[d]
NIA	857	1,500	1,960	4,142	4,211	5,196	8,054	11,848	21,456	28,830	34,048	32,691	40,760
NINCDS	2,314	2,333	2,422	2,844	4,960	5,427	6,243	8,678	11,700	12,826	14,030	13,427	15,900
NIMH	728	815	790	1,315	2,151	4,700	4,800	5,000	5,600	5,750	6,000	5,750	6,000
NIAID	—	—	—	1,381	1,775	1,394	1,256	1,041	1,336	1,211	1,247	1,192	1,412
DRR	—	—	—	—	—	—	—	604	709	1,034	1,055	1,010	1,062
AOA	—	—	—	—	—	—	—	—	164	1,128	900	627	600
HCFA	—	—	—	—	—	—	—	—	—	—	—	—	1,200
Total DHHS	3,899	4,648	5,172	9,682	13,097	16,717	20,353	27,171	40,965	50,779	57,280	54,697	66,934

[a]NIA (National Institute on Aging), NINCDS (National Institute on Neurological and Communicative Disorders and Stroke), NIMH (National Institute of Mental Health), NIAID (National Institute on Allergy and Infectious Diseases), DRR (Division of Research Resources, National Institutes of Health), AOA (Administration on Aging), and HCFA (Health Care Financing Administration). All agencies are in the U.S. Department of Health and Human Services.
[b]Appropriated by Congress in Public Law 99-178.
[c]Estimates following sequestration of funding under the Deficit Reduction Act of 1985.
[d]Estimates based on Continuing Resolution appropriations for Fiscal Year 1987 (P.L. 99-500), with individual figures taken from agency budget offices and direct appropriations.

SOURCE: National Institute on Aging Budget Office, 1986; National Institute of Mental Health Budget Office, 1986; and *Progress Report on Alzheimer's Disease: Volume II*, NIH Publication 84-2500, July 1984; modified by the Office of Technology Assessment in light of fiscal year 1987 appropriations. Estimates obtained from individual agency budget offices for years 1986 and 1987.

applications. Knowledge of the brain is still scant in comparison to the size of the task, and the study of the nervous system—neuroscience—is one of the most exciting areas in biology today. Support for research on dementing conditions will likely support work that will increase such knowledge in these disciplines. Research on dementia could, in fact, become a focus for neuroscience, just as cancer research led to many important advances in molecular biology and the spawning of biotechnology.

Major successes in biomedical research could also substantially reduce the costs and projected social and personal burdens of dementia. In other areas of research, successful prevention or treatment may actually lead to *increased* health care costs (e.g., a death prevented in middle age can increase aggregate costs because the person lives longer to have more episodes of ill health, each of which involves costs). Prevention or effective treatment of dementing disorders is likely to be highly cost-effective in the long term because the financial impact is severe, chronic, and occurs at the end of life. An effective means of preventing Alzheimer's disease would, for example, dramatically reduce the need for nursing homes and costly medical care without necessarily leading to substantially longer life or new medical problems. Other medical problems would likely cost less, rather than more.

An exclusive focus on biomedical research is unwise, however. Although increased funding makes scientific discoveries more likely, such discoveries will not necessarily lead to a means of prevention or cure, diagnostic tests, or even effective treatments. The consequences of new scientific findings may not be known for several decades, and may only much later improve clinical care. Scientific problems posed by disorders causing dementia are likely to yield to scientific inquiry, but public policy that presumes a revolution in care methods—based on discoveries not yet made —is not advisable.

Health Services Research

Health services research, as it applies to the subject of this report, is the multidisciplinary study of those with dementia and of the systems that serve them. It includes the community and family, but excludes biomedical research. Some types of research, such as epidemiology and patient assessment, bridge the gap between health services and biomedical research. Study of how to care for individuals, especially evaluation of methods that do not employ drugs or medical devices, is included in health services research, although some elements are also clinical. Topics range from studying how best to care for persons with dementia (at home, in nursing homes, or in day care centers) to evaluating different methods of paying for long-term care services.

Health services research tends to be supported by different agencies than biomedical research, although there is some overlap (NIMH and NIA, for example, mainly support biomedical research but are also among the agencies providing the most support for health services research on dementia). The type of information derived from health services research is crucial to rational planning of public policy and informed consumer choice. One analyst has observed, however, that "public policy is hampered by the woeful state of information about almost all social aspects of senile dementia and the deplorable quality of studies of intervention effects" (58).

Health services research related to dementia was the topic of an OTA workshop held in February 1986, cosponsored by the Subcommittee on Aging of the Senate Committee on Labor and Human Resources, the Human Services Subcommittee of the House Select Committee on Aging, and ADRDA. Results of that workshop are summarized here, and are discussed more fully in another document available through the Senate Committee on Labor and Human Resources and the House Select Committee on Aging. Discussions at that workshop revolved around six general topics:

1. epidemiology,
2. patient assessment,
3. service needs,
4. availability of and access to services,
5. cost of care, and
6. quality assurance and measurements of outcome.

Several points of consensus emerged at the workshop. First, dementing disorders are a substantial problem for the health care system, particularly in long-term care. Second, little is known about them in any setting. Third, data have been gathered that might shed light on current policies, but the data have not been analyzed with a view to discerning the needs of the large number of individuals who have dementia (71). Finally, there is a need to intensify the study of health care delivery to individuals with dementia and their families.

The few studies of health services that have focused specifically on the needs of individuals with dementia stand in stark contrast to the amount of information about treatment of specific groups of comparable size in acute care (e.g., persons with diabetes). That lack reflects both a general paucity of information about long-term care services, and a failure of long-term care studies to focus on the large subpopulation with dementia.

Many recent and ongoing efforts to gather data about long-term care do contain information about individuals with dementia. No single survey is ideal in assessing needs, disabilities, severity of cognitive impairment, and availability of informal supports, but "the breadth and depth of the information collected across the data sources . . . suggest that a substantial understanding of health service questions . . . could be acquired by analysis of the data sets" (73). Efforts to analyze such data sets would be much less costly than beginning extensive new surveys, and could answer some important questions and identify other key ones to address in future demonstrations. Some questions are not addressed, however, in available data sets (e.g., whether special care is effective or economical, or the long-term impact of respite care on family stress, functional disability, and costs). Analysis of such questions will require new demonstrations, but these should start from the most sophisticated understanding of current data available.

Several important questions about long-term care need to be resolved before prudent public policy on health services can be enacted. It is frequently argued, for example, that in-home services can help physically and cognitively impaired people to remain in their homes. Yet a growing body of evidence indicates that expanded use of in-home services does not generally reduce the need for nursing home beds (120). Such research has failed to separately analyze those with and without dementia, to focus on specific target groups (99), or to concentrate on long-stay patients whose needs are more supervisory than medical (52). Persons with dementia fall into the groups about which there is the least information—those needing supervisory care for long periods rather than "skilled" care for short periods. It is thus unclear whether in-home and other respite services will supplement, supplant, or increase nursing home care for those with dementia. Special attention to this group may prove crucial to designing long-term care services in general.

A large proportion of nursing home residents, particularly long-stay residents, are individuals with dementia who require 24-hour supervision, a service that is not generally offered in the home. Conversely, persons needing long-term care but not 24-hour supervision (e.g., those with arthritis or paralysis due to stroke) may benefit greatly from home care services but are less likely to be in a nursing home. The lack of correlation between availability of home services and reduction of nursing home care may thus be explained, at least in part, as use by different types of individuals. Only further study of long-term care service delivery in various settings can resolve that and other questions of interest to providers and policymakers.

Research on delivery of care can build on efforts by States, long-term care providers, and family support groups, but Federal coordination would be useful to reduce needless duplication of effort, to ensure wide dissemination of relevant results (a clearinghouse function), and to maintain sufficient focus on Federal issues (e.g., quality assurance, cost containment, and payment).

Health services research will determine the future basis for public and private activities in financing, quality assurance, training, and service delivery to persons with dementia. Research in this field does not necessarily depend on projects including only individuals with dementia. Evaluation of more general long-term care demonstrations can shed light on how those with dementia use such care. HCFA is supporting a study of reimbursement in the State of Texas, for example, that covers a sample of all nursing home patients, not just those with dementia. A part of the information gathered will include assessment of cognitive status that can be compared with existing studies on those with dementia in the community. That study should permit an evaluation of the influence of cognitive impairment per se, which has not been previously possible.

Federal spending for health services research in 1984 reached $200 million. That was one-twentieth of 1 percent of total health care spending that year ($387 billion), one-fifth of 1 percent of Federal health care spending ($111.9 billion), and 3.2 percent of the Federal budget for biomedical research ($6.15 billion). A survey of Federal agencies supporting health services research on dementia was conducted in April 1986 by the Congressional Research Service (81, cited in 119). The survey found that AOA was funding 12 projects, with the following spending history: $163,817 for two projects in fiscal year 1984; $1,127,618 for 12 projects in fiscal year 1985; and $431,400 continuing and $500,000 planned new spending in fiscal year 1986. NIA was planning $426,000 for fiscal year 1986. NIMH was funding three health service research projects that would include a component focused on dementia in fiscal year 1983, four in fiscal year 1984, seven in fiscal year 1985, and seven in fiscal year 1986, but the budget specific to dementia was not estimated. AOA, NIMH, and HCFA were each soliciting proposals for research that included analysis of health services for those with dementia. The National Center for Health Services Research (NCHSR) and Health Care Technology Assessment had not funded specific research and was not soliciting projects.

Estimated Federal spending on health services research related to dementia was thus in the range of $1.3 million to $2 million in 1986. That corresponds to roughly one-two-hundredth of 1 percent of the estimated national costs of dementing illness ($24 billion to $48 billion), one-thirtieth of 1 percent of Federal payments for long-term care of those with dementia ($4.4 billion), and 3 percent of biomedical research on dementia ($54 million).

The need for information about long-term care of those with dementia in order to plan national health policy has prompted Congress to fund research in this area. The final column in table 1-8 shows the estimated levels of research funding provided by the Continuing Appropriations for fiscal year 1987 (called the "continuing resolution"—Public Law 99-500). The bulk of funding is for basic and clinical research, but also includes $1.2 million for HCFA to develop and fund three demonstration projects on respite care for families of those with Alzheimer's disease and related disorders. The Omnibus Budget Reconciliation Act of 1986 (OBRA—Public Law 99-509) authorizes up to $40 million to create 5 to 10 regional centers to diagnose and treat individuals with Alzheimer's disease and related disorders. Funding will come from Medicare payments for those already Medicare eligible. (The continuing resolution limits funding for demonstration projects under Medicare, and a few experts contacted by OTA believe that this limit might apply to the Alzheimer's disease diagnosis and treatment centers. Most consulted, however, believed that the restrictive language would not apply, and the centers would be funded as specified in OBRA.) OBRA also authorized $1 million for fiscal year 1987, and $2 million in each of the three following years, to develop a respite care demonstration program in New Jersey under the State's Medicaid program.

HCFA funding for health services research will be supplemented by a group of projects supported by a combination of private and government sources. The Robert Wood Johnson Foundation, Administration on Aging, and ADRDA are jointly planning a competitive grants program. They intend to support the development of dementia service delivery demonstration projects in a number of communities throughout the Nation.

The last piece of legislation passed by the 99th Congress (Public Law 99-660) includes the Alzheimer's Disease and Related Dementias Services Research Act. This law establishes a Council on Alzheimer's Disease within the Department of Health and Human Services (making permanent the Task Force on Alzheimer's Disease), an Advisory Panel on Alzheimer's Disease (composed of 15 citizens appointed by the Director of the Office of Technology Assessment), a new group of awards for achievement in research to be bestowed by the Director of NIA, and an information clearinghouse to disseminate information about Alzheimer's disease—also administered by NIA. The act authorizes health services research to be conducted by NIA, NIMH, NCHSR/HCTA, and HCFA (beginning in October 1987) and mandates educational programs for the Social Security Administration (regarding disability policies related to dementia) and training of safety and transportation personnel about special problems in dealing with individ-

uals who have dementia. It also authorizes increased support for training in geriatrics. Several of the provisions of the new law can go into effect without further action. The research programs and other activities authorized by the act will, however, depend on new appropriations in the 100th Congress.

CHAPTER 1 REFERENCES

1. Almquist, E., and Bates, D., "Training Program for Nursing Assistants and LVNs in Nursing Homes," *Journal of Gerontological Nursing* 6:622-627, 1980.
2. Alzheimer Task Force, "Alzheimer Task Force Report," Long-Term Care Coordinating Council for the Elderly, Austin, Texas, Oct. 31, 1985.
3. Alzheimer's Disease and Related Disorders Association, *Advocacy Update*, July 31, 1985.
4. Alzheimer's Disease and Related Disorders Association, Ad Hoc Committee on Planning, Jan. 9 and 10, 1986 report.
5. Alzheimer's Resource Center, *Caring: A Family Guide To Managing the Alzheimer's Patient at Home*, New York City Alzheimer's Resource Center, 1986.
6. American Association of Retired Persons, "AARP Long-Term Care Research Study," survey conducted by the Gallup Organization, Jan. 30, 1986.
7. American Psychiatric Association, *Diagnostic and Statistical Manual of Mental Disorders*, 3d ed. (Washington, DC: 1980).
8. Arnett, R.H., McKusick, D.R., Sonnefeld, S.T., et al., "Projections of Health Care Spending to 1990," *Health Care Financing Review* 7:1-36, spring 1986.
9. Barclay, L.L., Zemcov, A., Blass, J.P., et al., "Survival in Alzheimer's Disease and Vascular Dementias," *Neurology* 35:834-840, 1985.
10. Battelle Memorial Institute, "The Economics of Dementia," contract report prepared for the Office of Technology Assessment, U.S. Congress, 1984.
11. Bloom, D.E., and Korenman, S.D., "The Spending Habits of American Consumers," *American Demographics* 8:23-25, 51-54, March 1986.
12. Brody, E.M., "Parent Care as a Normative Family Stress," Donald P. Kent Memorial Lecture, Gerontological Society of America, San Antonio, TX, Nov. 18, 1984. Reprinted in *The Gerontologist* 25:19-29, 1985.
13. Brody, E.M., Lawton, M.P., and Liebowitz, B., "Senile Dementia: Public Policy and Adequate Institutional Care," *American Journal of Public Health* 74:1381-1383, 1984.
14. Brody, E.M., and Brody, S.J., "Service Systems for the Aged," prepared for the *Encyclopedia of Social Work*, in press.
15. Brody, S.J., "The Thirty-to-One Paradox: Health Needs and Medical Solutions" *National Journal* 11:1869-1873, 1979.
16. Brody, S.J., and Magel, J.S., "LTC: The Long and Short of It," *Long-Term Care*, C. Eisdorfer (ed.) (Baltimore: Johns Hopkins Press, in press).
17. Chandra, V., Bharucha, N.E., and Schoenberg, B.S., "Conditions Associated With Alzheimer's Disease at Death: Case Control Study," *Neurology* 36:209-211, 1986.
18. Chandra, V., Bharucha, N.E., and Schoenberg, B.S., "Patterns of Mortality From Types of Dementia in the United States, 1971 and 1973-1978," *Neurology* 36:204-208, 1986.
19. Chavkin, D., "Interstate Variability in Medicaid Eligibility and Reimbursement for Dementia Patients," contract report prepared for the Office of Technology Assessment, U.S. Congress, March 1986.
20. Cicirelli, "Family Relationships and the Care/Management of the Dementing Elderly," *The Dementias: Policy and Management*, M.L.M. Gilhooly, S.H. Zarit, and J.E. Birren (eds.) (Englewood Cliffs, NJ: Prentice-Hall, 1986).
21. Cohen, D., and Eisdorfer, C., *The Loss of Self: A Family Resource for the Care of Alzheimer's Disease and Related Disorders* (New York: W.W. Norton, 1986).
22. Cohen, J., Holahan, J., and Liu, K., "Financing Long-Term Care for the Mentally Ill: Issues and Options," working paper # 3546-01, Urban Institute, Washington, DC, May 1986.
23. Colerick, E.J., and George, L.K., "Predictors of Institutionalization Among Caregivers of Patients With Alzheimer's Disease," *Journal of the American Geriatrics Society* 34:493-498, 1986.
24. "Coolfont Report: A PHS Plan for Prevention and Control of AIDS and the AIDS Virus," report of a Public Health Service meeting in Berkeley

Springs, WV, June 4-6, 1986, *Public Health Reports* 101:341-348, 1986.

25. Coons, D.H., "A Residential Care Unit for Persons With Dementia," contract report prepared for the Office of Technology Assessment, U.S. Congress, 1986.

26. Cornelius, E., Health Care Financing Administration, personal communication, April 1986.

27. Cross, P.S., and Gurland, B.J., "The Epidemiology of Dementing Disorders," contract report prepared for the Office of Technology Assessment, U.S. Congress, 1986.

28. *Danish Medical Bulletin*, Special Issue on Alzheimer's Disease, vol. 32, Gerontology Special Supplement No. 1, February 1985, pp. 1-111.

29. Doty, P., Liu, K., and Wiener, J., "Special Report: An Overview of Long-Term Care," *Health Care Financing Review* 6:69-78, 1985.

30. Dunn, L., "The Senior Respite Care Program," contract report prepared for the Office of Technology Assessment, U.S. Congress, 1986.

31. Fields, S.D., MacKenzie, C.R., Charlson, M.E., et al., "Cognitive Impairment: Can It Predict the Course of Hospitalized Patients?" *Journal of the American Geriatrics Society* 34:579-585, 1986.

32. Foley, W.J., "Dementia Among Nursing Home Patients: Defining the Condition, Characteristics of the Demented, and Dementia on the RUG-II Classification System," contract report prepared for the Office of Technology Assessment, U.S. Congress, 1986.

33. Folstein, M., Anthony, J.C., Parhad, I., et al., "The Meaning of Cognitive Impairment in the Elderly," *Journal of the American Geriatrics Society* 33:228-235, 1985.

34. Fox, P.J., Lindeman, D.A., and Benjamin, A.E., "Status of Alzheimer's Disease Diagnostic and Treatment Centers and Alzheimer's Disease Research Grants in California," Institute for Health and Aging, University of California, San Francisco, January 1986.

35. French, C.J., "Experiences in the Development and Management of the Community Services Program of the Atlanta Area Chapter of Alzheimer's Disease and Related Disorders Association, Inc.," contract report prepared for the Office of Technology Assessment, U.S. Congress, 1986.

36. Garfield, A., Alzheimer's Disease and Related Disorders Association, Chicago, IL, personal communication, April 1986.

37. George, L.K., "The Dynamics of Caregiver Burden," final report submitted to the American Association of Retired Persons—Andrus Foundation, Washington, DC, 1984.

38. Georgia Department of Human Resources, Office of Aging, Study Committee Report, "Alzheimer's Disease," Atlanta, GA, December 1985.

39. Geriatric Nursing Assistant Training Task Force, "Geriatric Nursing Assistant Training in Virginia," Final Report, Department of Education of the Commonwealth of Virginia, Richmond, VA, January 1982.

40. Gordon, N.M., Assistant Director for Human Resources and Community Development, Congressional Budget Office, statement before the U.S. House of Representatives, Committee on Energy and Commerce, Subcommittee on Health and the Environment, prepared by S.H. Long, J. Rodgers, and B. Vavrichek, Congressional Budget Office, Mar. 26, 1986.

41. Governor's Committee on Alzheimer's Disease, Commonwealth of Massachusetts, Boston, MA, 1985.

42. Governor's Task Force on Alzheimer's Disease and Related Disorders, "The Maryland Report on Alzheimer's Disease and Related Disorders," State of Maryland, Annapolis, MD, June 30, 1985.

43. Gurland, B.J., "Public Health Aspects of Alzheimer's Disease and Related Dementias," *Alzheimer's Disease and Related Disorders: Research and Management*, W.E. Kelley (ed.) (Springfield, IL: Charles C. Thomas, 1985).

44. Gwyther, L.P., *Care of Alzheimer's Patients: A Manual for Nursing Home Staff* (Chicago, IL: Alzheimer's Disease and Related Disorders Association, 1985).

45. Handschu, S.S., "Profile of the Nurse's Aide," *The Gerontologist* Part I, pp. 315-317, autumn 1973.

46. Heckler, M.M., "The Fight Against Alzheimer's Disease," *American Psychologist* 40:1240-1244, 1985.

47. Henderson, J.N., "Mental Disorders Among the Elderly: Dementia and its Sociocultural Correlates," *Modern Pioneers: An Interdisciplinary View of the Aged*, P. Silverman (ed.) (Bloomington, IN: Indiana University Press, 1986).

48. Heston, L.L., and White, J.A., *Dementia: A Practical Guide to Alzheimer's Disease and Related Disorders* (New York: W.H. Freeman, 1983).

49. Hogstel, M.O., "Auxiliary Nursing Personnel," *Management of Personnel in Long-Term Care*, M.O. Hogstel (ed.) (Bowie, MD: Robert J. Brady Co., 1983).

50. Hu, T.W., Huang, L.F., and Cartwright, W.S., "Evaluation of the Costs of Caring for the Senile Demented Elderly: A Pilot Study," *The Gerontologist* 26:158-163, 1986.

51. Huang, L.-F., Hu, T.-W., and Cartwright, W.S., "The Economic Cost of Senile Dementia in the

United States, 1983," contract report prepared for the National Institute on Aging, No. 1-AG-3-2123, 1986.

52. Hughes, S.L., "Apples and Oranges? A Review of Evaluations of Community-Based Long-Term Care," *Health Services Research* 20:461-488, 1985.

53. ICF, Inc., "Private Financing of Long-Term Care: Current Methods and Resources," final report submitted to the Assistant Secretary for Planning and Evaluation, U.S. Department of Health and Human Services, January 1985.

54. ICF, Inc., "The Role of Medicare in Financing the Health Care of Older Americans," submitted to American Association of Retired Persons, Washington, DC, July 1985.

55. Intergovernmental Health Policy Project, "Alzheimer's Initiatives Advance," *State Health Notes*, No. 56, September 1985, pp. 1-3.

56. International Classification of Diseases, 9th Revision Conference, 1975, (Geneva: World Health Organization), vol. 1, 1977 and vol. 2, 1978; modified by *Coding Clinics for ICD-9 CM*, American Hospital Association, various issues.

57. Jazwiecki, T., Director, Office of Reimbursement and Financing, American Health Care Association, Washington, DC, personal communication, April 1986.

58. Kane, R.A., "Senile Dementia and Public Policy," *The Dementias: Policy and Management*, M.L. Gilhooly, S.H. Zarit, and J.E. Birren (eds.) (Englewood Cliffs, NJ: Prentice-Hall, 1986).

59. Kane, R.L., "Acute and Long-Term Care: Decisions and Decisionmakers," paper prepared for the Conference on the Impact of Technology on Long-Term Care, Feb. 16-18, 1983, sponsored by the Office of Technology Assessment, U.S. Congress, Project HOPE, the George Washington University Health Policy Forum, and the Institute of Medicine, National Academy of Sciences, 1983.

60. Kansas Alzheimer's and Related Diseases Task Force, *Final Report to the Kansas Department on Aging*, Topeka, KS, 1986.

61. Katzman, R., "The Prevalence and Malignancy of Alzheimer's Disease: A Major Killer," *Archives of Neurology* 33:217-218, 304, 1976.

62. Katzman, R., "Aging and Age-Dependent Disease: Cognition and Dementia," *America's Aging: Health in an Older Society*, Committee on an Aging Society, Institute of Medicine and National Research Council (Washington, DC: National Academy Press, 1985).

63. Katzman, R., "Alzheimer's Disease," *New England Journal of Medicine* 314:964-973, 1986.

64. Katzman, R., Lasker, B., and Bernstein, N., "Accuracy of Diagnosis and Consequences of Misdiagnosis of Disorders Causing Dementia," contract report prepared for the Office of Technology Assessment, U.S. Congress, submitted for publication, 1986.

65. Larson, E.B., Reifler, B.V., Sumi, S.M., et al., "Diagnostic Tests in the Evaluation of Dementia: A Prospective Study of 200 Elderly Outpatients," Department of Medicine, University of Washington Medical Center, Seattle, WA, in press.

66. Levit, K.R., "Personal Health Care Expenditures by State: 1966-1982," *Health Care Financing Review* 6:1-49, 1985.

67. Lidoff, L., "Mobilizing Community Outreach to the High-Risk Elderly: The 'Gatekeepers' Approach," (Washington, DC: National Council on the Aging, Inc., 1984).

68. Light, Enid, U.S. Department of Health and Human Services, National Institute of Mental Health, Program on Aging, personal communication, Apr. 19, 1986.

69. Light, E., Lebowitz, B., and Bailey, F., "CMHCs and Elderly Services: An Analysis of Direct and Indirect Services and Services Delivery Sites," submitted for publication by the U.S. Department of Health and Human Services, National Institute of Mental Health, 1986.

70. Lindeman, D.A., Bliwise, N.G., Berkowitz, G., et al., "Development of a Uniform, Comprehensive Nomenclature and Data Collection Protocol for Brain Disorders," Institute for Health and Aging, University of California, San Francisco, June 1986.

71. Liu, K., "Analysis of Data Bases for Health Services Research on Dementia," contract report prepared for the Office of Technology Assessment, U.S. Congress, 1986.

72. Liu, K., and Manton, K. G., "The Length-of-Stay Pattern of Nursing Home Admissions," *Medical Care* 21:1211-1222, 1983.

73. Lockery, S.A., "Impact of Dementia Within Minority Groups," contract report prepared for the Office of Technology Assessment, U.S. Congress, 1986.

74. Mace, N., and Rabins, P., *The 36-Hour Day: A Family Guide To Caring for Persons With Alzheimer's Disease, Related Dementing Illnesses, and Memory Loss in Later Life* (Baltimore, MD: Johns Hopkins University Press; and New York: Warner, 1981).

75. Max, W., Lindeman, D.A., Segura, T.G., et al., "Estimating the Utilization and Costs of Formal and Informal Care Provided to Brain-Impaired Adults: A Briefing Paper," Institute for Health and Aging, University of California, San Francisco, June 1986.

76. McCall, N., Rice, T., and Sangl, J., "Consumer

Knowledge of Medicare and Supplemental Health Insurance Benefits," *Health Services Research* 20:633-657, 1981.

77. Minnesota Task Force on the Needs of Persons With Brain Impairment, "Final Report," submitted to the Commissioner of the Department of Human Services, State of Minnesota, December 1985.

78. Mortimer, J.A., "Epidemiology of Dementia—International Comparisons," *Epidemiology and Aging*, G. Maddox and J. Brody (eds.) (New York: Springer, 1986).

79. Mortimer, J.A., and Hutton, J.T., "Epidemiology and Etiology of Alzheimer's Disease," *Senile Dementia of the Alzheimer Type*, J.T. Hutton and A.D. Kenny (eds.) (New York: A.R. Liss 1985).

80. Mulley, G.P., "Differential Diagnosis of Dementia," *British Medical Journal* 292:1416-1418, 1986.

81. O'Shaughnessy, C., "Survey of Agencies Performing Health Services Research on Long-Term Care of Patients with Dementia," Congressional Research Service, Library of Congress, U.S. Congress, April 1986.

82. Ouslander, J.G., and Kane, R.L., "The Costs of Urinary Incontinence in Nursing Homes," *Medical Care* 22:69-79, 1984.

83. Petty, D., "The Family Survival Project," contract report prepared for the Office of Technology Assessment, U.S. Congress, 1986.

84. Powell, L.S., and Courtice, K., *Alzheimer's Disease: A Guide for Families* (Reading, MA: Addison-Wesley, 1983).

85. Price, D.L., "Basic Neuroscience and Disorders Causing Dementia," contract report prepared for the Office of Technology Assessment, U.S. Congress, 1986.

86. Private/Public Sector Advisory Committee on Catastrophic Illness, "Report to the Secretary of Health and Human Services," Aug. 19, 1986.

87. Prospective Payment Assessment Commission, personal communication, Apr. 17 and 18, 1986.

88. Radebaugh, T.S., Hooper, F.J., and Gruenberg, E.M., "The Social Breakdown Syndrome in a Community Residing Elderly Population," *British Journal of Psychiatry*, in press.

89. Raschko, R., "Systems Integration at the Program Level: Aging and Mental Health," Spokane Community Mental Health Center, Spokane, WA, in press.

90. Rees, K.C., "Legislative Advocacy and Alzheimer's Disease: The California Experience," presented at the National Conference on Alzheimer's Disease and Dementia, Detroit, MI, Apr. 10-12, 1986.

91. Reifler, B.V., and Orr, N., "*Alzheimer's Disease and the Nursing Home: A Staff Training Manual*," (Tacoma, WA: Westprint Division of Hillhaven Corp., 1985).

92. Rhode Island Legislative Commission, "Dementias Related to Aging," Providence, RI, May 1, 1984.

93. Risse, S.C., and Barnes, R., "Pharmacologic Treatment of Agitation Associated With Dementia," *Journal of the American Geriatrics Society* 34:368-376, 1986.

94. Ron, M.A., Toone, B.K., Garralda, M.E., et al., "Diagnostic Accuracy in Presenile Dementia," *British Journal of Psychiatry* 134:161-168, 1979.

95. Rovner, B.W., Kafonek, S., Filipp, L., et al., "Prevalence of Mental Illness in a Community Nursing Home," *American Journal of Psychiatry*, in press.

96. Rubenstein, L.Z., Josephson, K.R., Wieland, G.D., et al., "Differential Prognosis and Utilization Patterns Among Clinical Subgroups of Hospitalized Geriatric Patients," *Health Services Research* 20:881-895, 1986.

97. Sayetta, R.B., "Rates of Senile Dementia—Alzheimer's Type in the Baltimore Longitudinal Study," *Journal of Chronic Diseases* 39:271-286, 1986.

98. Schneider, D., Desmond, M., Foley, W., et al., "Long-Term Care Case Mix Reimbursement Using RUG-II" (Albany, NY: New York State Department of Health, December 1985).

99. Shaughnessy, P.W., "Long-Term Care Research and Public Policy," *Health Services Research* 20:489-499, 1985.

100. Stone, R., Cafferata, G.L., and Sangl, J., "Caregivers of the Frail Elderly: A National Profile," National Center for Health Services Research and Health Care Technology Assessment, U.S. Department of Health and Human Services, 1986.

101. Study Committee Report, 1985, "Alzheimer's Disease," Georgia Department of Human Resources, Office of Aging, December 1985.

102. Sulvetta, M.B., and Holahan, J., "Cost and Case-Mix Differences Between Hospital-Based and Freestanding Nursing Homes," *Health Care Financing Review* 7:75-84, spring 1986.

103. Texas Department of Health, *Alzheimer's Disease Initiative: Nursing Home Study* (Austin, TX, 1985).

104. U.S. Congress, House Select Committee on Aging, "Twentieth Anniversary of Medicare and Medicaid: Americans Still at Risk," Hearing Before the U.S. House of Representatives, 99th Congress, July 30, 1985, Comm. Pub. No. 99-538 (Washington, DC: U.S. Government Printing Office, 1986).

105. U.S. Congress, Office of Technology Assessment, *Technology and Aging in America*, OTA-BA-264 (Washington, DC: U.S. Government Printing Office, 1985).

106. U.S. Congress, General Accounting Office, "Con-

straining National Health Care Expenditures: Achieving Quality Care at an Affordable Cost," No. HRD-85-105 (Washington, DC: U.S. General Accounting Office, 1985).

107. U.S. Congress, General Accounting Office, *The Well-Being of Older People in Cleveland, Ohio*, No. HRD-77-70 (Washington, DC: U.S. General Accounting Office, 1977).

108. U.S. Department of Health and Human Services, "Alzheimer's Disease," vol. 32, Gerontology Special Supplement, No. 1, February 1985, pp. 1-111.

109. U.S. Department of Health and Human Services, "Report of the Secretary as Required by Section 16, Public Law 98-460," September 1985.

110. U.S. Department of Health and Human Services, *Alzheimer's Disease: Report on Secretary's Task Force on Alzheimer's Disease*, DHHS Pub. No. ADM 84-1323, (Washington, DC: U.S. Government Printing Office, 1984).

111. U.S. Department of Health and Human Services, Health Care Financing Administration, "Long-Term Care: Background and Future Directions," 1981.

112. U.S. Department of Health and Human Services, National Center for Health Statistics, "Characteristics of Nursing Home Residents, Health Status, and Care Received: National Nursing Home Survey, United States, May-December 1977," *Vital Health Statistics* Series 13, No. 51, DHHS Pub. No. (PHS) 81-1712, 1981.

113. U.S. Department of Health and Human Services, Task Force Report on Long-Term Care, "Report of the Under Secretary," April 1981.

114. U.S. Department of Health and Human Services, "Catastrophic Illness Expenses," Report to the President, November 1986.

115. U.S. Veterans Administration, *Caring for the Older Veteran*, (Washington, DC: U.S. Government Printing Office, 1984).

116. U.S. Veterans Administration, International Work Group, *The Veterans Administration and Dementia, Recommendations for Patient Care, Research, and Training*, Office of Geriatrics and Extended Care, Veterans' Administration Central Office, Kellogg International Scholarship Program on Health and Aging, Institute of Gerontology of the University of Michigan, and Institute of Social Medicine, University of Copenhagen (Washington, DC: October 1985).

117. U.S. Veterans Administration, Office of Geriatrics and Extended Care, Department of Medicine and Surgery, Veterans Administration Central Office, *Dementia: Guidelines for Diagnosis and Treatment* (Washington, DC: 1986).

118. Valle, R., "Natural Support Systems, Minority Groups, and the Late Life Dementias: Implications for Service Delivery, Research, and Policy," *Clinical Aspects of Alzheimer's Disease and Senile Dementia* (Aging, vol. 15), N.E. Miller and G.D. Cohen (eds.) (New York: Raven Press, 1981).

119. Vierck, E., "Health Services Research Related to Dementia," a report by the Subcommittee on Aging, U.S. Senate Committee on Labor and Human Resources, draft report, June 1986.

120. Weissert, W.G., "Seven Reasons Why It Is So Difficult to Make Community-Based Long-Term Care Cost-Effective," *Health Services Research* 20:423-433, 1985.

121. Whitehouse, P.J., "Alzheimer's Disease," *Current Therapy in Neurologic Disease, 1985-1986*, R.T. Johnson (ed.) (Philadelphia, PA: B.C. Decker, 1985).

122. Winograd, C.H., and Jarvik, L.F., "Physician Management of the Demented Patient," *Journal of the American Geriatrics Society* 34:295-308, 1986.

123. Yankelovich, Skelly, and White, Inc., "Caregivers of Patients With Dementia," contract report prepared for the Office of Technology Assessment, U.S. Congress, 1986.

124. Zarit, S.H., and Anthony, C.R., "Interventions With Dementia Patients and Their Families," *The Dementias: Policy and Management*, M.L.M. Gilhooly, S.H. Zarit, and J.E. Birren (eds.) (Englewood Cliffs, NJ: Prentice-Hall, 1986).

125. Zarit, S.H., Reever, K.E., and Back-Peterson, J., "Relatives of the Impaired Elderly: Correlates of Feelings of Burden," *The Gerontologist* 20:649-655, 1980.

Chapter 2
Characteristics of Persons With Dementia

CONTENTS

Characteristics of Persons With Dementia*

What happens to the mind when a dementing illness strikes? Families and professionals alike struggle to understand why persons with dementing illnesses act as they do, and what, if anything, can be done to modify the person's strange behaviors or support lost skills.

The burden of caring for individuals with dementia arises as much out of the need to protect them from their own lack of judgment and to restrain them from dangerous behaviors as it does from providing personal or medical care (22). The difficult behaviors, poor judgment, profound memory loss, and changes in cognition as the diseases progress significantly affect both family caregivers and those working in formal support systems (see box A and chs. 4 and 7).

*This chapter is a contract report by Nancy Mace, Consultant in Gerontology, Towson, MD.

This chapter will describe persons with dementia: the abilities they are losing, those that remain, and the ways in which these changing impairments affect the care these individuals need. The chapter:

- outlines the stages of decline of chronic dementing illnesses and discusses the usefulness of documenting stages in the illness;
- describes the symptoms of dementia and the impairments individuals experience;
- identifies the symptoms that are most readily alleviated; and
- considers the care needs of victims of dementia that arise from these symptoms.

While some causes of dementia are treatable (see ch. 3), only chronic and irreversible illnesses are discussed here.

Box A.—The Experience of the Victim

Dementing illnesses do not abruptly or uniformly disrupt a person's thinking: they gradually and selectively impair intellectual functions. In addition, other illnesses, a nonsupportive environment, fatigue, or stress can make persons with dementia even more impaired in function and intellect than they need be. The seemingly strange contradictions of impaired and spared areas of intellect are probably as frightening to persons with a dementia as they are to those who care for them.

At first, individuals may be aware of their failures and become deeply discouraged and frightened. They may fear that they are going insane. As the disease progresses, however, they will forget their forgetfulness and be unaware that they are ill. They will try to continue to do what they have always done—go to the office, prepare meals, or drive—unaware that they are getting lost or making dangerous mistakes.

People with dementia may be frustrated to the point of rage when they can no longer do simple tasks, such as button a dress or jacket or tie their shoes. Their environment becomes filled with inexplicable obstacles—once familiar tasks now lead to failure and embarrassment. Unable to understand why they fail, they may struggle to cover up their failures or they may not understand what is wrong. Their clumsiness can be humiliating. As the disease progresses, they may not know who they are and may experience extreme and ongoing terror. They may cling tenaciously to the one person who seems familiar. When individuals with dementia are no longer able to convey pain or fear, no one may respond to them, although they will be unaware that no one can understand them. Yet their ability to enjoy human companionship—and to give and receive love—appears to continue some time after they have lost the ability to talk clearly or to care for themselves.

Although most physicians and researchers agree on the definition of dementia, there is disagreement over the stages of an individual's decline, on the causes of behaviors, and on the treatability of symptoms. The course and symptoms vary among dementing diseases, and with patients thought to have the same disease. These variations, both in medical opinion and in knowledge of the diseases, have a significant impact on policy.

DEFINITION OF DEMENTIA

Several different methods are used to determine whether an individual has dementia. Clinicians increasingly use the criteria specified by the American Psychiatric Association in the third edition of its *Diagnostic and Statistical Manual of Mental Disorders* (DSM-III) (1). Many of the epidemiologic and clinical studies done since 1980 have also used these criteria. The DSM-III diagnostic classification provides a method for systematically grouping symptoms that affect mental function.

A similar set of criteria was developed in 1983 in a joint effort between the National Institute of Neurological and Communicative Disorders and Stroke and the Alzheimer's Disease and Related Disorders Association (ADRDA) (17,27).

Based on these two sets of criteria, dementia is defined as:

- a decline in intellectual function;
- global cognitive impairment, that is, memory impairment and at least one of the following:
  —impairment of abstract thinking;
  —impairment of judgment;
  —impairment of other complex capabilities such as language use, ability to perform complex physical tasks, ability to recognize objects or people, or to construct objects; and
  —personality change; and
- being in *clear consciousness* (i.e., awake and alert).

The definition differentiates dementia from mental retardation, in which there is no *decline* from a previous level. Thus a person with exceptional intelligence might have dementia if his or her intellectual ability declined to average. Similarly, a mentally retarded person can suffer from dementia when his or her intellectual limitations worsen.

That qualification requires that the individual's previous level of function be known. If no one can give a clear account of the person's past, the only way to determine if abilities are declining is to observe the individual over time. That necessity has implications for both epidemiology (7) and policy. If criteria for eligibility for services were to include documentation of change over time, individuals who require immediate assistance might be excluded. If, on the other hand, documentation of decline is not required, persons with lifelong impaired capacity might use limited services intended for persons with dementia. It is usually easy to document decline, based on the family's report. When someone has no close family, it is more difficult.

The next part of the definition, *global*, means that more than one area of intellectual function is impaired. Thus a person suffering only a memory impairment (e.g., caused by Korsakoff's syndrome) or only an impairment in the ability to speak (e.g., caused by some strokes) is usually not said to be suffering from a dementia (26). In practice, these individuals are often similarly handicapped and limited in their ability to function independently. They will need services and resources like those for persons with a dementing illness. In addition, many people with Alzheimer's disease suffer only memory loss at first. It is the expectation that other abilities will be lost that differentiates them from persons with pure amnesia.

The definition also distinguishes dementia from other mental states such as delirium, sleep, coma, stupor, and intoxication. The third major qualification, *in clear consciousness*, means that in contrast to delirium, the person is mentally impaired even when awake and alert. Several criteria distinguish delirium from dementia.

- **State of consciousness**: Persons with delirium have fluctuating or clouded consciousness, while those with dementia are as attentive as they can be.

- **Stability**: With delirium, the individual's ability to pay attention and respond varies over short periods, only minutes or hours, while dementia is relatively stable in comparison.
- **Duration**: Delirium is usually short-lived, while dementia has a more prolonged course.
- **Rate of onset**: Delirium usually appears abruptly, over days or weeks, while dementia, except for some vascular dementia, usually develops insidiously.
- **Cause**: Delirium usually can be traced to a recent source—head trauma, drugs, fever, infection—while dementia may not be linked to another cause.

These distinctions are usually easy to make in young persons, but the borders between dementia and delirium blur with age. Elderly people can remain delirious for prolonged periods and the cause can be obscure. Many of the physical insults that cause delirium in the young can produce symptoms that look very much like dementia in older people.

The elderly delirious patient can exhibit a full spectrum of psychiatric symptoms including delusions, hallucinations, depression, excitement, agitation, fear, anger, and apathy. A cognitive examination reveals disorientation, memory impairment, problems in writing, and inability to sustain a conversation (9). Thus delirious persons can easily be misdiagnosed as having a dementing illness, and the underlying cause of the delirium may be left untreated.

Elderly people are especially vulnerable to delirium caused by illness or reactions to medication. Some may have only a delirium; others may suffer from both a delirium and a dementia. Persons with dementing illnesses are prone to develop additional delirium when they develop any other illness (42). In such cases, the delirium may cause a further decline in the individual's cognitive abilities. Therefore, the presence of an underlying dementia cannot be determined until any concurrent delirium has disappeared (39).

Thus, eligibility for services based on the presence of dementia requires a careful search to exclude delirium. Any assessment of need for services would be difficult to determine for elderly persons who are acutely ill and confused. That is a particularly significant problem when such persons have been hospitalized. In order to avoid delays, plans for a patient's discharge are begun soon after admission, when the presence and severity of dementia may be difficult to determine.

Other Diagnostic Criteria

Several criteria that have been used in defining dementia are omitted from the DSM-III definition. DSM-III does not include any statement regarding the course of the illness (i.e., chronic or acute) or prospects for treatment (i.e., reversible or irreversible). It makes no statement regarding the cause of the dementia (e.g., Alzheimer's disease or stroke) (26). Nor does it require the presence of specific behaviors such as agitation or wandering. Its great advantage is that it allows the description of disabilities along several axes without using unproved assumptions about cause or classification to label an individual.

The absence of such labels has policy implications. In the past, elderly persons with memory loss or changed behaviors were said to be suffering from "chronic organic brain syndrome"—a label that consigned them to a hopeless category before their condition had been diagnosed, and that discouraged the search for treatable causes of the dementia. Although the most common disorders causing dementia—Alzheimer's disease and multi-infarct dementia—are not curable, that may not always be so. Therefore, a definition that includes irreversibility would be inappropriate. Excluding the cause of the dementia from the diagnosis also permits identification of an individual's characteristics and needs in the absence of a causal diagnosis. Behaviors such as wandering are not necessary for the diagnosis because they may disappear as the person's condition declines or when under treatment.

Variation in Symptoms

The specific cognitive functions that are lost and those that remain can vary from time to time and from person to person (17). These variations may be due to several factors:

- The progression (stage) of the disease or the length of time the person has had the disease

(18): Over time individuals gradually lose more and more cognitive ability. Because the speed at which these changes occur varies from person to person (from 1 to 20 years) (18), services need to be flexible if they are to meet changing impairments. (The limitations inherent in describing the course of the disease by stages are described later in this chapter.)

- The underlying disease causing the dementia (14): Some dementing illnesses affect gait, bladder control, or mood to a greater or lesser extent; other dementias affect reason, judgment, mathematical ability, and complex thought (26). These variations can affect the equitable distribution of resources. For example, eligibility criteria for Old Age Survivors Disability Insurance include evidence of deterioration of personal habits. One person's coherent speech and appearance of well-being may conceal very poor judgment and inability to hold a job, while another's apathetic and disheveled appearance may make him or her appear much more impaired. Furthermore, Alzheimer's disease and multi-infarct dementia can be difficult to distinguish, making the course of an individual's illness hard to predict.

- The presence of other illnesses or reactions to medication (18): As noted earlier, persons with dementia often experience a further impairment in their intellectual function when they also develop other illnesses or drug reactions. Even minor illness can temporarily cause worsened behavior or greater confusion (20).

- The idiosyncratic characteristics of the individual (19): One person with Alzheimer's disease may be agitated and combative, while another may be amiable and easily managed. The causes of these differences are not understood. The difference affects the services needed and the individual's ability to use services.

- The uneven impact of the illness on different areas of intellect (19): The ill person will be able to do some things better than others. This seeming paradox of intellectual function often leads to misunderstandings of a person's abilities. Families often mistakenly believe that ability to do one task indicates an ability to do an apparently similar task. For example, one woman could load her elder daughter's dishwasher but not the younger one's. The daughters attributed this to the mother's long-standing preference for the elder daughter, but an occupational therapist found that the elder daughter's dishwasher was old, and the mother had learned to operate it before she became ill. The younger daughter's dishwasher was new and the mother was unable to learn even the simple skill of opening it (19).

- The varied response of different symptoms to intervention: Symptoms vary in their responsiveness to treatment, regardless of whether the underlying disease is treatable. Angry outbursts or hallucinations may be controlled or prevented, for example, but an increasing memory loss may not be stopped.

Because of these variations, the ability and behavior of individuals with the same disease may differ widely, and the ability of one individual may vary through the day, or from week to week. Neuropsychological tests are being designed that more accurately measure these varied disabilities and changes over time. However, the relationship between the test results and the person's actual ability to function in familiar surroundings has not been standardized. Although useful in research, such tests are not sufficient by themselves to determine eligibility for services (see ch. 8).

STAGES OF THE DISEASE

The most common cause of dementia, Alzheimer's disease, is a chronic, progressive disorder. Its worsening course has been described in terms of stages of increasing severity. The course of the disease differs from that of multi-infarct dementia or other diseases, but the problems in accurately diagnosing Alzheimer's disease and multi-infarct dementia make it difficult to develop ways to describe these stages. This section will discuss the concept of identifying stages only for Alzheimer's disease.

Theoretical Advantages of Staging or Measures of Severity

The successful definition of a series of discrete and reliable stages describing Alzheimer's disease would have several advantages. Staging would enable a family to plan ahead for an individual's needs. It would enable researchers to compare different individuals at similar points in their illnesses. It would allow researchers to measure the effect of experimental interventions in postponing the next stage. Researchers could test the effects of experimental drugs by comparing treated persons with untreated persons at the same stage.

Staging would also allow planning for appropriate levels of service needed as individuals decline. Average lengths of time in each stage would allow planners to estimate costs of care. The stage of the individual's illness could be used as a criterion of eligibility for specific services.

Staging Instruments

The effort to develop accurate measures of stages has only begun. One of the classic descriptions of Alzheimer's disease, which has been used by many clinicians, has three stages. The first stage is marked by the onset of memory loss. The second stage is marked by problems in language, motor ability, and recognition of objects. The third or terminal stage shows profound dementia with loss of continence, loss of the ability to walk, and nearly complete loss of language (38).

Several more detailed theories of stages have been developed recently in an effort to characterize more specifically the predictable changes during the course of the disease. Although the validity of scales remains controversial, two examples are included here.

Table 2-1 shows the Brief Cognitive Rating Scale (32), which describes seven stages of the patient's illness on 10 axes: concentration, recent memory, past memory, orientation, functioning and self-care, speech, motor functioning, mood and behavior, practice of an art or skill, and calculation

ability. This scale has the advantage of describing declines in several areas of function. Also it is more detailed and specific than the three-stage model.

Table 2-2 shows the Global Deterioration Scale, which defines seven stages of deterioration, ranging from no cognitive decline to very severe cognitive decline, and their associated clinical phases and characteristics.

The Clinical Dementia Rating Scale (15) (table 2-3) uses five stages and six axes and is designed to measure the severity of major areas of cognition.

Use of Assessment Tools for Staging

Tests intended to diagnose the presence of dementia, to assess those areas of cognition that are more impaired than others, or to track the decline of individuals can be used to describe stages. These scales may rate person's abilities to perform familiar tasks (3), or several general kinds of functioning (10). Researchers have examined many other specific characteristics of intellect in search of those that show a consistent and reliable pattern of change in dementia (18).

Problems in the Use of Scales and Stages

Researchers do not agree about the validity of the scales. While some report consistent similarities in persons with dementia, others are struck by the degree of variability. Although one researcher states, "present investigations indicate that seven stages of progressive deterioration in normal aging and Alzheimer's disease can readily be described" (33), another maintains that: "although the patient with Alzheimer's disease or a related disorder undergoes a series of behavioral changes and losses, empirical data are still not available to describe the course of the illness. Cognitive skills and competency in life tasks appear to deteriorate at different rates in different people, but the losses are progressive until the individual ultimately dies" (4).

Alzheimer's disease is a gradually progressive disorder with no noticeable hallmarks that mark a person's passage from one stage to the next. Observers note that some individuals remain un-

Table 2-1.—Brief Cognitive Rating Scale

Part 1

Axis 1: Concentration
1. No objective or subjective evidence of deficit in concentration.
2. Subjective decrement in concentration ability.
3. Minor signs of poor concentration (e.g., subtraction of serials 7s from 100).
4. Definite concentration deficit for persons of their background (e.g., marked deficit on serial 7s; frequent deficit in subtraction of serial 4s from 40).
5. Marked concentration deficit (e.g., giving months backwards or serials 2s from 20).
6. Forgets the concentration task. Frequently begins to count forward when asked to count backwards from 10 by 1s.
7. Marked difficulty counting forward to 10 by 1s.

Axis II: Recent memory
1. No objective or subjective evidence of deficit in recent memory.
2. Subjective impairment only (e.g., forgetting names more than formerly).
3. Deficit in recall of specific events evident upon detailed questioning. No deficit in the recall of major recent events.
4. Cannot recall major events of previous weekend or week. Scanty knowledge (not detailed) of current events, favorite TV shows, etc.
5. Unsure of weather; may not know current president or current address.
6. Occasional knowledge of some recent events. Little or no idea of current address.
7. No knowledge of recent events.

Axis III: Past memory
1. No subjective or objective impairment in past memory.
2. Subjective impairment only, can recall two or more primary school teachers.
3. Some gaps in past memory upon detailed questioning. Able to recall at least one childhood teacher and/or childhood friend.
4. Clear-cut deficit, the spouse recalls more of the patient's past than the patient. Cannot recall childhood friends and/or teachers but knows the names of schools attended. Confuses chronology in reciting personal history.
5. Major past events sometimes not recalled (e.g., names of schools attended).
6. Some residual memory of past (e.g., may recall country of birth or former occupation; may or may not recall mother's name; may or may not recall father's name).
7. No memory of past (cannot recall country, State, or town of origin; cannot recall names of parents, etc.).

Axis IV: Orientation
1. No deficit in memory for time, place, identity of self or others.
2. Subjective impairment only, knows time to nearest hour, location.
3. Any mistake in time of 2 hours or more; day of the week of 1 day or more; date of 3 days or more.
4. Mistakes in month of 10 days or more; or year of 1 month or more.
5. Unsure of month and/or year and/or season; unsure of locale.
6. No idea of date. Identifies spouse but may not recall name. Knows own name.
7. Cannot identify spouse. May be unsure of personal identity.

Axis V: Functioning and self-care
1. No difficulty, either subjectively or objectively.
2. Complains of forgetting location of objects. Subjective work difficulties.
3. Decreased job functioning evident to co-workers, difficulty in traveling to new locations.
4. Decreased ability to perform complex tasks (e.g., planning dinner for guests, handling finances, marketing, etc.).
5. Requires assistance in choosing proper clothing.
6. Requires assistance in feeding, and/or toileting, and/or bathing, and/or ambulating.
7. Requires constant assistance in all activities of daily life.

SOURCE: B. Reisberg, S. Ferris, and M.J. deLeon, "Senile Dementia of the Alzheimer's Type: Diagnostic and Differential Diagnostic Features With Special Reference to Functional Assessment Staging," *Proceedings*, Second International Tropon-Bayer Symposium, 1984.

to order tests. There were trade-offs—some minor problems would be missed by the less costly strategies. The range of costs per patient was large, from $153.92 to $1,109.50 (182). The optimal diagnostic algorithm for dementia is likely to be as elusive as for other syndromes. Diagnostic processes will defy unanimity and become established slowly through large numbers of clinical investigations, medical textbooks, journal articles, and health professional conferences. Rigorous studies of comparative costs and benefits of different diagnostic approaches will, however, permit both greater certainty of diagnosis and more efficient delivery of care.

CHARACTERISTICS OF SPECIFIC DISEASES

This section describes briefly some of the major disorders that cause dementia, emphasizing those that are most common or have yielded most to scientific inquiry. Alzheimer's disease, which accounts for the majority of cases of dementia among the U.S. population, is the focus of most discussion because so little is known about its cause, prevention, or treatment. This discussion is followed by descriptions of multi-infarct dementia (the second most common cause of dementia) and other disorders that are scientifically or clinically instructive. The final part of this section considers disorders that may provide important scientific insights, present prospects for future research, or threaten to grow in magnitude and thus act as new sources of demand for long-term care.

Alzheimer's Disease

Alzheimer's disease refers to the disease process occurring in a patient who shows both the clinical symptoms of dementia and the characteristic microscopic changes in the brain. The clinical diagnosis is made on the basis of finding typical symptoms that progress over time and by eliminating other possible diagnoses that could explain those symptoms. (The symptoms have been described in the preceding section, and also in chs. 2 and 8.) Symptoms are only part of the picture, however; the definitive diagnosis of Alzheimer's disease requires biopsy or autopsy examination of brain tissue.

Microscopic Changes

Alois Alzheimer first noted microscopic changes that occurred in the brain of a woman patient with clinical dementia in 1906, and the following year he reported this first case of the disease that bears his name (2). The findings he described are still those used to make the diagnosis of Alzheimer's disease, although the microscopic features that define the disease continue to be refined (193).

The significance of the abnormal findings in Alzheimer's disease can best be understood by describing some aspects of the organization of the human brain. The brain is organized differently from other organs in several ways. It consists of at least 10 billion nerve cells, with 10 times as many "supporting" cells. The nerve cells are connected to each other, each connecting with hundreds or thousands of other nerve cells. Scientists have made significant progress in understanding the complex organization of the brain over the past decade, although what they do not know still overwhelms what they do. The relationship between disrupted brain cell organization and certain disorders is becoming clearer, and Alzheimer's disease is one such disorder.

Anatomy of Abnormal Changes.—Death of nerve cells occurs in several locations in brains of patients with Alzheimer's disease. Pathologists have long noted a loss of cells from parts of the brain called the cerebral cortex (constituting the outer layers of nerve cells covering the brain) and the hippocampus (a large, curved aggregation of nerve cells near the underside of the brain). The abnormal microscopic findings are found both within nerve cells and between cells (near specialized junctions with other cells). The locations of the microscopic abnormalities appear to correspond roughly to the distribution of cells that use the chemical acetylcholine for cell-to-cell communication (see following discussion).

More recently, investigators have found that nerve cells are lost from a number of brain regions in Alzheimer's disease. Loss of nerve cells from one group, called the nucleus basalis of Meynert (10,279,329), is thought to be especially relevant. These cells are believed to be part of a "circuit" of nerve cells that communicate with one another and are involved in the physiological processes that perform memory and other complex brain functions (70). The loss of the nerve cells in the nucleus basalis is increasingly believed to be an important feature of Alzheimer's disease.

The nerve cells of the nucleus basalis connect to the two areas where the microscopic changes, Alois Alzheimer originally noted, take place: the cerebral cortex and the hippocampus. The parts of the hippocampus that are destroyed in Alzheimer's disease are those generally thought to be involved in memory (149). Some researchers have even suggested that symptoms of the disease could be explained by the lesions in the hippocampus alone (13), although there is disagreement on this point (62). Recent advances in identifying specific hippocampal cells lost in Alzheimer's disease may further elucidate their role in causing symptoms (199).

Types of Microscopic Changes.—Two patterns of microscopic change are generally used to make the diagnosis of Alzheimer's disease. The first consists of an aggregation of abnormal filamentous proteins in nerve cells called neurofibrillary tangles (220), which do not dissolve in solvents that dissolve most other proteins (65,285), although they have recently been dissolved in special solvents (151,284,285). Neurofibrillary tangles are not the same as normal fiberlike proteins found in nerve cells (150), although they share some features with proteins involved in maintaining the cell's shape (174). Neurofibrillary tangles are not found exclusively in Alzheimer's disease, but are also found in several other diseases, and the relationship of tangles to other microscopic abnormalities typical of some other diseases is not yet clear (114).

The second type of change is found in the area between cells, near the points of contact at which a nerve cell receives signals from other cells. These abnormal clusters of proteins and associated components are called senile plaques or neuritic plaques.

Neurofibrillary tangles and senile plaques look quite different under the microscope, and their relation to one another is uncertain. Some studies suggest that they may be aggregates of similar types of protein (168), but preliminary characterizations of the protein components suggest significant biochemical differences (285). It also appears that the disease processes that have been known for years to affect the cortex and hippocampus are quite similar to those that affect cells in the nucleus basalis (279), suggesting that analogous processes may be taking place in many different parts of the brain.

Several other changes in the brain are often found in Alzheimer's disease, called granulovacuolar bodies, Lewy bodies, and Hirano bodies (248), but these are not generally used to identify patients with Alzheimer's disease, and may even suggest involvement of another disease (e.g., Parkinson's).

Neurofibrillary tangles and senile plaques are not found exclusively in the brains of patients with Alzheimer's disease. Both are found in most people as they age (33). One investigator found plaques or tangles in almost three-fourths of patients age 55 to 64 who did not have dementia (318). That may confuse those trying to understand the difference between normal aging and Alzheimer's disease, but the confusion is warranted only in a minority of cases. In most patients with this type of dementia, the plaques and tangles are found in dramatically increased numbers and their profusion is concentrated in the regions of the hippocampus and certain parts of the cerebral cortex (247,248). In aging patients who do not have dementia, the plaques and tangles are much less frequent and are dispersed. Physicians do occasionally encounter patients in whom there are mild symptoms of dementia combined with autopsy findings showing an intermediate number and distribution of plaques and tangles. It is difficult to be certain whether these individuals had Alzheimer's disease, but such patients are exceptions, rather than the norm.

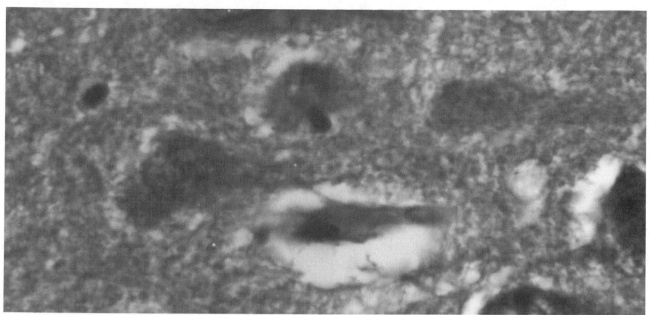

Photo credit: Office of Technology Assessment

Microscopic appearance of neurofibrillary tangles in nerve cells of the cerebral cortex of a 64-year-old man with Alzheimer's disease of 24 years' duration. The photo is taken at 400× magnification of tissue stained with standard techniques. Nerve cells are the dark pyramidal structures. The most prominent neurofibrillary tangle is found to the left of the nucleus of the cell just off center, and consists of deeply stained filaments extending from below the nucleus towards the upper tip of the cell.

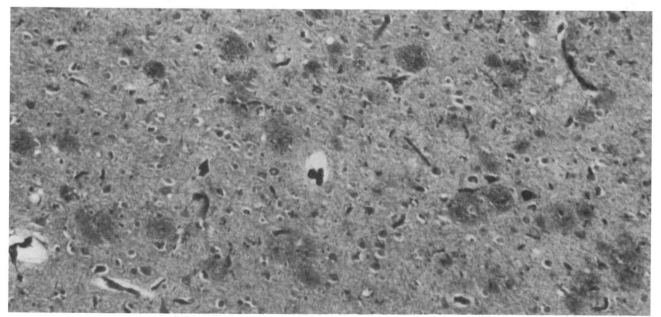

Photo credit: Office of Technology Assessment

Microscopic appearance of senile plaques, taken of brain tissue from the cerebral cortex of a 60-year-old woman with Alzheimer's disease of over 10 years' duration. The photo is taken at 100× magnification of tissue stained with a silver-containing dye that binds to the abnormal material associated with senile plaques. The plaques are dark areas dispersed throughout the photograph.

Heterogeneity of Alzheimer's Disease

Alzheimer's disease is primarily defined by its clinical symptoms and microscopic changes. It is quite likely, however, that this combination of clinical and microscopic findings actually refers to a *group* of disorders, each with possibly different causes.

Researchers in recent years have increasingly focused on identifying subtypes of patients with clinically diagnosed Alzheimer's disease. A consensus is beginning to form that there are several types (35,118,205,286). Several different findings have been suggested as defining important subtypes:

- familial aggregation (presence of many cases in one family);
- disturbance of reading, writing, and speaking ability;
- age at onset of symptoms;
- presence of uncontrollable abnormal movements; and
- severe personality disorders and psychoses.

Patients showing the brain changes typical of Alzheimer's disease can have a wide variety of symptoms (232). Investigators have found younger patients to have more severe cognitive deterioration (205), more severe behavioral disruption (14), and more severe disturbance of language use (56). Several other features differentiate early from late-onset cases. Younger patients have poorer results on psychological tests (190). They also show degeneration of additional groups of brain cells (36) and more "circuits" of nerve cells (272). PET scanning devices have been reported to detect differences between patients who develop the disease at younger ages and those who first show symptoms when older (175).

These differences may be due to the illness lasting longer for patients with younger age of onset (investigators could be measuring *duration* rather than finding real biological differences). The most recent studies have attempted to assess that issue and have concluded that there are differences in the disease process itself, rather than merely in stage of illness when patients are studied. Other variants may be due to atypical presentations

whose cause and relationship to more typical cases are unclear (289). Despite all the suggestions that there may be distinct subtypes of Alzheimer's disease, no single way of defining such groups has emerged, and conflicts between the different studies of subgroups must be resolved before the categories are widely accepted (156).

The diagnosis of Alzheimer's disease may thus be refined over the next several decades, as subtypes are better defined and their characteristics are codified into diagnostic practice. In the meantime, it is likely that work being done on patients with Alzheimer's disease is focused on a diverse group of disorders with different causes. The treatment and prevention of the illness will likely depend on identifying specific causes and characteristics that differ for the various subgroups. This dependence of new treatments and preventive strategies on understanding the etiology and biological processes of the disease reinforces the importance of finding the cause or causes of Alzheimer's disease.

Possible Causes of Alzheimer's Disease

Scientists have not identified a cause of Alzheimer's disease. But various hypotheses have been supported by different amounts and quality of supporting data. There is substantial evidence for some ideas (e.g., the loss of some chemicals used in nerve cell communication and the existence of familial clustering), while others are primarily working hypotheses. (For an overview about the possible causes, see ref. 338, or one of the books on the topic written for the lay audience: see refs. 57a,141,191). A recent scientific review is also available in *Neuroscience* (246).

The possible causes of Alzheimer's disease can be roughly divided into several groups. The groups overlap extensively, and one cause does not preclude others. They may even be directly linked. The disruption of nerve cell circuits often cited as a potential cause does not explain *why* the nerve cells die. Complete understanding of the etiology will thus need to elucidate the sequence of events that lead to the expression of disease, and is likely to involve many steps. The loss of specific nerve cells is not, for example, incompatible with the role of genetic factors, infectious agents, or environmental exposures that might explain why the cells die. One way of grouping possible causes is:

- genetic factors (e.g., familial aggregation, association with Down's syndrome, and altered DNA-binding proteins);
- exaggerated aging (i.e., the severe form of a normal process—discussed in ch. 2);
- environmental factors (e.g., metal exposures, head trauma, viruses, and other infectious agents);
- immunologic factors (e.g., special susceptibility to infectious agents or proclivity for reacting against one's own brain cells);
- disrupted nerve cell "circuits" (including loss of specific populations of nerve cells and disruption of communication between certain groups of brain cells), which is a causal hypothesis that would require a *further* explanation for cell death; and
- intrinsic metabolic factors (e.g., disruption of biochemical pathways in brain cells or in different types of cells throughout the body, disturbance of protein transport in nerve cells, and changes in cell membranes), which would also require a further explanation of why certain factors were lost.

Genetic Factors.—One of the questions about Alzheimer's disease most often asked of physicians and other health professionals is: Is it genetic? This is a common fear among relatives of affected patients. Unfortunately, the answer is not simple.

Clearly in some families Alzheimer's disease appears in a way that looks very much like a genetic trait. When a pattern suggests an inherited trait, the disease is called "familial Alzheimer's disease." The largest such family discovered so far, spanning seven generations, was reported in 1983 (233), and more than 100 smaller families had been reported in various medical journals (63,64,296).

In familial Alzheimer's disease, the children of an affected parent have been found to have a 50-50 chance of having the putative gene that leads to the disease (although a person carrying the disease gene may die before showing symptoms). The chances of eventually developing the disease are high if a person carries the gene and lives past age 85. This pattern of inheritance is called "au-

tosomal dominant" transmission by medical geneticists, and it suggests that the presence of a single gene confers predisposition to Alzheimer's disease in such families.

Although there is no longer any doubt that some families are affected by Alzheimer's disease in a way that suggests a single gene trait, substantial disagreement exists on how many cases of Alzheimer's disease can be traced to genetic factors and whether there is only one genetic form. Some researchers have found that early-onset cases (beginning before age 65) are more likely to be familial than late-onset (337), but this has not been confirmed by all investigators (56).

If genetic and nonfamilial forms exist, what can families be told about their genetic risks? One physician who has studied families with Alzheimer's disease extensively has developed a way to calculate risks (141, app. C) and suggests that a case is most likely to be genetic if it begins before age 65 and if there are two or more immediate relatives also affected (139). If the case is of the genetic form, then the risk to the patient's children depends on the age at which the disease began—later onset means lower risk to children. Some investigators have suggested that disturbance of language function might predict familial occurrence (38,40,96), but others have reported just the opposite (171). One group has constructed a mathematical model based on preliminary clinical studies. The model suggests that a single gene may predispose to Alzheimer's disease among patients with a specific set of clinical symptoms (41,42). The model also suggests that all such cases may be genetic, and account for 78 percent of all cases of Alzheimer's disease.

Many if not most people who develop Alzheimer's disease do not have relatives who are also affected. This evidence has been offered to suggest that fewer than a third of cases are genetic, but the data cannot be so simply interpreted. Most studies exclude investigation of cases over a certain age (often 69 or 79) because of the unreliable nature of medical information available about very old individuals. Yet such exclusion can unduly diminish the reported number of cases in relatives, particularly since Alzheimer's disease becomes increasingly common with age and is highly prevalent only among those over 80. Any age cut-off thus precludes investigation of the group most likely to be informative. A definitive answer about the prevalence of familial versus nonfamilial Alzheimer's disease thus awaits rigorous study of large families with longitudinal investigation of all patients into advanced old age.

Because of these uncertainties, the relative number of genetic and nonfamilial cases of Alzheimer's disease is difficult to estimate. Recent studies have shown familial rates as low as 25 percent (142), but most show higher familial prevalence (40,96, 140,312). One statistical analysis of patients with Alzheimer's disease estimated that over half of all cases may be of the genetic form (40,96), but this has not been uniformly accepted (258). Some confusion over the conflicting studies is due to the unusual genetic characteristics of Alzheimer's disease in affected families: Because of its late manifestation this trait should appear in only about one-third of predisposed individuals (39). When life expectancy is age 70 to 75, two-thirds of the people carrying the postulated Alzheimer's gene will die before they show symptoms, and only one-third would develop the disease. The child of an affected patient would thus stand a one in six chance of developing Alzheimer's disease. Yet life expectancy is rapidly increasing, especially among older age groups in the United States, and so the relative prevalence of the familial form of Alzheimer's disease may well increase.

In addition to the confusion caused by the delayed onset of Alzheimer's disease in affected families, many other uncertainties surround the prevalence and special characteristics of the genetic form of Alzheimer's disease. Some of these uncertainties are due to different scientists studying relatively small groups of patients that differ from one medical center to another. Other differences arise from varying measurement techniques for assessing the type, severity, and clinical characteristics of dementia in the studies. There may even be more than one genetic form of Alzheimer's disease (308).

The presence or absence of a single gene that predisposes people to developing Alzheimer's disease does not imply that other factors do not also play a role. The delay in onset of the disease caused by the postulated gene is difficult to explain, although this is also true of another genetic disease, Huntington's disease (discussed later). Other factors, including all other possible causes discussed in this section, could also play a role in the genetic form of Alzheimer's disease.

Uncertainty about the familial form of Alzheimer's disease should be resolved as soon as possible because of the importance of such information in counseling families. Some families are clearly affected by a familial form of the disease, and others are clearly affected by a form that is not primarily genetic. Many families, however, do not have enough information about their relatives to be sure whether the disease is genetic or not, and it is these people who most need guidance.

Environmental Factors.—Several scientists have attempted to identify personal or dietary habits, drug use, environmental toxins, or infectious agents that might cause Alzheimer's disease. Epidemiologic surveys of large numbers of patients have looked at many factors. One factor found by many studies is association with previous trauma to the head (100,143,223,340 citing 3,4). The age of the mother at birth of the affected patient, higher prevalence of thyroid disease, and risk of Down's syndrome in relatives have been reported by a few studies but not most; even the association with head trauma is not found in all studies (4,266).

The association of Alzheimer's disease with prior head trauma may simply be due to the family member's being more likely to remember a head injury for a patient with Alzheimer's disease than if the patient did not later develop the disease. Careful analysis of the data suggests this is unlikely, however (101,264). There are other reasons to suspect that the association of Alzheimer's disease with head trauma may be more than mere coincidence. First, the association has been uncovered in three independent studies that did not have other findings in common. Second, there have been several reports of individuals with severe head trauma who have subsequently (after years) developed Alzheimer's disease (reviewed in ref. 277). Third, the pathological changes that take place in Alzheimer's disease resemble those that have long been known to take place in boxers who live to old age. Most boxers sustain repeated and severe head trauma as part of their sport; the knockout is, after all, a form of concussion in which the brain temporarily fails to function normally because of acute trauma.

Many boxers who live to old age develop a clinical syndrome called dementia pugilistica (boxer's dementia) that includes tangles in the cerebral cortex and elsewhere (66,72). Dementia pugilistica has traditionally been classified separately from Alzheimer's disease because its cause is known, additional anatomical changes characteristic of previous trauma are usually absent in Alzheimer's disease, and the distribution of neurofibrillary tangles is not identical to that found in Alzheimer's disease. The evidence is equivocal at present, and the concept of head trauma causing Alzheimer's disease is controversial (277), but investigators are now reexamining the association to see if head trauma might not be a cause of Alzheimer's disease.

Viruses or other transmissible dementia agents have also been suggested as causes of Alzheimer's disease. Several disorders that cause dementia are known to be caused by viruses or unusual agents. The hypothesis that Alzheimer's disease might be caused by infection is based on such clinical associations, combined with additional scientific evidence. Plaques from patients with Alzheimer's disease are sometimes similar to those found in the animal disease scrapie, which is known to be infectious (268). Some patients also develop microscopic plaques in a part of the brain often affected in kuru, a transmissible human dementia (106,250).

The relationship between Alzheimer's disease and transmissible dementia is puzzling. Kuru is just one of several dementing conditions caused by an unusual group of slow-acting infectious agents unlike conventional viruses, bacteria, or other known microbes. Kuru was discovered on the island of New Guinea, where it was propagated by ritual cannibalism of those who died (106). Creutzfeldt-Jakob disease and Gerstmann-Strassler syndrome are two other dementing conditions caused by similar agents. The scientific work that elucidated the infectious cause and unusual characteristics of the agents causing kuru and Creutzfeldt-Jakob disease earned the 1976

Nobel Prize for Physiology and Medicine for D. Carleton Gajdusek.

Subsequent work has noted several associations between the microscopic plaques and protein constituents thought to be part of the infectious agents that cause these diseases—scrapie, Creutzfeldt-Jakob disease, Gerstmann-Strassler syndrome, and kuru (107,251,252,294). A gene whose expression is increased in mice infected with scrapie also binds to senile plaques of patients with Alzheimer's disease, providing another tantalizing association of unknown significance (332). Familial Alzheimer's disease was initially reported to be infectiously transmitted to primates, but these reports have not been replicated despite numerous attempts (44,120). Finally, some have questioned the evidence for the chemical similarity of Alzheimer's disease changes and the plaques associated with the unusual infectious disease scrapie (268). The hypothesis that unusual infectious agents cause Alzheimer's disease thus remains an intriguing but unconfirmed speculation.

It is also possible that a virus that acts in an unconventional way in some patients, causing a slow and insidious disease, may also cause Alzheimer's disease. The evidence for this is based primarily on knowledge that several other diseases believed to be caused by viruses can also cause dementia (e.g., progressive multifocal leukoencephalopathy and subacute sclerosing panencephalitis). On the other hand, no viruses have ever been consistently associated with Alzheimer's disease, despite extensive searches, and no immune reaction is found in the brains of patients with Alzheimer's disease comparable to that found in other viral dementias.

In summary, the possibility of a viral cause of Alzheimer's disease cannot be either ruled out or definitely confirmed by existing studies.

Several groups of scientists have found that the abnormal protein aggregations that make up plaques and tangles are also associated with high concentrations of aluminum and silicon. The elevation of silicon concentrations was first described in 1972 (11,235), and several groups found high aluminum content beginning in 1976 (71,241). The findings are not disputed, but their interpretation is not yet clear. Both aluminum and silicon are very common elements in the Earth's crust, and high exposure levels to dust containing both silicon and aluminum is normal. Recent studies have noted the association of aluminosilicates in damaged areas of the brain, and researchers postulate that these deposits are causing the alterations (50,51). Other studies show an association of several neurological diseases with aluminum deposition and trace mineral content in water supplies (234).

Many Alzheimer's disease researchers interpret the presence of aluminum and silicon as a result of cell death, rather than its cause. Their explanation is that the nerve cells die, or for some other reason insoluble abnormal protein aggregates begin to form in nerve cells and near nerve terminals. Aluminum and silicon, highly prone to forming insoluble complexes, then deposit on the protein moieties and are thereby concentrated. This explanation relegates the role of aluminum and silicon to a secondary and relatively unimportant function rather than serving as primary toxins. More work must be done, however, to determine whether silicon and aluminum deposition is a cause or a consequence of Alzheimer's disease.

Other metals may also play a role, particularly if absent from the diet. A disease process that resembles Alzheimer's disease in some respects is found in Guam, some islands in Japan, and a few other Pacific islands. This disease has clinical and microscopic overlap with Parkinson's disease, amyotrophic lateral sclerosis (Lou Gehrig's disease), and Alzheimer's disease. The factor common to each of these regions is a deficiency of calcium and magnesium in the water supply (107, 239).

Immunologic Factors.—Defects in the immune system have also been proposed as working hypotheses in explaining Alzheimer's disease. The involvement of the immune system theoretically could be independent of other factors, or could also involve infectious agents, genetic predisposition, or environmental toxins. Nerve cells share many surface features with cells of the immune system, and so might be affected by similar mechanisms (104,105). One study showed that the immune function of one type of cell—so-called T8$^+$ suppressor lymphocytes—is lower in patients with Alzheimer's disease than in control patients (293). Another showed diminished production of interleukin-1, a substance that stimulates immune cells, associated with Alzheimer's disease (167). Antibodies of a particular type, called IgG, are specifically increased in some patients with Alzheimer's disease (57,58,88,136). And a gene that controls a blood protein involved in immune function, factor C4B, has been associated with Alzheimer's disease (234). However, the significance of these findings is not clear. Several investigators have failed to find any significant decline in immune function or specific lymphocyte function that is predictive of Alzheimer's disease (136,155, 185,304).

Disrupted Nerve Cell Circuits.—Researchers in the last decade have correlated Alzheimer's disease with loss of specific groups of nerve cells and disrupted communication between nerve cells. Studies of the loss of cells in the nucleus basalis and hippocampus, noted earlier, are good examples of this work, but the story does not stop with the loss of nerve cells. Discovery of effects in the nucleus basalis and hippocampus was preceded by the work of several investigators who were studying cell-to-cell communication in the brains of patients who had died with Alzheimer's disease or other disorders. Investigators in the United Kingdom noted that there was a dearth of protein that makes the chemical acetylcholine in some parts of the brains of patients with Alzheimer's disease (reviewed in 16).

The relative absence of acetylcholine suggested that the cells using it to communicate with other cells might be dying off. Other evidence suggested that such a defect might explain the loss of memory in Alzheimer's disease (16,69), and researchers found that the cells lost from the nucleus basalis were a major source of acetylcholine for the cerebral cortex (69,329,330). Others were able to confirm that the nucleus basalis cells did indeed make acetylcholine (226), and transport it to the cortex (209). Taken together, the different studies began to present a coherent picture: Nerve cells that use acetylcholine were lost from the nucleus basalis and other areas, reducing the amount of acetylcholine released to cells in the cortex and hippocampus, and disrupting memory processes.

The story is not so simple, however, because nerve cells that use acetylcholine are not the only ones lost in Alzheimer's disease (245,295), and cell loss is not strictly correlated with the use of acetylcholine as a chemical transmitter (219). Several other regions of the brain suffer loss of nerve cells (193). Nerve cells that use the chemicals serotonin (73), somatostatin (78,116,178,272,287) and corticotropin-releasing factor (22,81,93,303) are also lost.

These discoveries represent a major advance in the understanding of Alzheimer's disease, but there are lingering complexities, and much is left unexplained (246). Some cell groups lost in Alzheimer's disease also die off in other disorders. Groups of cells that die off in some patients remain healthy in others (36,272), and different patients show contrasting patterns of cell loss and chemical defects (70,78). Some of the abnormal changes of Alzheimer's disease can also be induced in nerve cells grown in tissue culture by adding two chemicals—aspartate and glutamate—that are believed to be naturally used to communicate between cells (79), and these chemicals are found diminished in brain regions of patients dying with Alzheimer's disease (238,281). That finding suggests that cell communication involving these two chemicals may cause cell death in the brain, in addition to cells that use acetylcholine to communicate. Despite such evidence that other factors may be involved, the loss of acetylcholine does appear to be a consistent finding, affecting all subgroups (99). Some subgroups may have other defects in addition to the loss of cells that use acetylcholine.

Scientists do not appear near a complete explanation of why Alzheimer's disease occurs in some people and not others, or why only some cells die. Even if nerve cell circuits are involved, this provides only an intermediate explanation, and does not suggest an ultimate cause. Many questions remain unanswered. Are certain nerve cells genetically programmed to die in some people? Are they killed by viruses or toxins? Do they have specific biochemical or metabolic aberrations? Or are they mistakenly killed by the body's own immune defenses?

Intrinsic Metabolic Factors.—Several investigators have reported disrupted biochemical pathways and other metabolic abnormalities in patients with Alzheimer's disease. Enzymes are proteins that facilitate chemical reactions. Some researchers have found abnormal function of specific enzymes involved in sugar metabolism in brain cells (28,32,280), in patients' cells grown in tissue culture (293), and in red blood cells (29).

Others have found abnormalities of proteins that affect DNA or RNA, the genetic material of all cells. One group found that patients with Alzheimer's disease had less RNA in their brains at autopsy, and they traced the defect to more rapid degradation of RNA. The amount of a protein that slows RNA degradation was abnormally low, and so release from normal inhibition led to accelerated decay of RNA (278). That defect would make it difficult for cells to produce normal amounts of protein, and it might explain other biochemical abnormalities or cause cells to be vulnerable to insults. The specific metabolic features of RNA metabolism in Alzheimer's disease are still under study, and the results are not completely consistent from report to report (306). Other investigators have found slowed repair of DNA (189), increased sensitivity to damage of DNA (283), or changes in the proteins that stick to DNA (that might regulate which genes are turned on and off) (213,324).

Another focus of study has been the cell membrane—the thin layer of material that separates cells from one another and from body fluids. The cell membrane includes elements that determine its electrical properties (and the ability to transmit nerve cell impulses) and that allow other cells and proteins to recognize the cell from its exterior. Abnormalities of cell membranes could, therefore, have profound disrupting effects in nerve cell communication and recognition. Several researchers have produced preliminary evidence of such membrane changes (339,345).

Nerve cells need contact with other nerve cells or muscle cells in order to survive. The exact requirements for nerve cell survival are not known, but likely include "trophic factors" carried back to the nerve cell. One hypothesis suggests that trophic factors specific to particular nerve cell populations are lost in Alzheimer's disease, leading to loss of the nerve cells (8,9). Replacing the trophic factors might lead to partial clinical recovery or growth of new cells to replace those that are lost. This possibility of nerve cell regrowth has been supported by finding that some cells in certain regions of the brain do proliferate in Alzheimer's disease, but do not find their normal attachments (109). Recent studies of a protein called nerve growth factor (NGF) suggest that it may promote growth and sustenance of nerve cells that use acetylcholine in the nucleus basalis, and preliminary studies show improvement of learning-impaired rats in response to administration of NGF (reviewed in 198).

Some investigators have suggested that the nerve cells that die off in Alzheimer's disease do so because they cannot adequately move important structural proteins over long distances through the thin threadlike projections of the cell that conduct electrical impulses (107,121). These theories are based, in part, on the nature and location of abnormal protein aggregates (plaques and tangles) in the brain. Others interpret the location and composition of abnormal protein condensation as suggesting that proteins related to plaques and tangles accumulate around small blood vessels and impede the flow of oxygen and nutrients to nerve cells (112). That interpretation is supported by many reports of reduced metabolism in certain parts of the cortex of patients with Alzheimer's disease, but this condition could also be found if cells died from other causes. Finally, the abnormal protein aggregates in tangles share some features with proteins that are involved in maintaining the cell's shape (174).

Summary.—Many different causes of Alzheimer's disease have been postulated, and others may be suggested. It appears likely that genetic factors are important in some cases. Infectious agents, head trauma, immune dysfunction, toxins, and metabolic aberrations may also be involved and are being investigated vigorously. Research on Alzheimer's disease has become a priority only in the last decade, and the effort to track down a cause can succeed only with further work. That additional work will require substantial and sustained research support from Congress (see ch. 13).

Issues in Treatment of Alzheimer's Disease

No fully effective treatments or means of preventing Alzheimer's disease has been found. Although a few drugs can marginally alleviate some of the symptoms, the most effective way to manage patients is by adapting the environment to patient needs rather than prescribing a specific medical treatment. Medical options are limited, but much can be done to reduce the adverse impact of Alzheimer's disease on patients, families, and others (328).

A physician who makes a diagnosis of Alzheimer's disease must also make several related determinations. The health and safety of patients, their families, and those who come in contact with patients can be influenced by these considerations. Several issues commonly confronted are whether the patient:

- should continue to drive,
- can retain his or her job (especially difficult for those in highly skilled positions that involve substantial responsibility for others or affect public safety),
- can make decisions about financial and legal matters, and
- is eligible for special disability or health programs.

These determinations are not purely medical, but they involve a medical evaluation and assessment of the severity of illness. Physicians who care for a patient with dementia are therefore involved in these complex and difficult considerations (282). Correct determinations require understanding of the particular patient, the patient's environment, the family structure, the availability of outside supports, and eligibility criteria for government programs.

These nonmedical considerations become a part of patient management, although they are not commonly considered medical treatment. Other issues raised by the treatment of those with Alzheimer's disease are more directly linked to medical care.

Quackery.—Diseases that are common, devastating, and incurable attract crank remedies. Hope and desperation conspire to create a market that is open ground for opportunism. Many diseases are subject to this phenomenon: cancer, acquired immune deficiency syndrome (AIDS), and arthritis, among others. Alzheimer's disease, and many other dementing disorders, are among the targets for quackery. Bizarre treatments such as "chelation therapy" and "blue-green algae manna" have been promoted for those with Alzheimer's disease in the absence of evidence of efficacy (52), and there will doubtless be more such remedies proposed in the future.

Distinguishing legitimate treatment from quackery can be difficult. Quackery implies a cynical intent to profit from what is known to be useless, or failure to gather evidence that questions the legitimacy of a practice. The way that numerous accepted medical treatments work is only poorly understood, and many start out as accidents; few important treatments were expected, and many are irrational in their origins. A few characteristics of quack remedies, however, distinguish them from standard medical practice. Potential patients and families should ask several questions before embarking on a treatment regimen:

- How is it advertised? Quack remedies are often purveyed through popular magazines and are notably absent from medical journals.
- How accessible is it? Quack remedies are generally costly, and available only through special outlets. In contrast to experimental clinical trials, the promoters are not associated with universities, major medical centers, or reputable practitioners.
- What is in the treatment? Elixirs and miracle potions will not specify what they contain, while clinical trials involve clearly defined components.
- Are the practitioners qualified? Those involved in clinical trials will be licensed to practice medicine, and are likely to have specialty certification as well. Those with legitimate qualifications are not threatened by prospective patients asking about them. Those who lack qualifications cannot provide patients with the information and are more likely to take offense.
- What is the rationale behind the treatment? This may be difficult for someone not expert in the field to judge, but those explaining clinical experiments will be able to cite support in the medical literature, while quacks may refer only to a popular journal or offer no rationale.

- What evidence supports the effectiveness of the treatment? For early clinical trials, there will be evidence from animal testing; quack remedies will refer only to anecdotes of successful use. Another difference between them is the elaborate data-gathering methods and analysis for clinical trials. Remedies that have been used for years on many patients and yet lack rigorous scientific data on effectiveness are highly suspect.

False Hope and Preliminary Data.—The same factors that encourage charlatans can also generate problems for the most careful, well-meaning investigator. Preliminary reports of small increments of medical progress can be greeted by the release of pent-up emotions, leading to unjustifiably high hopes that are dashed in bitter disappointment.

That phenomenon has happened at least twice for preliminary reports of Alzheimer's disease treatments. One was a study on the use of naloxone, a drug that blocks the effect of heroin-like drugs, and the second a report on implantable drug pumps. Both were both picked up by the national press.

The story on naloxone resulted from a small clinical trial in a few patients that was published in a letter to the *New England Journal of Medicine* (259). The trial was carefully planned, but involved only seven patients. Such a small sample is common for treatments on the frontier of inquiry. The report was singled out by Margaret Heckler, then Secretary of Health and Human Services, at a press conference on the efforts of the Federal Government to address the problems of Alzheimer's disease. It then was widely publicized. The Secretary had merely cited it as an example of promising research, but the preliminary nature of the data could not support the onslaught of public attention. Subsequent trials of the agent belied the initial optimism (298).

The other episode attracted even wider publicity. A group at Dartmouth Medical School implanted drug pumps in four patients with Alzheimer's disease (diagnoses that were confirmed by biopsy at the time of insertion). The pumps were used to deliver a drug that simulates the action of acetylcholine, based on the theory that the reduction in acetylcholine might be corrected by direct replacement of the drug. The primary interest in doing the study was to test the feasibility of using such pumps to deliver drugs for patients with Alzheimer's disease, not to cure the disease in the four initial patients. The investigators did, however, distribute questionnaires to the patients' families to find out if they could detect any changes in the patients. The families did not know which drugs were infused into the pumps, and the investigators alternated between using the drug and a harmless fluid. The preliminary drug pump study is being followed up by studies at 10 centers across the United States.

A few members of the national press heard about the initial experiment and asked permission to cover the story. The investigators wrote a short description in the medical journal *Neurosurgery* (131). They also held a press conference because of the interest the story had generated. Although one reason for the press conference was to note the preliminary nature of the data (the title of the paper started with the words "preliminary report"), it had the opposite effect, making reporters believe there was a big story to cover (242). Reports on the pump therapy eventually reached the public through 160 newspapers, many national magazines (including *Newsweek*, *McCall's*, *Forbes*, and *Family Circle*), and most of the national television news services (PBS, NBC, CBS, and Cable News Network) (242). One result was that the "2,600 persons—many desperately trying to stop the dementia consuming their loved ones—who contacted Dartmouth Hitchcock officials in the weeks following the news all had to be told the same thing: there is no new treatment at Dartmouth for Alzheimer's disease, only a research program; it is unproven, however good-looking in principle" (242).

The article in *Neurosurgery* contained only passing reference to the beneficial effects reported by families, but the television and news services talked mainly to enthusiastic family members and doctors. The press release distributed at the news conference referred to patient benefits in the opening sentences, and added qualifications only in the third paragraph (242). Neither the medical article nor the press release noted that the psy-

chological tests that had been given to the patients throughout the trial had failed to show significant improvements. Although it is standard practice to "spice up" stories in public relations work—and the Dartmouth press release is not atypical—the result in terms of the effects on the hospital, the investigators, and the families who heard about the work and yearned for good news was far from the benign, good publicity intended.

The bloating of preliminary research data, whether by reporters, investigators, or research subjects, has several untoward effects. The ensuing publicity can impede the conduct of the very research being reported, endangering the validity of results and making life difficult for investigators who must split their time between doing their work and fielding questions from the media. Other investigators doing similar work are often irritated by such episodes. Some of that irritation might be due to jealousy, but it can also stem from adverse effects on their work and suddenly having to temper the unrealistic hopes of their own patients. Finally, the hopes of those desperately looking for progress are dramatically lifted, then suddenly dropped and shattered.

Recently, the problem of constraining public expectations has taken a new twist. Stories about scientific advances in finding biological markers for diagnostic purposes have appeared in *Time*, *Newsweek*, business publications, and many newspapers, resulting in many physicians being asked to do the diagnostic tests, yet the tests are clearly stated in the articles to be in experimental stages of development.

Even more instructive is the intense publicity surrounding the publication of the lead article in the November 13, 1986, issue of the *New England Journal of Medicine* (302a). The article reports encouraging results from testing of the drug tetrahydroaminoacridine (THA, first discovered in 1909, but newly applied to treatment of Alzheimer's disease) on 17 subjects with the diagnosis of Alzheimer's disease. The Associated Press report about the article reads "Researcher Fears Hysteria Over Alzheimer's Drug Discovery" (130a). The researchers in this case have clearly anticipated that their drug trial would be widely reported, and that the public would demand quick action to make the drug available. (THA is nonpatentable, raising yet another issue, because private firms state they are reluctant to manufacture it and push it through the expensive FDA approval procedure without any way to guarantee a profit.) Press hunger for new results is clear in this instance, where all the rules of careful reporting were followed. The study was carefully controlled, the results dispassionately displayed, and the steps leading to the trial were called a "triumph for the scientific method" in an accompanying editorial (78a). Yet many physicians learned of the story from their patients (the AP story was released on a Wednesday about the Thursday issue of the *Journal*, and most subscribers do not receive their copies until Friday or early the following week). People do in fact want to know the results of reliable studies as soon as they can, and the early news accounts of the THA article contain the important qualifiers, yet the scientists clearly anticipate widespread misunderstanding.

There is no simple way to prevent public relations disasters. Any institutional or regulatory solutions are likely to be worse than the problem. Reporters can work to be more objective, and investigators can be open but not unrealistic. The line between enthusiasm for work in progress and the creation of unjustified optimism is thin. Most researchers are working in this field, after all, just so they can contribute to the eradication of the blight of Alzheimer's disease. Progress is welcomed and feeds the emotional drives of investigators as well as patients and their families. Further, it is important that such events *not* inhibit the reporting of preliminary results. Preliminary reports are efficient ways to test new approaches to treatment, and reporting them when preliminary results are known—whether successful or not—can save other investigators time and wasted effort. But physicians and other scientists can be careful in how the results are reported.

Many family members are grasping for straws. In research on dementia, many such straws are reported each month, but most are buried in medical journals. Both the reports cited here were covered not only in the medical literature (where their significance was likely to be understood), but also heralded at press conferences (where it was likely to be misunderstood). It is safe to report failures,

but success must be handled carefully. Perhaps the most important preventive measure is for clinical investigators to anticipate the publicity, think through how to handle it, and at times eschew it. A delicate balance must be struck between informing the public and the risk of misinforming it.

Medical Management.—Health professionals can manage Alzheimer's disease in several ways. Some of their functions are:

- diagnosis of the disease causing dementia;
- the search for diseases of other organ systems that can be treated, which might improve the patient's mental function;
- assessment of the type and severity of the disease or diseases;
- management of those aspects of the disorder that *can* be treated (e.g., behavioral problems amenable to treatment by medication or to family education on avoidance or management);
- referral to medical supports (e.g., participation in clinical trials can be therapeutic not only for medical benefits but also in providing a feeling of contributing to the ultimate conquest of Alzheimer's disease);
- education of the patient and family about the disease (e.g., what to expect, genetic risks, drugs and foods to avoid); and
- referral to social and legal supports (e.g., family support groups, legal services, government programs).

The importance of family education, legal referral, and recommendation of family support groups is elaborated in several other chapters. The focus here is on management of the medical aspects of this dementing disease.

Some pharmaceutical agents have been reported to diminish the cognitive impairment of patients with Alzheimer's disease. Only one, however, has been approved for clinical use by the U.S. Food and Drug Administration (FDA) (based on several clinical trials). Although patient improvement is consistent, it is minimal. The agent in question, a mix of different drugs, has been in clinical use for three decades; it is marketed under the trade name Hydergine. Hydergine has been used in Europe for treating dementia for over a decade, and is increasingly being used in the United States.

Its mechanism of action is unknown. Hydergine was once thought to improve blood flow, but it is now called a "metabolic enhancer." It alters the biochemistry of nerve cells in several ways, but the reason for mild mental improvement is not known (47,180,328).

Medical management of behavioral symptoms can improve mental function of the patient, simplify the patient's care, or both (135,265). Many patients develop depression, which can be treated by both education and antidepressant medications. Care must be taken to avoid those antidepressant agents that inhibit the action of acetylcholine, which can worsen the patient's dementia, and to use agents less likely to exacerbate dementia (83, 154,239).

Management of hallucinations, anxiety, sleep disorders, agitation, aggression, and wandering often includes changing the patient's habits, adapting the environment, educating the family, and administering drugs targeted specifically at the behavior in question. One physician has suggested that the guidelines for treatment should be to *treat disability not abnormality*, to reverse associated curable illnesses, to limit troublesome symptoms, and to maintain continued support (27).

Most physicians with extensive practice in treating dementia occasionally use medications to control patients' behavior, but the drugs are carefully monitored, and a different selection of agents is usually tried than for other kinds of patients. The drugs used to manage behavioral symptoms, for example, are chosen to minimize their untoward effects on intellectual functions (333). Older individuals in general, and patients with dementia in particular, are more likely to develop adverse side effects from drugs affecting behavior. Thus special care must be taken to prescribe those medications least likely to worsen the dementia and to induce unwanted side effects (328).

This careful approach to medications contrasts with the situation found in some nursing homes. One study reported a more than 300-fold variation among different long-term care facilities in the dose and frequency of medications used to control patients' behavior (256). Such large differences cannot be explained by variations in accepted medical practice, and the pattern of use suggested that drugs were relied on in some facilities as substitutes for staff.

Difficulty in eating can be a major problem among dementia patients. It is not clear why patients with dementia have difficulty eating. They may forget how to eat, refuse to eat—expressing a wish to die—or lose their desire for food. One preliminary report of eating in a nursing home suggests that the cause may be difficulty in swallowing. That study found that of those who depended on caregivers to eat there was a strong correlation with poor mental function, but only a minority of those with very poor mental function had eating difficulties (290). This suggests that there may be a common factor linking eating difficulty to severity of dementia for a fraction of residents. If true, that common factor might also indicate that difficulty in swallowing is an organic symptom, and refusal to eat more involuntary than conscious.

For those experiencing eating difficulty, it is important to evaluate the cause of the difficulty. Is it confusion about how to eat, or tendency to gag or cough when swallowing? Training both family and institutional caregivers how to differentiate organic from voluntary refusal to eat, and how to deal with eating difficulty is the main avenue to treatment. Referral to a speech therapist may help to determine the nature of the eating difficulty, if ability to swallow is in question.

Incontinence of bowel and bladder is a significant problem for many of those with dementia. Half of all patients in nursing homes have urinary incontinence, and this group overlaps extensively with those suffering with dementia. The majority of those in nursing homes with urinary incontinence also have bowel incontinence (64 percent), and most showed severe mental impairment (57 percent). Despite the magnitude of the problem, fewer than 5 percent had a specific cause for the incontinence noted in their medical record (237). Many cases of incontinence can be either eliminated or compensated for using existing technologies, but require a careful evaluation of the cause of incontinence, use of appropriate drugs or devices, and staff training (237).

Many of the problems faced by those with dementia are probably susceptible to improvement by using current technologies with more rigorous application of existing knowledge. One hope for improved care of dementia patients—not only in nursing homes, but also in hospitals, clinics, homes, and day care centers—is knowledge that will be developed in special teaching nursing homes. The National Institute on Aging, the Robert Wood Johnson Foundation, and the Veterans Administration are supporting a new movement to affiliate nursing homes with centers of medical excellence such as nursing and medical schools. These facilities will be much more involved in testing new methods of treatment and management, and will in the long run likely set new standards for care of the chronically ill.

Prospects for Research on Drugs and Devices.—Although only one minimally effective agent has been approved by FDA to be marketed for use in dementia, many other drugs and devices are under investigation. These are too numerous to describe here, and the list changes rapidly as new ideas or agents emerge.

One promising route to discovering new drugs has been the study of chemical imbalances in Alzheimer's disease. The acetylcholine hypothesis suggests numerous possible treatments, and many have been tried or are under investigation. The rationale behind these trials has been extensively reviewed (see 25,54,119,132,200,255,271,341). Many agents are also being tested in relation to other theories of causation, such as the silicon-aluminum hypothesis, the viral hypothesis, the improvement of membrane characteristics, and the correction of immune deficiency. Other agents being tested in the United States have been used in other countries with some reported success (216). Some experimental therapies are directed at chemical imbalances in the brain that involve chemicals other than acetylcholine. These include very short proteins (called neuropeptides), nicotine, and drugs that oppose the action of opiate drugs (117). Advances in therapy may arise from these numerous clinical trials, but existing reports of successful treatment are either preliminary, have not been replicated by other investigators, are inconsistent, or result in only minimal clinical improvement.

Novel ways to deliver drugs to the brain are also important in treatment research. Many chemicals that are active in the brain are digested before they reach the bloodstream or cannot get into the brain even if they enter the blood. Many investigators are developing drug pumps or altering drug structure in attempts to circumvent these problems.

Use of nerve cells themselves for treatment of Alzheimer's disease or other brain diseases is an especially intriguing possibility. The technique involves directly placing nerve cells in the brain, where they grow and can release chemicals that communicate with other brain cells. The method has been used successfully in several animal model diseases—most recently in primates (257) and cell growth can be confirmed and behavioral deficits corrected by the new cells (23,68,95,199). Nerve cells from one species can also grow in another; they appear to be protected from the immune system of the recipient, but they do not function as well (23).

Investigators hope that nerve cell implantation (sometimes called "brain transplants" in the popular press) can eventually benefit patients with Alzheimer's disease (as well as those with Parkinson's disease) (23), but such therapies will hinge on extensive animal testing and preliminary human trials and are unlikely to be available within the next decade. Many technical problems must be overcome, and the appropriate source of nerve cells is not at all clear. Use of human fetal cells would be ethically objectionable to many, and cells from other species do not work as well and might also be rejected by some recipients on moral grounds (95). A neutral source of tissue (e.g., from a source in the patient) may yet be found.

Implantation of patients' own cells has already been tried in Swedish patients suffering from Parkinson's disease (described later in this chapter), but it yielded no clinical benefit (23). The cells were taken from the core of the adrenal gland, which contains nerve-like cells. None of the barriers to development of this technique now appears insurmountable, although it will likely take many years of research before practical treatments are found.

Dementia Caused by Blood Vessel Disease

Diseases of the blood vessels cause more deaths in the United States than any other group of disorders. Coronary heart disease and stroke are the most prominent examples. In addition to causing death, blood vessel disease can cause many other clinical syndromes, including dementia.

Vascular disease is believed to be the second most common cause of dementia. In one large study, it accounted for 17 percent of cases, and was found in combination with Alzheimer's disease in an additional 18 percent (310). The prevalence of pure vascular dementia is, however, now a topic of clinical debate (221). Current methods of classifying patients are being questioned, and some clinicians are uncertain about the relationship between symptoms of dementia and brain cell loss due to vascular disease. Some investigators beginning clinical trials specifically for patients with multi-infarct dementia are noting difficulty in identifying sufficient numbers of patients (31a).

The prevalence of vascular dementia can be resolved only with further rigorous longitudinal studies. Some answers may be found in the ongoing Systemic Hypertension in the Elderly Project, whose primary sponsor is the National Heart, Lung, and Blood Institute. The National Institute on Aging is sponsoring an analysis of the data that will track the incidence of multi-infarct dementia in response to treatment of high blood pressure.

Detection of vascular dementia is important for several reasons. If dementia is caused by large strokes, further deterioration may be prevented using standard treatments for stroke. Finding vascular disease in the brain can also alert the physician to look for damage to the heart, kidneys, or other organs. Evaluation of patients with vascular dementia may also disclose preventable or treatable underlying risk factors such as hypertension or diabetes. And risk to other family members is different if the dementia is caused by blood vessel disease rather than by Alzheimer's disease. (The genetic aspects of vascular disease are more indirect, generally related to underlying causes such as blood lipids, diabetes, or hypertension. Relatives may benefit from detection of such risk factors if they take action to reduce the chances of developing vascular disease themselves.)

The incidence of and mortality from stroke and heart disease have declined dramatically over the past two decades. Mortality from stroke decreased almost 50 percent from 1968 to 1982, for example (91). The decline is likely due to a combination of changing dietary patterns, other changes in personal habits, and improved medical care of the elderly—the major factors behind the parallel decline in mortality from heart disease (188). Most of the statistics on this decline are for large strokes, however, and do not yield direct information about vascular dementia. It is likely that this encouraging trend also pertains to vascular dementia, but that relationship has not been studied directly.

Dementia caused by blood vessel disease results from death of nerve cells in regions nourished by diseased vessels. The death of brain tissue due to poor delivery of blood is called *cerebral infarction*. Dementia may ensue after a certain total mass of brain tissue has been destroyed (273). Such damage can be caused by one or a few large strokes, several smaller ones, or many microscopic ones. Dementia may also result from death of brain cells due to lack of oxygen reaching the brain (following a heart attack or heart failure, or for other reasons) (46,320). Large strokes are not usually difficult to differentiate from other dementing conditions because they affect many brain functions in addition to mental activity.

When cerebral infarcts are smaller, however, dementia may be the main symptom—making it difficult to distinguish from Alzheimer's disease or other dementias. The precise symptoms and physical findings depend on which parts of the brain die, and attempts are being made to define more specifically the characteristics of vascular dementia (89,152,221,225,344).

When there are multiple infarcts, the diagnosis is called multi-infarct dementia (MID). The number can range from a few to over a dozen. On average, individual infarcts are about a half inch in diameter (1 centimeter), and symptoms are commonly absent until 100 to 200 cubic centimeters of brain tissue have been destroyed (160,273), unless the patient has another dementing condition.

Multi-infarct dementia can be distinguished from Alzheimer's disease and most other disorders by its association with:

- a relatively abrupt onset;
- progression of dementia in "steps" rather than gradual deterioration;
- history of previous strokes;
- symptoms or physical findings that can be anatomically traced to loss of specific nerve cells; and
- presence of diabetes, high blood pressure, or cardiovascular disease affecting other organs.

Poor blood flow in the major arteries feeding the brain can be directly detected and correlated with dementia (317). Such poor blood flow typically precedes symptoms in patients with MID, but is found only after symptoms arise in Alzheimer's disease (267). Rigidity of blood vessels in the brain can be indirectly measured, and corroborates the association with MID compared with controls or those with Alzheimer's disease (157).

The special features of MID are measured in standardized questionnaires developed to differentiate it from other dementias (108,128,270), and these are used in research studies to classify patients with dementia.

Life expectancy is somewhat shorter for patients with MID than for those with Alzheimer's disease (15). Patients with MID also tend to be older and more frequently have abnormal electrocardiograms (indicating higher likelihood of heart disease) (48), although one recent study found a 5 to 6 percent prevalence of dementia among young stroke victims (under 65) (176).

If MID is associated with high blood pressure, diabetes, or disease in other organs, the associated conditions can be treated. Some believe MID should be treated like stroke, but the treatment of stroke is itself controversial and variable when the stroke is not caused by identifiable factors. As with Alzheimer's disease, treatment of MID awaits new discoveries.

In addition to multi-infarct dementia, dementia can arise from occlusion of blood vessels by debris in the blood stream (emboli) (reviewed in 159). These emboli can arise from diseased heart valves, damage to cells lining the heart, dislodging of clots in large vessels, the release of fat from large bones, or large sudden infusions of air or other gases.

Death of cells due to loss of blood supply can also affect the white matter of the brain, rather than the cerebral cortex. The white matter contains relatively few nerve cell bodies; death of non-neural cells and nerve cell *processes* in these regions results in disconnection of different nerve cell groups rather than loss of nerve cells. This can nonetheless cause dementia. One name for this type of disease is Binswanger's disease, or subacute arteriosclerotic encephalopathy (236). Its prevalence may be higher than previously estimated—something newly discovered because MRI scanning makes its detection possible. One recent study described a number of patients with a disorder that is clinically difficult to distinguish from Binswanger's disease, but that appears to have a cause other than hypertension or arteriosclerosis (46). That new finding further demonstrates the uncertainty of classification and cause even among clinical subtypes of vascular dementia. Further studies employing MRI scanning may confirm that brain infarction is more common than previously believed, and should clarify the relationship between infarction and clinical symptoms of dementia (160).

Dementia can follow bleeding into the brain caused by diseased or malformed blood vessels. Blood vessels in the brain may also form balloon-like sacs, called aneurysms, that can disturb adjacent structures or rupture to cause bleeding. Both bleeding and aneurysm formation are relatively common, but patients presenting with just dementia only rarely have them. Finally, some very rare diseases of the brain's blood vessels, such as Moya-Moya disease or Takayasu's disease, can cause dementia.

Other Dementias

Parkinson's Disease

Parkinson's disease is a relatively common disorder, and some Parkinson's patients develop dementia. The prevalence of symptomatic dementia among Parkinson's patients is somewhat controversial (19). Some investigators have found a disproportionate fraction of patients with Parkinson's disease exhibit symptoms of dementia (87,184, 206), while others find that the rate of cognitive impairment has been inflated, and is actually no higher than the risk for the general population (45,183,305). Most neurologists now consider Parkinson's disease to be associated with dementia in a minority of patients even in those who do not have Alzheimer's disease or another dementia (148,245,300).

There is also a clear subset of patients whose brains show the changes of both Parkinson's and Alzheimer's diseases (34,186,276,331). That group of patients underscores the confusing relationship between the various disorders causing dementia. The dementia occurring in Guam and other Pacific islands combines features of Alzheimer's disease, Parkinson's disease, and other disorders, and is now thought to be historically (and probably causally) related to decreased calcium and increased levels of other minerals in local water supplies (107,240).

The primary symptoms of Parkinson's disease are involuntary movements, slowness, and rigidity. Speech is often slow, and movement is difficult to initiate. Most patients have a characteristic tremor (rapid shaking) of the fingers that is traditionally likened to pill-rolling.

Parkinson's disease is associated with loss of nerve cells located in the substantia nigra (black substance, so called because the cells contain dark pigment). Whereas the cells lost in Alzheimer's disease are believed to use acetylcholine or other chemicals to communicate with other cells, those lost in Parkinson's disease use primarily dopamine. The work on the biochemistry of Parkinson's disease in fact predates that on Alzheimer's disease by over a decade, and Parkinson's disease serves as the model for researchers studying Alzheimer's disease (245). Drugs that partially replace the function of dopamine have been discovered, and these substantially reduce the abnormal movements in most patients with Parkinson's disease. The advent of such drugs was welcomed as a therapeutic revolution in neurology in the 1970s.

There are several different varieties of Parkinson's disease. The cause of classic Parkinson's disease is not known. Another type, postencephalitic Parkinsonism, has been linked to previous brain infection with a virus. It is most often found among those who contracted brain infections during the influenza epidemic of 1918, but it can occur in others as well. One interesting feature of postencephalitic Parkinson's disease that distinguishes it from classic Parkinson's disease is the finding of neurofibrillary tangles in nerve cells of the substantia nigra. The tangles are similar to those found in other groups of cells in Alzheimer's disease.

Another interesting aspect of Parkinson's disease and its relation to dementia has emerged from an unfortunate experiment that began a few years ago in Stanford, CA. A former chemistry student began manufacturing a drug resembling heroin in his home. The process he used also yielded a side product that was ingested with the drug. This side product, called 1-methyl-4-phenyl-1,2,3,6-tetrahydropyridine (MPTP), caused him and others who took the drug to develop symptoms of Parkinson's disease. Administration of the drug to primates also induces a disease resembling Parkinson's disease, and the animals lose cells in the substantia nigra just as would a human patient with Parkinson's disease. The cells that die do not look like those found in classic Parkinson's disease, however, and the degree to which MPTP-induced Parkinson symptoms suggests the primary cause of classic Parkinson's disease remains unknown. MPTP-induced symptoms bear on the debate about whether Parkinson's disease can cause dementia in the absence of other diseases, because MPTP patients showed intellectual decline (301).

Progressive Supranuclear Palsy (PSP)

PSP is a disorder with several clinical similarities to Parkinson's disease. It was first described in 1904 (153). Half to two-thirds of the patients with PSP deteriorate intellectually (192). PSP was not clinically distinguished from Parkinson's disease until 1964 (297), and accounts for roughly 4 percent of patients with Parkinson's disease (343). It differs from Parkinson's disease in that patients lose the ability to gaze up or down, and it is usually not associated with a tremor. Recent reports have shown that the chemical imbalances in PSP, like Parkinson's disease, involve dopamine, but these same studies disagree on the extent to which there are also Alzheimer-like changes in acetylcholine (169,276).

An interesting group of recent findings bears on the relationship among these disorders. The pathological changes of PSP are anatomically located in places characteristic of Parkinson's disease, but microscopically they more closely resemble the neurofibrillary tangles of Alzheimer's disease (although they can be distinguished on careful inspection). Further, investigators have found some suggestive, but not conclusive, chemical similarities in the tangles found in Alzheimer's disease, PSP, postencephalitic Parkinson's disease, and several other rare disorders (82). These similarities represent one more of the mysterious and poorly understood relationships among the various disorders causing dementia.

Huntington's Disease

Huntington's disease is a genetic disorder that causes uncontrollable twisting and writhing movements and also leads to dementia. Most patients with Huntington's disease do not develop symptoms until late middle age, and the symptoms may vary from person to person even in the same family. The movement disorder is thought to be caused by a loss of nerve cells in brain regions called the caudate nucleus and putamen.

Children of an affected parent have a 50-percent risk of developing the disease. The social and long-term care needs of these patients are similar to those for Alzheimer's patients (325,326). A group of investigators recently tracked the gene from parents to children in large families, including one extended family living near Lake Maracaibo in Venezuela. Molecular genetic techniques were used to map human chromosomes (37) and were applied to families with Huntington's disease (126). The disease-causing gene is located on chromosome number 4, and the test can be used in some families to predict whether particular individuals will develop Huntington's disease (326).

The test is not available for clinical use and is not useful in many families (e.g., because tracking the gene usually requires that DNA from an affected parent be available). Even in the best studied families, the test is not always accurate (because it does not detect the Huntington's gene

itself, but rather one close to it), and so interpretation must be cautious. Such care is important in Huntington's disease because test results are fraught with serious social, emotional, economic, and financial problems (21,173,197,325,326).

Current experience with the Huntington's disease test will be relevant to genetic risks of familial Alzheimer's disease if an analogous test can be developed for Alzheimer's and other dementing disorders. Problems in techniques, information dissemination, and privacy protection encountered by Huntington's families will likely prove true for those concerned with familial Alzheimer's disease as well. The work on Huntington's disease is thus an important pioneering effort.

Dementias Caused by Infection

Infection by bacteria, viruses, fungi, or unconventional agents can all cause dementia, but do so only rarely. Two infectious dementias—transmissible dementia and AIDS dementia—are of special note because of their prevalence and scientific interest.

Other infections can cause dementia, but only rarely. Longstanding syphilis, for example, was once among the most common causes of dementia, but it is now quite rare in the United States.

Transmissible Dementia.—The transmissible dementias caused by unusual infectious agents—Creutzfeldt-Jakob disease, Gerstmann-Strassler syndrome, and kuru—have already been discussed in describing possible infections caused by Alzheimer's disease above. Several interesting features were not mentioned there, however. Transmissible dementias characteristically kill patients much more rapidly than Alzheimer's disease does, although the transmissible dementias are also clinically heterogeneous.

Creutzfeldt-Jakob disease has become a concern among those receiving hormone therapy for congenital short stature because several young patients who were treated with human growth hormone recently died with Creutzfeldt-Jakob disease; an additional four patients are being investigated to see if they too have transmissible dementia (43,304). The dementing disease in these young patients is thought to be linked to contamination of growth hormone by patients with Creutzfeldt-Jakob disease (110,172,309). Until mid-1985, growth hormone was only available from preparations purified from pooled human pituitary glands, but that supply has been terminated and a new source derived from genetically engineered bacteria has been approved. Current and future stocks of growth hormone should thus not be contaminated.

A related concern has emerged in connection with blood donations. Creutzfeldt-Jakob disease can be transmitted to animals from the blood of affected human patients (195). That finding has led one group to urge that patients with dementia refrain from donating blood, and that blood banks reject blood from dementia patients (202). The handling of tissues and fluids of patients with Creutzfeldt-Jakob disease and other transmissible dementias also requires special precautions (6).

The relationship between Alzheimer's disease and transmissible dementia has long been a topic of speculation. As with Alzheimer's disease, there is clustering of cases in some families (12,203). Familial cases of transmissible dementia can clearly infect primates (12,44,203). The microscopic changes of the transmissible dementias are quite different from those of Alzheimer's disease—loss of nerve cells, proliferation of nonnerve supporting cells, and a peculiar "spongy" appearance of defined brain regions under the microscope. In some patients, however, there is overlap of microscopic findings (64,203).

Attention has recently shifted from atypical transmissible dementias to infections caused by more conventional viruses as causes of Alzheimer's disease (195). Dementia caused by lingering brain infections with conventional viruses is also well known, but it was rare until recently except in patients whose immune systems were debilitated.

AIDS Dementia.—A most alarming cause of dementia has been recently identified in patients with acquired immune deficiency syndrome. AIDS is caused by a small virus that attacks and kills specific cells of the immune system, rendering the patient defenseless against micro-organisms. The AIDS virus causes infectious dementia through two mechanisms: the immune dysfunction of AIDS leads to brain infections by other organisms, and the AIDS virus also appears to cause dementia directly (24,144,229,230,246,262). Brains of patients who die with AIDS dementia—that directly caused by the AIDS virus—show clusters of immune cells in some areas, affecting primarily cells deep in the brain rather than in the cerebral cortex. AIDS dementia is now the most common cause of dementia caused by infection (161). A large fraction, probably most, of patients with AIDS develop dementia (245). The majority of such cases appear to be due to the AIDS virus itself, while a minority are caused by a variety of other organisms in addition to AIDS virus infection (230).

Researchers do not yet know whether the dementia also afflicts those who are infected by the virus and do not get full-blown AIDS (249). Dementia in such patients can precede other symptoms of AIDS, and at least some patients with this type of dementia do not fulfill all the criteria of AIDS (187,214). That is of concern for several reasons. Patients infected with AIDS virus who do not develop clinical AIDS far outnumber those who do. Those who succumb to AIDS invariably die under current therapies, but mortality rates among those who do not develop AIDS though infected with the virus are unknown. Children and infants infected with AIDS can also develop dementia and malformations of the brain (18). Investigations in this area are just beginning, and the magnitude of the problem of AIDS dementia will not be known until many more investigators are involved and more data accumulated.

Dementias Caused by Toxins

Alcohol.—Alcohol is associated with over a dozen forms of brain disease. The diseases may be due to direct effects of alcohol, to nutritional factors, or to indirect effects of damage to the liver or other organs. The most common alcohol-related dementia is Wernicke-Korsakoff syndrome. Korsakoff's syndrome is not found only among chronic alcoholics, but alcoholism is by far its most common cause.

Wernicke's encephalopathy—the early, short-term part of the Wernicke-Korsakoff syndrome—is characterized by disorders of eye movement, abnormal gait, and global confusion. If left untreated, it can progress to coma or permanent neurological damage, and severe cases can be fatal even if treated. Eighty percent of those who develop Wernicke's encephalopathy go on to develop Korsakoff's syndrome (263) although some patients develop Korsakoff's syndrome without ever showing Wernicke's encephalopathy. Korsakoff's syndrome is characterized by loss of recent memory, often attended by disorientation to time and place and other mental symptoms. Some cases of Korsakoff's syndrome have only memory loss, and represent a pure amnesia rather than dementia.

Wernicke-Korsakoff syndrome is related to deficiency of vitamin B-1 (thiamine), and the standard initial treatment is thiamine administration (122). The disease appears to be caused by poor nutritional intake in patients with a genetic predisposition to the disease (31). The chain of events leading to the syndrome is not fully understood, however, in part because animal models of thiamine deficiency are not exact duplicates of the human disease (122,263).

There is currently a debate in neurology and psychiatry about whether there is a dementia directly caused by long-term alcoholism, in the absence of nutritional problems or diseases of other organs (such as heart, liver, and endocrine glands) (49,115). Circumstantial evidence indicates that those who have a history of heavy drinking for 15 to 20 years develop a dementia that is distinct from either Alzheimer's disease or Wernicke-Korsakoff syndrome. Such patients typically show listlessness, poor judgment, carelessness, diminished attention, and slowing of thought processes. They do not usually have the language problems or difficulty drawing figures typical of Alzheimer's disease (115). The debate is about whether these changes are due to direct chronic toxicity of alcohol on the brain or to other factors.

Other Toxic Dementias.—Liver damage due to alcohol or severe liver disease can also cause dementia. The liver is responsible for clearing many toxins out of the body, and liver failure due to cirrhosis can cause accumulation of byproducts followed by dementia and even coma.

Chronic exposure to heavy metals (especially mercury and lead) at home or in the workplace can cause dementia. Many alcohol-related diseases in addition to Korsakoff's syndrome and liver disease can induce dementia. Dementia can result from excess blood lipids, exposure to toxic chemicals, and severe nutritional deficiencies.

Normal Pressure Hydrocephalus

Normal pressure hydrocephalus (NPH) is a relatively uncommon cause of dementia. Its importance lies not in its frequency, but in its potential for correction. The classic description of the findings is a combination of dementia with urinary incontinence, a slow and hesitant gait, and dilation of the fluid-filled spaces in the brain. Another symptom that suggests NPH is a history of bleeding in the brain or head trauma. In practice, NPH may lack some of these features or have characteristics of other dementing conditions (47).

Normal pressure hydrocephalus was first described in 1964 (210), and the condition began to be more widely noticed the following year (129). The treatment for NPH is to provide a surgically implanted conduit (shunting) for fluid to drain from the brain into another body cavity, usually the abdominal cavity (164). The efficacy of shunting varies widely, depending on severity, diagnostic accuracy, and duration of illness (success hinges on accurate detection and prompt treatment). Many studies find successful relief of symptoms in 40 percent of cases (127,164,291). When shunting works, it brings rapid clinical improvement.

One consideration in shunting for NPH is whether a sample of brain tissue should be taken for microscopic examination while inserting the shunt inside the skull. That procedure may permit a diagnosis of another dementia if the shunting procedure fails, but it does entail a slight added risk to the patient. A problem with current treatment for NPH is the high rate of major complications, estimated at 40 percent, and this emphasizes the need for careful selection of patients (164).

Down's Syndrome

There are several interesting relationships between Alzheimer's disease and Down's syndrome. First, the number of individuals affected with Down's syndrome among relatives of patients with Alzheimer's disease is greater than expected (137,

138,140,141). But even more curious is the similarity in brain changes that occur with age in Down's syndrome.

Young individuals with Down's syndrome have a reduced number of cells in the nucleus basalis, and these cells may die off with age (53). Patients with Down's syndrome who survive into middle age frequently develop a dementia, and the microscopic and anatomic features of the findings in the brain are visually indistinguishable from those that occur in Alzheimer's disease (194,247,327,334, 335). There may be some differences, however, in the detailed chemical composition of tangles and plaques between Alzheimer's disease and Down's syndrome (179). The similarities between Alzheimer's disease and premature aging in Down's syndrome have led to speculations about causal links between the two diseases (94).

Down's syndrome is usually caused by the presence of an extra chromosome 21 in the patient's cells. More rarely, it is caused by chromosomal rearrangements or malformations that lead to excess of only part of chromosome 21. These findings have led to investigation of whether there is a chromosome defect in Alzheimer's disease as well, but results are mixed, and no aberration is consistent (reviewed in 327). Many investigators are studying Down's syndrome as a model of Alzheimer's disease in a relatively homogeneous population, assuming that the brain changes that occur are part of the syndrome and might provide clues to the origin of Alzheimer's disease.

Pick's Disease

Pick's disease is a rare dementing disorder clinically similar to Alzheimer's disease. The diagnosis of Pick's disease is, in fact, most often made on autopsy of a patient with clinically diagnosed Alzheimer's disease. The cause of Pick's disease is mysterious and uncertain, and it also can occur in families.

The distinction between Pick's and Alzheimer's diseases rests on the microscopic appearance of the brain. While someone with Alzheimer's disease has plaques and tangles, a patient with Pick's disease has pale and swollen nerve cells that contain globules of protein that are designated "Pick bodies." Recent evidence suggests biochemical similarities between Alzheimer tangles and plaques and Pick bodies (254). The intriguing relationship between these two dementing disorders is underscored by a newly described genetic disease that combines features of both (222).

Dementia Without Detectable Brain Changes

One final category of dementia is defined by the absence of any abnormal findings in the brain despite clear clinical symptoms. Such cases constituted a small fraction (2 of 50 patients) of those in a classic autopsy study of dementia (311), and cases continue to be reported—5 of 99 patients in a recent study (134). One 91-year-old man whose brain revealed no plaques at all (despite extensive search) but who suffered from dementia is of particular interest (13) since most persons his age without dementia would have a few plaques. This mysterious group of patients has been called the "5 percent problem" (163). The condition has also been called "simple atrophy" or "idiopathic dementia" because its cause and mechanism are unknown.

CHAPTER 3 REFERENCES

1. Albert, M., Naeser, M.A., Levine, H.L., et al., "CT Density Numbers in Patients With Senile Dementia of the Alzheimer's Type," *Archives of Neurology* 41:1264-1269, 1984.
2. Alzheimer, A., "Uber Eine Eigenartige Erkrankung der Hirnrinde," *Gesamte Psychiatrie* 64:146-148, 1907.
3. Amaducci, L.A., Fratiglioni, L., Rocca, W.A., et al., "Risk Factors for Alzheimer's Disease (AD): A Case-Control Study on an Italian Population," (abstract) *Neurology* 35 (Supplement 1):277, 1985.
4. Amaducci, L.A., Fratiglioni, L., Rocca, W.A., et al., "Risk Factors for Clinically Diagnosed Alzheimer's Disease: A Case-Control Study of an Italian Population," *Neurology* 36:922-931, 1986.
5. American Medical Association, Council on Scientific Affairs, "Dementia," pending.

6. American Neurological Association, Committee on Health Care Issues, "Precautions in Handling Tissues, Fluids, and Other Contaminated Materials From Patients With Documented or Suspected Creutzfeldt-Jakob Disease," *Annals of Neurology* 19:75-77, 1986.

7. American Psychiatric Association, *Diagnostic and Statistical Manual of Mental Disorders*, 3d ed. (Washington, DC: 1980).

8. Anderson, B., "Is Alpha-MSH Deficiency the Cause of Alzheimer's Disease?" *Medical Hypotheses* 19:379-385, 1986.

9. Appel, S.H., "A Unifying Hypothesis for the Cause of Amyotrophic Lateral Sclerosis, Parkinsonism, and Alzheimer Disease," *Annals of Neurology* 10:499-505, 1981.

10. Arendt, T., Bigl, V., Tennstedt, A., et al., "Neuronal Loss in Different Parts of the Nucleus Basalis is Related to Neuritic Plaque Formation in Cortical Target Areas in Alzheimer's Disease," *Neuroscience* 14:1-14, 1985.

11. Austin, J.H., Rinehart, R., Williamson, T., et al., "Studies in Aging of the Brain, III. Silicon Levels in Postmortem Tissues and Body Fluids," *Progress in Brain Research* 40:485-495, 1973.

12. Baker, H.F., Ridley, R.M., and Crow, T.J., "Experimental Transmission of an Autosomal Dominant Spongiform Encephalopathy: Does the Infectious Agent Originate in the Human Genome?" *British Medical Journal* 291:299-302, 1985.

13. Ball, M.J., Hachinski, V., Fox, A., et al., "A New Definition of Alzheimer's Disease: A Hippocampal Dementia," *Lancet*, Jan. 5, 1985, pp. 14-16.

14. Barclay, L.L., Zemcov, A., Blass, J.P., et al., "Factors Associated With Duration of Survival in Alzheimer's Disease," *Biological Psychiatry* 20:86-93, 1985.

15. Barclay, L.L., Zemcov, A., Blass, J.P., et al., "Survival in Alzheimer's Disease and Vascular Dementias," *Neurology* 35:834-840, 1985.

16. Bartus, T.R., Dean, R.L., Beer, B., et al., "The Cholinergic Hypothesis of Geriatric Memory Dysfunction," *Science* 217:408-417, 1982.

17. Becker, P.M., Feussner, J.R., Mulrow, C.D., et al., "The Role of Lumbar Puncture in the Evaluation of Dementia," *Journal of the American Geriatrics Society* 33:392-396, 1985.

18. Belman, A.L., Ultmann, M.H., Horoupian, D., et al., "Neurological Complications in Infants and Children With Acquired Immune Deficiency Syndrome," *Annals of Neurology* 18:560-566, 1985.

19. Benson, D.F., "Subcortical Dementia: A Clinical Approach," *Advances in Neurology 38 (The Dementias)* (New York: Raven, 1983).

20. Besson, J.A.O., Corrigan, F.M., Foreman, I., et al., "Nuclear Magnetic Resonance (NMR). II. Imaging in Dementia," *British Journal of Psychiatry* 146:31-35, 1985.

21. Bird, S.J., "Presymptomatic Testing for Huntington's Disease," *Journal of the American Medical Association* 253:3286-3291, 1985.

22. Bissette, G., Reynolds, G.P., Kits, C.D., et al., "Corticotropin-Releasing Factor-Like Immunoreactivity in Senile Dementia of the Alzheimer Type," *Journal of the American Medical Association* 254:3067-3069, 1985.

23. Bjorklund, A., and Gage, F.H., "Neuronal Replacement After Traumatic or Age-Dependent Brain Damage," *International Journal of Technology Assessment in Health Care* 1:93-107, 1985.

24. Black, P.H., "HTLV-III, AIDS, and the Brain," *New England Journal of Medicine* 313:1538-1540, 1985.

25. Blackwood, D.H.R., and Christie, J.E., "The Effects of Physostigmine on Memory and Auditory P300 in Alzheimer-Type Dementia," *Biological Psychiatry* 21:557-560, 1986.

26. Blass, J.P., "Editorial: NIH Diagnostic Criteria for Alzheimer's Disease," *Journal of the American Geriatrics Society* 33:1, 1985.

27. Blass, J.P., "Pragmatic Pointers in Managing the Demented Patient," *Journal of the American Geriatrics Society* 34:548-549, 1986.

28. Blass, J.P., Gibson, G.E., Shamada, M., et al., "Brain Carbohydrate Metabolism and Dementia," *Biochemistry of Dementia*, P.J. Roberts (ed.) (London: John Wiley, 1980).

29. Blass, J.P., Hanin, I., Barclay, L., et al., "Red Blood Cell Abnormalities in Alzheimer Disease," *Journal of the American Geriatrics Society* 33:401-405, 1985.

30. Blass, J.P., and Barclay, L.L., "New Developments in the Diagnosis of the Dementias," *Drug Development Research* 5:39-58, 1985.

31. Blass, J.P., and Gibson, G.E., "Abnormality of a Thiamine-Requiring Enzyme in Patients With Wernicke-Korsakoff Syndrome," *New England Journal of Medicine* 297:1367-1370, 1977.

31a. Blass, J.P., Makesberg, W., and Whitehouse, P.J., comments at a meeting of the OTA advisory panel, June 1986.

32. Blass, J.P., and Zemcov, A., "Alzheimer Disease: A Metabolic Systems Degeneration?" *Neurochemistry and Pathology* 2:103-114, 1984.

33. Blessed, G., Tomlinson, B.E., and Roth, M., "The Association Between Quantitative Measures of Dementia and of Senile Change in the Cerebral Grey Matter of Elderly Subjects," *British Journal of Psychiatry* 114:797-811, 1968.

34. Boller, F., Mizutani, T., Roessmann, U., et al., *Annals of Neurology* 7:329-335, 1980.

35. Bondareff, W., "Age and Alzheimer Disease," *Lancet*, June 25, 1983, p. 1447.

36. Bondareff, W., Mountjoy, C.Q., and Roth, M., "Loss of Neurons of Origin of the Adrenergic Projection to the Cerebral Cortex (Nucleus Locus Coeruleus) in Senile Dementia," *Neurology* 32:164-168, 1982.

37. Botstein, D., White, R.L., Skolnick, et al., "Construction of a Genetic Linkage Map in Man Using Restriction Fragment Length Polymorphisms," *American Journal of Human Genetics* 32:314-333, 1980.

38. Breitner, J.C.S., "Aphasia/Apraxia and Familial Aggregation in Alzheimer's Disease," *Annals of Neurology* 15:614-615, 1984.

39. Breitner, J.C.S., "Familial Nature of Alzheimer's Disease," *New England Journal of Medicine* 311:1318-1319, 1984.

40. Breitner, J.C.S., and Folstein, M.F., "Familial Alzheimer Dementia: A Prevalent Disorder With Specific Clinical Features," *Psychological Medicine* 14:63-80, 1984.

41. Breitner, J.C.S., Folstein, M.F., and Murphy, E.A., "Familial Aggregation in Alzheimer Dementia—I. A Model for the Age-Dependent Expression of an Autosomal Dominant Gene," *Journal of Psychiatric Research* 20:31-43, 1986.

42. Breitner, J.C.S., Murphy, E.A., and Folstein, M.F., "Familial Aggregation in Alzheimer Dementia—II. Clinical Genetic Implications of Age-Dependent Onset," *Journal of Psychiatric Research* 20:45-55, 1986.

43. Brown, P., Gajdusek, D.C., Gibbs, C.J., et al., "Potential Epidemic of Creutzfeldt-Jakob Disease From Human Growth Hormone Therapy," *New England Journal of Medicine* 313:728-730, 1985.

44. Brown, P., Salazar, A.M., Gibbs, C.J., et al., "Alzheimer's Disease and Transmissible Dementia (Creutzfeldt-Jakob Disease)," *Annals of the New York Academy of Sciences* 396:131-144, 1982.

45. Brown, R.G., and Marsden, C.D., "How Common Is Dementia in Parkinson's Disease?" *Lancet*, Dec. 1, 1984, pp. 1262-1265.

46. Brun, A., and Englund, E., "A White Matter Disorder in Dementia of the Alzheimer Type: A Pathoanatomical Study," *Annals of Neurology* 19:253-262, 1986.

47. Brust, J.C.M., "Dementia and Cerebrovascular Disease," *Advances in Neurology 38 (The Dementias)* (New York: Raven, 1983).

48. Bucht, G., Adolfsson, R., and Winblad, B., "Dementia of the Alzheimer Type and Multi-Infarct Dementia: A Clinical Description and Diagnostic Problems," *Journal of the American Geriatrics Society* 32:491-498, 1984.

49. Butters, N., and Brandt, J., "The Continuity Hypothesis: The Relationship of Long-Term Alcoholism to the Wernicke-Korsakoff Syndrome," *Recent Developments in Alcoholism* 3:207-226, 1985.

50. Candy, J.M., Edwardson, J.A., Klinowski, J., et al., "Co-Localization of Aluminum and Silicon in Senile Plaques: Implications for the Neurochemical Pathology of Alzheimer's Disease," *Senile Dementia of Alzheimer Type*, J. Traber and W.H. Gispen (eds.) (Berlin: Springer-Verlag, 1985).

51. Candy, J.M., Klinowski, J., Perry, R.H., et al., "Aluminosilicates and Senile Plaque Formation in Alzheimer's Disease," *Lancet*, Feb. 15, 1986, pp. 354-356.

52. Cardelli, M.B., Russell, M., Bagne, C.A., et al., "Chelation Therapy: Unproved Modality in the Treatment of Alzheimer-Type Dementia," *Journal of the American Geriatrics Society* 33:548-551., 1985.

53. Casanova, M.F., Walker, L.C., Whitehouse, P.J., et al., "Abnormalities of the Nucleus Basalis in Down's Syndrome," *Annals of Neurology* 18:310-313, 1985.

54. Caulfield, M., and Smith, C., "British Pharmacological Society Symposium: Alzheimer's Disease —Central Cholinergic Mechanisms," *Neurobiology of Aging* 6:61-63, 1985.

55. Chase, T.N., Brooks, R.A., DiChiro, G., et al., "Focal Cortical Abnormalities in Alzheimer's Disease," *The Metabolism of the Human Brain Studied With Positron Emission Tomography*, T. Greitz (ed.) (New York: Raven, 1985).

56. Chui, H.C., Teng, E.L., Henderson, V.W., et al., "Clinical Subtypes of Dementia of the Alzheimer Type," *Neurology* 35:1544-1550, 1985.

57. Cohen, D., and Eisdorfer, C., "Serum Immunoglobulins and Cognitive Status in the Elderly: 1. A Population Study," *British Journal of Psychiatry* 136:33-39, 1980.

57a. Cohen, D., and Eisdorfer, C., *The Loss of Self* (New York: Norton, 1986).

58. Cohen, D., Eisdorfer, C., Prinz, P., et al., "Immunoglobulins, Cognitive Status and Duration of Illness in Alzheimer's Disease," *Neurobiology of Aging* 1:165-168, 1980.

59. Cohen, M.B., Graham, L.S., Lake, R., et al., "Diagnosis of Alzheimer's Disease and Multiple Infarct Dementia by Tomographic Imaging of Iodine-123 IMP," *Journal of Nuclear Medicine* 27:769-774, 1986.

60. Coleman, R.E., Blinder, R.A., and Jaszczak, R.J., "Single Photon Emission Computed Tomography (SPECT). Part II: Clinical Applications," *Investigations in Radiology* 21:1-11, 1986.

61. Colgan, J., "Regional Density and Survival in Senile Dementia. An Interim Report on a Prospective Computed Tomographic Study," *British Journal of Psychiatry* 147:63-66, 1985.

62. Collcrton, D., and Fairbairn, A., "Alzheimer's Disease and the Hippocampus," *Lancet*, Feb. 2, 1985, pp. 278-279.

63. Cook, R.H., Schneck, S.A., and Clark, D.B., "Twins With Alzheimer's Disease," *Archives of Neurology* 38:300-301, 1981.

64. Cook, R.H., Ward, B.E., and Austin, J.H., "Studies in Aging of the Brain. IV. Familial Alzheimer Disease: Relation to Transmissible Dementia, Aneuploidy, and Microtubular Defects," *Neurology* 29:1402-1412, 1979.

65. Cork, L.C., Sternberger, N.H., Sternberger, L.A., et al., "Phosphorylated Neurofilament Antigens in Neurofibrillary Tangles in Alzheimer's Disease," *Journal of Neuropathology and Experimental Neurology* 45:56-64, 1986.

66. Corsellis, J.A.N., "Posttraumatic Dementia," R. Katzman, R.D. Terry and K.L. Bick (eds.), *Aging, Volume 7: Alzheimer's Disease: Senile Dementia and Related Disorders* (New York: Raven, 1978).

67. Coull, B.M., "Neurologic Aspects of Dementia," *Geriatric Medicine*, vol. 1, C.K. Cassel and J.E. Walsh (eds.) (New York: Springer-Verlag, 1984).

68. Cowen, R., "Brain Cell Implants and Studies of Disease Mechanism Performed on Animal Models of Parkinsonism," *Research Resources Reporter* 10:1-5, February 1986, vol. X, pp. 1-5.

69. Coyle, J.T., Price, D.L., and DeLong, M.R., "Alzheimer's Disease: A Disorder of Cortical Cholinergic Innervation," *Science* 59:277-289, 1983.

70. Coyle, J.T., Singer, H., McKinney, M., et al., "Neurotransmitter Specific Alternations in Dementing Disorders: Insights From Animal Models," *Journal of Psychiatric Research* 18:501-512, 1984.

71. Crapper, D.R., Krishnan, S.S., and Quittkat, S., "Aluminum, Neurofibrillary Degeneration and Alzheimer's Disease," *Brain* 99:67-80, 1976.

72. Critchley, M., "Medical Aspects of Boxing, Particularly From a Neurological Standpoint," *British Medical Journal* 1:357-362, 1957.

73. Cross, A.J., Crow, T.J., Ferrier, I.N., et al., "The Selectivity of the Reduction of Serotonin S2 Receptors in Alzheimer-Type Dementia," *Neurobiology of Aging* 7:3-7, 1986.

74. Cummings, J.L., and Benson, D.F., "Dementia of the Alzheimer Type: An Inventory of Diagnostic Clinical Features," *Journal of the American Geriatrics Society* 34:12-19, 1986.

75. Cutler, N.R., Haxby, J.V., Duara, R., et al., "Brain Metabolism as Measured With Positron Emission Tomography: Serial Assessment in a Patient With Familial Alzheimer's Disease," *Neurology* 35:1556-1561, 1985.

76. Cutler, N.R., Haxby, J.V., Duara, R., et al., "Clinical History, Brain Metabolism, and Neuropsychological Function in Alzheimer's Disease," *Annals of Neurology* 18:298-309, 1985.

77. Cutler, N.R., Kay, A.D., Marangos, P.J., et al., "Cerebrospinal Fluid Neuron-Specific Enolase Is Reduced in Alzheimer's Disease," *Archives of Neurology* 43:153-154, 1986.

78. Davies, P., Katzman, R., and Terry, R.D., "Reduced Somatostatin-Like Immunoreactivity in Cerebral Cortex From Cases of Alzheimer Disease and Alzheimer Senile Dementia," *Nature* 288:279-280, 1980.

78a. Davis, K.L., and Mohs, R.C., "Cholinergic Drugs in Alzheimer's Disease," *New England Journal of Medicine* 315:1286-1287, 1986.

79. DeBoni, U., and McLachlan, D.R.C., "Controlled Induction of Paired Helical Filaments of the Alzheimer Type in Cultured Human Neurons, by Glutamate and Aspartate," *Journal of the Neurological Sciences* 68:105-118, 1985.

80. DeLeon, M.J., and George, A.E., "Computed Tomography in Aging and Senile Dementia of the Alzheimer Type," *Advances in Neurology 38 (The Dementias)* (New York: Raven, 1983).

81. DeSouza, E.B., Whitehouse, P.J., Kuhar, M.J., et al., "Reciprocal Changes in Corticotropin-Releasing Factor (CRF)-Like Immunoreactivity and CRF Receptors in Cerebral Cortex of Alzheimer's Disease," *Nature* 319:593-595, 1981.

82. Dickson, D.W., Kress, Y., Crowe, A., et al. "Monoclonal Antibodies to Alzheimer Neurofibrillary Tangles. 2. Demonstration of a Common Antigenic Determinant Between ANT and Neurofibrillary Degeneration in Progressive Supranuclear Palsy," *American Journal of Pathology* 120:292-303, 1985.

83. DiGiacomo, J., and Prien, R., "Pharmacologic Treatment of Depression in the Elderly," *Physicians' Guide to the Diagnosis and Treatment of Depression in the Elderly*, T. Crook and G.D. Cohen (eds.) (New Canaan, CT: Mark Powley and Associates, 1983).

84. Drachman, D.A., "Alzheimer's Disease: Diagnos-

tic Dilemmas," *Proceedings of the National Conference on 'Alzheimer's Disease: A Challenge for Care,' "* J.E. Hansan (ed.) (Memphis, TN: Hillhaven Foundation, 1985).

85. Drayer, B.P., Heyman, A., Wilkinson, W., et al., "Early-Onset Alzheimer's Disease: An Analysis of CT Findings," *Annals of Neurology* 17:407-410, 1985.

86. Duara, R., Grady, C., Haxby, J., et al., "Positron Emission Tomography in Alzheimer's Disease," *Neurology* 36:879-887, 1986.

87. DuBois, B., Hauw, J.J., Ruberg, M., et al., "Demence et Maladie de Parkinson: Correlations Biochimiques et Anatomo-Cliniques," *Revue Neurologique* 141:184-193, 1985.

88. Eisdorfer, C., and Cohen, D., "Serum Immunoglobulins and Cognitive Status in the Elderly: 2. An Immunological-Behavioral Relationship?" *British Journal of Psychiatry* 136:40-45, 1980.

89. Erkinjuntti, T., Sulkava, R., and Tilvis, R., "HDL Cholesterol in Dementia," *Lancet*, July 6, 1985, p. 43.

90. Eslinger, P.J., Damasio, A.R., Benton, A.L., et al., "Neuropsychologic Detection of Abnormal Mental Decline in Older Persons," *Journal of the American Medical Association* 253:670-674, 1985.

91. Feinleib, M., "The Magnitude and Nature of the Decrease in Coronary Heart Disease Mortality Rate," *American Journal of Cardiology* 54:2C-6C, 1984.

92. Ferris, S.H., de Leon, M.J., Wolf, A.P., et al., "Positron Emission Tomography in Dementia," *Advances in Neurology 38 (The Dementias)* (New York: Raven, 1983).

93. Fine, A., "Peptides and Alzheimer's Disease," *Nature* 319:537-538, 1986.

94. Fishman, M.A., "Will the Study of Down Syndrome Solve the Riddle of Alzheimer Disease?" *Journal of Pediatrics* 108:627-629, 1986.

95. Fishman, P.S., "Neural Transplantation: Scientific Gains and Clinical Perspectives," *Neurology* 36:389-392, 1986.

96. Folstein, M.F., and Breitner, J.C.S., "Language Disorder Predicts Familial Alzheimer's Disease," *Johns Hopkins Medical Journal* 149:145-147, 1981.

97. Folstein, M.F., Folstein, S.E., and McHugh, P. R., " 'Mini-Mental State': A Practical Method of Grading the Cognitive State of Patients for the Clinician," *Journal of Psychiatric Research* 12:189-198, 1975.

98. Foster, N.L., Chase, T.N., Patronas, N.J., et al., "Cerebral Mapping of Apraxia in Alzheimer's Disease by Positron Emission Tomography," *Annals of Neurology* 19:139-143, 1986.

99. Francis, P.T., Palmer, A.M., Sims, N.R., et al., "Neurochemical Studies of Early-Onset Alzheimer's Disease," *New England Journal of Medicine* 313:7-11, 1985.

100. French, L.R., Schuman, L.M., Mortimer, J.A., et al., "A Case-Control Study of Dementia of the Alzheimer Type," *American Journal of Epidemiology* 121:414-421, 1985.

101. French, L.R., Schuman, L.M., Mortimer, J.A., et al., (reply to letter), "The Authors Reply," *American Journal of Epidemiology* 123:753-754, 1986.

102. Friedland, R.P., Brun, A., and Budinger, T.F., "Pathological and Positron Emission Tomographic Correlations in Alzheimer's Disease," *Lancet*, Jan. 26, 1985, p. 228.

103. Friedland, R.P., Budinger, T.F., Brant-Zawadzki, M., et al., "The Diagnosis of Alzheimer-Type Dementia," *Journal of the American Medical Association* 252:2750-2752, 1984.

104. Fudenberg, H.H., Whitten, H.D., Arnaud, P., et al., "Is Alzheimer's Disease an Immunological Disorder? Observations and Speculations," *Clinical Immunology and Immunopathology* 32:127-131, 1984.

105. Fudenberg, H.H., Whitten, H.D., Arnaud, P., et al., "Immune Diagnosis of a Subset of Alzheimer's Disease With Preliminary Implications for Immunotherapy," *Biomedicine and Pharmacotherapy* 38:290-297, 1984.

106. Gajdusek, D.C., "Unconventional Viruses and the Origin and Disappearance of Kuru," Nobel Lecture, Dec. 13, 1976, reprinted in *Science* 197:943-960, 1977.

107. Gajdusek, D.C., "Hypothesis: Interference With Axonal Transport of Neurofilament as a Common Pathogenetic Mechanism in Certain Diseases of the Central Nervous System," *New England Journal of Medicine* 312:714-719, 1985.

108. Gauthier, S., "Practical Guidelines for the Antemortem Diagnosis of Senile Dementia of the Alzheimer Type," *Progress in Neuro-Psychopharmacology and Biological Psychiatry* 9:491-495, 1985.

109. Geddes, J.W., Monaghan, D.T., Cotman, C.W., et al., "Plasticity of Hippocampal Circuitry in Alzheimer's Disease," *Science* 230:1179-1181, 1985.

110. Gibbs, C.J., Joy, A., Heffner, R., et al., "Clinical and Pathological Features and Laboratory Confirmation of Creutzfeldt-Jakob Disease in a Recipient of Pituitary-Derived Human Growth Hormone," *New England Journal of Medicine* 313:734-738, 1985.

111. Gibson, C.J., Logue, M., and Growdon, J., "CSF

Monoamine Metabolite Levels in Alzheimer's and Parkinson's Disease," *Archives of Neurology* 42:489-492, 1985.

112. Glenner, G.G., "On Causative Theories in Alzheimer's Disease," *Human Pathology* 16:433-435, 1985.

113. Glosser, G., Wexler, D., and Balmelli, M., "Physicians' and Families' Perspectives on the Medical Management of Dementia," *Journal of the American Geriatrics Society* 33:383-391, 1985.

114. Goldman, J.E., Yen, S.H., "Cytoskeletal Protein Abnormalities in Neurodegenerative Diseases," *Annals of Neurology* 19:209-223, 1986.

115. Goldstein, G., "Dementia Associated With Alcoholism," *Alcohol and the Brain: Chronic Effects*, R.E. Tarter and D.H. van Thiel (eds.) (New York: Plenum, 1985).

116. Gomez, S., Davous, P., Rondot, P., et al., "Somatostatin-Like Immunoreactivity and Acetylcholinesterase Activities in Cerebrospinal Fluid of Patients With Alzheimer Disease and Senile Dementia of the Alzheimer Type," *Psychoneuroendocrinology* 11:69-73, 1986.

117. Goodnick, P., and Gershon, S., "Chemotherapy of Cognitive Disorders in Geriatric Subjects," *Journal of Clinical Psychiatry* 45:196-209, 1984.

118. Gottfries, C.G., "Alzheimer's Disease and Senile Dementia: Biochemical Characteristics and Aspects of Treatment," *Psychopharmacology* 86:245-252, 1985.

119. Gottfries, C.G., "Critique: Transmitter Deficits in Alzheimer's Disease," *Neurochemistry International* 7:565-566, 1985.

120. Goudsmit, J., Morrow, C.H., and Asher, D.M., "Evidence for and Against the Transmissibility of Alzheimer Disease," *Neurology* 30:945-950, 1980.

121. Gray, E.G., "Spongiform Encephalopathy: A Neurocytologist's Viewpoint With a Note on Alzheimer's Disease," *Neuropathology and Applied Neurobiology* 12:149-172, 1986.

122. Greenberg, D.A., and Diamond, I., "Wernicke-Korsakoff Syndrome," *Alcohol and the Brain: Chronic Effects*, R.E. Tarter and D.H. van Thiel (eds.) (New York: Plenum, 1985).

123. Grundke-Iqbal, I., Iqbal, K., Tung, Y.C., et al., "Alzheimer Paired Helical Filaments: Immunochemical Identification of Polypeptides," *Acta Neuropathologica* (Berlin) 62:259-267, 1984.

124. Gurland, B., Golden, R.R., Teresi, J.A., et al., "The SHORT-CARE: An Efficient Instrument for the Assessment of Depression, Dementia, and Disability," *Journal of Gerontology* 39:166-169, 1984.

125. Gurland, B., and Toner, J., "Differentiating Dementia From Nondementing Conditions," *Advances in Neurology 38: The Dementias*, (New York: Raven, 1985).

126. Gusella, J.F., Wexler, N.S. Conneally, P.M., et al., "A Polymorphic DNA Marker Genetically Linked to Huntington's Disease," *Nature* 306:234-238, 1983.

127. Haase, G.R., "Differential Diagnosis and Clinical Features of the Dementing Illnesses," Annual Course No. 215, *Dementia and Aging* (S.A. Schneck, course director), American Academy of Neurology, April 27-May 3, 1986.

128. Hachinski, V., Iliff, L., Shilkha, E., et al., "Cerebral Blood Flow in Dementias," *Archives of Neurology* 32:632-637, 1975.

129. Hakim, S., and Adams, R.D., "Clinical Problem of Symptomatic Hydrocephalus With Normal Cerebrospinal Fluid Pressure. Observations on CSF Hydrodynamics," *Journal of Neurological Sciences* 2:307-327, 1965.

130. Hammerstrom, D.C., and Zimmer, B., "The Role of Lumbar Puncture in the Evaluation of Dementia," *Journal of the American Geriatrics Society* 33: 397-400, 1985.

130a. Haney, D.Q., "Researcher Fears Hysteria Over Alzheimer's Drug Discovery," Associated Press Newswire, Nov. 12, 1986.

131. Harbaugh, R.E., Roberts, D.W., Coombs, D.W., et al., *Neurosurgery* 15:514-518, 1985.

132. Hardy, J., Adolfsson, R., Alafuzoff, I., et al., "Review: Transmitter Deficits in Alzheimer's Disease," *Neurochemistry International* 7:545-563, 1985.

133. Hayden, M.R., Martin, W.R.W., Stoessel, et al., "Positron Emission Tomography in the Early Diagnosis of Huntington's Disease," *Neurology* 36:888-894, 1986.

134. Heilig, C.W., Knopman, D.S., Mastri, A.R., et al., "Dementia Without Alzheimer's Pathology," *Neurology* 35:762-765, 1985.

135. Helms, P.M., "Efficacy of Antipsychotics in the Treatment of the Behavioral Complications of Dementia: A Review of the Literature," *Journal of the American Geriatrics Society* 33:206-209, 1985.

136. Henschke, P.J., Bell, D.A., and Cape, R.D.T., "Immunologic Indices in Alzheimer Dementia," *Journal of Clinical and Experimental Gerontology* 1:23-37, 1979.

137. Heston, L.L., "Alzheimer's Disease, Trisomy 21, and Myeloproliferative Disorders: Associations Suggesting and Genetic Diathesis," *Science* 196:322-323, 1977.

138. Heston, L.L., "Alzheimer's Dementia and Down's

Syndrome: Genetic Evidence Suggesting an Association," *Annals of the New York Academy of Sciences* 396:29-38, 1982.

139. Heston, L.L., "Ask the Doctor: Genetics and Dementia of the Alzheimer Type," *ADRDA Newsletter* 5:4, 1985.

140. Heston, L.L., Mastri, A.R., Anderson, V.E., et al., "Dementia of the Alzheimer Type: Clinical Genetics, Natural History and Associated Conditions," *Archives of General Psychiatry* 38:1085-1090, 1981.

141. Heston, L.L., and White, J.A., *Dementia: A Practical Guide to Alzheimer's Disease and Related Illnesses* (New York: W. H. Freeman, 1983).

142. Heyman, A., Wilkinson, W.E., Hurwitz, B.J., et al., "Alzheimer's Disease: Genetic Aspects and Associated Clinical Disorders," *Annals of Neurology* 14:507-515, 1983.

143. Heyman, A., Wilkinson, W.E., and Stafford, J.A., et al., "Alzheimer's Disease: A Study of Epidemiological Aspects," *Annals of Neurology* 15:335-341, 1984.

144. Ho, D.D., Rota, T.R., Schooley, R.T., et al., "Isolation of HTLV-III From Cerebrospinal Fluid and Neural Tissues of Patients With Neurologic Syndromes Related to the Acquired Immunodeficiency Syndrome," *New England Journal of Medicine* 313:1493-1497, 1985.

145. Hoffman, R.S., "Diagnostic Errors in the Evaluation of Behavioral Disorders," *Journal of the American Medical Association* 248:964-967, 1982.

146. Holman, B.L., "Perfusion and Receptor SPECT in the Dementias—George Taplin Memorial Lecture," *Journal of Nuclear Medicine* 27:855-860, 1986.

147. Holman, B.L., Gibson, R.E., Hill, T.C., et al., "Muscarinic Acetylcholine Receptors in Alzheimer's Disease: In Vivo Imaging With Iodine 123-Labeled 3-Quinuclidinyl-4-Iodobenzilate and Emission Tomography," *Journal of the American Medical Association* 254:3063-3066, 1985.

148. Huber, S.J., Shuttleworth, E.C., Paulson, G.W., et al., "Cortical Versus Subcortical Dementia," *Archives of Neurology* 43:392-394, 1986.

149. Hyman, B.T., van Hoesen, G.W., Damasio, A.R., et al., "Alzheimer's Disease: Cell Specific Pathology Isolates the Hippocampal Formation," *Science* 225:1168-1170, 1984.

150. Ihara, Y., Abraham, C., and Selkoe, D.J., "Antibodies to Paired Helical Filaments in Alzheimer's Disease Do Not Recognize Normal Brain Proteins," *Nature* 304:727-730, 1983.

151. Iqbal, K, Grundke-Iqbal, I., Zaidi, T., et al., "Are Alzheimer's Neurofibrillary Tangles Insoluble Polymers?" *Life Sciences* 38:1695-1700, 1986.

152. Ishii, N., Nishihara, Y., and Imamura, T., "Why Do Frontal Lobe Symptoms Predominate in Vascular Dementia With Lacunes?" *Neurology* 36: 340-345, 1986.

153. Jankovic, J., "Progressive Supranuclear Palsy: Clinical and Pharmacologic Update," *Neurology Clinics* 2:473-486, 1984.

154. Jenike, M.A., "Monoamine Oxidase Inhibitors as Treatment for Depressed Patients With Primary Degenerative Dementia (Alzheimer's Disease)," *American Journal of Psychiatry* 142:763-764, 1985.

155. Jonker, C., Eikelenboom, P., and Tavermier, P., "Immunological Indices in the Cerebrospinal Fluid of Patients With Presenile Dementia of the Alzheimer Type," *British Journal of Psychiatry* 140:44-49, 1982.

156. Jorm, A.F., "Subtypes of Alzheimer's Dementia: A Conceptual Analysis and Critical Review," *Psychological Medicine* 15:543-553, 1985.

157. Judd, B.W., Meyer, J.S., Rogers, R.L., et al., "Cognitive Performance Correlates With Cerebrovascular Impairments in Multi-Infarct Dementia," *Journal of the American Geriatrics Society* 34: 355-360, 1986.

158. Kahn, R.L., Goldfarb, A.I., Pollack, M., et al., "Brief Objective Measures for the Determination of Mental Status in the Aged," *American Journal of Psychiatry* 117:326-328, 1960.

159. Kaplan, J.G., Katzman, R., Horoupian, D.S., et al., "Progressive Dementia, Visual Deficits, Amyotrophy, and Microinfarcts," *Neurology* 35:789-796, 1985.

160. Kase, C.S., "'Multi-Infarct' Dementia: A Real Entity?" *Journal of the American Geriatrics Society* 34:482-484, 1986.

161. Katzman, R., University of California at San Diego, personal communication, Dec. 24, 1985.

162. Katzman, R., Brown, T., Fuld, P., et al., "Validation of a Short Orientation-Memory-Concentration Test of Cognitive Impairment," *American Journal of Psychiatry* 140:734-739, 1983.

163. Katzman, R., Lasker, B., and Bernstein, N., "Accuracy of Diagnosis and Consequences of Misdiagnosis of Disorders Causing Dementia," contract report prepared for the Office of Technology Assessment, U.S. Congress, 1986.

164. Kawas, C., and Wolfson, L., "Normal Pressure Hydrocephalus," *Current Therapy in Neurologic Disease, 1985-1986*, R.T. Johnson (ed.) (Philadelphia: B.C. Decker, 1985).

165. Kerzner, L.J., "Diagnosis and Treatment of Alz-

heimer's Disease," *Advances in Internal Medicine* 29:447-470, 1984.

166. Khachaturian, Z.S., "Diagnosis of Alzheimer's Disease," *Archives of Neurology* 42:1097-1105, 1985.

167. Khansari, N., Whitten, H.D., Chou, Y.K., et al., "Immunological Dysfunction in Alzheimer's Disease," *Journal of Neuroimmunology* 7:279-285, 1985.

168. Kidd, M., Allsop, D., and Landon, M., "Senile Plaque Amyloid, Paired Helical Filaments, and Cerebrovascular Amyloid in Alzheimer's Disease Are All Deposits of the Same Protein," *Lancet*, Feb. 2, 1985, p. 278.

169. Kish, S.J., Chang, L.J., Mirchandani, L., et al., "Progressive Supranuclear Palsy: Relationship Between Extrapyramidal Disturbances, Dementia, and Brain Neurotransmitter Markers," *Annals of Neurology* 18:530-536, 1985.

170. Klein, L.E., Roca, R.P., McArthur, J., et al., "Diagnosing Dementia: Univariate and Multivariate Analyses of the Mental Status Examination," *Journal of the American Geriatrics Society* 33:483-488, 1985.

171. Knesevich, J.W., Toro, F.R., Morris, J.C., et al., "Aphasia, Family History, and the Longitudinal Course of Senile Dementia of the Alzheimer Type," *Psychiatry Research* 14:255-263, 1985.

172. Koch, T.K., Berg, B.O., DeArmond, S.J., et al., "Creutzfeldt-Jakob Disease in a Young Adult With Idiopathic Hypopituitarism," *New England Journal of Medicine* 313:731-733, 1985.

173. Koller, W.C., and Davenport, J., "Genetic Testing in Huntington Disease," *Annals of Neurology* 16:511-512, 1984.

174. Kosik, K.S., Duffy, L.K., Dowling, M.M., et al., "Microtubule-Associated Protein 2: Monoclonal Antibodies Demonstrate the Selective Incorporation of Certain Epitopes Into Alzheimer Neurofibrillary Tangles," *Proceedings of the National Academy of Sciences, USA* 81:7941-7945, 1984.

175. Koss, E., Friedland, R.P., Ober, B.A., et al., "Differences in Lateral Hemispheric Asymmetries of Glucose Utilization Between Early- and Late-Onset Alzheimer-Type Dementia," *American Journal of Psychiatry* 142:638-642, 1985.

176. Kotila, M., Waltimo, O., Niemi, M.L., et al., "Dementia After Stroke," *European Neurology* 25:134-140, 1986.

177. Kuhl, D.E., Metter, E.J., Riege, W.H., et al., "Patterns of Cerebral Glucose Utilization in Dementia," *The Metabolism of the Human Brain Studied With Positron Emission Tomography*, T. Greitz (ed.) (New York: Raven, 1985).

178. Kulmala, H.K., and Hutton, J.T., "Role of the Senile Plaque in Neuropeptide Deficits of Alzheimer's Disease," *Progress in Neuro-Psychopharmacology and Biological Psychiatry*, 9:625-628, 1985.

179. Kumar, M., Eisdorfer, C., and Cohen, D., "Serum IgG Antineurofilament Antibodies in Alzheimer's Disease and Down's Syndrome, submitted.

180. *Lancet*, "Editorial: Ergot for Dementia?" Dec. 8, 1984, pp. 1313-1314.

181. Larson, E.B., Reifler, B.V., Sumi, S.M., et al., "Diagnostic Evaluation of 200 Elderly Outpatients With Suspected Dementia," *Journal of Gerontology* 40:536-543, 1985.

182. Larson, E.B., Reifler, B.V., Sumi, S.M., et al., "Diagnostic Tests in the Evaluation of Dementia: A Prospective Study of 200 Elderly Outpatients," in press.

183. Lees, A.J., "Parkinson's Disease and Dementia," *Lancet*, Jan. 5, 1985, pp. 43-44.

184. Lees, A.J., and Smith, E., "Cognitive Deficits in the Early Stages of Parkinson's Disease," *Brain* 106:257-270, 1983.

185. Leffell, M.S., Lumsden, L., and Steiger, W.A., "An Analysis of T Lymphocyte Subpopulations in Patients With Alzheimer's Disease," *Journal of the American Geriatrics Society* 33:4-8, 1985.

186. Leverenz, J., and Sumi, S.M., "Parkinson's Disease in Patients With Alzheimer's Disease," *Archives of Neurology* 43:662-664, 1986.

187. Levy, J.A., Shimabukuro, J., Hollander, H., et al., "Isolation of AIDS-Associated Retroviruses from Cerebrospinal Fluid and Brain of Patients With Neurological Symptoms," *Lancet*, Sept. 14, 1985, pp. 586-588.

188. Levy, R.I., "Causes of the Decrease in Cardiovascular Mortality," *American Journal of Cardiology* 54:7C-14C, 1984.

189. Li, J.C., and Kaminskas, E., "Deficient Repair of DNA Lesions in Alzheimer's Disease Fibroblasts," *Biochemical and Biophysics Research Communications* 129:733-738, 1985.

190. Loring, D.W., and Largen, J.W., "Neuropsychological Patterns of Presenile and Senile Dementia of the Alzheimer Type," *Neuropsychologia* 23:351-357, 1985.

191. Mace, N.L., and Rabins, P.V., *The 36-Hour Day: A Family Guide to Caring for Persons With Alzheimer's Disease, Related Dementing Illness, and Memory Loss in Later Life* (Baltimore: Johns Hopkins University Press, 1981).

192. Maher, E.R., Smith, E.M., and Lees, A.J., "Cognitive Deficits in the Steele-Richardson-Olszewski Syndrome (Progressive Supranuclear Palsy),"

Journal of Neurology, Neurosurgery, and Psychiatry 48:1234-1239, 1985.

193. Mann, D.A., "The Neuropathology of Alzheimer's Disease: A Review With Pathogenetic, Aetiological and Therapeutic Considerations," *Mechanisms of Aging and Development* 31:213-255, 1985.

194. Mann, D.M.A., Yates, P.O., and Marcyniuk, B., "Alzheimer's Presenile Dementia, Senile Dementia of Alzheimer Type and Down's Syndrome in Middle Age Form an Age-Related Continuum of Pathological Changes," *Neuropathology and Applied Neurobiology* 10:185-207, 1984.

195. Manuelidis, E.E., "Presidential Address: Creutzfeldt-Jakob Disease," *Journal of Neuropathology and Experimental Neurology* 44:1-17, 1985.

196. Manuelidis, E.E., Kim, J.H., Mericangas, J.R., et al., "Transmission to Animals of Creutzfeldt-Jakob Disease from Human Blood," *Lancet*, Oct. 19, 1985, pp. 896-897.

197. Martin, J.B., "Editorial Comment: Genetic Testing in Huntington Disease," *Annals of Neurology* 16:512-513, 1984.

198. Marx, J.L., "Nerve Growth Factor Acts in Brain," *Science* 232:1341-1343, 1986.

199. Marx, J.L., "Lost Neurons Identified in Alzheimer's Disease," *Science* 232:1500, 1986.

200. Mash, D.C., Flynn, D.D., and Potter, L.T., "Loss of M2 Muscarine Receptors in the Cerebral Cortex in Alzheimer's Disease and Experimental Cholinergic Denervation," *Science* 228:1115-1117, 1985.

201. Massachusetts General Hospital Newsletter, "Should Lumbar Puncture Be Part of the Workup for Dementia?" *Topics in Geriatrics* 4:21,23, December 1985.

202. Massachusetts General Hospital Newsletter, "Dementia: A Contraindication to Donation of Blood," *Topics in Geriatrics* 4:27, February 1986.

203. Masters, C.L., Gajdusek, D.C., and Gibbs, C.J., Jr., "The Familial Occurrence of Creutzfeldt-Jakob Disease and Alzheimer's Disease," *Brain* 104:535-558, 1981.

204. Mattis, S., "Mental Status Examination for Organic Mental Syndrome in the Elderly Patient," *Geriatric Psychiatry*, R. Bellack and B. Karasu (eds.) (New York: Grune and Stratton, 1976).

205. Mayeux, R., Stern, Y., and Spanton, S., "Heterogeneity in Dementia of the Alzheimer Type: Evidence of Subgroups," *Neurology* 35:453-461, 1985.

206. McCarthy, R., Gresty, M., and Findley, L.J., "Parkinson's Disease and Dementia," *Lancet*, Feb. 16, 1985, p. 407.

207. McCartney, J.R., and Palmateer, L.M., "Assessment of Cognitive Deficit in Geriatric Patients: A Study of Physician Behavior," *Journal of the American Geriatrics Society* 33:467-471, 1985.

208. McGeer, P.L., Kamo, H., Harrop, R., et al., "Positron Emission Tomography in Patients With Clinically Diagnosed Alzheimer's Disease," *Canadian Medical Association Journal* 134:597-607, 1986.

209. McGeer, P.L., McGeer, E.G., Suzuki, J., et al., "Aging, Alzheimer's Disease, and the Cholinergic System of the Basal Forebrain," *Neurology* 34:741-745, 1984.

210. McHugh, P.R., "Occult Hydrocephalus," *Quarterly Journal of Medicine* 33:297-308, 1964.

211. McKeel, D.W., "The Autopsy's Untimely Demise: Physicians Are Neglecting a Vital Medical Resource," *The Sciences* 26:30-35, July/August 1986.

212. McKhann, G., Drachman, D., Folstein, M., et al., "Clinical Diagnosis of Alzheimer's Disease," *Neurology* 34:939-944, 1984.

213. McLachlan, D.R.C., Lewis, P.N., Lukiw, W.J., et al., "Chromatin Structure in Dementia," *Annals of Neurology* 15:329-334, 1984.

214. Medical World News, "AIDS Virus Casts Another Shadow," May 13, 1985, pp. 11-15.

215. Medical World News, "Pathologists Build Case for More Autopsies, Oct. 14, 1985, pp. 73-74.

216. Medical World News, "New Drug May Improve Memory," May 12, 1986, p. 37.

217. Medical World News, "New Alzheimer's Neurologic Link," June 9, 1986, p. 35.

218. Mesulam, M.M., "Dementia: Its Definition, Differential Diagnosis, and Subtypes," *Journal of the American Medical Association* 253:2559-2561, 1985.

219. Mesulam, M.M., Volicer, L., Marquis, J.K., et al., "Systematic Regional Differences in the Cholinergic Innervation of the Primate Cerebral Cortex: Distribution of Enzyme Activities and Some Behavioral Implications," *Annals of Neurology* 19:144-151, 1986.

220. Miller, C., Haugh, M., Kahn, J., et al., "The Cytoskeleton and Neurofibrillary Tangles in Alzheimer's Disease," *Trends in Neurosciences*, February 1986, pp. 76-81.

221. Molsa, P.K., Paljarvi, L., Rinne, J.O., et al., "Validity of Clinical Diagnosis in Dementia: A Prospective Clinicopathological Study," *Journal of Neurology, Neurosurgery, and Psychiatry* 48:1085-1090, 1985.

222. Morris, J.C., Cole, M., Banker, B. Q., et al., "Hereditary Dysphasic Dementia and the Pick-Alzheimer Spectrum," *Annals of Neurology* 16:455-466, 1984.

223. Mortimer, J.A., French, L.R., Hutton, J.T., et al.,

"Head Injury as a Risk Factor for Alzheimer's Disease," *Neurology* 35:264-267, 1985. (Also letter and reply, *Neurology* 35:1530-1531, 1985).

224. Moss, M.B., Albert, M.S., Butters, N., et al., "Differential Patterns of Memory Loss Among Patients With Alzheimer's Disease, Huntington's Disease, and Alcoholic Korsakoff's Syndrome," *Archives of Neurology* 43:239-246, 1986.

225. Muckle, T.J., and Roy, J.R., "High-Density Lipoprotein Cholesterol in Differential Diagnosis of Senile Dementia," *Lancet*, May 25, 1985, pp. 1191-1192.

226. Nagai, T., McGeer, P.L., Peng. J.H., et al., "Choline Acetyltransferase Immunohistochemistry in Brains of Alzheimer's Disease Patients and Controls," *Neuroscience Letters* 36:195-199, 1983.

227. National Institutes of Health Conference, "Brain Imaging: Aging and Dementia," *Annals of Internal Medicine* 101:355-369, 1984.

228. National Institute on Aging, Task Force Report, "Senility Reconsidered. Treatment Possibilities for Mental Impairment in the Elderly," *Journal of the American Medical Association* 244:259-263, 1980.

229. Navia, B.A., Eun-Sook, C., Petito, C.K., et al., "The AIDS Dementia Complex: II. Neuropathology" *Annals of Neurology* 19:525-535, 1986.

230. Navia, B.A., Jordan, B.D., and Price, R.W., "The AIDS Dementia Complex: I. Clinical Features," *Annals of Neurology* 19:517-524, 1986.

231. Neary, D., Snowden, J.S., Bowen, D.M., et al., "Cerebral Biopsy in the Investigation of Presenile Dementia due to Cerebral Atrophy," *Journal of Neurology, Neurosurgery, and Psychiatry* 49:157-162, 1986.

232. Neary, D., Snowden, J.S., Bowen, D.M., et al., "Neuropsychological Syndromes in Presenile Dementia due to Cerebral Atrophy," *Journal of Neurology, Neurosurgery, and Psychiatry* 49:163-174, 1986.

233. Nee, L.E., Polinsky, R.J., Eldridge, R., et al., "A Family With Histologically Confirmed Alzheimer's Disease," *Archives of Neurology* 40:203-205, 1983.

234. Nerl, C., Mayeux, R., and O'Neill, G.J., "HLA-Linked Complement Markers in Alzheimer's and Parkinson's Disease: C4 Variant (C4B2) A Possible Marker for Senile Dementia of the Alzheimer Type," *Neurology* 34:310-314, 1984.

235. Nikaido, T., Austin, J.H., Trueb, L., et al., "Studies in Aging of the Brain, II. Microchemical Analyses of the Nervous System in Alzheimer Patients," *Archives of Neurology* 27:549-554, 1972.

236. Olszewski, J., "Subcortical Arteriosclerotic Encephalopathy: Review of the Literature on the So-Called Binswanger's Disease and Presentation of Two Cases," Resume 374, *World Neurology* 3:359-373, 1982.

237. Ouslander, J.G., Kane, R.L., and Abrass, I.B., "Urinary Incontinence in Elderly Nursing Home Patients," *Journal of the American Medical Association* 248:1194-1198, 1982.

238. Palmer, A.M., Procter, A.W., Stratmann, G.C., et al., "Excitatory Amino Acid-Releasing and Cholinergic Neurones in Alzheimer's Disease," *Neuroscience Letters* 66:199-204, 1986.

239. Passeri, M., Cucinotta, D., De Mello, M., et al., *Lancet*, April 6, 1985, p. 824.

240. Perl, D.P., "Relationship of Aluminum to Alzheimer's Disease," *Environmental Health Perspectives* 63:149-153, 1985.

241. Perl, D.P., and Brody, A.R., "Alzheimer's Disease: X-Ray Spectrometric Evidence of Aluminum Accumulation in Neurofibrillary Tangle-Bearing Neurons," *Science* 208:297-299, 1980.

242. Petit, C., "Dartmouth's Big Story: How It Got Pumped Up—And Then Deflated," *Newsletter of the National Association of Science Writers* 33:1-5, February 1985.

243. Pfeffer, R.I., Kurosaki, T.T., Harrah, C., et al., "A Survey Diagnostic Tool for Senile Dementia," *American Journal of Epidemiology* 114:515-527, 1981.

244. Pfeiffer, E., "A Short Portable Mental Status Questionnaire for the Assessment of Organic Brain Deficits in Elderly Patients, *Journal of the American Geriatrics Society*, 23:433-441, 1975.

245. Price, D.L., "Basic Neuroscience and Disorders Causing Dementia," contract report prepared for the Office of Technology Assessment, U.S. Congress, 1986.

246. Price, D.L., "New Perspectives on Alzheimer's Disease," *Annual Review of Neuroscience* 9:489-512, 1986.

247. Price, D.L., Whitehouse, P.J., Struble, R.G., et al., "Alzheimer's Disease and Down's Syndrome," *Annals of the New York Academy of Sciences* 396:145-164, 1982.

248. Price, D.L., Whitehouse, P.J., and Struble, R.G., "Cellular Pathology in Alzheimer's and Parkinson's Diseases," *Trends in Neurosciences*, January 1986, pp. 29-33, 1986.

249. Price, R., Memorial Sloan Kettering Cancer Center, personal communication, October 1985.

250. Pro, J.D., Smith, C.H., and Sumi, S.M., "Presenile Alzheimer Disease: Amyloid Plaques in the Cerebellum," *Neurology* 30:820-825, 1980.

251. Prusiner, S.B., "Prions," *Scientific American* 251:50-59, 154, October 1984.

252. Prusiner, S.B., "Some Speculations About Prions,

Amyloid, and Alzheimer's Disease," *New England Journal of Medicine* 310:661-663, 1984.

253. Rabins, P.V., "Reversible Dementia and the Misdiagnosis of Dementia," *Hospital and Community Psychiatry* 34:830-835, 1983.

254. Rasool, C.G., and Selkoe, D.J., "Sharing of Specific Antigens by Degenerating Neurons in Pick's Disease and Alzheimer's Disease," *New England Journal of Medicine* 312:700-705, 1985.

255. Rathmann, K.L., and Conner, C.S., "Recent Advances in Alzheimer's Disease," *Pharmacy International* 5:193-195, August 1985.

256. Ray, W.A., Federspiel, C.F., and Schaffner, W., "A Study of Anti-Psychotic Drug Use in Nursing Homes: Epidemiologic Evidence Suggesting Misuse," *American Journal of Public Health* 70:485-491, 1980.

257. Redmond, D.E., Sladek, J.R., Roth, R.H., et al., "Fetal Neuronal Grafts in Monkeys Given Methylphenyltetrahydropyridine," *Lancet*, May 17, 1986, pp. 1125-1127.

258. Reisberg, B., DeLeon, M.J., and Ferris, S.H., "Familial Nature of Alzheimer's Disease?" *New England Journal of Medicine* 311:1318-1319, 1984.

259. Reisberg, B., Ferris, S.H., Anand, R., et al., "Effects of Naloxone in Senile Dementia: A Double-Blind Trial," *New England Journal of Medicine* 308:721-722, 1983.

260. Reisberg, B., Ferris, S.H., Anand, R., et al., "Functional Staging of Dementia of the Alzheimer Type," *Annals of the New York Academy of Sciences* 435:481-483, 1984.

261. Reisberg, B., Ferris, S.H., de Leon, M.J., et al., "Age-Associated Cognitive Decline and Alzheimer's Disease: Implications for Assessment and Treatment," *Thresholds in Aging* (London: Academic Press, 1985).

262. Resnick, L., DiMarzo-Veronese, F., Schupbach, J., et al., "Intra-Blood-Brain-Barrier Synthesis of HTLV-III-Specific IgG in Patients with Neurologic Symptoms Associated with AIDS or AIDS-Related Complex," *New England Journal of Medicine* 313:1498-1504, 1985.

263. Reuler, J.B., Girard, D.E., and Cooney, T.G., "Wernicke's Encephalopathy," *New England Journal of Medicine* 312:1035-1039, 1985.

264. Rimm, A.A., "Re: 'A Case-Control Study of Dementia of the Alzheimer Type,'" (letter) *American Journal of Epidemiology* 123:753, 1986.

265. Risse, S.C., and Barnes, R., "Pharmacologic Treatment of Agitation Associated With Dementia," *Journal of the American Geriatrics Society* 34:368-376, 1986.

266. Rocca, W.A., Amaducci, L.A., and Schoenberg, B.S., "Epidemiology of Clinically Diagnosed Alzheimer's Disease," *Annals of Neurology* 19:415-424, 1986.

267. Rogers, R.L., Meyer, J.S., Mortel, K.F., et al., "Decreased Cerebral Flow Precedes Multi-Infarct Dementia, but Follows Senile Dementia of Alzheimer Type," *Neurology* 36:1-6, 1986.

268. Rohwer, R.G., "Scrapie-Associated Fibrils," *Lancet*, July 7, 1984, p. 36.

269. Rosen, W.G., Mohs, R.C., and Davis, K.L., "A New Rating Scale for Alzheimer's Disease," *American Journal of Psychiatry* 141:1356-1364, 1984.

270. Rosen, W.G., Terry, R.D., Fuld, P.A., et al., "Pathological Verification of Ischemic Score in Differentiation of Dementias," *Annals of Neurology* 7:486-488, 1980.

271. Rossor, M.N., "Critique: Transmitter Deficits in Alzheimer's Disease," *Neurochemistry International* 7:567-570, 1985.

272. Rossor, M.N., Iversen, L.L., Reynolds, et al., "Neurochemical Characteristics of Early and Late Onset Types of Alzheimer's Disease," *British Medical Journal* 288:961-964, 1984.

273. Roth, M., "Senile Dementia and Its Borderlands," Paul Hoch Award Lecture, *Psychopathology in the Aged*, J.O. Cole and J.E. Barrett (eds.) (New York: Raven, 1980).

274. Rovner, B.W., Kafonek, S., Filipp, L., et al., "Prevalence of Mental Illness in a Community Nursing Home," in press.

275. Ruberg, M., Ploska, A., Javoy-Agid, F., et al., "Muscarinic Binding and Choline Acetyltransferase Activity in Parkinsonian Subjects With Reference to Dementia," *Brain Research* 232:129-139, 1982.

276. Ruberg, M., Javoy-Avid, F., Hirsch, E., et al., "Dopaminergic and Cholinergic Lesions in Progressive Supranuclear Palsy," *Annals of Neurology* 18:523-529, 1985.

277. Rudelli, R., Strom, J.O., Welch, P.T., et al., "Post-traumatic Premature Alzheimer's Disease: Neuropathologic Findings and Pathogenetic Considerations," *Archives of Neurology* 39:570-575, 1982.

278. Sajdel-Sulkowska, E.M., and Marotta, C.A., "Alzheimer's Disease Brain: Alterations in RNA Levels and in a Ribonuclease-Inhibitor Complex," *Science* 225:947-949, 1984.

279. Saper, C.B., German, D.C., and White, III, C.L., "Neuronal Pathology in the Nucleus Basalis and Associated Cell Groups in Senile Dementia of the Alzheimer's Type," *Neurology* 35:1089-1095, 1985.

280. Saraiva, A.A., Borges, M.M., Madeira, M.D., et al., "Mitochondrial Abnormalities in Cortical Dendrites From Patients With Alzheimer's Disease," *Journal of Submicroscopic Cytology* 17: 459-464, 1985.

281. Sasaki, H., Muramoto, O., Kanazawa, I., et al., "Regional Distribution of Amino Acid Transmitters in Postmortem Brains of Presenile and Senile Dementia of Alzheimer Type," *Annals of Neurology* 19:263-269, 1986.

282. Schneck, S.A., "Overview: Aging and Dementia," Annual Course No. 215, *Dementia and Aging*, (S.A. Schneck, course director), American Academy of Neurology, April 27-May 3, 1986.

283. Scudiero, D.A., Polinsky, R.J., Brumback, R.A., et al., "Alzheimer Disease Fibroblasts are Hypersensitive to the Lethal Effects of a DNA-Damaging Chemical," *Mutation Research* 159:125-131, 1986.

284. Selkoe, D.J., "Recent Advances in the Molecular Basis of Alzheimer-Type Dementia," Annual Course No. 215, *Dementia and Aging* (S.A. Schneck, course director), American Academy of Neurology, April 27-May 3, 1986.

285. Selkoe, D.J., Ihara, Y., and Salazar, F.J., "Alzheimer's Disease: Insolubility of Partially Purified Paired Helical Filaments in Sodium Dodecyl Sulfate and Urea," *Science* 215:1243-1245, 1982.

286. Seltzer, B., and Sherwin, I., "A Comparison of Clinical Features in Early- and Late-Onset Primary Degenerative Dementia," *Neurology* 40: 143-146, 1983.

287. Serby, M., Richardson, S.B., and Twente, S., "CSF Somatostatin in Alzheimer's Disease," *Neurobiology of Aging* 5:187-189, 1984.

288. Sharp, P., Gemmell, H., Cherryman, G., et al., "Application of Iodine-123-Labeled Isopropylamphetamine Imaging to the Study of Dementia," *Journal of Nuclear Medicine* 27:761-768, 1986.

289. Shuttleworth, E.C., "Atypical Presentations of Dementia of the Alzheimer Type," *Journal of the American Geriatrics Society* 32:485-490, 1984.

290. Siebens, H., Trupe, E., Siebens, A., et al., "Correlates and Consequences of Eating Dependency in Institutionalized Elderly," *Journal of the American Geriatrics Society* 34:192-198, 1986.

291. Simon, D.G., and Lubin, M.F., "Cost-Effectiveness of Computerized Tomography and Magnetic Resonance Imaging in Dementia," *Medical Decision Making* 5:335-354, 1986.

292. Sims, N.R., Finegan, J.M., and Blass, J.P., "Altered Glucose Metabolism in Fibroblasts From Patients With Alzheimer's Disease," *New England Journal of Medicine* 313:638-639, 1985.

293. Skias, D., Bania, M., Reder, A.T., et al., "Senile Dementia of Alzheimer's Type (SDAT): Reduced T8$^+$-Cell-Mediated Suppressor Activity," *Neurology* 35:1635-1638, 985.

294. Somerville, R.A., "Ultrastructural Links Between Scrapie and Alzheimer's Disease," *Lancet*, Mar. 2, 1985, pp. 504-506.

295. Sparks, D.L., Markesbery, W.R., and Slevin, J.T., "Alzheimer's Disease: Monoamines and Spiperone Binding Reduced in Nucleus Basalis," *Annals of Neurology* 19:602-604, 1986.

296. Spence, M.A., Heyman, A., Marazita, M. L., et al., "Genetic Linkage Studies in Alzheimer's Disease," *Neurology* 36:581-584, 1986.

297. Steele, J.C., Richardson, J.C., and Olszewski, J., "Progressive Supranuclear Palsy: A Heterogeneous Degeneration Involving the Brainstem, Basal Ganglia, and Cerebellum with Vertical Gaze and Pseudobulbar Palsy, Nuchal Dystonia, and Dementia," *Archives of Neurology* 10:333-359, 1964.

298. Steiger, W.A., Mendelson, M., Jenkins, T., et al., "Effects of Naloxone in Treatment of Senile Dementia," *Journal of the American Geriatrics Society* 33:155, 1985.

299. Steinberg, E.P., Sisk, J.E., and Locke, K.E., "X-Ray CT and Magnetic Resonance Imagers: Diffusion Patterns and Policy Issues," *New England Journal of Medicine* 313:859-864, 1985.

300. Stern, M.B., Gur, R.C., Saykin, A.J., et al., "Dementia of the Parkinson's Disease and Alzheimer's Disease," *Journal of the American Geriatrics Society* 34:475-478, 1986.

301. Stern, Y., and Langston, J.W., "Intellectual Changes in Patients With MPTP-Induced Parkinsonism," *Neurology* 35:1506-1509, 1985.

302. Storandt, M., Botwinick, J., Danziger, W.L, et al., "Psychometric Differentiation of Mild Senile Dementia of the Alzheimer Type," *Archives of Neurology* 41:497-499, 1984.

302a. Summers, W.K., Majovski, L.V., Marsh, G.M., et al., "Oral Tetrahydroaminoacridine in Long-Term Treatment of Senile Dementia, Alzheimer Type," *New England Journal of Medicine* 315: 1241-1245, 1986.

303. Swanson, I.W., "Alzheimer's Disease and Corticotropin-Releasing Factor," *Journal of the American Medical Association* 254:3085-3086, 1985.

304. Tavolato, B., and Argentiero, V., "Immunological Indices in Presenile Alzheimer's Disease," *Journal of Neurological Sciences* 46:325-331, 1980.

305. Taylor, A., Saint-Cyr, J.A., and Lang, A.E., "Dementia Prevalence in Parkinson's Disease," *Lancet*, May 4, 1985, p. 1037.

306. Taylor, G.R., Carter, G.I., Crow, T.J., et al., "Re-

covery and Measurement of Specific RNA Species from Postmortem Brain Tissue: A General Reduction in Alzheimer's Disease Detected by Molecular Hybridization," *Experimental and Molecular Pathology* 44:111-116, 1986.

307. Thal, L.J., Grundman, M., and Golden, R., "Alzheimer's Disease: A Correlational Analysis of the Blessed Information-Memory-Concentration Test and the Mini-Mental State Exam," *Neurology* 36:262-264, 1986.

308. Thienhaus, O.J., Hartford, J.T., Skelly, M.F., et al., "Biologic Markers in Alzheimer's Disease," *Journal of the American Geriatrics Society* 33: 715-726, 1985.

309. Tintner, R., Brown, P., Hedley-Whyte, E.T., et al., "Neuropathologic Verification of Creutzfeldt-Jakob Disease in the Exhumed American Recipient of Human Pituitary Growth Hormone: Epidemiologic and Pathogenetic Implications," *Neurology* 36:932-936, 1986.

310. Tomlinson, B.E., Blessed, G., and Roth, M., "Observations on the Brains of Non-Demented Old People," *Journal of Neurological Sciences* 7:331-336, 1968.

311. Tomlinson, B.E., Blessed, G., and Roth, M., "Observations on the Brains of Demented Old People," *Journal of Neurological Sciences* 11:205-270, 1970.

312. Traub, R., Gajdusek, D.C., Gibbs, C.J., et al., Transmissible Virus Dementia: the Relation of Transmissible Spongiform Encephalopathy to Creutzfeldt-Jakob Disease," *Aging and Dementia*, M. Kinsbourne and W.L. Smith (eds.) (New York: Spectrum, 1977).

313. Tune, L., Gucker, S., Folstein, M., et al., "Cerebrospinal Fluid Acetylcholinesterase Activity in Senile Dementia of the Alzheimer Type," *Annals of Neurology* 17:46-48, 1985.

314. Tyler, K.L., and Tyler, H.R., "Differentiating Organic Dementia," *Geriatrics* 39:38-52, March 1984.

315. U. S. Congress, Office of Technology Assessment, *Nuclear Magnetic Imaging Technology: A Clinical Industrial, and Policy Analysis*, Health Technology Case Study 27, OTA-HCS-27 (Washington, DC: U.S. Government Printing Office, 1984).

316. U. S. Congress, Office of Technology Assessment, *Technologies for Managing Urinary Incontinence*, Health Technology Case Study 33, OTA-HCS-33 (Washington, DC: U.S. Government Printing Office, 1985).

317. Uematsu, S., and Folstein, M.F., "Carotid Blood Flow Measured by an Untrasonic Volume Flowmeter in Carotid Stenosis and Patients with De-

mentia," *Journal of Neurology, Neurosurgery, and Psychiatry* 48:1230-1233, 1985.

318. Ulrich, J., "Alzheimer Changes in Nondemented Patients Younger Than Sixty-Five: Possible Early Stages of Alzheimer's Disease and Senile Dementia of the Alzheimer Type," *Annals of Neurology* 17:273-277, 1985.

319. Vitaliano, P.P., Breen, A.R., Russo, J., et al., "The Clinical Utility of the Dementia Rating Scale for Assessing Dementia Patients," *Journal of Chronic Diseases* 37:743-753, 1984.

320. Volpe, B.T., and Petito, C.K., "Dementia With Bilateral Medial Temporal Lobe Ischemia," *Neurology* 35:1793-1797, 1985.

321. Wang, G.P., Grundke-Iqbal, Kascsak, R.J., et al., "Alzheimer Neurofibrillary Tangles: Monoclonal Antibodies to Inherent Antigen(s)," *Acta Neuropathologica* (Berlin) 62:268-275, 1984.

322. Wellman, H.N., Gilmor, R., Hendrie, H., et al., "Dual Head HIPDM SPECT Imaging in the Differential Diagnosis of Dementia With MR and CT Correlation," *Journal of Nuclear Medicine* 26:P106, 1985.

323. Wells, C.E., (ed.), *Dementia*, 2d ed. (Philadelphia: Davis, 1971), pp. 1-14, 247-276.

324. Wetmur, J.G., Casals, J., and Elizan, T.S., "DNA Binding Protein Profiles in Alzheimer's Disease," *Journal of Neurological Sciences* 66:201-208, 1984.

325. Wexler, N.S., 1983, recorder at the Mary Jennifer Selznick Mini-Workshop, Hereditary Disease Foundation, Bethesda, MD, Nov. 30-Dec. 1, 1983.

326. Wexler, N.S., Conneally, P.M., and Gusella, J.F., *Huntington Disease "Discovery" Fact Sheet* (Santa Monica, CA: Hereditary Disease Foundation, May 1, 1984).

327. Whalley, L.J., "The Dementia of Down's Syndrome and Its Relevance to Aetiological Studies of Alzheimer's Disease," *Annals of the New York Academy of Sciences* 396:39-54, 1982.

328. Whitehouse, P.J., "Alzheimer's Disease," *Current Therapy in Neurologic Disease, 1985-1986*, R.T. Johnson (ed.) (Philadelphia: B. C. Decker, 1985).

329. Whitehouse, P.J., Price, D.L., Clark, A.W., et al., "Alzheimer Disease: Evidence for Selective Loss of Cholinergic Neurons in the Nucleus Basalis," *Annals of Neurology* 10:122-126, 1981.

330. Whitehouse, P.J., Price, D.L., Struble, R.G., et al., "Alzheimer's Disease and Senile Dementia: Loss of Neurons in the Basal Forebrain," *Science* 215:1237-1239, 1982.

331. Whitehouse, P.J., Hedreen, J.C., White, C.L., III, et al., *Annals of Neurology* 13:243-248, 1983.

332. Wietgrefe, S., Zupanic, M., Haase, A., et al., "Cloning of a Gene Whose Expression Is Increased in Scrapie and in Senile Plaques in Human Brain," *Science* 230:1177-1179, 1985.

333. Winograd, C.H., and Jarvik, L.F., "Caregivers of Patients With Dementia," *Journal of the American Geriatrics Society* 34:295-308, 1986.

334. Wisniewski, K.E., Dalton, A.J., McLachlan, D.R.C., et al., "Alzheimer's Disease in Down's Syndrome: Clinicopathologic Studies," *Neurology* 35:957-961, 1985.

335. Wisniewski, K.E., Wisniewski, H.M., and Wen, G.Y., "Occurrence of Neuropathological Changes and Dementia of Alzheimer's Disease in Down's Syndrome," *Annals of Neurology* 17:278-282, 1985.

336. Wolozin, B.L., Pruchnicki, A., Dickson, D.W., et al., "A Neuronal Antigen in the Brains of Alzheimer Patients," *Science* 232:648-650, 1986.

337. Wright, A.F., and Whalley, L.J., "Genetics, Aging and Dementia," *British Journal of Psychiatry* 145:20-38, 1984.

338. Wurtman, R.J., "Alzheimer's Disease," *Scientific American* 252:62-74, 120, January 1985.

339. Wurtman, R.J., Blusztajn, J.K., and Maire, J.C., "'Autocannibalism' of Choline-Containing Membrane Phospholipids in the Pathogenesis of Alzheimer's Disease—A Hypothesis," *Neurochemistry International* 7:269-372, 1985.

340. Wyngaarden, J.B., "Risk Factors for Alzheimer's Disease, 'From the NIH' " *Journal of the American Medical Association* 255:1105, 1986.

341. Yates, C.M., "Critique: Transmitter Deficits in Alzheimer's Disease," *Neurochemistry International* 7:571-573, 1985.

342. Yen, S.H., Crowe, A., and Dickson, D.W., "Monoclonal Antibodies to Alzheimer Neurofibrillary Tangles. 1. Identification of Polypeptides," *American Journal of Pathology* 120:282-291, 1985.

343. Young, A.B., "Progressive Supranuclear Palsy: Postmortem Chemical Analysis," *Archives of Neurology* 18:521-522, 1985.

344. Zanetti, O., Rozzini, R., Bianchetti, A., et al., "HDL Cholesterol in Dementia," *Lancet*, July 6, 1985, p. 43.

345. Zubenko, G.S., Cohen, B.M., Growden, J., et al., "Cell Membrane Abnormality in Alzheimer's Disease," *Lancet*, July 28, 1984, p. 235.

Chapter 4
The Family

CONTENTS

The Family*

Families provide most of the care of the impaired elderly and act as the advocates for persons with dementia (1,30,65). They are appealing for relief from the burdens of patient care (1,74). Their appeals coincide with efforts to control public health care expenditures, including determining how much financial responsibility families should assume for the care of the elderly ill. Caregiving families are also receiving attention, as recent studies begin to show that the characteristics of a family are as important as those of the person with dementia in determining which individuals will be institutionalized (16).

This chapter examines the impact of dementing diseases on caregiving families and discusses

the potential effect of policy options. The first section asks:

- Who provides how much of what kinds of care and services to individuals with dementia?
- What is the impact of the disease on the family?
- Are the burdens caused by dementia unique to the condition or similar to those created by other long-term chronic illnesses?
- How will changing patterns of family life affect the availability of caregivers in the future?

The second section focuses on helping families and considers whether the family can be assisted to provide more care at a savings to the taxpayer. The last section examines six options available to the Federal Government to assist or support families.

---

*This chapter is a contract report by Nancy Mace, consultant in gerontology, Towson, MD.

A PROFILE OF FAMILY CARE

Who Provides How Much and What Kind of Care in Which Families?

Extent of Care

Studies of the dependent or frail elderly show that family caregivers provide 80 to 90 percent of the care of these individuals (10). Even though the United States is a mobile society, most elderly persons live near at least one family member and see that person frequently (66). Families do not abandon the ill to institutions; they avoid placing their relatives in nursing homes as long as possible, often at great cost to themselves. Indeed, many nursing home placements are not only appropriate, but should have been made sooner (51).

Studies that focus on caregivers of persons with dementia confirm that families also provide the majority of care. The Secretary's Task Force on Alzheimer's Disease reported that most people with dementing illnesses are cared for by their families for the majority of their illness (77). The tasks of caring for a person with dementia are

constant. A significant number of caregivers of dementia victims spend more than 40 hours a week in direct personal care (54). In fact, a popular book refers to caregiving as "the 36-hour day" (44).

At the same time, persons with dementia are overrepresented in nursing homes (8). Many are placed there after having exhausted those caring for them:

> In the overwhelming majority of cases, nursing home placement occurs only after responsible family caregivers have endured prolonged, unrelenting strain (often for years), and no longer have the capacity to continue their caregiving efforts (12).

Others have outlived their caregivers. Individuals who have no children or whose spouse becomes ill or dies are much more likely than those with families to be in nursing homes (8,45).

To learn more about family caregivers and how they obtain help, OTA surveyed 2,900 persons on the Alzheimer's Disease and Related Disorders

Association (ADRDA) mailing list. (See ref. 82; the study is referred to in this chapter as the OTA study.) Table 4-1 indicates the living arrangements of those with dementia identified in this study. Although 39 percent were currently living with a family caregiver, 50 percent had lived with relatives at some point in their illness. (This figure does not include those living in their own home and cared for by a spouse.) Thus, over the long course of a dementing illness, many people will be at home for part of their illness and in a nursing home or similar residential setting for part of the time.

Care Providers Within Families

One definition of the family is:

. . . that group of individuals [who] are related by blood or marriage. . . . The family may include those persons somewhat distantly related by blood or marriage, such as cousins of various degrees or in-laws, all of whom may be perceived as family members. Further, for any one person the family network is not static. It may expand to include even more distant relatives as a need arises for information, services, or help from these relatives (66).

A "family caregiver" may include individuals unrelated by blood or marriage but sharing in a relationship of intimacy and support. "Family" does not necessarily refer to persons sharing a household or living nearby—it may include someone living at great distance who is in close communication.

Within the white middle-class family, one individual usually assumes most of the tasks of car-

ing (51). Studies show that when the disabled individual is married, the caregiver will most often be the spouse (one-third to one-half of all caregivers—most of whom are women); when there is no available spouse, adult daughters or daughters-in-law assume the role. (One-quarter to one-third of the caregivers are adult children.) The remainder are other family members or unrelated persons. In the absence of immediate family members, often a sibling or the adult child of a sibling will assume primary responsibility for the patient (18,26,83). Even friends and neighbors occasionally act as primary caregivers (68). The patterns of family caregiving may be different for other socioeconomic or cultural groups (33,37,42).

Little is known about the ways in which other family members—whether living nearby or far away—help the primary caregiver, although it is clear that they do help (59,71). Anecdotal information reveals that many family members who live further away also are actively involved in care plans.

More women than men are primary caregivers. This is in part because of women's traditional roles and in part because wives tend to be younger than their husbands. (Men are closely involved in care, but often their tasks and investments of time are different.) Nevertheless, many husbands and sons are providing around-the-clock intensive personal care.

Most caregivers are middle-aged. The 1982 Long-Term Care Survey found that the average age of caregivers was 57 years, with one-quarter aged 65-74, and 10 percent aged 75 or over (69). They are persons with numerous responsibilities, which may include the care of other dependent elderly, children, grandchildren, and spouses. Thus the difficulties they experience by helping a relative with dementia may affect many lives. Caregivers are often employed, and they often are beginning to experience chronic illnesses associated with their own aging (10). The Long-Term Care Study found that one-third of caregivers rated their health as fair or poor (69). Spouse caregivers are often as old as or older than the ill person and may have chronic illnesses of their own. They may be unable to meet the physical demands of caregiving. One program found that caregivers

Table 4-1.—Where The Person With Dementia Lives

Where the person with dementia lives:	Total respondents
With primary caregiver (if other than you) or with you	39%
In a nursing home	33%
Patient now deceased	17%
Alone	4%
In a foster, personal care, or boarding home	3%
In a Veterans Administration home or hospital	1%
With someone else	1%
Not applicable	1%

NOTE: Percentages rounded to nearest whole number.

SOURCE: Yankelovich, Skelly, & White, Inc., "Caregivers of Patients With Dementia," contract report prepared for the Office of Technology Assessment, U.S. Congress, 1986.

using home respite care were much older than the average recipients of all programs (56).

Although this profile encompasses the majority of caregivers, the diversity among caregivers is striking (34). A few elderly parents are caring for middle-aged sons and daughters with a dementing illness and a significant number of younger spouses are caring for both a young victim and young children. More information about how families provide care is needed if successful services for them are to be developed. The diversity among caregivers indicates that no one service will serve all families.

Kinds of Care

Families provide a wide range of care: from giving advice and acting as a confidant, to providing financial help and total personal care. Family care is highly flexible. Unlike formal support services, families provide care at night, over weekends, and on demand. The care they give is individualized to meet the idiosyncratic needs of the person with dementia (23).

The care provided changes as the illness progresses. Early in the course of the disease, families must make decisions for the individual and take over shopping, meal preparation, banking, and legal and financial responsibilities (44). Later, families must assume responsibility for personal tasks such as dressing, bathing, and eating. Because the individual is usually ambulatory but has impaired judgment, round-the-clock supervision is necessary. Many persons with dementia are awake and active at night—the OTA study found that 17 percent were out of bed most nights—and therefore their caregivers must also be awake. After a time, caregivers must assist persons with dementia to walk (or must lift those who become bedfast)—8 percent of the individuals in the OTA study were living with family and were bedfast. Many must help these persons use the toilet; others manage complete incontinence (14 percent of the persons in the OTA study were incontinent and were living with family caregivers).

For most of the illness, persons with dementia appear unaware of their need for help and may respond to assistance with anger or resistance. They may accuse a caregiver of stealing from them or trying to harm them. Many patients are unable to express any appreciation for their care. They may fail to recognize a spouse or child, or may exhibit bizarre behaviors that complicate the tasks of personal care. Families report a long list of difficult and upsetting behaviors (see table 4-2). In addition, the tasks of caring remind the caregiver

Table 4-2.—Patient's Behavior Problems Cited by Families

Behavior	Number of families reporting	Families reporting the behavior No. (%)	Families reporting the behavior and citing it as a problem No. (%)
Memory disturbance	55	55 (100)	51 (93)
Catastrophic reactions	52	45 (87)	40 (89)
Demanding/critical behavior	52	37 (71)	27 (73)
Night waking	54	37 (69)	22 (59)
Hiding things	51	35 (69)	25 (71)
Communication difficulties	50	34 (68)	25 (74)
Suspiciousness	52	33 (63)	26 (79)
Making accusations	53	32 (60)	26 (81)
Needing help at mealtimes	55	33 (60)	18 (55)
Daytime wandering	51	30 (59)	21 (70)
Bathing	51	27 (53)	20 (74)
Delusions	49	23 (47)	19 (83)
Physical violence	51	24 (47)	22 (92)
Incontinence	53	21 (40)	18 (86)
Cooking	54	18 (33)	8 (44)
Hitting	50	16 (32)	13 (81)
Driving	55	11 (20)	8 (73)
Smoking	53	6 (11)	4 (67)
Inappropriate sexual behavior	51	1 (2)	0 (0)

SOURCE: Adapted from P.V. Rabins, N.L. Mace, and J.T. Rabins, "The Impact of Dementia on the Family," *Journal of the American Medical Association* 248:334, 1982.

of the deterioration of a loved one. The experience of ongoing grief was described by one family member as "the funeral that never ends" (29).

Even after someone has been placed in a nursing home, families continue to visit, assist staff, wash and mend clothing, dress the person, take him or her for walks, pay bills, handle money, and, finally, continue to give love and affection (18). For many caregivers, the year following placement in a nursing home may be as stressful as the years of caregiving (27).

Many families cover all the expenses of a relative placed in a home: half the total cost of nursing home care is borne by patients and their families (4). That figure does not include extras such as laundry, haircuts, toiletries, and sometimes medication.

Families That Provide Care

Because there is no known racial or socioeconomic variation in the prevalence of Alzheimer's disease (47), the families that provide care are believed to represent all groups. Racial and socioeconomic differences have been found by clinical practice and in voluntary organizations, but these may reflect variations in knowledge of the disease, access to services, and ways of obtaining help rather than real variations in prevalence.

Little is known about patterns of elder care among minority groups. In States where the demand for nursing home beds exceeds the supply, facilities are able to selectively exclude "undesirable" patients—those who are receiving Medicaid, for example, or those who are difficult to care for (72). Since individuals with dementing illnesses are perceived by nursing home staff as difficult to care for, and since minorities are overrepresented among the poor, these persons are least likely to find a nursing home (38).

Other characteristics of the caregiving situation also influence the decision to place an individual in a nursing home (16). Spouses who depend on the patient's pension or who cannot afford a nursing home have little choice except to care for the person at home. These economic realities may operate in concert with strong cultural values of the importance of caring for family.

Many patients do not have family members available who can provide care. An estimated 7 million older people have no family, have families that are not nearby, or have family relationships that have long been impaired (8). As many as half the people living in unlicensed (and therefore uncounted) boarding homes, hotel rooms, "foster homes," and single-room occupancy hotels have dementing illnesses (8). These individuals also are less likely to have family members who could care for them or oversee the quality of the care they are given. Thus, a significant group of persons with dementia are at risk of exploitation, abuse, or neglect because they have no relatives to speak for them.

What Effect Does Caring for a Dementia Patient Have on the Family?

Reports from families of dementia victims are filled with accounts of the severe pressures created by these illnesses (30). The Secretary's Task Force on Alzheimer's Disease stated that:

> . . . the extremely debilitating and chronic nature of Alzheimer's disease places a tremendous financial and social burden on family caregivers (77).

One observer found that:

> . . . persons with dementing disorders contribute to the community burden disproportionately. This demonstrates . . . that the observations in clinical settings represent only the tip of an iceberg of unknown shape and size (68).

Several studies have sought to measure and describe the impact on families. Researchers unanimously report enormous and prolonged demands. Caring for a person who has a dementia often has an adverse effect on:

- the caregiver's physical and mental health (28,61),
- the caregiver's participation in recreation and social activities (62),
- the family living arrangements (26),
- the caregiver's employment status (73), and
- the caregiver's financial security (73).

Some of these and other studies have sought to identify the aspects of care that influence a caregiver's feelings of burden. They have found that the burden a caregiver experiences may be influenced by the person's relationship (husband, wife, son, daughter) to the person with dementia (26), by whether caregiver and patient share a residence (10), and by the emotional support the caregiver receives from other members of the family (84). Symptoms of mental impairment, disruptive or "acting out" behaviors, extent of need for personal care, and the number of disruptive behaviors all increase the caregiver's stress (59). There is no direct relationship between stress and a family's decision to use a nursing home, although stress may be a factor (see below).

Further study is needed to answer several questions:

* To what extent do the problems families face—poverty, the presence of children who need care, the demands of jobs, divorce, crowded living arrangements, unhappy family relationships, loss of a caregiver's income —interact with and compound their burden?
* In what ways is the burden of caring for a person with primarily mental or behavioral symptoms different from caring for a person with a physical disability?
* Why do a few families not report distress?
* Why do some persons with dementia not exhibit the disturbed behaviors commonly reported?
* Do some families have better resources that allow them to manage? If so, what are they— money; health; coping strategies such as religious faith, humor, cognitive restructuring skills?
* Does the duration of the illness affect feelings of burden?
* What are the special needs or problems of rural, minority, or socioeconomically disadvantaged families?

There are significant weaknesses in the design of some of the studies to date. For instance, most have examined white middle-class families. Little is known about the effects of caregiving on rural, minority, and impoverished families.

Physical and Mental Health

Because dementia is most prevalent late in life, caregivers are often elderly spouses or adult sons and daughters who are themselves entering early old age, with their own age-related health problems (10). One report noted that three-fourths of the adult sons and daughters of dependent elderly entering the Philadelphia Geriatric Center were in their fifties or sixties (8).

Caregivers report that the tasks of caring have a deleterious effect on their health (61). One-third of the caregivers in a national study of people caring for the frail or disabled elderly rated their own general health as fair or poor (69). They report illnesses resulting from exhaustion and stress, as well as injuries resulting from the physical tasks of caregiving (17). When caregivers are compared with groups of similar individuals who are not caring for an ill relative, those living with an ill person tended to have poorer health. Men with ill wives are more likely than an aged-matched control to die prematurely of stress-related diseases (26). The OTA study found that 12 percent of the caregivers who were living with the person with dementia reported becoming physically ill or being injured as a result of caring for the person. That is a significant hazard, especially for wife caregivers who are smaller than a husband who has dementia.

Studies report high levels of depression among caregivers (25,40,60,62,81). These studies also find that many caregivers feel angry and guilty and are grieving. They report increased levels of family conflict. People caring for someone with dementia have three times as many stress symptoms as people of the same age who are not caregivers, and they report lower life satisfaction. Caregivers used more psychotrophic drugs (sleeping medications, tranquilizers, and antidepressants) and more alcohol than comparison groups (28). Women who have given up a job to care for a parent experience poorer physical and mental health than other women (10). In the OTA study, 35 percent of caregivers who were living with the patient reported becoming very stressed and 11 percent of the primary caregivers sought the help of a counselor or psychiatrist.

Participation in Recreation and Social Activity

Closely related to mental health is the time caregivers spend in recreation and social activity and their feelings of satisfaction from leisure activities. Often the tasks of giving care fill their days, allowing no time for recreation (62). The patient's bizarre behaviors and need for constant supervision further limit opportunities for social activity. Caregivers lose friends and give up hobbies. They become isolated by the need to provide full-time caregiving.

Yet a caregiver's need for social contact is underscored by studies showing that his or her feeling of burden is related to the amount of support given by others. Caregivers who felt well supported by friends and family had fewer feelings of burden than those who did not feel supported by others (7,84). One study reported that support from others had a greater effect on caregiver's feelings of burden than did any other factor, including patient behavior and level of cognition (84).

Living Arrangements

Neither elderly individuals nor their adult children prefer living in three-generation households. Instead, where possible, at least one adult child lives near the parents (65). However, the situation may be different for the families of persons with dementia. Unlike many other chronically ill persons who can be left alone for brief periods of time, individuals with dementia need constant supervision. Therefore, the family may have no choice but to share a household in order to watch the person day and night. Data tend to support this hypothesis: The greatly or extremely impaired are more likely to be in shared households (65). And shared households have been linked with the symptoms common to dementia (63). The OTA study found only 4 percent of persons with dementia living alone. The 1982 National Long-Term Care Survey found that almost three-quarters of caregivers in a nationally representative sample of people helping frail and/or disabled persons lived with the care recipient (69).

Sharing a household with the impaired elderly may lead to increased family conflict, poorer caregiver health, and greater caregiver stress (10,26). Shared households more often include children of the caregiver. The demands of a behaviorally disturbed elder and the needs of children may interact to increase the caregiver's stress.

Employment Status

Twenty-eight percent of the nonworking women in one study had quit their jobs in order to care for an aging parent, and an equal percentage of working women were considering doing so (10). The women who had left employment had parents who were older. They more often shared their household with a parent, and the parents more often were cognitively impaired (i.e., had symptoms of dementia and scored lower on a standard mental status test). Caring for a parent had resulted in a greater deterioration in these women's physical and mental health, and their families had lower incomes.

The OTA study found that there was an employed person in 14 percent of households and that in 12 percent someone, almost always the primary caregiver, had stopped working in order to care for the person with dementia. The Travelers Insurance Co. conducted a study of employees at its Hartford, CT, headquarters and found that 28 percent of the full-time employees spent an average of 10.2 hours a week caring for an aged relative, while 8 percent devoted 35 hours a week to care (49). Those who quit work are only part of a much larger group. The 1982 National Long-Term Care Survey found that:

> . . . among the one million caregivers who had been employed sometime during the caregiver's experience, one-fifth cut back on hours, 29.4 percent rearranged their schedules, and 18.6 percent took time off without pay to fulfill caregiver obligations (69).

Another study (52) found that higher percentages of the adult-child caregivers with children in the household were employed either part-time or full-time, particularly when the caregiver was divorced or separated. It is likely that the costs of child rearing necessitate the employment of many middle-aged women in three-generation households. Despite their multiple roles as spouse, parent, and primary caregiver, half these women were also in the labor force. In the summer of 1986, the Family Survival Project conducted a study of employed caregivers of persons with dementia. Preliminary data from that study indicate that many caregivers are leaving employment to provide care (24).

Financial Impact

The Maryland Report on Alzheimer's Disease and Related Disorders states that:

... the financial burdens of dementing disorders can be particularly devastating . . . the caregiver is faced with the prospect of wearing himself or herself out or spending large amounts of money for home nursing aides or nursing home placement (30).

The financial burdens include loss of the ill person's salary; denial of his or her disability or retirement income; loss of the caregiver's salary; the costs of home or respite care (which are generally not covered by insurance, Medicare, or Medicaid); and the costs of nursing home care (also rarely covered by insurance or Medicare). The 1982 National Long-Term Care Survey found that almost one-third of caregivers had incomes within the poor or near poor category (69).

Many families lose the salary of the person with dementia. Although the disease is more common among people who are likely to be retired, it strikes many people during their peak earning years. The percent of individuals who lose a job due to a dementia is not known and can only be inferred from epidemiologic data. The OTA study found that 11 percent of the persons with dementia had applied for Old Age and Survivors' Disability Insurance (OASDI) and 7 percent had applied for disability pension from an employer, one indicator of employment status at the time of the onset of the illness. In addition, many women with dementia had been homemakers at the onset of their illness (18). Since someone else must assume housekeeping tasks or a homemaker must be hired, that loss must also be considered in economic terms.

The onset of the disease is gradual and insidious, often going unnoticed or misunderstood. Therefore there may be a substantial number of individuals who leave employment or are asked to take an early retirement because of inadequate job performance. Some people have lost a job, only to try several more jobs unsuccessfully before the dementing illness is discovered (18).

Researchers and disability examiners both report a long litany of problems caregivers face in obtaining disability and retirement benefits on be-

half of an ill person (18,21). Some individuals have been fired because the disease was not recognized; others quit their jobs before a diagnosis had been made. Thus, an unknown number of persons with dementia may sometimes be denied disability or retirement benefits. In addition, some families, already exhausted by caregiving, have had to make repeated appeals to obtain benefits (18).

People with a dementing illness are often unable to learn a new, less difficult skill, and therefore may be totally disabled early in the illness. An Institute of Gerontology study mentioned one man who "was reduced from supervisor to work crew, then to janitor" but who was unable to function successfully at any level (18). Farm and unskilled laborers may be disabled as completely and quickly as persons with technical or professional skills. The same study described a farmer who:

... would take hours to do simple chores. He wouldn't be able to find farms where he was contracted to haul cattle and other livestock. He didn't know what to do when he got there. He needed help getting to the stockyard and doing routine things when he got there.

As indicated earlier, a significant number of family members give up jobs to care for the patient. Families with lower incomes are more likely to experience the loss of a caregiver's salary (10). Table 4-3, taken from the OTA study, shows the amount of salary lost by those who quit a job to care for a person with dementia. These data agree with reports that low-income women are more likely than higher-income women to quit a job to care for an aged parent (10). Families face the financial burdens of care that extend over many years. Insurance or Medicare usually covers the

Table 4-3.—Amount of Salary Lost by Family Members Who Quit a Job to Care for a Person with Dementia

Approximate amount of salary lost	Total respondents
Less than $4,999	23%
$5,000 to $9,999	17%
$10,000 to $14,999	12%
$15,000 to $19,999	18%
More than $20,000	11%
Did not answer	20%

NOTE: Percentages rounded to nearest whole number.

SOURCE: Yankelovich, Skelly, & White, Inc., "Caregivers of Patients With Dementia," contract report prepared for the Office of Technology Assessment, U.S. Congress, 1986.

costs of diagnosis and physician care, but that represents only part of the total. The financial burden on family caregivers has been widely documented (18,30,75).

In addition to the loss of income, individuals with dementia often give away, hide, or spend money needed for their long-term care.

Half the total costs of nursing home care are borne by residents and families (4). Most respite and home care programs, when available, depend on client fees or private sources (30). The care of persons with dementia in such programs usually does not qualify as medical (skilled nursing) care and therefore is not reimbursed by Medicare; nor is it tax deductible. Day care programs that focus on service to people with dementia report less use of Medicaid than programs that serve other frail elderly, and almost no use of Medicare (46).

The OTA study found that no respondents had been reimbursed by either Medicaid or Medicare for a visiting nurse or day care program. Many families in the OTA survey (11 to 31 percent by program) did not use *available* services because they were too expensive. Families caring for a person with dementia also pay for renovations to make their home safe for the resident and for over-the-counter medications, diapers, special diets, and supportive devices, many of which are not covered by Medicare.

Although the ill person's own income and assets appear to be used first, 29 percent of the respondents report that a spouse was contributing to the cost of care, and one in five report that children and other relatives contribute to the cost of care (see table 4-4). One family in four reports that all the patient's savings had already been spent on care (table 4-5) and half expected that all or most of the patient's savings would eventually be spent (table 4-6). Those who had been ill longer were more likely to have expended their savings.

The financial impact on family varies. Half report that there has been no impact thus far or that they had been able to handle extra expenses fairly easily. However, 22 percent report not being able to make ends meet or having to cut back sharply on expenses (table 4-7). Nearly 20 percent

of families had spent all or at least half the family's savings on care; another 21 percent had spent less than half (table 4-8).

Spouse caregivers are more likely to be impoverished than other family members. One-third of families report that the person with dementia relies on the spouse for support, and 15 percent report that very little of the couple's income was left for the well spouse (table 4-9). That agrees with the finding of another study that spouse caregivers are disproportionately impoverished (26).

Between one-fourth and one-third of families surveyed in the OTA study reported that they were facing the early stages of the relative's illness when financial drains are not so great as when he or she is in a nursing home. When families were surveyed by another study 2 years later, more reported a serious financial impact (26). Thus more families in the OTA sample can be expected to become impoverished or experience a significant impact of the cost of care in coming years. Programs that provide assistance and see families after they have provided care for many years report higher percentages who are severely affected by the burdens of care. A Massachusetts study found that two-thirds of individuals and one-third of couples aged 66 and older would spend themselves into poverty within 13 weeks if stricken by a chronic illness that required long-term care (74). Clearly, not only does the impact fall most heavily on spouses, but it is also heaviest when the person must be cared for in an institution.

Because persons on the ADRDA mailing list cannot be assumed to be representative of all persons caring for someone with a dementing illness, the findings of the OTA study must be regarded as preliminary. Furthermore, many of the caregivers who responded to the survey did not answer the questions about expenses, making these findings on costs much less reliable (see table 4-9). For these reasons, it is likely that the data in these tables underreport the financial impact on families.

The OTA study also asked families what sources of funds helped support the person with dementia or pay for the person's care and what percent of care was provided by each source (see table 4-4). Of all families surveyed, 70 percent report

Table 4-4.—Sources of Income Used To Support Person With Dementia[a]

Source	Percent of total respondents reporting this source[b]	Mean contribution[c]
Patient's Social Security	70%	38%
Patient's own savings, income from assets	53%	46%
Other retirement/pension income of patient	32%	34%
Patient's spouse	30%	11%
Medicare	29%	19%
Medicaid	15%	9%
Patient's children	15%	24%
SSI (Supplemental Security Income)	6%	37%
Veterans Administration	5%	67%
OASDI or other disability payment	4%	23%
Contributions from other relatives	4%	13%
Other	4%	37%

[a]Most families report having more than one source of income.
[b]Does not indicate percent of contribution by source.
[c]Respondents were asked what percent of the person's overall support was from each source. These responses were summed to obtain a mean.

SOURCE: Yankelovich, Skelly, & White, Inc., "Caregivers of Patients With Dementia," contract report prepared for the Office of Technology Assessment, U.S. Congress, 1986.

Table 4-5.—Amount of Patient's Savings Spent on Care Since Becoming Ill

How much of patient's savings spent	Total respondents (%)[a]
All or most	23%
A large amount (at least half)	16%
Some but less than half	28%
None	14%
Patient had no savings	9%
Did not answer	12%

[a]Percent based on total sample.
NOTE: Percentages rounded to nearest whole number.
SOURCE: Yankelovich, Skelly, & White, Inc., "Caregivers of Patients With Dementia," contract report prepared for the Office of Technology Assessment, U.S. Congress, 1986.

Table 4-6.—Proportion of Patient's Income/Savings Expected to Eventually Go for Care

How much expected to go for care	Total respondents (%)[a]
All or most	51%
At least half	15%
Less than half	8%
None	7%
Did not answer	20%

[a]Percent based on total sample.
NOTE: Percentages rounded to nearest whole number.
SOURCE: Yankelovich, Skelly, & White, Inc., "Caregivers of Patients With Dementia," contract report prepared for the Office of Technology Assessment, U.S. Congress, 1986.

that the patient's social security is a source of income. Among those who receive social security, it accounts for an average of 38 percent of their income. On the other hand, Veterans Administration funds account for an average of 67 percent of a person's income, but only 5 percent of individuals rely on VA funds. Few patients rely on financial help from their children, but those who do report that an average of one-fourth of the ill-person's income comes from the children.

Thus, families do make major contributions to care and are able and willing to share in the cost of care. At the same time, government funding sources are an essential resource. Not all families rely on sources such as Medicaid for patient care, but financial demands increase with the progression of the disease. The burden of care can quickly exhaust the resources of persons with dementia and impoverish their families, especially those most vulnerable—spouses, female heads of household, and minorities (see ch. 12)—and ultimately have a significant effect on the resources of many families.

Families have charged that Medicaid and Medicare standards contain biases and restrictions that mitigate against persons with dementia, against women caregivers, and against home care as opposed to nursing home care (13,18,30,51,70).

Except for physician care and medications, most persons with a dementing illness do not need the medically oriented care Medicare/Medicaid call "skilled" until late in their illnesses. The care they need is termed "custodial" by Medicare and Medicaid; it does not qualify them for Medicare coverage in nursing homes, or for home health care.

Table 4-7.—Financial Impact on Family Paying for Patient's Care

Which statement best describes the financial impact on your family?	Total respondents[a]
We have had to cut back sharply on expenses and still can't make ends meet	5.7%
We have had to cut back sharply on expenses but have been able to make ends meet	16.2%
We have had to do without some things but are getting by	7.5%
We have been able to pick up the extra expenses fairly easily	14.5%
So far there has been no impact; we have not had to contribute to the patient's support	34.5%
Did not answer	28.0%

[a]More than one response was allowed.

SOURCE: Yankelovich, Skelly, & White, Inc., "Caregivers of Patients With Dementia," contract report prepared for the Office of Technology Assessment, U.S. Congress, 1986.

Table 4-8.—Proportion of Family Savings Spent for Patient Care

Portion of family savings	Total respondents
All or most	9%
More than half	10%
Less than half	21%
None	47%
No answer	14%

NOTE: Percentages rounded to nearest whole number.

SOURCE: Yankelovich, Skelly, & White, Inc., "Caregivers of Patients With Dementia," contract report prepared for the Office of Technology Assessment, U.S. Congress, 1986.

Table 4-9.—Proportion of Income/Savings Left for Patient's Spouse After Paying for Care

Proportion of income/savings left	Total respondents
All or most	17%
About half	19%
Some but very little	15%
Patient has no living spouse	7%
Did not answer	43%

NOTE: Percentages rounded to nearest whole number.

SOURCE: Yankelovich, Skelly, & White, Inc., "Caregivers of Patients With Dementia," contract report prepared for the Office of Technology Assessment, U.S. Congress, 1986.

In some States it means that the care of persons with dementia in nursing homes is reimbursed at lower rates by Medicaid. Families and professionals have argued that considerable skill is needed to care for these persons successfully (30) and "custodial" rates are too low to provide the care needed by people with dementia.

Certain groups are especially vulnerable to the financial biases of some government programs. Although the financial well-being of the elderly in general has improved, aged female heads of households remain impoverished (79). It is these women who are most likely to give up a job to provide care for a person with dementia (11) and who can least afford to lose income. Women are much more likely than men to receive no retirement pension or only Supplemental Security Income (SSI)—$325/month—because many older women did not work outside the home or worked only as domestics (18). Women are more likely than men to be widowed and therefore to have lost the pension on which they depended. Daughters caring for an aged parent in a household without a male wage-earner and retired couples on a fixed income also report high levels of financial burden.

The Maryland State Office on Aging found that Medicaid policy is inadvertently biased against wives (13). Since many women in the older cohorts of the elderly were never employed, they depend on their husband's retirement income, almost all of which must be paid for his nursing home care if he is to qualify for Medicaid. The wife then becomes eligible for SSI, at a much lower standard of living, often after she has devoted years to her husband's care. In contrast, when a wife with no income of her own is institutionalized, 23 States do not require the husband who continues living in the community to spend his pension on her care. He can continue to live at his previous standard of living (see ch. 11).

Efforts to encourage alternatives to nursing home care can also result in inadvertent discrimination. Programs that fund in-home care often require clients to meet criteria for skilled nursing care. That requirement is to ensure that home care replaces institutional care and does not become an add-on service. Persons with dementia, excluded by the skilled-nursing language, are thereby unable to use these programs until they are too severely ill to be managed at home.

In some States, Medicaid considers room and board provided by a caregiving family to be part of the applicant's income. That effectively makes the income of persons living with family members higher than that of comparable persons living alone or in a nursing home. Family caregivers complain that this method of calculation is inequitable since persons with dementia cannot live alone.

Families report being given incorrect or conflicting information when they have applied for Medicaid. Such problems produce further stress, and may have resulted in the unnecessary impoverishment of caregivers. The extent of this problem is difficult to document, although complaints are common (14).

Medicaid law is convoluted and difficult to understand. It is a mix of Federal and State statutes and varies from State to State (14). The minutes of the Governor's Task Force on Alzheimer's Disease in Maryland reveal that even experts disagreed on their interpretations of that State's Medicaid law (30). Anecdotal reports tell of different Medicaid offices within a State giving different information, nursing home staff giving incorrect information about eligibility, families being required to pay private rates for nursing home care after being incorrectly told that the patient was not eligible for Medicaid, and families being required to make a donation to nursing homes or to sign agreements to pay at private rates.

The OTA study found that of the 164 families who had applied for Medicaid, 38 percent had encountered problems; 22 percent could not get a clear explanation of the eligibility rules, and almost 9 percent said they were treated rudely.

Of those who applied for Medicaid, 38 percent were told by the Medicaid office that the spouse must provide support, although 23 States do not hold spouses responsible for long-term care. ADRDA chapters report numerous spouses who were required to support a patient in nursing homes, often for many years, even in States in which spouses are not responsible for support after the first month (2,3).

Among families who sought to place relatives in a nursing home, the OTA study found that 12 percent were told they must make a donation to the home—a practice that violates Federal policy in homes accepting Federal funds. One-third were asked to sign agreements to pay privately. (Eleven different attorneys general in States with Federal support have issued opinions holding that Federal law makes it a felony to require a person who is Medicaid-eligible to agree to pay privately) (15).

Varying Impact on Spouses, Adult Children, and Young Children

Although studies have shown that men and women, adult children, and spouses experience burden in different ways, the research has covered only a narrow socioeconomic subgroup. Differences between economic or racial groups may be greater than those between the sexes or by relationship. Much more significant than these differences is the number of caregivers of all types who are significantly distressed. Nevertheless, if supportive services are to be targeted effectively, the differences among caregivers must be better understood.

Little is known about the number of children living with or near a person with dementia or about the impact of these diseases on children. Younger persons with dementia often still have young children or adolescents at home. Many individuals live in three-generation families, where grandchildren grow up in the presence of a person with dementia; a national survey of caregivers of the frail or disabled elderly found that one-quarter of the caregiving sons and daughters had children in the household (69).

One commentator has stated, "problems and role changes experienced by one family member affect every other family member and each person in the family feels the repercussions" (9). Thus even children not living with the ill person may experience the effects of their parent's burden.

The 36-Hour Day (44), a guide for families of persons with dementia, identifies some of the common problems encountered when children or adolescents share a home with a person with dementia. When the child's parent is the primary caregiver, parenting roles may be diminished by the demands on the exhausted caregiver. Caregivers often cannot leave a person with dementia in another room for even a few minutes, so finding time to talk alone with a worried child can be difficult. Family activities may cease because no sitter can be found for the ill person; family meals and sleep may be disrupted by disturbed behavior during the years a child is growing up. Many caregivers are also employed—often of necessity—adding to the burdens of both caregiver and child (52).

Disoriented and distressed people with dementia may punish a child unjustly, or may berate an adolescent for being a "hippie," "lazy," or "a thief." They may yell or curse. Their behavior may make a child too embarrassed to bring friends home. Because the person cannot control his or her behavior or learn not to act that way, children may have no choice but to put up with it—and with little support from their exhausted and depressed parent.

The number of children touched by a dementing illness may be quite high. The OTA study found that 6 percent of persons with dementia currently living in a family household shared the home with children. Many more children may have shared a household with a person with dementia at some point. The Travelers Insurance Co. surveyed its employees who were caring for an elder family member and found "that 52 percent of those giving care were adults between the ages of 41 and 55, many of whom were attempting to satisfy the needs not only of elderly parents but also those of their own children" (49). A study of schoolchildren found that 25 percent had an elderly family member who was not mentally alert and that these children had more negative attitudes toward aging than other young people did (67).

Although many schools now offer courses in family life, many have little or no material about abnormal aging. The Maryland Report on Alzheimer's Disease and Related Disorders, for example, found no material in the Maryland school curriculum about abnormal aging (30). In 1986 Maryland (HB173) and Virginia (HJR105) introduced legislation to correct that lack. It is the current generation of schoolchildren who will have to assume responsibility for vast numbers of the elderly with dementing illnesses.

Varying Impact on Different Socioeconomic Groups

As indicated, little information exists on the effect of dementing diseases on minority populations or on different socioeconomic groups. Studies of the minority aged indicate that the burden of a dementing illness may be experienced differently by different socioeconomic groups. Two general theories are postulated: that minority groups have stronger family ties and are more willing to keep their aged at home; or that the combined burdens of minority status, poverty, and age exacerbate the problems faced by these families.

Minority groups tend to have lower incomes and more single women as heads of household. As mentioned earlier, both factors point to higher levels of caregiver stress. Such multiple disadvantages probably compound the struggle these families face. Blacks and Hispanics are underrepresented in nursing homes (42), which implies that informal caregivers are providing extensive amounts of care. It may also reflect the shorter life expectancy of blacks and significant inequalities in access to resources.

Burdens Related to Public Policy or Access to Services

Families report that there are few services to assist them in caring for a person with a dementing illness, that the services that do exist will not accept persons with dementia, or that staff members of these services are not trained in the special care of persons with dementia (70).

The OTA survey of ADRDA members asked several questions about use of services. Table 4-10 shows caregiver's subjective assessment of health care for persons with a dementing illness. High proportions reported dissatisfaction with the service, a position consistent with the concerns expressed publicly and through ADRDA.

The responses in tables 4-11 and 4-12 show that these persons made considerable use of physicians (although this sample cannot be assumed to the representative). Many respondents reported that professional caregivers were not knowledgeable

Table 4-10.—Assessment of Health Care Professional's Role in Caring for Patients With Alzheimer's or Another Dementing Illness

What is your reaction to these statements?	Strongly agree	Agree	Disagree	Strongly disagree	Not sure/ not applicable	No answer
The assistance I've received from health care professionals—in caring for an individual with Alzheimer's disease—has been excellent.............	8	29	23	12	19	9
In my experience, most health care professionals know little about *managing* patients who have Alzheimer's disease..	21	36	20	2	13	9
From what I have seen, a patient who is ill with dementia receives *worse* care from health professionals than patients who are ill with something else	15	24	30	4	20	7
I have found it difficult to find satisfactory paid professionals to assist in caring for an Alzheimer's patient at home..	25	26	8	1	29	11
I really don't know where to go to get help in caring for an Alzheimer's patient at home	20	28	21	3	17	11
In my view, the existing nursing homes where Alzheimer's patients might live are inadequate in the care they provide	20	30	20	4	19	8

NOTE: Percentages rounded to nearest whole number.

SOURCE: Yankelovich, Skelly, & White, Inc., "Caregivers of Patients With Dementia," contract report prepared for the Office of Technology Assessment, U.S. Congress, 1986.

Table 4-11.—Number of Physicians Seen by Patient To Diagnose or Treat the Dementia

Number of physicians seen	Total respondents
1....................................	18%
2 to 3..............................	46%
More than 3	20%
Don't know/no answer	17%

NOTE: Percentages rounded to nearest whole number.

SOURCE: Yankelovich, Skelly, & White, Inc., "Caregivers of Patients With Dementia," contract report prepared for the Office of Technology Assessment, U.S. Congress, 1986.

Table 4-12.—Frequency of Patient Visits to a Physician Who Treats Patients With Dementia

Frequency	Total respondents
At least once a month	25%
Several times a year	19%
Only occasionally	27%
Never...............................	16%
No answer	12%

NOTE: Percentages rounded to nearest whole number.

SOURCE: Yankelovich, Skelly, & White, Inc., "Caregivers of Patients With Dementia," contract report prepared for the Office of Technology Assessment, U.S. Congress, 1986.

Table 4-13.—Amount of Trouble Finding a Doctor To Care Adequately for Patient With Dementia

How much trouble had	Total respondents
A great deal of trouble	17%
A moderate amount	25%
Only a little........................	16%
None at all	30%
No answer	12%

NOTE: Percentages rounded to nearest whole number.

SOURCE: Yankelovich, Skelly, & White, Inc., "Caregivers of Patients With Dementia," contract report prepared for the Office of Technology Assessment, U.S. Congress, 1986.

Table 4-14.—Level of Satisfaction With Care Patient Currently Receives From Doctor(s)

How satisfied are you?	Total responses
Very satisfied........................	25%
Moderately satisfied	33%
Only somewhat satisfied	21%
Not satisfied at all	9%
No answer	12%

NOTE: Percentages rounded to nearest whole number.

SOURCE: Yankelovich, Skelly, & White, Inc., "Caregivers of Patients With Dementia," contract report prepared for the Office of Technology Assessment, U.S. Congress, 1986.

about care of patients with dementia, or that they had trouble finding a physician to care adequately for the patient (tables 4-13 and 4-14). While these figures represent a serious knowledge gap, equal numbers of respondents who used a family doctor for care reported satisfaction with physician expertise (table 4-15). These findings may be an indication that some sectors are responding to the

Table 4-15.—Caregiver Rating of Family Doctor's Knowledge of Care of Persons With Dementia

Doctor's rating	Total respondents[a]
Very knowledgeable	17%
Somewhat knowledgeable	53%
Not knowledgeable	16%
Don't know/no answer	14%

[a]Among caregivers reporting that the patient sees a family doctor; base is 88 percent of those surveyed.
NOTE: Percentages rounded to nearest whole number.
SOURCE: Yankelovich, Skelly, & White, Inc., "Caregivers of Patients With Dementia," contract report prepared for the Office of Technology Assessment, U.S. Congress, 1986.

demand for improved care of these individuals. However, the group surveyed may be better able to locate services than others who do not receive ADRDA newsletters and information. The informed family physician plays an important role in maintaining patient function (31) (see ch. 2). Pathologists (who conduct autopsies), ophthalmologists, podiatrists, and dentists who are knowledgeable about the care of confused persons are also important to families.

The OTA report found that 64 percent of persons with dementia have been hospitalized at least overnight since becoming ill with dementia, but of these, only 41 percent of caregivers felt hospital care had been good. Twenty-six percent reported receiving fair care, and 21 percent said care was poor. Nineteen percent of families felt that the patient had been discharged from the hospital prematurely.

The Family Survival Project in San Francisco, CA, points out that families often report a need for legal and financial advice and counseling. Families need help with wills, insurance, and property disposition (56). Lawyers and financial advisors received criticism for their lack of knowledge about the illness. OTA found that 60 percent of families had consulted a lawyer to obtain power of attorney or guardianship, but only 27 percent of them felt that the attorney was informed about the disease. Thirty-eight percent of families sought professional financial advice, with 29 percent of these reporting they found a knowledgeable consultant.

Family members may work hard to get a confused person to visit a physician or lawyer. When that professional fails to offer appropriate help,

families may be unable to persuade the confused person to visit a second professional.

Caregivers gave nursing homes mixed marks. Fifty-four percent of families had applied for admission to a nursing home at some time; 30.5 percent of the patients had been in more than one home. Ten percent of these patients had been asked to leave a nursing home, usually due to their behavior. That response by nursing homes places great burdens on the caregiver who must find another resource for a hard-to-place and often severely ill individual. Such requests are often made suddenly; families have only a few days to find a new facility or arrange for care at home.

Of those families using nursing homes, 18 percent say the care the patient received was excellent; 37 percent reported it to be good; 27 percent say care was "average"; and 16 percent said care was poor or very poor. Families who had placed a patient in a nursing home in the preceding year experienced greater stress than families who were providing care at home (33).

Caregivers report a great need for services (ch. 6 discusses the availability and use of supportive services). Sixty-four percent of caregivers said that having the services of a paid companion in the home for a few hours a week to give the caregiver a rest is essential. However, more than 40 percent of the families ranked all services except domiciliary care as "essential/most important." The rank order may be of less significance than the families' overall need for a range of services.

Many respondents reported that services were not available, but a surprising number were unsure about availability. Although that uncertainty may reflect a need for case management (see discussion of issue 3, "Issues and Options" section, below), it may also indicate absence of services. Almost half of caregivers report that visiting nurses or paid companions were available, but fewer than one in four thought that overnight respite, adult day care, or domiciliary care was available. Many reported that available services were too expensive (see table 7-4, ch. 7).

In summary, the minimal availability of services, the difficulty in locating services, cost, and the absence of informed professionals can add significantly to the burdens experienced by caregivers.

For some family members, providing information about resources is not sufficient. Family members may be so demoralized that they are unable to negotiate the bureaucracy in search of help. The OTA study revealed that half of families ranked "help in locating people or organizations that provide care for the patient" as "most important" and 47 percent of families ranked "assistance in applying for Medicare, OASDI, etc.," as "most important" (see table 4-16).

Day care, home care, and other programs report large amounts of staff time spent helping families find other needed resources or giving short-term, problem-oriented counseling even though their funding sources do not provide for such assistance. Typically, a day care program may offer the following services to one caregiver over a period of about 2 years: referral to a support group, referral to a dentist who cares for people with dementia, advice on behavior management, assistance in better coordinating the help of other family members, referral to a lawyer, referral to a private home health aide, short-term counseling, and, finally, help in selecting a nursing home. Thus, the current fragmented nature of the service providing system compounds the caregiver's burden.

The Impact Over Time

For many caregivers the tasks of care may extend over 10 years or more (85). In this way dementing illnesses differ from many others. During such a long period, many changes may occur in the caregiver's own status—employment, marriage, personal health, and children—that can affect that person's ability to provide care. The nature of the illness and the demands it makes also change over time. The burden on families shifts but does not necessarily increase (86). Some families report that it is easier to care for a bedfast patient than for an agitated and wandering one. Others find that the physical effort of providing total personal care is more difficult.

Such factors affect the family's continued ability to care at home. (Some of the hypotheses regarding the family's ability to care over time are discussed later.) Little is known, however, about the impact such prolonged caregiving has on the

Table 4-16.—Assessment of Importance of Certain Services To Be Provided to Patients With Dementia, Regardless of Cost and Current Availability

How important is it that these services be provided?	Essential, very/most important %	Very important %	Important %	Not so important %	No answer %
A paid companion who can come to the home a few hours each week to give caregivers a rest	64	19	7	3	7
Assistance in locating people or organizations that provide care for the patient	50	26	12	3	9
Assistance in applying for Medicaid, OASDI, SSI, etc.	47	20	15	5	12
Paid companion—overnight care	48	23	13	7	9
A home health aide—a person paid to provide personal care for a patient, such as bathing, dressing, or feeding in the home	46	27	13	6	8
Support groups of others who are caring for persons with dementia	45	26	14	5	10
Nursing home care—special nursing home programs only for persons with dementia	43	22	17	8	11
Respite care—temporary round-the-clock care in a nursing home or hospital to care for the patient while the caregiver is away or takes some rest	43	25	16	7	9
A visiting nurse—a registered nurse paid to provide nursing care to the patient at home	36	23	19	19	9
Adult day care—a group program that provides out-of-the-home activity and supervision during the day	36	22	19	12	11
Domiciliary or boarding care—a living arrangement that provides residential care but not nursing care either in another family's home or in a group home	21	15	24	26	14

NOTE: Percentages rounded to nearest whole number.
SOURCE: Office of Technology Assessment, 1987.

family members themselves. Nor is there adequate information on how easily people return to normal social activities, employment, and good health at the end of their work as caregivers.

Are the Burdens Caused by Dementia Unique to the Condition?

In 1985, Secretary of Health and Human Services Margaret Heckler stated that:

> . . . the pattern of care for persons with Alzheimer's disease is not unlike the long-term care required for many other adults with multiple numbers of chronic physical and mental impairments (78).

In contrast, one expert claimed that those with dementia are more likely to be institutionalized because:

> . . . senile dementia is the most socially disruptive ailment of all, placing a particularly severe burden on families (8).

The position of the Department of Health and Human Services (DHHS) was based on studies that showed that functional ability, how much a person can do for him- or herself, is a better measure than a diagnosis for determining the amount of care the individual will need. (One person with a diagnosis of cancer may be able to dress, eat, and bathe while another person with the same diagnosis might need total care.)

For several reasons, it is difficult to carry that assumption to dementia. DHHS relied on findings that applied to the costs of institutional care, not to the burdens of families, which might be quite different. And, as discussed in chapter 7, the care needs of persons with impaired thinking may be quite different from those with a physical handicap. Studies such as the Resource Utilization Group Survey based their findings on measurements made in traditional nursing homes (22), where the physical care model might be inappropriately applied to people who have dementia.

Many believe that caregiving is made more difficult by the unique characteristics of a dementing illness that affect the relationship between the caregiver and the care receiver, impede communication, cause a lack of cooperation or apprecia-

tion for care, require constant supervision, and lead to bizarre behaviors. Since dementia is characterized by changes in behavior, it may be more appropriate to compare the problems of caring for a person with dementia to those of caring for a person with mental retardation, brain damage, or mental illnesses.

Greater caregiver stress has been noted in those who care for persons with more personal care dependencies, more symptoms of mental impairment, and more disruptive or "acting out" behaviors (19,41,52,59). Of these, one study found disruptive behavior to be most stressful for families (59).

Caregivers of persons with a dementing illness have been compared with those who care for equally impaired, nondemented elderly:

> Caring for the physically disabled versus the mentally disabled are unique situations . . . . The mean number of hours spent providing care was remarkably similar, . . . but the personal stress and negative feelings were significantly higher for the dementia group . . . and caregivers of dementia victims were more likely to be considering placement (7).

How Will Changing Patterns of Family Life Affect the Availability of Caregivers in the Future?

Increasing Numbers of the Very Old

The oldest age groups are among the fastest growing segments of the population. It is these groups that are most at risk of developing a dementia (12). They are also more vulnerable to multiple health problems, increasing the amount of care they may need, and reducing the likelihood that family members can provide it. The very old are more often widowed or have a spouse too frail or ill to care for a person with dementia (8). Their children are entering old age themselves. One study found that 40 percent of those admitted to a nursing home had an adult son or daughter over 60, and that half the applications for admission to a nursing home were precipitated by the death or severe illness of the spouse or adult child (8). Thus age makes this cohort both more vulnerable to dementia and less likely to have caregivers available.

As more people live into old age, four-generation families become more common. From the point of view of the younger potential care provider, the family tree is exceedingly top heavy (9). Over time, an individual caregiver may provide care to several dependent family members: an in-law, a parent, and a spouse. In addition, the declining birth rate reduces the ratio between potential caregivers and the elderly. Other changes—including the increasing number of women working outside the home, rising divorce rates, mobility, and smaller families—also contribute to the number of persons without available caregivers.

Return of Women to the Work Force

The number of working women has quadrupled in the past 50 years, with women between the ages of 45 and 64 accounting for the largest increase in the labor force (80). It is women in this age group who are most likely to be called on to provide care for a parent or spouse with a dementing disease. Although women of all ages agree that care of a frail elderly relative becomes the responsibility of daughters, the majority also feel that a woman should not adjust her work schedule to care for aging parents (10).

Women face conflicting demands on their time—work, parents, children, an aging spouse—a conflict that has been called the "woman in the middle" (9). Often women in older cohorts give up time for rest or recreation for themselves. Some point out that there is a limit to the amount these women can do (9). Others argue that the "baby boom" women have entered the labor force and are raising children, with fathers assuming a more active role in child care (51). Currently working women are more willing than those of previous generations to purchase child care while they work, and they may follow the same pattern in care of their parents, with sons assuming increasing responsibility for aging parents and with families becoming more willing to purchase care for elderly family members. Single women heads of households and low-income women, however, have fewer options for sharing or purchasing care (52).

Increasing Numbers of Single Persons Living Alone

The number of single-person households is increasing (76). These individuals lack the most common source of caregivers should they become impaired—others members of a household. Since individuals with dementia generally need a person living in the home to provide supervision, the growing number of persons living alone is of particular concern. The OTA study found that 4 percent of persons with a dementing illness were living by themselves. That figure is probably a significant underestimate because the sample was taken from those who had taken action to join ADRDA—unlikely in the case of an individual with dementia living alone.

The insidious onset of Alzheimer's disease is often overlooked in persons who continue to live by themselves although significantly impaired. They are at risk of accidents, robbery, and severe personal neglect, and they pose dilemmas for social agencies who are asked to assist them.

High Divorce Rates and Changing Patterns of Remarriage and Cohabitation

The current frequency of divorce and remarriage can be expected to have an impact on the number of caregivers available to persons with dementia. Single adults often have multiple responsibilities for children, employment, and homemaking and may have little time for the added demands of caring for the elderly. Divorced women frequently have lower incomes and are thus less able to purchase care. In fact, many such women depend on their parents, if they are healthy, to provide both financial help and child care.

Remarried families have complex and varied loyalties and feelings of obligation that complicate plans for coordinated patient care. The number of unmarried couples living together is also increasing and these people may have different concepts of responsibility for "in-law" care (9).

Increasing Mobility of Families

One study found that most elderly persons have at least one child living near them, and that child's proximity has been stable for over 20 years (66). But often only one child assumes responsibility for the majority of parental care because siblings live out of town. The role of these more distant adult children in caregiving is unknown. However, it is known that caregivers who feel well supported by their families feel less burdened by care. This feeling of support may be more important to the caregiver than even the severity of patient behaviors (85). Isolated caregivers thus may be additionally burdened by the limited support of other family members imposed by geographic distance.

Changing Attitudes About Family Responsibility

Some commentators believe that the spouses of persons with dementia demonstrate exceptional loyalty to the ill partner, remaining in the marriage and providing care for many years (36). Whether future cohorts of caregiving spouses will display a similar loyalty is not known. Most of the present group of elderly Americans are in first marriages of long duration at the time of the onset of the disease. In addition, this cohort entered marriage with a commitment to a lifelong relationship. Future cohorts with marriages of shorter duration or different commitments may show different patterns.

HELPING FAMILIES

A major concern for those who shape policy for persons with dementia and their families is identifying services that will assist caregivers and at the same time control government costs. Respite care has been identified as a key element in helping families and has been proposed as a means of reducing costs by enabling families to continue to care at home rather than turn to more costly nursing home care. Respite care is any formal program that cares for the person with dementia on a part-time basis so that the caregiver can rest, remain employed, seek medical care, etc. Respite programs include in-home companion care, in-home personal care, adult day care, and short-term stays in a nursing home, hospital, or boarding home.

A Duke University survey of families (26) and the OTA survey (see table 4-16) both found that families preferred care in the home to other forms of respite. The OTA study also found that families called several options for respite care "urgently needed." That finding, rather than the ranking of those options, may be the most significant: A family's choice of services may change as the patient's disease progresses and the family's ability to provide care changes.

The Family Survival Project has described the characteristics of respite it has found to be workable. This description points out that respite is intended to be temporary, is not to replace other services, and describes what works with family caregivers.

- Respite services work best when the family (and, if possible, the patient) works with the service provider to structure the care plan. Before a program is set up, the ages and traditional values of both the disabled person and the caregiver (and others in the home) should be considered, as should the home environment and the relationship between the patient/disabled person and the caregiver. The patient's functional level and behavioral status should be assessed in conjunction with the caregiver's health status and needs for relief.
- Any amount of respite seems to work for those who accept it as an option. Ten hours a week of home care, 1 day a week in day care centers, an occasional weekend, 2 weeks in a foster home—all achieve some degree of relief and help to postpone or avoid institutional placement and family breakdown.

- In cases where the patient or caregiver faces a deteriorating situation, usually because of failing health, respite must be seen as a temporary solution. It is not a substitute for the family but for a much needed community-based and coordinated long-term care program.
- As many community resources as possible should be utilized in designing and providing a respite service. What works in a respite program will depend on what supports it in the community: volunteer programs, day care centers, nursing homes, companion programs, etc.
- Training of family members in physical patient care, behavioral problem management (particularly for persons with dementing illness or mental disability), financial management, and stress reduction all enhance the potential for success of respite. At the same time, self-care training for disabled persons will increase opportunities for independence. Respite is, after all, temporary and time controlled and should be offered together with other caregiving education.
- All situations will not be served by respite care. Many family members do not seem to give up their care role easily, even when 24-hour care exceeds 10 to 20 years. For some caregivers, the concept of respite is simply an unknown and, once the new term is explained, they seek the service readily. Others fear that one small vacation will disrupt their ability to continue as they did before. Some fear that once the patient is out of the home for even a short period, the door to permanent institutional placement will be opened. As in home health care, strangers in the home present problems to some families. Many patients are too ill or disabled (given the declining health of the caregiver) to be cared for at home, and respite will help only in a short-term, limited way. Appropriateness of respite must be considered for each situation (58).

Will Improving Supports for Caregivers Ease the Burdens on Families?

Although the burden families experience is well established, and some things are known about the groups most at risk (28), the relationship between providing respite or support and reducing family burdens may not be straightforward. For example, increased respite will not alleviate the grief that adds to the caregiver's experience of burden. Also, the level of either distress or burden may not correlate with family use of nursing homes. Families may choose to keep a person at home despite their burden, or because a satisfactory nursing home may not be available. There may be no relationship between burden and placement, or the relationship may be a complex one, involving behavioral symptoms, prior relationship, the needs of the family, and access to suitable care.

Two conflicting theories about family needs sometimes influence policy. The "wear and tear" theory holds that families are fragile and unstable, and that unless they are assisted they will become exhausted, overburdened, unable to provide adequate care to the frail elderly, and impaired as a family unit (subject, for example, to divorce, delinquency, substance abuse, chronic illnesses of caregivers, or suicide). The "adaptation" theory, on the other hand, assumes that families have a great capacity for change and therefore will adjust to the demands of care, through sharing of tasks, purchase of care, personal growth, and so on.

Neither theory has been proven. Either can be argued effectively on the basis of existing data. Equally significant is the fact that either can be intuitively accepted, based on one's knowledge of families. Thus they both influence public thinking about the kinds of services and government assistance families need.

Although researchers disagree about the kinds of care needed and the nature of the burden experienced, no one claims that most families are *not* burdened. Evidence of increased substance abuse and indications of poor mental health support the position that at least some families are vulnerable to the pressures of care.

The fact that the majority of caregivers continue to provide care for years and to juggle the many demands of caregiving, employment, and the needs of other family members does not entirely support the hypothesis of adaptation, for it does not reveal the damage done by concealed stress.

One study found that husbands who provided care complained less about the burden of care but tended to die prematurely (26).

The most reasonable assumption is that both theories are correct. Some families adapt successfully to the demands of caregiving for at least part of a relative's illness, and others show symptoms of distress (26). In fact, a family may adapt successfully for part of the illness but experience problems during other periods. One study found that caregivers were more stressed in the year following nursing home placement than were those caring for a patient at home (26) but bereaved caregivers experienced increased well being. This indicates that relief from caregiving does not necessarily bring relief from the emotional burden of care.

Research has identified some ways in which family burden or distress can be alleviated (32,35,64). Counseling and support groups decrease caregivers' feelings of loneliness and of being misunderstood. They also help caregivers better adapt to the demands of caregiving. Families and respite care staff both report that respite from caregiving plays a vital role in reducing family stress and burden. Families are enthusiastic in their praise of respite programs and many report that a program "saved my life" or "kept me sane." Family concern over the urgent need for respite has led ADRDA chapters to set up successful grassroots programs (see ch. 7). However these elements may not influence the family decision to place a person in a nursing home (86).

A controlled, prospective study (funded by the American Association of Retired Persons and the Andrus Foundation and carried out at Duke University—George and Gwyther, principal investigators) is looking at the effects of home care on the family, the patient, and the provider. Such studies will identify the kinds of services that help families most or predict which services are most urgently needed.

Will Respite Care Reduce Use of Costly Nursing Homes at a Savings to the Taxpayer?

Families clearly need respite. The role of respite in reducing the use of nursing homes and the cost to the taxpayer of institutionalizing, however, is not so clear. In fact, when respite postpones placement, it may also result in the admission of sicker persons, resulting in a more costly case mix. There are several other reasons why provision of respite may not influence cost of institutionalization to the taxpayer.

- Patients without caregiving families will continue to need institutional care.
- Persons with serious multiple illness—including cognitive impairment—will need more care than respite can provide.
- Families may choose to keep ill persons at home despite the burden caused.
- Nursing homes may not be available to some persons.
- Studies that report that respite postpones placement may not have measured what families would actually do in the absence of respite.
- Families now receiving few services may be more willing to use respite than nursing home care.

Half the residents of nursing homes have no family, and those who do have fewer caregivers, or have caregivers who are ill or have sensory impairments (12). The death or serious illness of a caregiver clearly predicts placement (45). Thus more than half the residents of nursing homes have no one to care for them at home. Savings to taxpayers from enabling a family to keep a patient at home longer cannot be calculated on the basis of institutional costs, but only on that fraction of the institutional costs expended on patients with available families. Since the sizes of the oldest cohorts are growing rapidly and since these people are the most vulnerable both to developing a dementia and to loss of caregivers, the need for institutional care for patients without families can be expected to grow.

Many people in nursing homes have multiple illnesses, including dementia or delirium, and need more care than respite can give. The severity of illness, not the presence of dementia or the family's need for respite is the cause of nursing home placement.

In addition, families who do not have close bonds to the person with dementia or who are poorly equipped to provide care can be expected to turn to nursing homes. This group includes families in which the caregiver is not a close relative, the caregiver is seriously or chronically ill, there is a long history of family discord, the caregiver is psychiatrically or intellectually impaired, or the patients' needs are not met because the family is so disorganized. There may be no financial incentive that will make ill-equipped or unavailable kin provide care (51).

Conversely, are there incentives that would encourage more families to keep patients at home longer? One study found that 42 percent of patients who had caregivers lived with that caregiver until the patient died (26). The OTA study found that 74 percent of families felt that a person with a severe dementia should be in a nursing home, but only 45 percent had placed a family member and 48 percent felt that nursing homes did not provide high-quality care. Thus many families never use placement.

Some families chose to keep patients at home, despite the burden; or place loved ones too late rather than too early. Dedication to the ill person and barriers to nursing home use combine to keep people at home. Testimony from the Maryland Governor's Task Force on Alzheimer's Disease and handwritten comments attached to the OTA survey questionnaires included many reports of a frail or exhausted caregiver continuing to care at home for a person who needed skilled nursing care. Respondents indicated that the cost of the nursing home would impoverish both the caregiver and the ill person.

As stated, 48 percent of the respondents to the OTA survey felt that nursing homes provided unacceptably poor quality care. Families also resist nursing home care because they have much less control of their relatives' quality of life or type of care after placement, especially when Medicaid funds are used (33). Caregiver attitudes about the quality of care nursing homes provide has been found to be at least as important to placement as the ill person's physical and emotional health (20).

Nursing homes may not be available to some people. The General Accounting Office found that persons with dementia are less likely than other individuals to be admitted to nursing homes and, if admitted, less likely to receive quality care (72). Cost saving ceilings on nursing home beds, imposed by some States, create a situation in which nursing home bed use is artificially low. Difficult dementia patients are less likely to be admitted than other patients.

While certain incentives such as tax credits might help a subgroup of affluent families, the commitment families show to continue providing care despite the stress it causes indicates that further incentives would have a limited impact on caregiving. In addition, there may be negative implications to incentives: Is it desirable to encourage an employed head of household to give up a job to provide more hours of care? Should incentives encourage a frail wife to continue to care for a violent husband? Should incentives encourage a caregiver who is abusing tranquilizers to continue providing care? How can a caregiving wife care for an ill husband much larger than she is? If the caregiver becomes ill from caregiving, both persons may need institutionalization—at a greater cost.

Discouraging nursing home use further may compromise patient care and family survival. Since families are already providing almost all care, the effect of further incentives may be limited by families' ability to do more. Virtually the only resources available to families are nursing homes and family support groups.

Furthermore, there may be many families needing extensive care that are not now using nursing homes due to bed shortages, cost, poor quality care, etc. These families may be more willing to use respite resources than existing nursing home services, especially if a plan for shared payment allows the family to remain partially in control of care and if such services are readily accessible, are individualized, and provide better care than families believe is available in nursing homes.

Will Providing Supports for Caregivers Cause Them To Do Less for the Recipient?

There has long been a debate over whether formal supports tend to supplant informal support (friends, family, or neighbors). Much of the evidence, however, indicates that both formal and informal care, working together, would best serve persons with dementia. For example, the object of respite care is to provide care for some of the hours a family would otherwise cover. Replacement of family care is intended in this case, and should be expected. In other cases, caps on respite reimbursement stretch programs' limited resources. Such caps also control runaway costs. The Family Survival Project, which offers respite care, reports that 59 percent of families in the respite program supplemented cost out of pocket in 1984-85 (57). Counseling and family support groups offer caregivers improved caregiving skills, reassurance, and other assistance, supplementing informal services rather than supplanting them.

The current behavior of families supports the belief that they will continue to care for family members. Despite the fact that Medicaid encourages institutionalization over home care for some people, families have resisted use of nursing homes until they can no longer manage. Indeed, a common complaint in nursing homes is that some caregivers continue to spend many hours a week with patients and are not reestablishing their other social relationships.

Studies have shown that families do not decrease the care they provide when alternative services are available. Many of the services families provide are individualized and are offered at all hours and on weekends (23). The family "contribution" includes emergency assistance for short periods (28). In addition, important components of the family contribution include love, financial advice, and someone to talk to—things no formal support service is likely to supply. And given the magnitude of the need for supportive care resources, it is unlikely that a program large enough to supplant the family could be established. Some caregivers provide all care and refuse offers of assistance such as day care even when clearly overburdened. The thrust of public policy will be most effective if it aims to supplement, not supplant, family care.

Factors Leading a Family To Seek Nursing Home Placement

Research has sought to identify the factors that lead to placing someone in a nursing home. If re-

searchers could identify a specific behavior that is likely to trigger placement, better treatment of that symptom might result in fewer placements. Unfortunately no such factor has been identified. Incontinence, violence, extreme mood swings, and night wandering are suspected as precipitants of placement, but the data neither confirm nor refute this belief. Severity of physical disability as well as severity of mental impairment both add to caregiver stress (19,41,53,59) and perhaps to the decision to place a person in the nursing home. Rather than seeing specific problems (such as incontinence) as overwhelming, the experience of families is variable, with many factors, not just behavior, causing burden (86).

The characteristics of caregivers influence placement decisions at least as much as the characteristics of the person with dementia. A prospective study identified caregivers who are more likely to turn to nursing home care. They are often younger women, and more often the adult child of the ill person than the spouse. They report high levels of stress, used more psychotropic drugs in the year before placement, and had higher incomes (16). Caregivers who are isolated or have sensory impairments may also be more likely to use placement (33).

Studies That Examine the Relationship of Respite and Placement

Some studies have looked at patients already in nursing homes and asked questions about why they were admitted. For example, the New York State Respite Demonstration Project found that families receiving services were less inclined than before to place patients in nursing homes (48); another study reported that families found daycare postpones placement (55). These studies are subject to bias; the weakness of retrospective research is that there may be a difference between what families think they would have done, and what they actually have done.

Several studies funded by the Health Care Financing Administration (HCFA) under so-called 2176 waivers have matched families receiving care with a control group who did not receive respite care (see ch. 11 for a discussion of 2176 waivers). These studies looked at the frail elderly in general, not just those with dementia. But to ensure that the intervention was directed at persons who really were at risk of placement, the studies required that all persons in the experimental and control groups be eligible for Medicare's skilled nursing care (a medically oriented definition that excludes the kind of care needed by people in the middle stages of dementia). These studies did not find significant differences in placement rates between those using and not using respite care. One possible explanation is that the skilled care requirements meant that interventions were offered too late (i.e., when the patient already needed more care than the family could provide) and that if family stress is to be reduced, or placement postponed, the intervention must be made earlier. Also, selection for those requiring skilled care would exclude most people with dementia unless they also have other serious illnesses or are in the late phases of their dementia.

A study at Duke University found that families who used formal community services were more likely to turn to placement within a year (26). This finding supports the hypothesis that families who actually need nursing home care turn to respite when they are desperate, but are reluctant to think about nursing home care. The involvement of a professional may reassure families of their need for more help with care. Respite may be a temporary bridge—the Family Survival Project originally named its program "Bridges to Survival"—between total family care and institutionalization. Such a bridge may be necessary for families and it needs to be provided before it is too late to help (33). It may be inappropriate to consider respite as a solution to the high public costs of nursing homes. Policies that place cost saving as the primary goal of respite care may be likely to fail.

The OTA survey asked families who had used respite care why they had stopped using it (see ch. 7). The most common reason was that the person had entered a nursing home. The other major reasons are that the service is too expensive, the patient died or became worse, or the caregivers found they did not need the service. These findings support the hypothesis that nursing home care is a needed part of the continuum of care for many families, and that after a certain point other services do not prevent its use. (These data do *not* tell whether respite postponed nursing home placement.) The finding that many families in the survey did not feel the need for respite services does not indicate that these resources are not needed in general. Respite care is probably most needed in the middle phases of a dementing illness. Many respondents were caring for people who were too ill to use programs such as day care or who were too early in the course of their illness to need constant supervision. That finding may also explain the number of families who avoid using formal services.

Provision of family support may postpone placement, though studies have not yet confirmed that hypothesis. Recent studies do point to interventions that should be tested: providing additional emotional support to caregivers, using information to reduce difficulties in providing care, case management, assistance, equipment, or respite (16,20,50). Interventions to reduce disruptive and socially inappropriate behavior and to enable management of incontinence are also needed.

In summary, the reasons behind placement may lie with the characteristics of the family and its support system:

> When physicians assess a patient's need for nursing home care, it is not enough to evaluate symptoms or to know how long the patient has been ill or functioning at the current level. The structure and characteristics of the caregiver support system are also important—and, in fact, are better predictors of institutional placement than patient characteristics (20).

The combined stress of multiple role demands, problems in caring for the patient, the caregivers' perception of burden, the absence of support or help, the lack of information about how to care for the patient, and high cost, poor quality, and limited capacity may all be factors in nursing home placement. The final straw may be less significant than the years of attrition that have finally exhausted the caregiver (12).

ISSUES AND OPTIONS

ISSUE 1: Should the Government Encourage Families To Assume Additional Responsibility for Their Relatives Who Have a Dementing Illness?

Option 1. Make no change in the current division of responsibility for persons with dementia between government and families.

Option 2. Encourage greater family responsibility for persons with dementia.

Option 3. Assume a greater share of the task of caring for persons with dementia.

Examples of the government shouldering more of the burden (option 3) include tax breaks to caregivers, allowing services on the basis of caregiver need as well as patient need, reimbursing respite programs, and correcting inequities in Medicaid laws.

Examples of encouraging increased family responsibility (option 2) include holding sons and daughters responsible for parent care in a nursing home, encouraging purchase of insurance coverage, reverse mortgage plans, etc. The complex issue of the responsibility of government and families is discussed in chapter 12. This chapter has pointed out some of the issues raised about families.

1. Families already provide the majority of care.
2. Families provide kinds of care that formal services cannot or do not provide.
3. Current policies create inequities in the financial burden imposed on families; for example, spouses, particularly women, are more likely to be impoverished by care than other family members.
4. Efforts to control government expenditures can result in inequitable access to services; persons who are dependent on Medicaid, have a dementia, and who have behavior problems are less likely to be admitted to nursing homes.
5. Current funding policy encourages use of nursing homes but does not support use of other services.
6. Respite care cannot be assumed to be a substitute for nursing home care, but is needed by families to assist them in the burdens of care and to reduce caregiver exhaustion and burnout.
7. Families prefer to share the costs and burdens of care. The present system, however, requires families to impoverish themselves and to give up control and involvement in patient care in order to receive help with the cost of institutionalization.
8. Current funding is based on medical need for care. This approach excludes many patients and their families from appropriate assistance until late in their illness.
9. Families contribute about half the costs of nursing home care and most of the costs of respite care, as well as large amounts of in-kind services and room and board.

Efforts to obtain further contributions from families may be difficult and costly to enforce. Such steps could harm some caregivers and families (by leading to increased drug use, poor health, inattention to children, loss of employment) or push families to neglect the person with dementia.

If government assumes a greater role in caring for persons with dementia (option 3), it will probably cost more than the current government share of care (see ch. 12 for a more complete discussion).

ISSUE 2: Should the Government Include the Caregiver in the Definition of the Care Recipient?

Option 1. Continue to consider eligibility for services based only on the needs of the patient.

Option 2. Modify existing programs to provide services that are more social and less narrowly medical in defining eligibility.

Option 3. Modify existing programs so that individuals with dementia are eligible for services geared to the caregiver.

Option 4. Develop new programs that provide both care for the patient and care aimed at giving respite to the caregiver.

Current criteria for eligibility for most services is based on the needs of the ill person. However, it is clear that caregivers of persons with dementia also need services to enable them to continue to provide care and to reduce the negative effects of burden. Option 1, maintaining current criteria for eligibility for services, will help to contain costs, but places severe and in some cases harmful burdens on families and includes inequities of access.

Providing services to other than ill persons (option 4) would require a major shift from current policy. It would also create difficult issues in determining which caregivers should be eligible for service. A compromise would be to broaden patient eligibility for social or psychosocial services (option 2). These are the kinds of services most often needed by persons with dementia and their families and include case management (or case coordination, or information and referral), adult day care, in-home respite care, and short-term respite care. Support for this approach comes from preliminary findings that both the individual and the caregiver benefit from psychosocial interventions (see ch. 7.)

Option 3, modifying existing program so that individuals with dementia are eligible for services geared to the caregiver, would limit additional costs to those people who are now eligible for services. However, this option would exclude services to those families in which it is the caregiver's need for help, rather than the patient's need for service, that precipitates placement or caregiver morbidity. Since access to services is already limited for persons not needing skilled nursing care, this plan would restrict help for the caregiver except when the patient is severely ill. Many providers believe that if interventions are to be effective, they must be provided early enough to avoid caregiver burnout.

While option 4 would require a shift of policy, it has the major advantage of being flexible enough to allow the system to respond either to the needs of the patient or of the caregiver.

Options 2, 3, and 4 would probably increase costs. In most instances, they will not replace existing services, which are generally limited to the patient's need for skilled nursing care. In addition, an unknown number of persons in the community who are not now using funded services will use respite or home care services. The ex-tent to which interventions aimed at the caregiver will postpone or prevent placement is not known. It is almost certain that additional services will reduce caregiver burden, may reduce caregiver morbidity, and may enable caregivers to remain productively employed.

ISSUE 3: Should the Government Assist in Coordination or Selection of Services

Option 1. Leave case management a State, local, or informal system.

Option 2. Link case coordination or case management to services it provides or funds.

Option 3. In place of case management or case coordination, require that programs using Federal funds establish and use efficient coordination with other existing programs.

Information about available service is a primary need for caregivers. The OTA survey found that many families need help finding services and negotiating the system to obtain needed services. Families also need information on a variety of topics: how and where to get help, what the implications of a diagnosis of dementia are, what the genetic risks are, what costs and burdens they will face and should plan for (39,43). Families and service providers report that existing services are fragmented and that families and patients cannot move easily from one to another.

Case management has been proposed as one method of assisting families. One accepted definition of case management describes functions in terms of long-term care:

> The principal functions of case management in long-term care are the following: 1) screening and determining eligibility; 2) assessing the need for services and related needs; 3) care planning (developing a care plan); 4) requisitioning services; 5) implementing the service plan, coordinating service delivery and following up; and 6) reassessing, monitoring, and evaluating services periodically (6).

The lack of available information, services, and limited and uneven case management resources have been well documented. The existing services are not well coordinated in many areas. Those providing services frequently do not know about or refer families to complementary resources. And there are major gaps in the range of services available. The need for better referral to services and coordination of services is clear; the solution is less clear.

Case management is rarely mentioned as a critical part of any respite program although many programs offer some form of case management despite the absence of funding for it. Many argue that case management is essential to efficient service delivery (33). OTA previously reviewed the effectiveness of cases management systems such as ACCESS, TRIAGE, and channeling (73). The effect of such programs on persons with dementia or their families is not known. However, families rarely seek and use as many services on their own as case managers would prescribe.

There may be great variations in the amount of case management a family will need. Some families may be so overwhelmed by the demands of care that they cannot seek help for themselves, even when given the necessary information. Individuals with dementia who have no family member to coordinate services are especially disadvantaged. Service providers often do not help such people obtain appropriate care. Other families may be capable of coordinating care if supplied with information, and many would prefer to do so rather than use the services of a stranger.

Case management can have several objectives, and they will affect its success. Case management helps persons with dementia and their families use available services. It may enable them to make financial plans for future care needs. It may also permit more efficient use of services. Case management may ensure that individuals are not placed prematurely. It can be used to guarantee that the least restrictive environment be available to those who have no family members to advocate for them. However, when case management is a required part of programs whose goal (or financial objective) is to prevent placement, it can cause further delays and suffering for caregivers already exhausted by care.

The effectiveness of case management is limited when important services are not available. While it can efficiently use services that are available,

case management does not address the related problem, lack of resources.

Case management, or case coordination, can have several kinds of beneficial indirect effects. Formal providers who are reluctant to accept a person with dementia are more likely to do so when they are assured that others are continuing to assist the patient and family. Case managers sometimes informally train providers in care in order to gain admission for a person with dementia. Thus case managers increase the community response. Families are often reluctant to use respite resources, even when their own health or the patient's well being is in jeapordy. Case managers report that an important part of their role is to gain the trust of caregivers and thus enable them to accept services. Case managers can work with a family to reduce conflict and enable family members to better support the caregiver. When little family support is available, the case manager may serve as a substitute, providing necessary encouragement and sympathy to the caregiver.

Because management has strengths and weaknesses, it will be needed by some families and not by others. Families clearly wish to remain in control of the patient's care. Case management must be designed to assist when families are too overwhelmed to seek proper care for themselves or the patient but it must not usurp the family's role.

The existing system (option 1) does not provide needed information about services or ensure that additional case management services are available to those who need them. Option 2, including case coordination or case management in Federal programs, may improve access to services. It would also increase Federal costs, due to both the added service and the tendency of case management to increase the total number of services used. Further, case management must be designed so that it does not usurp family responsibility or create new problems. An effective and efficient method of delivering case management services must be identified.

Whether case management or case coordination is provided or not, more coordinated access to appropriate resources could be achieved by requiring that programs using government funds establish effective liaisons with other nearby programs so that they all routinely inform caregivers of other services that might help them (option 3). Federal agency policies could be reviewed for their impact on "issues related to overlapping and conflicting responsibilities. Federal funds could be directed toward communities that have established interagency cooperation and have resolved issues of duplication of services.

ISSUE 4: Should the Government Provide Respite Services?

Option 1. Leave provision or purchase of respite care to the States, the private sector, and to families.

Option 2. Fund a limited number of model respite programs.

Option 3. Provide some or all respite care through direct provision of services, by paying for services, or by such things as tax credits.

Families urgently need low cost, readily available noninstitutional services. These services must not take control away from the family; they must be flexible and varied enough to meet the needs of different families and patients. They should be convenient and offer families options. Passage from one service to another must be smooth, and gaps in service must be eliminated. For at least some families, the caregiver's physical and mental well-being may depend on respite programs. However, not all families use respite when it is available. There appear to be many reasons for this, including the quality and cost of the service, and caregiver's reluctance to turn over even part of care. Families are concerned that their resources will be depleted and seek to postpone purchase of any care, even at reasonable cost, in order to conserve funds. If a continuum of services at known costs were available, families could project their long-term expenses and budget accordingly.

Providing such programs is unlikely to save money, however, either through preventing placement or sustaining the caregiver. And such a program would be costly. Meeting the need for nonin-

stitutional care for large numbers of persons with dementia is probably beyond the capabilities of at least some States (option 1), and programs such as block grants have repeatedly been shown to underserve this population. Many families are unable to purchase the services they need.

However, there is insufficient information about what kinds of services are needed, what services families will use, how much they can afford to pay for services, what care techniques are beneficial to patients and families, and what other barriers to service delivery exist for this group. This lack of information impedes planning a federally funded service package, although a few centers could provide information for later national implementation. Some models do exist: the Family Survival Project has been a notably successful program, and California has initiated studies that will generate answers to some of these questions. If the Federal Government were to support research into care delivery for persons with dementia (option 2), costs of open-ended programs would be avoided, data would be gathered to answer vital questions about services, and some families would benefit directly from the use of pilot programs.

ISSUE 5: Should the Government Make Access to Reimbursable Resources Easier, More Equitable, or Available Sooner?

Option 1. Leave access to Federal programs as is.

Option 2. Change accessibility to, for example, Medicare and Medicaid.

Access to Medicare and Medicaid is discussed in chapters 11 and 12. Extensive modification of these programs could make problems of access even worse for some groups or could significantly increase costs. However, relatively minor changes in these two programs could greatly assist families (option 2). The government could establish a policy requiring all services using Federal funds to make clear and complete information about eligibility and the application process readily available to the public. There is considerable anecdotal information that information given to families is erroneous, or that families have difficulty getting this information. Easy access to such information would reduce the stress families experience in getting help, would assist those families who are given erroneous information, and would encourage families to plan ahead for major health expenditures.

Medicare could expand the coverage for certain home care services to include preventive nursing care. Such visits are not now covered. For example, some clinicians report that many cases of incontinence can be reduced by medical and nursing interventions and by training the family. Nursing visits might therefore reduce incontinence, which is known to be a source of severe burden to caregivers. Severe agitation and hallucinations are also known to respond to medical interventions. Nurses trained in managing these symptoms could greatly reduce the burdens families face. Home visits by a nurse may be preferable to physician office visits because assessment of the patient in the home allows an appraisal of the environmental factors that trigger behavior (see ch. 7).

These are but two examples of many possible. Further discussion of specific options is found in chapter 12. Further information about the care needs of people with dementia (ch. 7) and about respite programs will provide needed data for modifying these programs.

ISSUE 6: Should the Government Provide Family Support Groups or Information Centers for Caregivers?

Option 1. Provide information and support directly to families.

Option 2. Support the private sector in provision of these services.

It is clear that support groups and information are critical for families. The voluntary sector (primarily ADRDA) has been effective in establishing support groups and in disseminating information. However, their efforts have reached primarily the white middle classes. It may be most efficient for government to encourage the endeavors of the private sector (option 2) and focus government skill on research to identify how to reach the hard-to-reach socioeconomic groups. Information dissemination efforts should include the considerable resources of the Federal agencies with relevant expertise, such as the National Institute on Aging, National Institute on Mental Health, Health Care Financing Administration, Administration on Aging, National Center for Health Services Research, and others. A Federal mechanism for centrally collecting relevant information would facilitate both government and private efforts.

In addition, families continue to have difficulty obtaining support and information from the professionals to whom they turn. The government's role in educating these professionals is discussed in chapter 9.

CHAPTER 4 REFERENCES

1. Alzheimer's Disease and Related Disorders Association, *A National Program To Conquer Alzheimer's Disease*, Chicago, IL, 1986.
2. Alzheimer's Disease and Related Disorders Association, Central Maryland Chapter, personal communication, November 1984.
3. Alzheimer's Disease and Related Disorders Association, Greater Philadelphia Chapter, personal communications, November 1984.
4. American Health Care Association, *Trends and Strategies in Long-Term Care*, Washington, DC, 1985.
5. American Medical News, "Senior Citizen Agencies Don't Help Enough," Mar. 21, 1986.
6. Austin, C.D., "Case Management in Long-Term Care: Options and Opportunities," *Health and Social Work*, p. 16, 1983.
7. Birkel, R.C., "Sources of Caregiver Strain in Long-Term Home-Care," contract report prepared for the National Center for Health Services Research, U.S. Department of Health and Human Services, unpublished.
8. Brody, E.M., "The Formal Support Network: Congregate Treatment Settings for Residents With Senescent Brain Dysfunction," N.E. Miller and G.D. Cohen (eds.) *Clinical Aspects of Alzheimer's Disease and Senile Dementia, Aging*, vol. 15 (New York: Raven Press, 1981).
9. Brody, E.M., "Women in the Middle and Family Help to Older People," *The Gerontologist* 21:471-480, 1981.
10. Brody, E.M., "Parent Care as a Normative Stress," *The Gerontologist* 25:19-29, 1985.
11. Brody, E.M., Johnson, P.T., Fulcomer, M., et al.,

"Women's Changing Roles and Help to Elderly Parents: Attitudes of Three Generations of Women," *Journal of Gerontology* 38:597-607, 1983.

12. Brody, E.M., Lawton, M.P., and Liebowitz, B., "Senile Dementia: Public Policy and Adequate Institutional Care," *American Journal of Public Health* 74:1381-1383, 1984.

13. Caplis, J., "Financial Effects of Nursing Home Placement on the Community Spouse," Maryland State Office on Aging, Annapolis, MD, Aug. 1, 1980.

14. Chavkin, D., "Interstate Variability in Medicaid Eligibility and Reimbursement for Dementia Patients," contract report prepared for the Office of Technology Assessment, U.S. Congress, 1986.

15. Chavkin, D., Directing Attorney, Maryland Disability Law Center, personal communication, Aug. 28, 1986.

16. Colerick, E., and George, L.K., "Predictors of Institutionalization Among Caregivers of Alzheimer's Patients," *Journal of the American Geriatrics Society* 34:493-498, 1986.

17. Coons, D., "A Residential Care Unit for Persons With Dementia," contract report prepared for the Office of Technology Assessment, U.S. Congress, 1986.

18. Coons, D., Chenoweth, B., Hollenshead, C., et al., *Final Report of Project on Alzheimer's Disease: Subjective Experiences of Families* (Ann Arbor, MI: Institute of Gerontology, University of Michigan, 1983).

19. Deimling, G.T., and Bass, D.M., *Symptoms of Mental Impairment Among Aged and Their Effects on Family Caregivers* (Cleveland, OH: Benjamin Rose Institute, in press).

20. Deimling, G.T., and Poulshock, S.W., "The Transition From Family In-Home Care to Institutional Care," *Research on Aging* 7:563-576, 1985.

21. Fanning, J., President, National Association of Disability Examiners, personal communication, Oct. 12, 1983.

22. Foley, W.J., "Dementia Among Nursing Home Patients: Defining the Condition, Characteristics of the Demented, and Dementia on the RUG-II Classification System," contract report prepared for the Office of Technology Assessment, U.S. Congress, 1986.

23. Frankfather, D., Smith, M., and Caro, F., *Family Care of the Elderly* (Toronto: Lexington Books, 1981).

24. Friss, L., and Enright, R., "Employed Caregivers of Brain Impaired Adults," Family Survival Project, San Francisco, CA, unpublished.

25. George, L.K., "The Burden of Caregiving," *Center Reports on Advances in Research* 8(2):1-7, 1984.

26. George, L.K., "The Dynamics of Caregiver Burden," Report Submitted to the American Association of Retired Persons, Andrus Foundation, 1984.

27. George, L.K., "The Dynamics of Caregiver Burden: Changes in Caregiver Well-Being Over Time," paper presented at the Gerontological Society of America, November 1984.

28. George, L.K., and Gwyther, L.P., "Caregiver Well-Being: A Multidimensional Examination of Family Caregivers of Demented Adults," *The Gerontologist* 26:253-259, 1986.

29. Glaze, R., Testimony, Joint Hearing Before the Subcommittee on Aging, Senate Committee on Labor and Human Resources, and the Subcommittee on Labor, Health, Education, and Welfare, July 1980 (Washington, DC: U.S. Government Printing Office, 1980).

30. Governor's Task Force on Alzheimer's Disease and Related Disorders, *The Maryland Report on Alzheimer's Disease and Related Disorders*, Annapolis, MD, 1985.

31. Gwyther, L.P., and Blazer, D.G., "Family Therapy and the Dementia Patient," *Family Physician* 29:149-156, 1984.

32. Gwyther, L.P., "Caring for Caregivers: A Statewide Family Support Program Mobilizes Mutual Help," *Center Reports in Advances in Research* 16(4):1-8, 1982.

33. Gwyther, L.P., Director, Family Support Program, Center for the Study of Aging and Human Development, Duke University, personal communication, March 1986.

34. Gwyther, L.P., and George, L.K., "Symposium: Caregivers for Dementia Patients: Complex Determinants of Well Being and Burden: Introduction," *The Gerontologist* 26:245-247, 1986.

35. Harel, Z., and Townsend, A., "Health Vulnerability, Service Needed and Service Use Among the Aged," paper presented at Gerontological Society of America, November 1985.

36. Heckler, M., Secretary of Health and Human Services, presentation to Alzheimer's Disease and Related Diseases Association, Chicago, IL, Sept. 29, 1984.

37. Henderson, J.N., "Mental Disorders Among the Elderly: Dementia and Its Sociocultural Correlates," *Modern Pioneers: An Interdisciplinary View of the Aged*, P. Silverman (ed.) (Bloomington, IN: Indiana University Press, in press).

38. Institute of Medicine, *Improving the Quality of Care in Nursing Homes* (Washington, DC: National Academy Press, 1986).

39. Kahan, J., Kemp, B., Staples, F.R., et al., "Decreasing the Burden, Families Caring for a Relative With

a Dementing Illness," *Journal of the American Geriatrics Society* 23:664-669, 1985.

40. Lezak, M.D., "Living With the Characterologically Altered Brain Injured Patient," *Journal of Clinical Psychiatry* 39:592-598, 1978.

41. Livingston, M., "Families Who Care," *British Medical Journal* 29:919-920, 1985.

42. Lockery, S.A., "Impact of Dementia Within Minority Groups," contract report prepared for the Office of Technology Assessment, U.S. Congress, 1986.

43. Mace, N.L., "Self-Help for the Family," *Alzheimer's Disease and Related Disorders*, W.E. Kelly (ed.) (Springfield, IL: Charles Thomas, 1984).

44. Mace, N.L., and Rabins, P.V., *The 36 Hour Day: A Family Guide to Caring for Persons With Alzheimer's Disease, Related Dementing Illnesses, and Memory Loss in Later Life* (Baltimore, MD: The Johns Hopkins University Press, 1981).

45. Mace, N.L., and Rabins, P.V., "Areas of Stress on Families of Dementia Patients: A Two Year Follow-up," paper presented at the Gerontological Society of America, Boston, MA, Nov. 21, 1982.

46. Mace, N.L., and Rabins, P.V., "A Survey of Day Care for the Demented Adult in the United States," National Council on Aging, Washington, DC, 1984.

47. Mortimer, J.A., and Hutton, J.T., "Epidemiology and Etiology of Alzheimer's Disease," J.T. Hutton and A.D. Kenny (eds.) *Senile Dementia of the Alzheimer's Type* (New York: A.R. Liss 1985).

48. New York State Department of Social Services, Respite Demonstration Project, report to the Governor and members of legislature, Albany, NY, 1985.

49. Freudenheim, M., "Business and Health: Help in Caring for the Elderly," New York Times, Jan. 6, 1986, p. 2.

50. Noelker, L.S., "Incontinence in Elderly Cared for by Family," paper presented at the Gerontological Society of America, San Francisco, CA, Nov. 21, 1983.

51. Noelker, L.S., "Family Care of Elder Relatives: The Impact of Policy and Programs," paper presented at Conference on Families, InterAge; Minneapolis, MN, September 1984.

52. Noelker, L.S., and Wallace, R.W., "The Organization of Family Care for Impaired Elderly," *Journal of Family Issues* 6(1):23-44, 1985.

53. Noelker, L.S., Townsend, A.L., and Deimling, G.T., *Caring for Elders and the Mental Health of Family Members* (Cleveland, OH: Benjamin Rose Institute, 1984).

54. Ory, M.G., Williams, T.F., Emr, M., et al., "Families, Informal Supports and Alzheimer's Disease: Current Research and Future Agendas," working document by the Work Group of Families, Informal Supports, and Alzheimer's Disease, Department of Health and Human Services Task Force on Alzheimer's Disease, 1984.

55. Pannella, J.J., Lilliston, B.A., Brush, D., et al., "Day Care for Dementia Patients: An Analysis of a Four Year Program," *Journal of the American Geriatrics Society* 32:883-886, 1984.

56. Petty, D., Executive Director, Family Survival Project, San Francisco, CA, personal communication, 1986.

57. Petty, D., "The Family Survival Project," contract report prepared for the Office of Technology Assessment, U.S. Congress, 1986.

58. Petty, D., "Respite Care: A Growing National Alternative," *The Coordinator* 34-36, October 1984.

59. Poulshock, S.W., *The Effects on Families of Caring for Impaired Elderly in Residence* (Cleveland, OH: Benjamin Rose Institute, 1982).

60. Poulshock, S.W., and Deimling, G.T., "Families Caring for Elders in Residence: Issues in the Measurement of Burden," *Journal of Gerontology* 39:230-239, 1984.

61. Pratt, C.C., Schmall, V.L., Wright, S., et al., "Burden and Coping Strategies of Caregivers to Alzheimer's Disease Patients," *Family Relations* 34:27-33, 1985.

62. Rabins, P.V., Mace, N.L., and Lucas, M.J., "The Impact of Dementia on the Family," *Journal of the American Medical Association* 848:333-335, 1982.

63. Schorr, A., "Thy Father and Thy Mother: A Second Look at Filial Responsibility and Family Policy," U.S. Department of Health and Human Services, DHHS Pub. No.13-11953, Washington, DC, 1980.

64. Scott, J.P., Robert, R.A., Hutton, J.T., et al., "Families of Alzheimers Victims," *Journal of the American Geriatrics Society* 34:348-354, 1986.

65. Shanas, E., "The Family as a Social Support System in Old Age," *The Gerontologist* 19:169-183, 1979.

66. Shanas, E., "Social Myth as Hypothesis: The Case of the Family Relations of Old People," *The Gerontologist* 19:3-9, 1979.

67. Siegle, K., untitled article, *The Caregiver* (Newsletter of the Duke Family Support Network) 4(3):2, 1984.

68. Sluss-Radbaugh, T., "Families, Informal Supports and Alzheimer's Disease," position paper submitted to National Institute on Aging, National Institutes of Health, U.S. Department of Health and Human Services, Bethesda, MD, September 1983.

69. Stone, R., Caffarata, G., and Sangl, J., "Caregivers of the Frail Elderly: A National Profile," U.S. Department of Health and Human Services, National Center for Health Services Research, 1986.

70. Testimony of Family Caregivers at the National Conference for Families, U.S. Department of Health and Human Services, National Institutes of Health; and Alzheimer's Disease and Related Disorders Association, May 2, 1985.

71. Townsend, A., and Poulshock, S.W., *Caregiving and Decisionmaking Networks of Impaired Elders* (Cleveland, OH: Benjamin Rose Institute, 1983).

72. U.S. Congress, General Accounting Office, "Medicaid and Nursing Home Care: Cost Increases and the Need for Services are Creating Problems for the States and the Elderly," Washington, DC, Oct. 21, 1983.

73. U.S. Congress, Office of Technology Assessment, *Technology and Aging in America*, OTA-BA-264 (Washington, DC: U.S. Government Printing Office, June 1985).

74. U.S. Congress, Select Committee on Aging, "Caring for America's Alzheimer's Victims," hearing, May 21, 1985 (Washington, DC: U.S. Government Printing Office, 1985).

75. U.S. Congress, Special Committee on Aging, "Endless Night, Endless Morning," hearing, Sept. 12, 1983 (Washington, DC: U.S. Government Printing Office, 1983).

76. U.S. Department of Commerce, Bureau of Census, "Household and Family Characteristics," Series T-20, Washington, DC, March 1984.

77. U.S. Department of Health and Human Services, "Alzheimer's Disease," Report of the Secretary's Task Force on Alzheimer's Disease DHHS 84-1323, Washington, DC, September 1984.

78. U.S. Department of Health and Human Services, "Alzheimer's Disease," A Report to Congress, February 1985.

79. U.S. Department of Health and Human Services, Public Health Service, National Center for Health Statistics, "Money, Income, and Poverty Status of Families and Persons in the United States," Advanced data, P-60 series, March 1984, from Vital and Health Statistics, National Center for Health Statistics.

80. U.S. Department of Labor, Bureau of Labor Statistics, *U.S. Working Women: A Data Book* (Washington, DC: U.S. Government Printing Office, 1977).

81. Wilder, D.E., Teresi, J.A., and Bennett, R., "Family Burden and Dementia," *The Dementias*, R. Mayeux and W.G. Rosen (eds.) (New York: Raven Press, 1983).

82. Yankelovich, Skelly, & White, Inc., "Caregivers of Patients With Dementia," contract report prepared for the Office of Technology Assessment, U.S. Congress, 1986.

83. Zarit, J.M., "Family Role, Social Supports and Their Relation to Caregivers' Burden," paper presented at Western Psychological Association, Sacramento, CA, 1982.

84. Zarit, J.M., Gatz, M., and Zarit S., "Family Relationships and Burden in Long-Term Care," paper presented at Gerontological Society of America, November 1981.

85. Zarit, S.H., Reever, K., and Bach-Peterson, J., "Relatives of the Impaired Elderly, Correlates of Feelings of Burden," *The Gerontologist* 20:649-654, 1980.

86. Zarit, S.H., Todd, P.A., and Zarit, J.M., "Subjective Burden of Husbands and Wives as Caregivers: A Longitudinal Study," *The Gerontologist* 26:3, 260-266, 1986.

Making Decisions for Those With Dementia

CONTENTS

Tables

Making Decisions for Those With Dementia

Carolyn, 63, is in her second year in a nursing home. She has Alzheimer's disease and is no longer cognizant of her family or her surroundings. She is still remembered and loved by family members, who visit her regularly to check on her care and to assure themselves that she is nursed properly and made comfortable. The family is aware of the progression of the disease and has requested that the nursing home withhold life-sustaining measures when the time for such action arrives. When Carolyn contracts pneumonia and it becomes serious, the nursing home is faced with the decision to withhold treatment and balks. The nursing staff feels that death from pneumonia is painful and difficult; Carolyn contracted it accidently and withholding treatment does not seem either right or natural. They call the local hospital and transfer Carolyn to it; there she begins to receive the treatment the nursing home was asked to withhold. The family is then faced with a new dilemma in carrying out what they feel to be a humane decision. They must again appeal to the medical staff, this time to withdraw treatment that has been started on Carolyn. Withdrawal of treatment, they find, is more difficult to obtain, and the legal process with which they are faced is becoming increasingly more complex. The State Carolyn lives in has family consent provisions, but no clear-cut guidelines on the authority to make termination of treatment requests.

Robert is in the early stages of Alzheimer's disease. Even though he experiences fewer and fewer moments of lucidity, he knows what illness he has and what will eventually happen to his mind and his body. He talks about it with his wife and children, expressing his horror at being kept alive beyond his ability to be aware of life. Robert also has a chronic kidney condition that worsens and finally causes his hospitalization. An examination results in the medical conclusion that Robert must be operated on in order to save his life from imminent renal failure. Robert is told about the medical decision, but he refuses to give permission for the operation. The specialists, however, appeal to his wife and children for permission to operate; they also refuse, stating that they feel Robert has made a rational decision. The surgeons disagree. They are bound by oath and tradition to save Robert's life and they ponder the consequences of going ahead with the operation, declaring Robert incompetent to make the choice. Robert has executed a durable power of attorney, naming his wife attorney-in-fact, but laws in his State of residence are unclear as to whether attorneys-in-fact can make critical care decisions.

Jane, a 73-year-old, cheerful, vigorous female in the early stages of a progressive dementia, falls ill and is bedridden in her apartment. During her illness, her sister attempts to shop and cook for her, but Jane's condition deteriorates and she becomes incoherent and incontinent. Her sister immediately petitions for, and is granted guardianship over Jane's person and property. With Jane's condition steadily worsening, her sister also arranges for her entry into the hospital. The hospital tells her sister that Jane will have to undergo major surgery. Her sister requests that the surgery not be performed, in accordance with wishes stated by Jane at an earlier time. The hospital, pointing out that Jane has no formal advance directive for nontreatment, and that the State laws are unclear about guardians having the authority to make critical care decisions, goes ahead with the surgery. Jane survives surgery but shortly thereafter goes into an irreversible coma. When medically appropriate, arrangements are made for nursing home care. With her nutrition and hydration provided by tubes running into her nose and stomach, Jane may live for many years in this fashion (14).

These sketches bring painful clarity to several legal and practical problems that arise when individuals with a progressive dementia are no longer capable of making decisions regarding their own health and welfare. Each case involves a "surrogate decisionmaker," or someone who is empowered to make certain decisions on behalf of another person considered incompetent to make the judgment personally. This chapter will examine some of the issues surrounding surrogate decisionmaking, particularly as it relates to the medical care of incompetent individuals.

As part of this assessment, OTA commissioned papers entitled "Surrogate Decisionmaking for Elderly Individuals Who Are Incompetent or of Questionable Competence," and "Withholding and Withdrawing of Life-Sustaining Treatment for Elderly Incompetent Patients: A Review of Court Decisions and Legislative Approaches." These papers were discussed at an OTA workshop in Washington, DC, September 23, 1985. As a result of the workshop, OTA commissioned an additional paper on "Legal Perceptions and Medical Decisionmaking." These three papers, which contain an extensive analysis of the surrogate decisionmaking questions discussed in this chapter, will be published in 1987 by Milbank Memorial Fund as a supplement of *The Milbank Quarterly* and by OTA (see contract appendix for more information).

Surrogate decisionmakers are responsible for making decisions about an individual's health care, lifestyle, and estate. The limits on and types of decisions made depend on the type of surrogate and manner of appointment, as constrained by the laws of the State in which the incompetent individual resides.

Surrogates may be chosen by an individual before he or she becomes incompetent, appointed by a judge after an individual is incompetent, or identified by laws in certain States that automatically grant family members surrogate decisionmaking powers. Surrogates may have detailed decisionmaking instructions the individual wrote before becoming incompetent, or they may have no instructions whatsoever. Although circumstances may mandate the need for a surrogate decisionmaker, the designation of one calls more into question than the single decision needed in response to a specific problem. The determination of incompetence sets into motion an exploration of such fundamental issues as an individual's autonomy and a surrogate's ability to make decisions for another human being.

DETERMINING COMPETENCE

American society is based on the recognition of individual liberty. Competent individuals have the common law fundamental right to control their property, manage their personal affairs, and give or withhold consent for any bodily invasions such as medical treatment.

As early as 1905, an Illinois court held that "under a free government at least, the free citizen's first and greatest right which underlies all others—the right to the inviolability of his person, in other words, his right to himself—is the subject of universal acquiescence, and this right necessarily forbids a physician . . . to violate without permission the bodily integrity of the patient" (54). This concept of bodily integrity has been defined by the courts to provide that, for a patient's consent to be valid, the physician must provide him or her with enough information about the proposed treatment that the patient can give an "informed consent" (12).

As clear-cut as these basic rights appear, they pertain only to persons assumed competent to make decisions. Questions surrounding a possibly incompetent individual remain: What makes a person competent in the first place? What standard of decisionmaking ability should be used to determine whether an individual is competent? Who should decide whether an individual retains personal liberties?

Background and Precedents

Society's role in questioning a person's competence and assigning him or her a surrogate decisionmaker is not a new one. Guardianship, and its concurrent notion of decisionmaking by a surrogate, dates back at least to ancient Rome. It was apparently conceived as a means of protecting the ward, or individual in question, and that person's property (7). That authority, based on the State's police power and traditional role as *parens patriae*, imposes court-supervised external control over individuals not deemed capable of making informed autonomous decisions, such as minors or insane and incompetent persons (50).

State statutes govern incompetency and surrogate decisionmaking, resulting in multiple approaches. In general, however, standards prompting the need for a surrogate can be divided into three types (50):

1. **The Causal Link**. Once the most popular standard, it is still used in some States. Fundamentally, it entails diagnosis of a condition —i.e., a cause—that creates the socially improper behavior exhibited by the ward. That diagnosis generally precludes guardianship hearings for those who are perfectly capable of caring for themselves and their property adequately but who do not choose to do so (e.g., an eccentric person who decides never to bathe).
2. **The Uniform Probate Code**. This standard is more concerned with the health, well-being, and safety of the individual than his or her property management. It also emphasizes an individual's ability to both make and communicate decisions as the litmus test for competency. Notably, some State variations on this standard limit a finding of incompetence to situations where the health, safety, and physical necessities of an individual are endangered.
3. **The Therapeutic Approach**. This approach is increasingly favored in gerontological and mental health circles. It defines a defendant's incapacity as a legal rather than a medical state, measured by his or her functional limitations. Thus, a court's finding is based more on a person's capacities than on a medical diagnosis, and specific dysfunctions must be proved.

Defining Competence

Competence to make decisions is not like a light switch that turns on or off. Many elderly persons may be partially competent, or able to make some decisions but not others. They may be intermittently competent—more lucid and able to make

decisions on some days than on others. Ideally, all individuals would be allowed to retain their autonomy and make decisions for as long as possible. Those who are partially competent would make decisions they are competent to make; those who are intermittently competent would make decisions when they were capable of making them. However, this ideal requires that "the task of competence clarification" (11,60) be of the greatest importance. It has been argued that:

> The point of a competence determination is to sort people into two classes: those whose decisions must be respected, and those whose decisions will be set aside and for whom others will be designated as surrogate decisionmakers. Competence, then, is not a matter of degree—a person either is, or is not, competent to make a particular decision . . . . [But] no single standard for competence is adequate for all decisions. The standard depends in large part on the risk involved, and varies along a range from low/minimal to high/maximal. The more serious the expected harm to the patient from acting on a choice, the higher should be the standard of decisionmaking capacity, and the greater should be the certainty that the standard is satisfied (11).

An individual either is or is not competent for a specific task, i.e., to make a specific decision regarding, for example, health care, living arrangements, or financial affairs. For competent decisionmaking, a person should have the capacity for communication, understanding, reasoning, and deliberation, plus a relatively stable set of values. Appropriate standards for competence should focus on the process by which a decision is reached, and not on the decision itself (11,20).

Determinations of competence—whether viewed as a matter of degree of capability or as an either/or matter—invoke two important values. First, the standard of competence must protect and promote an individual's well-being; second, it must respect an individual's right to self-determination (11). (For more discussion of this issue, see ch. 8.)

Functional assessment has been suggested as an aid in determining incompetence and subsequent delineation of decisionmaking powers by a surrogate (50). Functional assessment does not provide a diagnosis, only a description of behaviors; a judge may then evaluate whether such behavior indicates the need for a surrogate decisionmaker. It is a tool to use in assessing an individual's physical and emotional ability to function on a daily basis, and, consequently, his or her need for a surrogate. One problem associated with the functional assessment standard of competence is that, without a medical diagnosis, an individual with a treatable condition may unnecessarily be judged incompetent.

One advantage of using functional assessment for individuals with dementia is that these disorders do not necessarily impair all areas of the brain equally, or even at the same rate. Thus, an assessment might support a person retaining some decisionmaking abilities, even if he or she is incompetent in other matters. However, some form of standardized functional assessment is needed—with a failure to attain basic levels of physical and intellectual sufficiency leading to a legal verdict of incompetency.

If an assessment takes place, the evaluator should apply the State's objective standards; the ward's previous mental and physical capacity are irrelevant. Assessments should be conducted by employees of community senior citizen centers, schools of nursing and social work, or public health departments, and presented to the court during surrogate appointment proceedings (16, 17, 50).

Consequences of Incompetence

An individual found incompetent—by a doctor, a family member, or a judge—may be moved from home, have money and property managed, and be unable to refuse medical treatment. He or she will lose most decisionmaking rights.

Not everyone is competent to make the fundamental decisions faced by sick and elderly Americans. Who has a right to make decisions for another? What kinds of decisions can be made by one person for another? Should the surrogate have the right to make critical care decisions? How should a surrogate decisionmaker be chosen? What happens if a surrogate decisionmaker is not selected before an individual becomes incompetent? What can and cannot be accomplished through advance directives? What happens if there is no advance directive when someone becomes incompetent? How have the courts and the medical community responded to the issues raised by surrogate decisionmaking and advance directives? Who, if anyone, is liable for decisions made by a surrogate?

These are the issues that are triggered by a determination of incompetence and form the basis for this chapter. There are no easy answers, and the questions themselves often act as lightning rods for controversy. In this largely undefined legal territory, highly personal family dilemmas can become public test cases.

Forums of Competence Adjudication

Strictly speaking, competence is a legal concept, but the legal and clinical standards differ considerably (30). Legally, an individual is presumed competent until a court declares otherwise and appoints a guardian (30). Practice differs from theory, however, in many cases of questionable competence. The determination of competence is usually made informally first by family or friends. The next informal determination is often made, with varying degrees of expertise, by the person's doctor, banker, or lawyer, who acquiesces to family requests to take responsibility for medical, fiscal, or legal matters.

Legal competency proceedings are rarely initiated for medical reasons. Instead,

> . . . if an elderly person is deemed incompetent by caregivers, they usually turn to family members to make decisions on behalf of the patient. It is not clear why clinical practice so diverges from legal standards. Physicians may be ignorant about the precise legal definition of competency or may regard legal proceedings as too cumbersome and time-consuming, with insufficient benefits to justify the cost (30).

Families prefer to consult informally with the doctor in making decisions rather than go through the time, trauma, and cost of having someone declared incompetent. This is an efficient, if not extralegal, way of coping with the competency issues. Moreover, all parties may be happy with the arrangement—as long as they continue to agree on what constitutes appropriate treatment (13).

When mental status examinations are given, examiners check a patient's orientation, memory, and ability to perform simple calculations (see ch. 8). However, mental status exams may not be able to assess a person's ability to comprehend medical treatments and alternatives, or their risks, benefits, and consequences. If a person's competence is questioned, a psychiatrist's input is more likely to be sought than a court's. Such informal competency determinations, while often effective, do not provide due process of law and may unfairly prevent individuals from making personal decisions. The scope of this potential problem is unknown, but general consensus seems to be that almost all competence determinations are the result of genuine concern of families or friends.

Courts also make competence determinations. Adjudications of competence, however, occur most frequently when competence is disputed. For instance, a doctor may feel that an operation is necessary for the health of a patient who refuses to consent. If there is reason to believe the patient is incompetent, the doctor may initiate court involvement. Likewise, a family who is concerned over a relative's aberrant behavior may seek a court determination of incompetence and appointment of guardianship.

SURROGATE DECISIONMAKING

When a determination of incompetence is made, either formally or informally, the surrogate decisionmaker assumes power to act for the incompetent individual. Surrogates may be selected by someone in advance of incompetence, self-appointed, or appointed by a court.

Advance Selection

Persons with clear personal, medical, and estate preferences may issue an advance directive. Advance directives are designed to allow a competent individual's choices and instructions to be recorded, and then followed after the person becomes incompetent. However, few people thus far have planned for future incompetence by instructing someone on how they would like to be treated in the event they are unable to make their own decisions about health care (56, app. B). Many are ignorant of their options, reluctant to face the thought of disability, or intimidated by the legal system. Recently, however, various consumer groups have begun publicizing the advantages of identifying a surrogate and writing advance directives for extending a person's autonomy and obviating reliance on the courts (41). However, ambiguity in State statutes and the relevance of health care facilities make it uncertain that an individual's advance directive will be followed.

Durable Power of Attorney

Durable power of attorney (DPA) is a modification of the standard power of attorney that permits an individual (principal) to transfer specified powers to another person (attorney-in-fact). The power may be broad in scope or limited. The fundamental difference between standard and durable power of attorney is that the former loses its validity when the principal becomes incompetent, and thereby is not useful for persons with a dementing illness. Durable power of attorney, authorized by State statute everywhere in the United States except in the District of Columbia, provides a means of surrogate decisionmaker designation that survives the incompetence of the principal (46).

There are two types of durable power of attorney. The first takes effect on being signed by the principal and continues, unless revoked while the principal still has capacity, until death. The second, called a "springing" durable power, takes effect when the principal becomes incapacitated. In both types, the principal determines which powers are delegated to the surrogate. Concerned parties may petition a court to review the surrogate's actions.

The use of durable powers to transfer decisionmaking authority avoids many of the legal fees and court costs associated with a conservatorship or guardianship, and does not require bonding or supervision. Additionally, it can fully represent the principal's choices and perspectives. Individuals may not be ready psychologically to execute this document before, or at the onset of, a dementia. For that reason and because of the generally progressive nature of impaired decisionmaking capacity, many lawyers recommend that already incapacitated individuals be brought to them during any reasonably lucid moment for explanatory purposes and signature (36,40).

There are other problems with durable power of attorney. Many banks and lending institutions are unfamiliar with it and may not accept a durable power as legal proof that the principal's finances are now under the control of another individual, unless the institution's own forms are used. That is impossible where the principal is already incompetent. Also, the validity of both types of durable power as applied to critical care decisions has been questioned in the courts and at patient bedsides (38,41,48).

Durable Power of Attorney for Health Care

California in 1983 passed legislation that created a new entity, the Durable Power of Attorney for Health Care (DPAHC). That power, also now available in several other States, attempts to address some of the issues surrounding the use of durable powers of attorney for critical care decisions (see table 5-1). It specifically empowers the attorney-in-fact to make medical care decisions. The DPAHC, which is a springing power, allows the principal to state, in detail, what kinds of medical intervention or life-sustaining systems are acceptable (22,24,36,41).

DPAHCs and living wills are the first legal measures that give individuals the ability to direct treatment decisions after incompetence. For people to make informed decisions, they need to be educated regarding their rights. They need to know what legal devices are available, under what circumstances they apply, and how to take advantage of them.

Living Wills

Living wills are another mechanism for expressing the principal's intent while competent and for honoring his or her desires once he or she is incompetent and death is imminent. A living will may declare the principal's intent on the use or refusal of life-sustaining procedures in the event the person cannot be reasonably expected to recover from extreme physical or mental disability. Statutes protect health care providers from civil and criminal liability for withholding or withdrawing life-sustaining treatment in compliance with a living will, and state that refusal of life-sustaining treatment by a terminally ill patient does not constitute suicide for insurance or other purposes. In most States, a physician who is unable to comply with a patient's directive for religious or personal reasons is obliged to transfer the patient to the care of someone who can comply. Failure to transfer such a patient may constitute unprofessional conduct on the part of the doctor or hospital (47,63).

However, living wills are frequently ambiguous, lacking specific instructions tailored to specific medical needs, and may request something that the State is unwilling to countenance. For instance, uncertainty exists regarding an individual's right to refuse artificial food or hydration through the living will (30). The legality of living wills may be unclear, and the document may draw uncertain responses from physicians. Nevertheless, or perhaps in response to these problems, the number of States with legislation on living wills is growing (see table 5-2). The States that did not recognize living wills as of July 1986 were Kentucky, Massachusetts, Michigan, Minnesota, Nebraska, New Jersey, New York, North Dakota, Ohio, Pennsylvania, Rhode Island, and South Dakota.

State-by-State variations include requirements for executing a valid living will and conditions making one applicable (see table 5-3). A document that is legally valid in the State where it was signed, for example, may not always be useful elsewhere. Most States provide a form that may be used to create a living will, but also permit individual variations as long as specific State requirements are

Table 5-1.—Special Requirements for Creating a Durable Power of Attorney for Health Care

State	Notary required	Filing required	Other
Arkansas	Yes (or approval of Probate Court)	Probate Court	
California[a]	Yes (or signed by two witnesses)		If patient is in nursing home, one witness must be patient, advocate, or ombudsman Must be accompanied by statutory notice or signed by an attorney
Connecticut	Yes		Must be accompanied by statutory notice
Florida	No		Only a spouse, parent, adult child, sibling, niece, or nephew may be appointed
Minnesota	Yes		
Missouri	Yes	Recorder of deeds	
New York	Yes		Must be accompanied by statutory notice
North Carolina	Yes	Register of deeds (copy with clerk of Superior Court)	
Oklahoma	No	Clerk of State District Court	Must be approved by judge of State District Court
Rhode Island[a]	No		At least one witness must not be related by blood, marriage, or adoption and must not be entitled to any part of the maker's estate
South Carolina	Yes	Register of Mesne Conveyance	Requires three witnesses
Wyoming	No	Clerk of District Court (copy with clerk of county court where principal resides)	Must be approved by judge of State District Court

[a]California and Rhode Island have statutory forms for durable powers of attorney for health care which include a notice or warning to persons executing the document.

SOURCE: B. Mishkin, "A Matter of Choice: Planning Ahead for Health Care Decisions," Senate Special Committee on Aging, 1986.

met. To avoid difficulties at the precise time the document is most needed, living wills are best drawn by a well-informed attorney. The States received some direction from the National Conference of Commissioners on Uniform State Laws in August 1985, when proposed uniform living will legislation was ratified, but there is still no consensus. Knowledgeable observers expect a more standard approach to be adopted by a significant number of States in the next few years (1).

States also differ in the conditions they set for a living will to become effective. Many States, for example, require a person to be "terminally ill" in order to activate a living will. However, there is no clear definition of when an illness becomes terminal. As two observers note:

Some people may consider a person who is expected to live six months terminal, while others may regard a patient as terminal only when survival is expected to be one month or one week. Some physicians consider patients terminally ill only when they are moribund and will die in a few days no matter what treatment is given. Some people may consider a patient terminal when cancer is first diagnosed, while others apply this label only after metastases develop or a relapse occurs after treatment (30).

If the diagnosis of "terminally ill" is taken to mean imminent death—as it frequently is—then such

Table 5-2.—Special Limitations on Living Wills (table complete as of September 1986)

State	Not valid during pregnancy	Categorically may not withhold food or fluids	Effective only for given number of years	Must sign after terminal diagnosis to be binding
Alabama	X			
Alaska	X[a]			
Arizona	X[a]	X		
California	X		5	X
Colorado	X[a]	X		
Connecticut	X	X		
Delaware	X			
Florida	X	X		
Georgia	X	X		
Hawaii	X			X
Illinois	X	X		
Indiana	X	X[b]		
Iowa	X[a]	X		
Kansas	X			
Maine		X		
Maryland	X	X		
Mississippi	X			
Missouri	X	X		
Montana	X[a]			
Nevada	X			
New Hampshire	X	X		
Oklahoma		X		X
Oregon		X[c]		
South Carolina	X	X		
Tennessee		X		
Texas	X			
Utah	X	X[d]		
Washington	X			
Wisconsin	X	X		
Wyoming	X	X		

[a]If fetus could develop to point of live birth.
[b]May not withhold "appropriate" nourishment and hydration.
[c]May withhold if patient cannot tolerate.
[d]Unless declarant specifically authorizes.
SOURCE: B. Mishkin, "A Matter of Choice: Planning Ahead for Health Care Decisions," Senate Special Committee on Aging, 1986.

a requirement negates an incompetent individual's ability to direct medical care through a living will until the last few days or weeks (i.e., victims of serious accidents or strokes, who are in a persistent vegetative state, may not be considered "terminally ill" even if they would not wish to live for years in a coma if recovery were impossible). The living will also might apply in the case of elderly persons who are in an irreversible decline, suffering from deterioration of various organ systems or the combined effects of degenerative disorders. Some States (California, Idaho, and Oklahoma) require living wills to be signed *after* a terminal diagnosis; thus, a living will would not help any of the patients just mentioned. Many of these people would not want to be kept on life-sustaining systems if they no longer had any awareness of life, but a living will statute relying

Table 5-3.—Witness Requirements for Living Wills (table complete as of September 1986)

State	Witness may not be: Related by blood or marriage	Heir/claimant to the estate	Declarant's physician	Employed by declarant's health care facility	Responsible for declarant's health care costs	Nursing home patient requires special witness
Alabama	X	X	. . . . . .	. . . . . .	X	
Alaska	X	. . . . . .	. . . . . .	. . . . . .	. . . . . .	
Arizona	X	X	. . . . . .	. . . . . .	X	
Arkansas	. . . . . .	. . . . . .	. . . . . .	. . . . . .	. . . . . .	
California	X	X	X	X	. . . . . .	Patient advocate or ombudsman
Colorado	. . . . . .	X	or any M.D.	or co-patient	. . . . . .	
Connecticut	. . . . . .	. . . . . .	. . . . . .	. . . . . .	. . . . . .	
Delaware	X	X	. . . . . .	X	X	Patient advocate or ombudsman
District of Columbia	X	X	X	X	X	Patient advocate or ombudsman
Florida	one of two witnesses	. . . . . .	. . . . . .			
Georgia	X	X	X	X	X	Medical director
Idaho	X	X	X	X	. . . . . .	
Illinois	X	X	. . . . . .	. . . . . .	X	
Indiana	only parents, spouse, and children	X	. . . . . .	. . . . . .	X	
Iowa	. . . . . .	. . . . . .	. . . . . .	. . . . . .	. . . . . .	
Kansas	X	X	. . . . . .	. . . . . .	X	
Louisiana	X	X	X	or co-patient	. . . . . .	
Maine	. . . . . .	. . . . . .	. . . . . .	. . . . . .	. . . . . .	
Maryland	X	X	X	X	X	
Mississippi	X	X	X	. . . . . .	. . . . . .	
Missouri	. . . . . .	. . . . . .	. . . . . .	. . . . . .	. . . . . .	
Montana	. . . . . .	. . . . . .	. . . . . .	. . . . . .	. . . . . .	
Nevada	X	X	X	X	. . . . . .	
New Hampshire	X	X	X	. . . . . .	. . . . . .	Medical director
New Mexico	. . . . . .	. . . . . .	. . . . . .	. . . . . .	. . . . . .	
North Carolina	X	X	X	X	. . . . . .	
Oklahoma	X	X	X	or co-patient	X	
Oregon	X	X	X	X	. . . . . .	Individual designated by Department of Human Resources
South Carolina[a]	X	X	X	X	X	Hospital or nursing home resident requires ombudsman
Tennessee	X	X	X	X	. . . . . .	
Texas	X	X	X	or co-patient	. . . . . .	
Utah	X	X	X	X	X	
Vermont	X	X	X	. . . . . .	. . . . . .	
Virginia	X	. . . . . .	. . . . . .	. . . . . .	. . . . . .	
Washington	X	X	X	X	. . . . . .	
West Virginia	X	X	X	X	X	
Wisconsin	X	X	X	X	. . . . . .	
Wyoming	X	X	. . . . . .	. . . . . .	X	

[a]South Carolina requires three witnesses and notary.

SOURCE: B. Mishkin, ''A Matter of Choice: Planning Ahead for Health Care Decisions,'' Senate Special Committee on Aging, 1986.

on "terminal illness" would not permit them to direct their own care and treatment after incompetence (47).

Informal, or Self-Selection

De facto surrogate decisionmaking, which is frequent, consists of an individual's assumption of the normal financial and personal decisions of another without formally being charged to do so through legally recognized proceedings. De facto surrogates usually are a person's close relatives or friends. For many elderly individuals who do not plan ahead by appointing a surrogate through a durable power of attorney, de facto surrogate decisionmaking is easier and less traumatic than the guardianship process. In effect, de facto surrogates act on another's behalf in the same way that court-appointed surrogates do—until such rare time as someone challenges their authority. The use of de facto surrogates eases the potential burden on the court system, but it also places people's liberties at risk. Legal advance appointment of a surrogate allows the principal a choice of surrogate that may differ from the de facto surrogate.

Many people rely on their physicians to make decisions for them. In most cases, particularly where there are also sympathetic family members involved, that approach is adequate. It is time-tested and remains the favorite of a vast majority of physicians (23). However, it presumes a strong concordance of views between physician, family, and facility. Also, nursing home residents are frequently transferred to acute care hospitals shortly before death (see ch. 10). Thus, the individual's regular nursing home physician, who may have agreed to a wish for nontreatment, might not be the physician responsible for the person's hospital care.

De facto surrogate decisionmaking is also more easily abused, as it occurs without a court's involvement. Only a legal challenge to the de facto surrogate's authority can initiate court review, and the decision to make that challenge can be traumatic and costly to the person bringing suit—an individual who may feel it is not his or her place to intervene. The dilemma is how to protect people who do not appoint or instruct a surrogate personally, without encumbering the court system or the emotional and financial resources of families. It is unclear if this is a problem; the number of persons affected is unknown and there is no available data.

Selection by Formal Appointment

Conservatorship and Guardianship

Conservatorships and guardianships are determined and supervised by the court. Specific State statutes and practices vary. There are two types: conservatorship (or guardianship) of estate covers finances; conservatorship (or guardianship) of person covers residency, certain kinds of health care and social service decisions, and other personal matters. The appointment is obtained by petitioning the court and presenting evidence of a person's relevant incapacity.

A guardianship proceeding generally requires two steps. First, a proposed ward must have a specified diagnosis or disability. Second, as a result of that disability, the proposed ward must be unable to make decisions on his or her own behalf. The Uniform Probate Code defines an "incapacitated person" as one "who is impaired by reason of mental illness, mental deficiency, physical illness or disability, advanced age, chronic use of drugs, chronic intoxication, or other cause (except minority) to the extent that he lacks sufficient understanding or capacity to make or communicate responsible decisions concerning his person" (58).

Courts and legislatures increasingly recognize that competence may wax and wane over time, and that patients may have the capacity to make some choices, but not others. In response, a growing number of States now permit limited or partial guardianship, in which surrogate decisionmaking authority is confined to specific areas. Some statutes allow courts to structure guardianship to fit the needs of an individual ward, while others require only that the guardian's powers be drawn as narrowly as possible (47).

Conservatorships and guardianships provide an incapacitated individual with as much legal protection, through court involvement, as possible. On the other hand, they can incur high and continuous legal fees (15), increase demands on the judicial system, and offer no guarantee that decisions always will be made in the best interest of the incompetent person or in keeping with that person's desires.

Guardian ad Litem

Another form of guardianship occurs when a specific problem, such as authorization for surgery, must be solved by the court and one of the concerned parties needs representation. In this instance, a "guardian ad litem" may be appointed to represent an arguably incompetent person in that specific matter.

Representative Payee

A representative payee is, in effect, guardian of a patient's social security or other government benefits. Neither conservatorship nor power of attorney is recognized by the Social Security Administration, Veterans Administration, or many other government agencies as a legal basis for transferring benefit payments to a person other than the beneficiary. Many agencies specify that an individual wishing to act as a "representative payee" for someone must obtain a physician's written statement that the beneficiary is incapable of handling his or her financial affairs.

The procedure for the appointment of a representative payee is much less formal than that entailed in a court competency hearing, the determination resting solely within the discretion of the head of the appropriate agency. In many cases the physician—whose recommendation will carry great credence—sees the patient only in stressful settings like the hospital or doctor's office, and communicates with the patient only about medical care, not the handling of financial affairs. Government agencies may transfer payment monies to a representative payee even if the principal has not been deemed incompetent by a court (28,29, 53,74). Further, although empowered to request an accounting, government agencies do not ordinarily audit the activities of the 4 million to 5 million representative payees to ensure that the transferred monies are being spent in the interests of the principal.

This practice of nonscrutiny led to a 3-year lawsuit, instigated by a woman in Oklahoma, whose Supplemental Security Income payments had been fraudulently used by her representative payee sister for several years. In 1983, the U.S. District Court for the Western District of Oklahoma did find, among other things, that the due process clause of the fifth amendment required that the Social Security Administration implement mandatory, periodic accounting procedures. Margaret Heckler, Secretary of Health and Human Services and the defendant in the case, submitted a plan whereby 0.025 percent of representative payees would have their accounting short form reviewed (74). In 1984, the court found that the substantial interest of Social Security beneficiaries for whom representative payees have been appointed could be adequately protected only by requiring universal annual accountings. Although initially acquiescent, the Department of Health and Human Services (DHHS) returned to the court in April 1986 and requested, once again, that it not be required to request or review representative payee accountings pending further court decisions. The court granted that stay, and the future of accountings by representative payees remains in question (19, 28,62,70).

Further complicating this issue is the Social Security Disability Benefits Reform Act of 1984 (Public Law No. 98-460), Section 16 of which provides that where payment is made to a person other than the entitled individual, an annual accounting is required, with the Secretary establishing and implementing "statistically valid procedures for reviewing such reports." DHHS has not implemented this requirement. Section 16 also sought a report to be prepared for Congress in 1985. That report was to examine the systems by which accountings would be reviewed, the problems inherent in the systems, and the problems inherent in the representative payee system. A six-page report was submitted in September 1985, containing no data on rates of auditing, no details about ascertaining mental competence for purposes of assigning representative payees, no description of procedures for identifying misuse of funds, and no special safeguards for those judged mentally incompetent who are cared for outside State mental institutions (19,68).

Family Consent Statutes

Under family consent statutes, a surrogate is identified in advance by the State and is automatically vested with certain powers, unless an individual has previously designated a different surrogate decisionmaker. Seventeen States have enacted laws clearly authorizing family members to make health care decisions on behalf of incapacitated adults—at least for those who are terminally ill (see table 5-4). Case law in California, Connecticut, Florida, Georgia, and New Jersey supports the right of family members to make health care decisions, including decisions to forgo treatment, for terminally ill or comatose patients. The family consent statutes remove doubts surrounding the legal basis for such decisions and permit doctors and other health care providers to follow the directions of family members without fear of subsequent civil or criminal liability (47). The provisions become effective when a patient is incompetent, but the majority of statutes do not at-

Table 5-4.—Family Consent Provisions

Provisions	State	Statute
Family may make health care decisions for incapacitated adults	Arkansas ....Ark. Stat. § 82-363 (1976)	
	Georgia...........Ga. Code § 31-9-1 (1982)	
	Idaho.............Idaho Code § 49-4303 (1985)	
	Louisiana ....La. Rev. Stat. Ann. tit. 40, § 1299.53 (1977)	
	Maine ....Me. Rev. Stat. Ann. tit. 24, § 2905 (1985)	
	Maryland[a].........Md. Ann. Code § 20-107(d) (1984)	
	Mississippi ....Miss. Code Ann. § 41-41-3 (1985)	
	Utah ....Utah Code Ann. § 78-14-5(4) (1977)	
Family may make health care decisions for terminally ill and incapacitated adults (including termination of treatment)	Florida ....Fla. Stat. Ch. 84-85, § 765.0 (1984)	
	Iowa ....Iowa Code Ch. 144A.1-144A.12 (1985)	
	Louisiana ....La. Rev. Stat. tit. 40, § 1299.58.5(A) (H.B. 795, 1985)	
	New Mexico .......N.M. Stat. Ann. § 24-7-5, as amended by S.B. 15 (1984)	
	North Carolina[b].....N.C. Gen. Stat. § 90-322(b), as amended by S.B. 240 (1983)	
	Oregon[b] ....Ore. Rev. Stat. § 97.083(2), as amended by H.B. 2963 (1983)	
	Texas ....Tex. Civ. Stat. Art. 4590h, as amended by H.B. 403 (1985)	
	Virginia...........Va. Code Ann. § 54-325.8:6 (1984)	
	Utah[c].............Utah Code Ann. §§ 75-2-1101-1118 (1985)	

[a]Except for sterilization, abortion, and treatment or hospitalization for a mental disorder.
[b]Patient must be comatose.
[c]Original law, passed in 1977, specified only incapacitated adults.
SOURCE: B. Mishkin, "A Matter of Choice: Planning Ahead for Health Care Decisions," Senate Special Committee on Aging, 1986.

tempt to define incompetence or require a formal competency hearing. Thus, the competency determination generally is made by the physician. Since most of these provisions are built into living will statutes, only families of the terminally ill are eligible to use them (see table 5-5).

The National Conference of Commissioners on Uniform State Laws adopted a Model Health Care Consent Act in 1982 (67). The model act states that when a patient is incompetent to consent to or refuse treatment, and has not designated a surrogate decisionmaker, decisions may be made by a spouse, adult child, parent, or adult sibling. Unlike some State statutes giving priority to one family member over another, the model act does not differentiate between family members, nor does it suggest how to proceed if family members disagree. It does emphasize that surrogate decisionmakers should base their decisions, inasmuch as possible, on the patient's previously expressed preferences. Thus far, the model act has had little effect on actual State legislation.

Alternative Forms of Surrogate Decisionmaking

Public guardianship programs vary somewhat from State to State, but typically are overseen by a county office of the public guardian, ombudsman, or court investigator. These offices supervise and manage guardianship cases, sometimes appointing private individuals as conservators where there are substantial estates. In these cases, it is not uncommon for a financially sophisticated "friend of the court" to be appointed (48).

The private practice of surrogate management is also becoming more common. Here, bonded individuals manage estates on behalf of their clients for a fee. Because of difficulties in some public guardianship programs, private for-profit programs are gaining some favor in the legal community. As a safeguard, it has been suggested that these private programs be subject to regular reporting requirements (10,39,49).

Table 5-5.—Individual State Provisions of Family Consent Laws

State	Patient must be		Family members					Priority given	Consent not valid for		
	Terminally ill	Comatose	Spouse	Adult child	Parent	Adult sibling	Other		Abortion	Sterilization	Mental health care
Arkansas			X	X	X	nearest relative	grandparent				
Florida	X		X	X^b	X		nearest relative	X			
Georgia			X		X^a	X^a	grandparent	X	X		
Idaho			X		X		any competent relative				
Iowa	X		X	X^b	X	X			X	X	X
Louisiana			X		X^a	X^a	grandparent^a		X	X	X
Louisiana^c	X		X	X^b	X^b	X^b	other ascendents or descendents^c	X			
Maine			X		X		nearest relative				
Maryland			X	X	X	X	grandparent	X	X	X	X
Mississippi			X	X	X	X	grandparent				
New Mexico	X or	X	X	X	X	X	family members^d	X			
North Carolina	X and	X	X	X	X	X		X			
Oregon	X and	X	X	X^b	X	X					
Texas	X		X	X^b	X		nearest relative	X^e			
Utah			X	X	X^a	X^a	grandparent^a				
Virginia	X		X	X	X		nearest relative	X			

a For minor child.
b Majority of this class required (if available).
c Louisiana has two family consent laws.
d All who can be contacted must agree on what patient would choose.
e Requires consent of at least two family members, if reasonably available.

SOURCE: B. Mishkin, ''A Matter of Choice: Planning Ahead for Health Care Decisions,'' Senate Special Committee on Aging, 1986.

There are also numerous private social service organizations that assist in establishing eligibility for public benefits. They generally support family members who may live too far away to be of help on a daily basis. Families may use this method to avoid the trauma and cost of a court hearing on conservatorship.

Hospitals and nursing homes also designate surrogates, such as patient advocates or ombudsmen. However, because the nature and philosophy of each facility can vary, defining the role of surrogates designated in this way is difficult. These surrogates typically act more as advocates than decisionmakers or case managers. In addition, because the surrogate is employed by the hospital or nursing home rather than the patient or resident a conflict of interest may occur. Cases of financial abuse where surrogates are employed by a facility have been documented (3,5,23,25,26,69, 71).

Occasionally, when an individual has no surrogate decisionmaker or when there is disagreement between family members and caretakers, an institutional ethics committee (IEC) may be used to assist in making a decision. Ethics committees are becoming a popular means of considering difficult medical treatment situations on behalf of an incompetent individual. They received their initial stamp of approval when the New Jersey Supreme Court proposed that such a group play a role in the decision about whether to disconnect Karen Anne Quinlan's respirator. In that instance the committee was to provide a prognosis for Quinlan's recovery, the outcome of which would help determine the court's decision (35,59, 72).

These committees have faced numerous operational questions, however (64,65). In 1983, only 1 percent of the Nation's nearly 2,000 acute care hospitals had a functioning IEC. That same year, the first national conference on IECs was held (Institutional Ethics Committees: Their Role in Medical Decision Making, sponsored by the American Society for Law and Medicine and Concern for Dying, Washington, DC, Apr. 21-23, 1983). In addressing what role an IEC may play, one law professor drew up three possible models:

1. in the "optional-optional" model, the committee acts on a standby basis, with no one being required to make use of its services or abide by its recommendations;
2. in the "mandatory-optional" model, physicians would have to consult the IEC when faced with a critical decision, but would not be required to adhere to its recommendations; and
3. in a "mandatory-mandatory" model, physicians would be compelled to consult the IEC when faced with a critical decision, and compelled to carry out its decision (61).

One underlying dilemma of IECs has been put this way:

> Either ethics committees will have well-grounded criteria for making recommendations in particularly difficult cases, or they will not. If such criteria are widely accepted, the committee seems redundant; why not appeal directly to the criteria? And if such criteria are not widely accepted, the committee's recommendation may seem arbitrary and fail to persuade some of those whose decisions the committee is reviewing (Callahan, as quoted in 34).

Despite these lingering questions, ethics committees are increasingly used in the hospital setting. There is some support, at least in the nursing community, for IECs having the authority to make legally binding critical care decisions (31,44).

Several other unrestrictive, extralegal alternatives to conservatorship of person are referral, case work, and case management. (For more information on these nonlegal alternatives, see ch. 6.)

The Influence of Setting

How a surrogate is chosen depends, in part, on the person needing the surrogate and his or her environment. Those choosing a surrogate from home frequently rely on family, friends, the local banker, the personal physician, and others who compose the informal support network.

In domiciliary care facilities (DCF) or board and care homes, the operator or a staff member may be acting as the surrogate—with or without formal legal appointment or even informal approval of the patient. That is problematic. These facilities generally are not as well defined or visible in a community as a nursing home. They frequently are supervised haphazardly if at all, by government agencies. Many are unlicensed and lack the benefit of ombudsman involvement. Because reporting responsibilities are few, surrogate decisionmaking generally devolves to the DCF operator with no external oversight (26,53,69).

Special problems may exist for those residents of nursing homes who have no interested relatives or friends. For those individuals, medical decisionmaking often consists of informally turning to a doctor or the nursing home staff, with some input from any available relatives. That is particularly true of Medicaid patients without concerned families, who lack large material assets to attract potential surrogate managers. Decisions are quite often made by physicians with some input from any members of the family who are available.

In hospital settings, patients may be in rapidly failing health, clearly incompetent, diagnosed as "terminal," or headed for a nursing home. Hospital administrators are wary about encouraging patients to sign documents appointing surrogate decisionmakers and about giving what may be considered self-serving advice. They have expressed concern that the acute care environment is inconsistent with the concept of competency and that they will be charged with the responsibility of certifying competence in all cases. Additionally, they worry that liability insurance coverage will be jeopardized by their delving into an area that is not formally part of their health care mandate (23).

The incompetent or questionably competent person in these health care settings has a role in selecting a surrogate. Even when there is some question as to the individual's capacity for decisionmaking, courts tend to respect that individual's decision. Nevertheless, patients, family members, caretakers, and social workers need to be educated and encouraged regarding the prompt identification of a surrogate (45).

DECISIONS MADE BY A SURROGATE

The previous section identified the various types of surrogates, explained how they are selected, and detailed the extent of their powers and limitations. Once a surrogate is in place, he or she must begin the sometimes difficult task of making decisions. How does a surrogate make crucial decisions for an incompetent person? What criteria does the surrogate take into account? What conflicts of interest might the surrogate encounter in making a decision? Who is liable for decisions made by the surrogate?

Criteria for Making Decisions

Once a patient has been deemed incompetent to make all or some decisions, some complex issues arise. Who should decide for the incompetent patient? By what set of principles should decisions be made? These questions have been addressed in dramatically different ways. Answers to the first question have been sought from a legal perspective, but answers to the second tend to be explored from an ethical framework. Thus, decisionmaking no longer is clarified by court rulings and State legislation; it operates in the ambiguity of what is right, or good, or ethical.

Briefly, various ethical principles can guide a surrogate in making a decision. The most fundamental of these are:

Ethical value principles identify the basic ethical values to be used in dealing with incompetent individuals. These values include respect for autonomy, concern for well-being, and justice in a patient's access to care and resources. Guidance principles give hints or direction as to how decisions should be made. These principles include: 1) substituted judgment, or choosing the way the individual, if competent, would choose; 2) best interest, or choosing what most benefits the individual; 3) advance directive, or choosing the way the individual has expressed in a previously written directive, such as a living will (11).

It is useful to compare and contrast these three guidance principles to understand how the use of one or another may vastly alter the outcome of the surrogate's decision.

The Best Interest Principle states that a surrogate is to choose what will best serve the patient's interests. The qualifier "best" indicates two important factors: some interests are more important than others in that they make a larger contribution to the patient's good, and a particular decision may advance some of the patient's interests while frustrating others. Thus, according to the Best Interest Principle, the surrogate must try to determine the net benefit to the patient of each option, after assigning weights reflecting the relative importance of various interests affected when subtracting the "costs" from the "benefits" for each option.

In contrast, the Substituted Judgment Principle states that a surrogate is to choose as the patient would choose if the patient were competent and aware both of the medical options and of the facts about his or her condition, including the fact that he or she is incompetent. Thus a surrogate who must decide whether antibiotics should be given to an unconscious man with terminal cancer might consider the following as a test of the Substituted Judgment Principle: "If the patient miraculously were to awaken from his coma for a few moments, knowing that he would soon lapse back into it, would he choose to have antibiotics administered?"

[The Advance Directive Principle] states that where a clear and bona fide advance directive is available, it is to be followed. There are two broad types of advance directives: *instructional* and *proxy* .... An instructional advance directive is an instrument whereby the patient when competent, specifies, perhaps only in rather general terms, which types of treatments he or she wishes to have or, more commonly, not have, under certain circumstances, should the person become incompetent .... In a proxy advance directive, a competent individual designates some other individual or individuals to serve as the surrogate should the person become incompetent. These two types of advance directive may be combined: An individual might designate his or her spouse as proxy but include instructions that place limits upon that person's discretion to decide the individual's fate (11).

Which principle is followed may make a life-and-death difference to the patient. For example, acting in the patient's best interest may not be the same as acting on substituted judgment or following an advance directive. Simply put, competent people sometimes make choices contrary to their own best interests, so these principles can be incompatible at times.

Further, following substituted judgment may lead to a different decision than following an advance directive. What a person would choose if he or she were competent during an illness may be different from what the person would choose at an earlier time, projecting ahead to a time of incompetence and illness.

Since following different principles may yield different results, it is necessary to assign them some priority in resolving situations where more than one principle could be used. In addressing this issue, the President's Commission for the Study of Ethical Problems in Medicine and Biomedical and Behavioral Research proposed that where a valid and clear advance directive applies, it should take precedence over any other guidance principle, including best interest and substituted judgment (57).

Why Surrogate Decisions Are Not Always Respected

Despite the legally approved role of surrogate decisionmakers, their decisions may not be followed. There is no single explanation why decisions by court-appointed or de facto surrogates are not necessarily implemented. The uneasy coexistence of law and medicine, the perceived and actual authority of physicians, the emergence of medical technologies that prolong life, quality-of-life issues, a nationally heightened sensitivity to individual autonomy, an increasingly litigious society, and a growing population of incompetent elderly Americans all have contributed to the current legal, ethical, medical, and moral confusion over critical care decisionmaking by surrogates. Questions raised by surrogate decisionmaking have been present all along, but now they are complicated by new options for medical treatment, the multitude of decisions to be made at each step in a disease, and the sheer number of cases.

The Chairman of the President's Commission addressed this issue in a report on decisions to forgo treatment:

Although our study has done nothing to decrease our estimation of the importance of this subject to physicians, patients, and their families, we have concluded that the cases that involve true ethical difficulties are many fewer than commonly believed and that the perception of difficulties occurs primarily because of misunderstandings about the dictates of law and ethics. Neither criminal nor civil law precludes health care practitioners or their patients and relatives from reaching ethically and medically appropriate decisions about when to engage in or to forgo efforts to sustain the lives of dying patients (57).

Nonetheless, misunderstandings about the dictates of law persist, and can strongly influence medical decisionmaking and action:

Undue concern with imagined legal requirements and consequences may cause the physician to neglect or disvalue other, seriously significant factors that should figure prominently in the calculus of withholding or withdrawing life-prolonging treatment (30).

The assessment of a patient's competence and the allocation of decisionmaking authority also may become hopelessly lost in the context of medical practice. Three separate studies of decisionmaking in "do not resuscitate" orders of patients found that 18 to 20 percent of competent patients, and 19 percent of the families of incompetent patients, did not participate in decisionmaking (37). A study conducted later at three other teaching hospitals found that for 78 percent of patients who were to be resuscitated, the decision was made without either patient or family input (21). Yet there is evidence that physicians are unable to determine accurately patient preferences about resuscitation without asking them directly. Reasons given by physicians for not involving either patient or family in such decisions include family requests that the patient not be involved, patient requests that the family not be involved, the belief that the doctor already knows what the patient wants, physician awkwardness in broaching the subject with the family, and the physician's belief that medical indications were decisive (4).

Physician uncertainty over the authority of advance directives is evidenced by data showing that most doctors would not resuscitate their patient in the event of cardiac or respiratory arrest if the patient had left written instructions not to prolong life through artificial means. However, if a patient left written instructions to do everything possible to prolong life, only about half the physicians polled said they would resuscitate (56). If some physicians question the authority of advance directives, still others appear to be unaware of their patients' treatment preferences. Several studies indicate that physicians often do not have a good understanding of their patients' wishes concerning resuscitation, and that although they agree that such matters should be discussed with their patients, they actually do so infrequently (4). A recent report on State Medical Disciplinary Boards by the American Medical Association includes physician "failure to comply with natural death act or failure to transfer patient care when physician cannot comply with patient's request to withhold life-sustaining treatment" as grounds for disciplinary action (63).

Questions of Liability in Medical Decisionmaking

. . . Traditionally, law and medicine did not occupy an antagonistic relationship. Rather, this relationship was fundamentally a symbiotic, mutual, and cooperative one. In fact, the medical profession has aggressively co-opted the legal system over the years and used the law's authority to serve its own ends. Illustrations of this interaction include the medical profession's traditional power to determine for itself the standards of care to be applied in a malpractice action, the standards of information disclosure that constitute informed consent, and licensure/discipline standards for determining who is allowed to be a part of the medical profession. The role of government in influencing such standards has historically been negligible (30).

A physician or other health care provider may not administer treatments, diagnostic tests, or surgical interventions without the consent of the patient. If medical interventions are administered without consent, the doctor and health care facility may be sued for assault and battery or for negligence (47,55). That precept was upheld in a recent case, when relatives of a patient who was placed on a life-sustaining system after she suffered a respiratory-cardiac arrest that left her in a chronic vegetative state filed action seeking damages for the time the patient was on life-

sustaining systems. Although the trial court dismissed the motion, the Court of Appeals of Ohio, Summit County, reversed the decision and held that "a cause of action exists for wrongfully placing and maintaining a patient on life-support systems, contrary to the express wishes of the patient and her family" (33). The second trial was decided in favor of the doctor, and the hospital privately reached a financial settlement with the family before the verdict was reached. During a second appellate proceeding, the doctor also privately settled with the family (73).

Complicating matters, however, is the distinction often cited between withholding (not starting) treatment and withdrawing or removing it. Although philosophers have argued that there is no significant moral difference between the two acts, many caregivers continue to worry that stopping existing treatment—like a mechanical ventilator or chemotherapy—may be considered direct action that entails higher liability risk (6,18,27,30, 66).

Grayer still is the question of whether doctors recommend treatment in these cases because they believe it is clinically indicated or because they are concerned about their liability if they do not—no matter what the family wants (30). Ironically, although unwanted cessations of treatment theoretically may lead to lawsuits, there are numerous cases of families seeking a court order to stop treatment, but court orders to continue treatment have been sought only rarely and in unusual circumstances (1).

Physicians, however, perceive themselves in a double bind. On one hand, families increasingly request that treatment be withheld or withdrawn; on the other hand, in 1982 two California physicians were charged with first degree murder after discontinuing mechanical ventilation and intravenous fluids to a persistently vegetative patient—even though the family had asked that this treatment be discontinued (2). Although that case was dismissed by a court of appeals and remains one of a kind, it made a deep impression on physicians (30). More recently, the Massachusetts Supreme Court upheld the right of an incompetent patient not to receive nutrition and hydration through a gastrostomy tube. Although it was widely agreed that the patient would not have wanted such treatment, his health care facility refused to discontinue it. The court, which respected the facility's decision, ruled that the patient must be transferred either to his home or another facility willing to comply with his wishes (9).

Questions of Abuse of Surrogate Decisionmaking Powers

Theoretically, a person with a dementing illness has the same right as any other individual to bring suit against those associated with his or her care. In practice, however, that may prove difficult. Where an individual has been formally deemed incompetent, has a history of confused behavior, or has depended on a de facto surrogate or attorney-in-fact, that person's views and statements are seriously discredited both in the courts and in the community. Moreover, people with dementing conditions may be suspicious, paranoid, and argumentative as part of the normal course of their diseases. Thus, while a person has ample theoretical recourse against abuse, those suffering from dementia are poorly situated to avail themselves of it. They must rely on the concern and advocacy of others.

The legal options against abuse of surrogate powers vary. De facto surrogates, with no formal power, could be challenged by another person. Where power of attorney has been granted and the principal is still competent, the principal may revoke the status of the attorney-in-fact. Although the ordinary power of attorney is not legally recognized where the principal is no longer competent, it may continue in fact until challenged by a concerned individual. A durable power of attorney could also be challenged in court by another person on the basis of abuse. For guardians or conservators, another individual or the court (under its continuing jurisdiction to review conduct) might challenge an abuse of decisionmaking power.

Individuals as Research Subjects

Progressive dementias—and especially Alzheimer's disease—can be difficult to diagnose, understand, and treat. There is compelling justification for research directed at understanding and controlling or preventing these diseases. The nature of the illnesses limits the use of animal research models, and human subjects are necessary for even the early stages of scientific research. Thus, the social value of finding a cure or prevention for progressive dementias must be balanced against the protection and best interests of individuals who cannot understand or consent to research participation (42,52).

Until the early 1970s, individuals in prisons, mental health facilities, and nursing homes were readily used as research subjects.

These groups presented unique research opportunities because of the researcher's ability to carefully control and monitor the subject and his environment and to find subjects who willingly or unwillingly could participate in studies. The research projects, which ranged from the nonintrusive to the very intrusive, included a wide variety of studies aimed at obtaining information on medical and psychological problems. Few bothered to question the propriety of using the mentally disabled for these purposes. By the early 1970s the public's attention was focused on certain research projects that were difficult to categorize as anything but abusive. For example, it was disclosed that some retarded residents at Willowbrook State Hospital in New York had been deliberately infected with viral hepatitis and that many of the residents then contracted this illness. It was also revealed that 22 geriatric patients at the Jewish Chronic Disease Hospital were injected with foreign cancer cells without their knowledge or consent (8).

These revelations led to public concern over unconsenting mentally disabled individuals being used in any research, and to the congressional establishment of the National Commission for the Protection of Human Subjects of Biomedical and Behavioral Research in 1974. Some restrictions on when the mentally disabled may be used as research subjects, along with measures to protect the disabled who do participate in research, resulted from the Commission's and the public's concern over this issue. Federal guidelines provide little specific legal and ethical guidance, however, as applied to elderly individuals with dementia.

Even if an elderly person with a dementing illness could give prior valid consent, as an advance directive in a durable power of attorney or through a decision made by a surrogate, there would still be the question of continuing consent: As research experimentation grows and changes, would the incompetent subject or surrogate still be in favor of any specific experiment and what kind of mechanism would enable him or her to choose to participate on a case-by-case basis (51)?

In November 1981, the National Institute on Aging held a conference on the ethical and legal issues related to informed consent for Alzheimer patients. That meeting led to the creation of a task force to formulate guidelines for use by researchers, policymakers, and institutional review boards (IRBs) concerned with experimentation regarding Alzheimer's disease or involving Alzheimer patients (43). In addition to proposing guidelines, the task force suggested that IRBs might want to encourage: 1) the development of a Federal policy on minimal-risk research that could guide State efforts to draft legislation regarding surrogate decisionmaking for research participation by incompetent individuals, and 2) the establishment of a national research ethics advisory body with authority to endorse or prohibit specific research protocols. Endorsement would be evidence of compliance with Federal regulations.

The suggested guidelines were supplied by the task force with these aims:

> . . . 1) to express a preference for research with patients who are competent or who are otherwise relatively less vulnerable to potential abuse; 2) to identify individuals who are favorably inclined to participation in research and to provide mechanisms for their participation now and in the future, subject to necessary safeguards; 3) to assure that all research protocols involving [Alzheimer] patient-subjects have adequate mechanisms to assess competence, assure the adequacy of the consent process, and assure the continued ability of the subjects to decline to participate or withdraw; 4) to indicate special considerations in and limitations on research involving patients who are not capable of granting legally effective consent on their own behalf (43).

Ten guidelines on these issues were drawn up. Among other recommendations, the task force suggested that IRBs be particularly sensitive to protocol design and methodology involving sub-

jects who lack capacity to give consent, who do not object to consent, or who have not given prior consent through a durable power of attorney or otherwise. Research involving such individuals may be roughly classified into three different groups:

1. nonintrusive, noninvasive data collection and observation, and invasive research posing no more than minimal risk to subjects;
2. invasive research posing more than minimal risk that offers some realistic possibility of direct therapeutic benefit to the subject; and
3. invasive research posing more than minimal risk that does not offer some realistic prospect of direct therapeutic benefit to the subject.

The task force suggested that, where applicable, subjects should be selected in the following order of preference:

1. noninstitutionalized, still-competent individuals with Alzheimer's disease who decide whether or not to participate;
2. noninstitutionalized individuals with Alzheimer's disease and with impaired competence who had earlier competently expressed, and still express, a willingness to participate in research;
3. noninstitutionalized individuals with Alzheimer's disease and with impaired competence who express a current willingness, with family support, to participate in research; and
4. other noninstitutionalized individuals with Alzheimer's disease and with impaired competence who express a current willingness to participate in research.

The task force maintained that consent forms and other appropriate IRB safeguards be required for subjects with Alzheimer's disease who have the capacity to provide or refuse legally effective consent. Long-range protocols should be developed in which valid subject consent could be obtained during the early stages of dementia. For individuals with a dementing illness, greater scrutiny of the subject's capacity to provide consent should occur. Other factors to consider include the risks posed by specific research, the likelihood that the subject is to receive direct benefits, and the complexity of the research. The task force also recommended that IRBs ensure that research protocols include a mechanism to designate a "legally authorized representative" or surrogate decision-maker when a subject lacks the capacity to provide valid consent to participate in research, but does not object to participating.

ISSUES AND OPTIONS

It has been said that laws function best when they are the end product of social consensus (30). Laws that precede consensus on divisive issues often act as lightning rods for continued unrest and controversy. Furthermore, action by the Federal Government that is later overturned by the courts only serves to confuse the public, and put into limbo the lives of directly affected individuals.

Consensus on the issues raised by surrogate decisionmakers is slowly forming in the courts and State legislatures. Allowing this consensus to mature is perhaps the only way to ensure lasting constituent support and agreement on these issues. Some of the issues presented here may be more quickly and easily resolved than others, and might be safely legislated upon at this time; others might more wisely be left to further public debate. Most options detailed in this section could be accomplished by State, as opposed to Federal legislation, except where noted.

ISSUE 1: Should a standard method of determining competence to make health care decisions be adopted, or institutional checks on such determinations be introduced?

Option 1: People could lose their right to self-determination upon diagnosis of a dementing disorder.

Option 2: Let physicians decide whether a patient with a dementing disorder is competent to make decisions.

Option 3: Base the determination of competence on a patient's demonstrated understanding of a treatment and its consequences—and of a refusal of treatment and its consequences.

Option 4: Consider competence to be decision-relative.

Option 5: Require court hearings for each person whose competence to make health care decisions is questioned.

Option 6: Form institutional committees to review the competence of a patient if competence is questionable or there is disagreement between physician and patient.

Option 7: Rely on a standing body of physicians, nurses, social workers, lawyers, mediators, laypeople, and others to act as an informal court, making competency determinations on a community or regional basis.

Option 8: Encourage health care facilities, such as hospitals and nursing homes, to develop and announce institutional policies and procedures for determining competence.

Option 1 would obliterate the rights of individuals who are diagnosed early in their diseases, yet permit self-determination for other individuals who have long since become incompetent but never had the benefit of diagnosis.

Letting physicians determine competence (option 2) is, for the most part, the status quo. One of the difficulties here is that a physician's religious, cultural, and moral beliefs and preferences may conflict with those of a patient. Often physicians deem patients competent when they consent to treatment, but incompetent when they refuse to continue the same treatment at a later date (32). This option also denies the patient due process of law before stripping him or her of decisionmaking powers.

Physician assessment of a patient should not be disregarded as an option, however. Frequently the physician (or other professional caretaker) is the most objective member of the patient-physician-family triangle, and has motives that are less clouded by grief, trauma, or guilt. The physician is likely to have the most experience in assessing individuals with dementia. Option 2 does not incur the expense or time of a court competency hearing. If family members and other professional caretakers agree that the patient is incompetent, this approach generally is suitable.

Option 3 focuses on a patient's understanding of the consequences of a health care decision, not on whether the person agrees or disagrees with the physician or with family members. Safeguards might be instituted to ensure that adequate information to aid an informed consent or refusal is given to each patient prior to a treatment decision. A patient's comprehension of a proposed treatment is crucial to a competent decision, yet physicians have not always given sufficient time and effort to explaining treatments and consequences clearly. Devising adequate informational safeguards (e.g., peer review) would be challenging, but could result in better informed decisions.

The more important the decision and its ramifications, the more careful should be the assessment of competence—a point acknowledged by option 4. If the decision and its ramifications are not life-threatening or particularly vital, the patient's preferences might be more readily upheld. Guidelines for evaluating the difficulty of decisions in relation to a patient's decisionmaking capacity could be created either by government or individual health care facilities. Devising and implementing such guidelines would take effort, but the advantage of option 4 is that such a system protects an individual's autonomy for as long as possible while still safeguarding health and safety.

Option 5, although it might safeguard the rights of some patients, is time-consuming, expensive, and traumatic for patients, family, and physicians. The judicial process often proceeds too slowly for medical needs. Such a proposal could also unduly burden the courts. However, if the judicial system could be streamlined to review competence effectively and efficiently, then a mandatory court hearing when a person's competence is questioned might present the enormous advantage of assuring each person the benefit of due process before losing the right to make decisions.

Institutional review committees—option 6— might be similar to the institutional ethics committees discussed earlier. Organization and operational questions regarding IECs, however, also would apply to this sort of competency review.

The advantage of such a committee would be that the patient's right to self-determination might be better protected. A committee with members having diverse beliefs and values might make the decision regarding a patient's competence a more neutral and balanced one.

The disadvantage of option 7 lies in the unknown composition and funding of a standing review group, although many health care facilities, insurance companies, and other institutions might agree to fund and staff it. There also may be questions regarding the group's expertise, methodology, and authority. The advantages include the independence of the group's members. Moreover, the assessment resources offered by such a group might be greater than those of an individual physician, hospital, or nursing home. A standing review group might also be an appropriate mechanism for determining competence to make nonmedical (e.g., financial) decisions. The group might be used for all competence determinations, or only when competence is questionable or in dispute. It might also recommend judicial action when unable to determine an acceptable resolution itself.

Option 8 could include developing a list of who is responsible for determining competence, effective safeguards against error and abuse, and an indication of when court intervention is appropriate. Many facilities already have such policies but either do not formally advise prospective patients of them or do not adhere to them. There is also a possible conflict of interest if health care facilities not only determine competence but also prescribe care. The advantage of option 8 is that patients and families could act as consumers— judging the stated policies and procedures of each facility and choosing the one most closely aligned with their own preferences. More importantly, patients and families have a right to know and understand the policies of their health care facility. Armed with that knowledge, the determination of competence for a given patient might be demystified, and patients and families might be better able to make informed consents or refusals.

ISSUE 2: Should a uniform definition of terminal illness be adopted?

Option 1: Refrain from adopting a uniform definition of terminal illness.

Option 2: Define terminal illness as the few days or weeks when death is imminent.

Option 3: Define terminal illness as occurring at some stage earlier than a few weeks preceding imminent death.

Option 4: Amend living will statutes to apply to health care decisions at any time, not solely at the point defined as "terminal illness."

The disadvantages of option 1, which is the status quo, have been discussed previously. The advantage of doing nothing now is that a societal consensus on this issue may form which law could then be enacted to embody.

Option 2 would give physicians, rather than patients, almost exclusive right to make treatment decisions until the very end of life. Further, it would strip most decisionmaking powers from surrogates and directive powers from advance directives.

A broader definition—option 3—would allow patients wishing to do so to execute advance directives to ensure withholding or withdrawing of treatment. It also would allow surrogates to act on the desires of the patient at an earlier stage.

Option 4 would allow incompetent patients who previously executed clearly defined directives or legally appointed a surrogate to have their medical treatment desires met through the course of their illness.

Living wills, family consent provisions, and durable powers of attorney mainly revolve around critical care decisions. Many statutes pertaining to these mechanisms, including living will statutes, depend on the diagnosis of a patient as terminally ill. With no standard definition of that term, confusion surrounds the application of these legal devices.

ISSUE 3: Could the identification of surrogate decisionmakers be encouraged?

Option 1: Require people to identify a surrogate decisionmaker when their tax status changes, or periodically.

Option 2: Give tax credits or deductions for the identification of a surrogate, or penalize people who have not identified a surrogate by a certain age.

Option 3: Require people claiming deductions for home or day care of their parents or spouses to document that a surrogate decisionmaker has been identified.

Option 4: Make enrollment into social service, health, and income maintenance programs contingent on identification of a surrogate.

Option 5: Encourage hospitals, nursing homes, other health care facilities, and board and care homes to institute procedures requiring or identifying surrogates of all entering persons.

Option 6: Expand the family consent provisions in State law.

Option 7: Encourage States to define precisely what powers are accorded surrogate decisionmakers.

Option 8: Impose sanctions against caretakers, facilities, or even family members who refuse to follow a surrogate's decisions.

People might be required to appoint a surrogate decisionmaker for health and estate purposes when their tax status changes from employed to retired, and to document that appointment with the submission of their taxes (option 1). One disadvantage of this method lies in relying on, and further burdening, the country's tax collection system. It also does not account for individuals who become incompetent before they retire, those who do not retire, and those for whom emergency decisions must be made. The advantage is that more people would designate, and communicate their wishes to, a surrogate while still competent. People could be required to appoint a surrogate or surrogates every 10 years, through forms filed with their taxes, voter registration, health insurance, or doctor. However, that approach excludes individuals who do not pay taxes, vote, or purchase health insurance. It also excludes those who never see a doctor or for whom emergency decisions must be made.

The disadvantages of option 2—giving tax credits or deductions—include the necessity for new tax laws, as well as the potential loss of tax revenue. Emergencies might also preclude the ability of a health care facility to find out the identity of the surrogate.

People claiming deductions for home or day care could be required to document that a surrogate has been identified (option 3). However, many individuals are already incompetent by the time they require tax-deductible care, so they would be unable to designate surrogates themselves. Other problems with option 3 include the increased burden on the tax review process, and the situation of people who do not have related caretakers.

Case managers might assist in or require the identification of a surrogate. If enrollment is not contingent on the identification of a surrogate (option 4) it might at least trigger the encouragement or counseling of the family on how to identify a surrogate. Again, however, by the time some assistance programs are used, many persons already are incompetent. Option 4 also increases the burden of reviewing eligibility for these programs.

The disadvantage of option 5 is that many board and care homes are unregulated. Also, health care facilities are not currently equipped to help identify surrogates.

Family consent provisions, creating an automatic surrogate decisionmaker for an incompetent individual are frequently tied to advance directives such as living wills and therefore may not be used until the individual is terminally ill. Under option 6, therefore, given the confusion over the definition of terminal illness, a family member may not be able to act as a surrogate until the last few days before an individual's death.

Option 7 would require States to tackle some possibly contentious issues head on, and legislators' decisions would likely be made without benefit of community consensus. The advantage of

this option is that, once powers were clearly determined, patients, families, surrogates, and administrators of health care facilities would have greater guidance in protecting the rights of an incompetent patient. Uniform guidelines for surrogate health care decisions could be adopted, making it easier for surrogates to act across State lines.

The advantage of option 8 is that treatment disputes could be circumvented, and surrogates with some evidence of what individuals would have wanted could carry out their wishes. However, surrogates, if appointed by the court or even by the individual, may not know the values and preferences of the individual.

Physicians and health care facilities not wishing to comply with the health care decisions of a surrogate could be compelled to refer the surrogate to alternate physicians or facilities that would comply. Surrogates could be given assistance in advocating an individual's wishes, and the occasionally combative situation when a physician disagrees about a surrogate's decision would be alleviated.

Surrogate decisionmakers are a living extension of a person's right to self-determination. The greater awareness of surrogates—the need to appoint them, and the need to use them—has encouraged individuals to think about how they want to be medically treated. If people take the time to think about these issues and communicate their desires, not only is their own treatment course clearer, but society also gains by moving toward an informed consensus on how to treat persons with dementia.

Numerous methods are already in place for identifying surrogate decisionmakers. Existing methods are adequate; what appears inadequate is the use of those methods. Therefore, the challenge lies less in identifying surrogates than in stimulating and promoting their use.

The increasing number of elderly individuals with dementia makes the early identification and timely use of surrogates vital. However, steps must be taken to lessen the cost, ignorance, and fear associated with surrogate decisionmaking. Lawyers (and other individuals) formally assisting in this process need sufficient, current information, as does the general public.

A number of these options might be used in concert, creating multiple opportunities for the early identification of a surrogate, and requiring—after a grace period, and with grandfather clauses—that individuals who have not complied seek a court order for treatment to be withheld or withdrawn.

ISSUE 4: Should the use of advance directives be stimulated?

Option 1: Use advance directives solely as a guide to what treatment an individual would have wanted.

Option 2: Require people to execute advance directives when their tax status changes, or periodically.

Option 3: Introduce uniform State statutes on advance directives.

Option 4: Require attorneys who prepare advance health care directives to have specific training in this field.

Option 5: Permit nonlawyers who have received special training to prepare advance directives.

Option 6: Make compliance with advance directives mandatory, with punishment for failure to follow them.

Under option 1, compliance with advance directives would not be mandatory, and the extent to which one would be followed would be determined by the aggressiveness of the physician or the family if the directive were disputed. That is basically the status quo. The main disadvantage of the status quo is the individual's uncertainty about whether his or her wishes will be respected. The advantage is that a societal consensus may continue to form in support of making compliance with advance directives mandatory.

Option 2, requiring people to prepare and sign advance directives, has the same advantages and disadvantages mentioned earlier with regard to identifying surrogate decisionmaking (issue 3, above). A percentage of people would not be reached through option 2.

States now have widely different statutes and interpretations. While option 3 might force States to legislate in advance of a clear-cut societal consensus, one advantage would be that advance directives executed in one State could be respected in another. Also, the public's participation in the legislative process leading to adoption of uniform statutes might go a long way toward the formation of a societal consensus.

Attorneys specifically trained to draft and execute advance directives (option 4) are likely to do so in a way that would be less open to subsequent medical, legal, or familial arguments. Again, a clarification of the decisionmaking powers of individuals appointed to carry out advance directives would be enormously helpful in knowing how to prepare such directives.

Additionally, advance directives could be prepared by other persons specifically educated in this field (option 5). Social workers, nurses, physicians, the staff of senior citizens centers, and others might be empowered to execute these directives after receiving appropriate education. While nonlawyers are not trained to craft legal documents, if living wills are viewed as a guide, as opposed to a mandate, then nonlegal personnel might be able, with training, to prepare them adequately. By allowing someone other than a lawyer to draft advance directives, they might become less daunting, more accessible, and less expensive for the average person.

One problem with option 6 is that many advance directives lack enough specificity regarding patient preferences and therefore are difficult to follow or may be subject to a variety of interpretations. The advantage of making them mandatory is a greater likelihood that the autonomy of individuals would be respected after their own incompetence. The stress and anxiety of the dying process might be alleviated if individuals knew they would not be treated in a personally offensive way.

Physicians and health care facilities not wishing to comply with an individual's advance directive could be compelled to refer family members to alternate physicians or care facilities that would comply. They could also be required to assist family members in transferring patients with advance directives to those alternative caregivers. As noted, many States and care facilities already have a policy on transfer, but do not follow it. Option 6 would give families assistance in carrying out a family member's instructions, and it would ease the occasional disagreement between physicians and families over adherence to an advance directive.

ISSUE 5: Should standard procedures for resolving disputes about treatment be adopted?

Option 1: Use an Institutional Ethics Committee as a resolving body.

Option 2: Employ trained mediators to settle treatment disputes.

Option 3: Establish a standing body of physicians, nurses, social workers, ethicists, lawyers, laypeople, and others to act as an alternative to court resolution on a community or regional basis.

Option 4: Require health care facilities to assist the families in transferring the patient to a doctor or facility more sympathetic to their wishes in cases of unresolvable dispute.

Option 5: Require family members who disagree among themselves to sign documents releasing the facility and physician from liability.

The advantage of option 1, reliance on an IEC, is that it creates an alternative arena in which cases might be decided without resort to the courts. IECs might allow family members and physicians who are unhappy with a treatment decision to air their concerns outside, rather than inside, a courtroom.

Mediators (option 2) could suggest alternate solutions that might be acceptable to both physician and family. Such mediators would need to be medically educated in order to understand the individual's prognosis, whether the physician has operated in the spirit of informed consent, and if all options had already been examined by physician and family. Operational and funding issues for this process would need to be worked out, but mediators offer the promise of resolving problems short of costly and time-consuming legal battles.

The disadvantages of option 3, as with the option of using such a group to determine patients' competence (issue 1, option 7, above), lie in the unknown composition and funding. Again, health care facilities, insurance companies, and other institutions might agree to fund and staff a group to resolve disputes, particularly as an alternative to court involvement. The advantages of such a standing body are the group's objectivity in arriving at alternate solutions, and its ability to recommend that certain cases go to the courts for resolution.

Option 4 will not help resolve disputes if no sympathetic alternative provider can be found or when the dispute is between family members, but it would allow many families and physicians to resolve their disputes peacefully.

Physicians and facilities may not want to raise the suggestion of a possible lawsuit, but a release from liability (option 5) might free the physician to suggest treatment based on medical decisions about the individual rather than on the physician's fear of a lawsuit. Clearer, more decisive, and bolder treatment decisions might result from a deemphasis on defensive medicine.

Treatment disputes sometimes arise between physicians and family members. Most of these disputes can be avoided. If a surrogate decisionmaker with clearly defined powers has been appointed in advance of an individual's incompetence, or if a clear directive has been executed, then many treatment disputes will be prevented. Until advance directives and surrogate decisionmaking powers are more clearly defined and widely used, however, methods to resolve treatment disputes are needed.

ISSUE 6: Should there be a distinction between unwanted treatment that sustains life and the unwanted cessation of such treatment?

Option 1: Consider unwanted treatment that prolongs life less objectionable than the unwanted cessation or withholding of treatment that would prolong life.

Option 2: Consider unwanted treatment that prolongs life just as objectionable as the unwanted cessation of treatment that prolongs life.

Option 1 errs on the side of life-sustaining treatment. Yet unwanted prolongation of life may be seen as just as objectionable as the unwanted cessation of life-sustaining treatment.

Under option 2, physicians would be less inclined to practice defensive medicine, as they could be held liable for refusing to withdraw or withhold unwanted treatment.

Legal clarification of the status of unwanted treatment would be useful. As noted, once advance directive and surrogate decisionmaking powers are more clearly delineated, many existing sources of tension would be eradicated.

ISSUE 7: Should States include the decision to withhold or withdraw medical treatment in advance directives or in powers given to surrogate decisionmakers?

Option 1: States could decide not to act, leaving resolution of disputes regarding the withholding and withdrawing of treatment up to the courts.

Option 2: Direct that critical health care decisions fall outside the purview of surrogate decisionmakers or advance directives.

Option 3: Grant surrogates and those following advance directives clear power to require the withholding or withdrawing of treatment.

Option 1, the current situation, has the disadvantages of forcing many more surrogates and family members through the trauma of court involvement, and of encouraging unwanted treatment of many individuals. The advantage of this option is that it allows States to await formation of a societal consensus.

The advantage of option 2 is that an extremely small percentage of incompetent individuals with unscrupulous surrogates would be protected. The disadvantages include the obliteration of individuals' right to determine critical health care treatment for themselves or to delegate that authority to a surrogate.

Granting surrogates and those following advance directives the power to withhold or withdraw treatment (option 3) might allow unscrupulous surrogates to make decisions only for their own motives, but it would also allow most individual preferences to be more easily respected, and might circumvent disputes between doctors, family members, and the patient.

Once again, a clarification of powers in the context of statutes on living wills, family consent, guardianship, conservatorship, durable powers of attorney, and durable powers of attorney for health care, is one of the best ways to stem the confusion and combativeness surrounding the issue of withholding or withdrawing life-sustaining treatment.

ISSUE 8: Should special precautions be taken when persons with a dementing illness are involved in biomedical research?

Option 1: Adopt the guidelines suggested in 1985 by the National Institute on Aging Task Force.

Option 2: Encourage the use of special informed consent forms or interview procedures when persons with dementia are involved in research.

Researchers and institutions receiving funding from the National Institutes of Health could be required to abide by the 10 provisions of the National Institute on Aging Task Force guidelines. Among other protections, option 1 would ensure that research protocols include a mechanism for designating a legally authorized surrogate decisionmaker when a patient-subject lacks decisionmaking capacity but does not object to participation in the research.

Forms for elderly persons should have short, clear sentences, large print, and simple explanations. Option 2 could entail having the forms critiqued by elderly consultants rather than by clinical researchers before they are given to the proposed patient-subjects. Researchers also could revise the traditional one-on-one, single interview process of obtaining an informed consent. Instead, they could leave a copy of the informed consent form with potential subjects and let them study it at leisure and in the security of their own residences; encourage friends and relatives of the individual to be present during the interviews; use informational aids, such as tape recorders, slides, or sketches, to further explain the research; and cosign the form with the patient-subject as an affirmation that the research is an ethically invested and mutual service.

The enormous impact that dementing diseases have on individuals, families, and society probably justifies the continued use of incompetent persons as research subjects in attempts to find a cure or prevention. However, these vulnerable individuals must be protected from experimentation that is unsafe, unnecessary, or irrelevant. One approach is to encourage individuals to give their informed consent or refusal to research participation prior to becoming incompetent. As a study changes, surrogates should constantly reevaluate whether an incompetent person would still wish to take part in the study.

CHAPTER 5 REFERENCES

1. Annas, G.J., Boston University, School of Medicine, personal communication, January 1986 and Mar. 31, 1986.
2. *Barber and Nedjl* v. *Superior Court*, 195 Cal Rptr. 484, 147 Cal App 3d 1054, 1983.
3. Beck, C.M., and Phillips, L.R., "The Unseen Abuse: Why Financial Maltreatment of the Elderly Goes Unrecognized," *Journal of Gerontological Nursing* 10(12):26-30, 1984.
4. Bedell, S.E., and Delbanco, T.L., "Choices About Cardiopulmonary Resuscitation in the Hospital," *New England Journal of Medicine* 310:1089-1093, 1984.
5. Bellotti, F.X., "Investigating and Prosecuting Patient Abuse and Neglect in Nursing Homes: The Massachusetts Perspective," Attorney General's Office, Medicaid Fraud Control Unit, Commonwealth of Massachusetts, February 1985.
6. Billings, A.J., "Comfort Measures for the Terminally Ill: Is Dehydration Painful?" *Journal of the American Geriatrics Society* 33:808-810, 1985.
7. Brackel, S.J., and Rock, R.S., *The Mentally Disabled and the Law* (Chicago, IL: University of Chicago Press, 1971).
8. Brackel, S.J., Parry, J., and Weiner, B.A., *The Mentally Disabled and the Law*, 3rd ed. (Chicago, IL: American Bar Foundation, 1985).
9. *Brophy* v. *New England Sinai Hospital, Inc.*, Massachusetts State Supreme Court, Sept. 11, 1986.
10. Brown, B., University of Detroit Law School, personal communication, May 3, 1985.
11. Buchanan, A., Gilfix, M., and Brock, D., "Surrogate Decisionmaking for Elderly Individuals Who Are Incompetent or of Questionable Competence," contract report prepared for the Office of Technology Assessment, U.S. Congress, 1986.
12. *Canterbury* v. *Spence*, 464 F.2d 772, D.C. Circuit 1972.
13. Cohen, E.S., "Autonomy and Paternalism: Two Goals in Conflict," *Law, Medicine & Health Care* 13(4):145-150, September 1985.
14. Cohen, E.S., Mace, N., and Myers, T.S., consultants and staff, Office of Technology Assessment, in collaboration, 1985.
15. Collin, F.J., Jr., Lombard, J., Moses, A., et al., *Drafting a Durable Power of Attorney: A Systems Approach* (Lexington, SC: R.P.W. Publishing, 1984).
16. Drane, J.F., "Competency To Give an Informed Consent: A Model for Making Clinical Assessments," *Journal of the American Medical Association* 252:925-927, 1984.
17. Drane, J.F., "The Many Faces of Competency," *Hastings Center Report* 15(2):17-21, 1985.
18. Dresser, R., "When Patients Resist Feeding: Medical, Ethical, and Legal Considerations," *Journal of the American Geriatrics Society* 33:790-794, 1985.
19. Dudowitz, N., National Senior Citizens Law Center, California, personal communications, Oct. 21, 1985, and Apr. 21, 1986.
20. Dyer, A.R., "Assessment of Competence To Give Informed Consent," *Alzheimer's Dementia—Dilemmas in Clinical Research*, V.J. Melnick and N.N. Dubler (eds.) (Clifton, NJ: Humana Press, 1985).
21. Evans, A.L., and Brody, B.A., "The Do Not Resuscitate Order in Teaching Hospitals," *Journal of the American Medical Association* 235:2236-2239, 1985.
22. Gilfix, M., Gilfix Associates, Palo Alto, CA, personal communication, December 1985.
23. Gilfix, M., Gilfix Associates, Palo Alto, CA, personal papers, 1985.
24. Gilfix, M., "Legal Issues and Alzheimer's Disease," testimony prepared for the California State Task Force on Alzheimer's Disease, March 1986.
25. Hynes, C.J., "Protecting Patients' Personal Funds: Failures and Needed Improvements" [A Report on the Assets of Patients in Residential Health Care

Facilities], Office of the Attorney General Investigating Nursing Homes, Health and Social Services, May 1977.

26. Hynes, C.J., "Private Proprietary Homes for Adults: Their Administration, Management, Control, Operation, Supervision, Funding & Quality of Care" [A Second Investigative Report], Office of the Attorney General Investigating Nursing Homes, Health and Social Services, Mar. 31, 1979.

27. In re Quinlan, 70 NJ 10, 355 A.2d 647, cert. denied, 429 US 922, 1976.

28. *Jordan v. Heckler*, United States District Court for the Western District of Oklahoma, CIV-79-994-W, Jan. 18, 1985.

29. *Jordan v. Schweiker*, United States District Court for the Western District of Oklahoma, CIV-79-994-W, Mar. 17, 1983.

30. Kapp, M.B., and Lo, B., "Legal Perceptions and Medical Decisionmaking," contract report prepared for the Office of Technology Assessment, U.S. Congress, 1986.

31. Kjervik, D., American Association of Colleges of Nursing, personal communication, Apr. 26, 1985.

32. *Lane v. Candura*, 376 NE2d, 1232, Mass. App. 1978.

33. *Leach v. Shapiro*, Court of Appeals of Ohio, Summit County, 469 N.E.2d 1047 (Ohio App. 1984), May 2, 1984.

34. Levine, C., "Hospital Ethics Committees: A Guarded Prognosis," *Hastings Center Report* 22-27, June 1977.

35. Levine, C., "Questions and (Some Very Tentative) Answers About Hospital Ethics Committees," *Hastings Center Report* 14 (Towson, MD, personal communication, May 3, 1985).

36. Lew, J., "The Health Care Decision-Making Process: Selected Legal Issues," speech delivered to the California State Task Force on Alzheimer Disease, March 1986.

37. Lo, B., Saika, G., and Strull, W., "Do Not Resuscitate Decisions: A Prospective Study at 3 Teaching Hospitals," *Archives of Internal Medicine* 145:1115-1117, 1985.

38. Lombard, J.J., Jr., and Emmert, W.W., "The Durable Power of Attorney: Underused Tool," *The National Law Journal* 15-19, Oct. 29, 1984.

39. Mace, N.L., consultant in gerontology, Towson, MD, personal communication, May 3, 1985.

40. Mace, N.L., and Rabins, P.V., *The 36 Hour Day: A Family Guide To Caring for Persons With Alzheimer's Disease, Related Dementing Illnesses, and Memory Loss in Later Life* (Baltimore, MD: Johns Hopkins University Press, 1981).

41. McKay, J.B., "Protective Services Give Elders More Autonomy," *Generations* 8(3), Spring 1984.

42. Melnick, V.J., *Alzheimer's Dementia: Dilemmas in Clinical Research*, V.J. Melnick and N.N. Dubler (eds.) (Clifton, NJ: Humana Press, 1985).

43. Melnick, V.J., Dubler, N.N., and Weisbard, A., "Clinical Research in Senile Dementia of the Alzheimer Type: Suggested Guidelines Addressing the Ethical and Legal Issues," *Journal of the American Geriatrics Society* 32:531-536, 1984.

44. Michels, K.A., American Nurses Association, personal communication, April 26, 1985.

45. Mishkin, B., "Making Decisions for the Terminally Ill," *Business and Health*, June 1985, pp. 13-16

46. Mishkin, B., "Giving Someone the Power To Choose Your Medical Care," *Washington Post Health Section*, Aug. 7, 1985.

47. Mishkin, B., "A Matter of Choice: How To Maintain Control Over Health Care Decisions," Senate Special Committee on Aging, 1986.

48. Nathanson, P., "Future Trends in Aging & the Law," *Generations* 8(3):7-9, Spring 1984.

49. Nathanson, P., Director, Institute of Public Law, Albuquerque, NM, personal communication, May 3, 1985.

50. Nolan, B.S., "Functional Evaluation of the Elderly in Guardianship Proceedings," *Law, Medicine & Health Care* 12:5, 210-218, October 1984.

51. Otten, A.L., "New 'Wills' Allow People To Reject Prolonging of Life in Fatal Illness," *Wall Street Journal*, July 2, 1985.

52. Otten, A.L., "Research Into Alzheimer's Disease Is Frustrated by Ethical Dilemma," *Wall Street Journal*, May 3, 1985.

53. Owens, P., "When the Trustee Gets SSI Check," *Newsday*, Jan. 9, 1984.

54. *Pratt v. Davis*, 118 Ill. App. 161, 1905 (aff'd Ill. 30, 79 N.E. 562, 1905)

55. President's Commission for the Study of Ethical Problems in Medicine and Biomedical and Behavioral Research, *Making Health Care Decisions, Vol. One: Report* (Washington, DC: U.S. Government Printing Office, 1982).

56. President's Commission for the Study of Ethical Problems in Medicine and Biomedical and Behavioral Research, *Making Health Care Decisions, Vol. Two: Appendices* (Washington, DC: U.S. Government Printing Office, 1982).

57. President's Commission for the Study of Ethical Problems in Medicine and Biomedical and Behavioral Research, *Deciding To Forgo Life-Sustaining Treatment* (Washington, DC: U.S. Government Printing Office, 1983).

58. Probate Code 5-103, 8 *Uniform Law Annals* 437, West Supplement 1983.

59. Randal, J., "Are Ethics Committees Alive and Well?" *Hastings Center Report* 13(6):10-12, 1983.

60. Regan, J.J., "Process and Context: Hidden Factors

in Health Care Decisions for the Elderly," *Law, Medicine & Health Care* 13(4):151-152, September 1985.

61. Robertson, J., Address to American Society for Law and Medicine, Concern for Dying Conference, Washington, DC, April 1983.

62. Social Security Disability Amendment of 1984, Calendar No. 899, Report 98-466, 98th Cong., 2d sess.

63. State Health Legislation Report, American Medical Association Department of State Legislation, vol. 14, No. 3, August 1986.

64. Suber, D.G., and Tabor, W.J., "Withholding of Life-Sustaining Treatment From the Terminally Ill, Incompetent Patient: Who Decides?" [Part 1], *Journal of the American Medical Association* 248:2250-2251, 1982.

65. Suber, D.G., and Tabor, W.J., "Withholding of Life-Sustaining Treatment From the Terminally Ill, Incompetent Patient: Who Decides?" [Part 2], *Journal of the American Medical Association* 248:2431-2432, 1982.

66. *Superintendent of Belchertown State School* v. *Saikewicz*, 370 N.E. 2d 417, Massachusetts Superior Judicial Court, 1977.

67. Uniform Law Commissioners' Model Health Care Consent Act, 9 *Uniform Law Annals* 332, West Supplement 1984.

68. U.S. Department of Health and Human Services, "Report of the Secretary as Required by Section 16, Public Law 98-460," September 1985.

69. U.S. Department of Health and Human Services, Office of the Inspector General, *Revised Nursing Home Inspection Guide; Health Care Provider Fraud: Technical Assistance Services*, Washington, DC, March 1984.

70. U.S. Department of Health and Human Services, Office of the Inspector General, *Supplemental Security Income Fraud: Technical Assistance Manual*, Washington, DC, November 1983.

71. U.S. Department of Health and Human Services, Office of the Inspector General, "Board and Care Homes," Washington, DC, April 1982.

72. Veatch, R.M., "Hospital Ethics Committees: Is There a Role?" *Hastings Center Report* 7(3):22-27, 1977.

73. Wilson, D., attorney to Leach, personal communication, Apr. 29, 1986.

74. Witt, S., "Disabled Easily Bilked of Support Checks," *The Tulsa Tribune* Mar. 20, 1984.

Long-Term Care Services and Settings: An Introduction

CONTENTS

Tables

Figure

Long-Term Care Services and Settings: An Introduction

The availability, appropriateness, quality, and cost of long-term care services for persons with dementia are major concerns for their families, for health care and social service providers, and for Federal, State, and local government. Many residents of nursing homes and board and care facilities and many recipients of long-term care services at home are persons with dementia. Yet families complain that long-term care services are frequently not available for such persons or, when available, are of poor quality, inappropriate for the needs of the person with dementia, and/or too expensive (122). Many health care and social service providers agree.

Government concerns about long-term care for persons with dementia arise from the complaints and urgent requests for help from families and others who care for them. On the other hand, the current and potential cost of providing appropriate long-term care services for the growing number of persons with dementia in this country is a grave concern. The congressional letters of request for this OTA assessment reflect both concerns.

This and the following six chapters take up these concerns. This chapter presents an overview of existing long-term care services and settings and the Federal Government's current role in long-term care. Chapter 7 discusses the relatively recent but growing phenomenon of long-term care services designed specifically for people with dementia, including special care units in nursing homes and board and care facilities and adult day care and home care services tailored to their needs. Other chapters consider aspects of long-term care that are most directly affected by Federal legislation and regulations, and thus most likely to be addressed by Congress:

- patient assessment and eligibility for publicly funded services (ch. 8);
- the training of health care and social service providers who treat individuals with dementia (ch. 9);
- quality assurance procedures for nursing homes, board and care facilities, and home care services (ch. 10);
- Medicare and Medicaid coverage of long-term care (ch. 11); and
- overall financing of services for persons with dementia (ch. 12).

Although an increasing number of long-term care facilities and agencies are providing services designed specifically for individuals with dementia, OTA estimates that fewer than 2 percent of such persons are receiving special services. The vast majority who receive any formal long-term care services are cared for by facilities and agencies that provide essentially the same services for everyone. Thus, the description of services and care settings in this chapter reflects what is currently available to most people with dementia. It also provides a basis for understanding why families and health care and social service providers are complaining to Congress and why many of them are so enthusiastic about the development of special services for these patients.

WHAT SERVICES ARE NEEDED FOR PERSONS WITH DEMENTIA?

Services for people with dementia include a wide variety of medical, social, rehabilitative, and legal services (see table 6-1). While some of those listed are not usually considered long-term care services—for example, physician, legal, and dental services—they are needed intermittently over the prolonged period of illness that characterizes many dementing conditions.

Table 6-1.—Care Services for Persons With Dementia

Physician services: Diagnosis and ongoing medical care, including prescribing medications and treating intercurrent illness.

Patient assessment: Evaluation of the individual's physical, mental, and emotional status, behavior, and social supports.

Skilled nursing: Medically oriented care provided by a licensed nurse, including monitoring acute and unstable medical conditions; assessing care needs; supervising medications, tube and intravenous feeding, and personal care services; and treating bed sores and other conditions.

Physical therapy: Rehabilitative treatment provided by a physical therapist.

Occupational therapy: Treatment to improve functional abilities; provided by an occupational therapist.

Speech therapy: Treatment to improve or restore speech; provided by a speech therapist.

Personal care: Assistance with basic self-care activities such as bathing, dressing, getting out of bed, eating, and using the bathroom.

Home health aide services: Assistance with health-related tasks, such as medications, exercises, and personal care.

Homemaker services: Household services, such as cooking, cleaning, laundry, and shopping, and escort service to accompany patients to medical appointments and elsewhere.

Chore services: Household repairs, yard work, and errands.

Supervision: Monitoring an individual's whereabouts to ensure his or her safety.

Paid companion/sitter: An individual who comes to the home to provide supervision, personal care, and socialization during the absence of the primary caregiver.

Congregate meals: Meals provided in a group setting for people who may benefit both from the nutritionally sound meal and from social, educational, and recreational services provided at the setting.

Home-delivered meals: Meals delivered to the home for individuals who are unable to shop or cook for themselves.

Telephone reassurance: Regular telephone calls to individuals who are isolated and often homebound.

Personal emergency response systems: Telephone-based systems to alert others that an individual who is alone is experiencing an emergency and needs assistance.

Transportation: Transporting people to medical appointments, community facilities, and elsewhere.

Recreational services: Physical exercise, art and music therapy, parties, celebrations, and other social and recreational activites.

Mental health services: Psychosocial assessment and individual and group counseling to address psychological and emotional problems of patients and families.

Adult day care: A program of medical and social services, including socialization, activities, and supervision, provided in an outpatient setting.

Respite care: Short-term, in- or out-patient services intended to provide temporary relief for the primary caregiver.

Dental services: Care of the teeth, and diagnosis and treatment of dental problems.

Legal services: Assistance with legal matters, such as advance directives, guardianship, power of attorney, and transfer of assets.

Protective services: Social and law enforcement services to prevent, eliminate, or remedy the effects of physical and emotional abuse or neglect.

Case management: Client assessment, identification and coordination of community resources, and followup monitoring of client adjustment and service provision.

Information and referral: Provision of written or verbal information about community agencies, services, and funding sources.

Hospice services: Medical, nursing, and social services to provide support and alleviate suffering for dying persons and their families.

SOURCE: Office of Technology Assessment, 1987.

Some of the services are defined primarily in terms of who provides them (e.g., physician and dental services, and physical, occupational, and speech therapy). Others are defined by the government programs that pay for them (e.g., skilled nursing and home health aide services paid for by Medicaid and Medicare); by the needs of recipients (e.g., supervision and paid companion); or by their intent (e.g., respite care and hospice services). Because they are defined in different ways, they overlap conceptually. For example, adult day care, respite care, and hospice services each include many of the others, and adult day care can be a form of respite care.

People with dementing illnesses live at home or in nursing homes, in board and care facilities, or, to a lesser extent, in State mental hospitals. Most of the services listed in table 6-1 can be provided

in any of these settings. A few apply only to patients living at home, such as home-delivered meals and home health aide services, but basically the same services (meals and assistance with medications, exercises, and personal care) are also provided to residents of nursing homes, board and care facilities, and State mental hospitals.

The list of the services in table 6-1 represents an ideal that is seldom realized. Many services are not available at all in some localities or are available in insufficient quantity to meet local needs. Moreover, some services are not available in certain settings. For example, mental health services are seldom available in nursing homes, in board and care facilities, or at home.

The ideal for services and settings is sometimes described as a continuum of care, implying that the services and settings can be ordered to correspond to the increasing disability and care needs of patients. Such ordering may be valid for physically impaired patients. However, current knowledge of the course of dementia-causing diseases and the care needs of persons with dementia at different stages of their illnesses is insufficient at present to serve as a basis for specifying an order for long-term care services and settings. For example, nursing homes are usually placed at one end of the continuum of care—indicating that they are appropriate for severely disabled persons—while adult day care and home care are services closer to the other end—indicating that they are appropriate for less severely disabled individuals. Yet some people in the early or middle stages of dementia may need institutional care, and some families and adult day care centers are managing extremely debilitated dementia patients at home. Therefore, although the goal of providing a full range of services and settings for persons with dementia remains, the criteria for ordering them in a continuum of care are unknown.

Later sections of this chapter discuss the four settings in which persons with dementia live—the home, nursing homes, board and care facilities, and State mental hospitals—and two nonresidential settings—adult day care centers and community mental health centers. Each section reviews what is known about the number of such persons in the setting, the services they receive, and the problems they experience in obtaining services.

Hospitals provide acute medical care for dementia patients, and some also provide care for prolonged periods for such patients, often because no other care setting is available. However, incentives for shorter length of stay associated with the Medicare Prospective Payment System and other government and private cost containment measures are expected to decrease the use of acute care hospital beds for long-term care. At the same time, in response to these and other changes in health care delivery, a growing number of hospitals are developing home care and adult day care services, and a few are converting acute care beds to chronic or long-term care. In addition, hospitals continue to play a pivotal role in referring patients to other community agencies for long-term care (11). This aspect of their role in long-term care is discussed later in this chapter.

Inpatient hospice units are a potential care setting for persons with dementia. They primarily serve terminally ill cancer patients, however. Persons with dementia are seldom treated, partly because they may be more difficult to manage than other patients; and partly because of fears about malpractice litigation since persons with dementia may not be competent to consent to withholding or withdrawal of treatment (115,116). To increase the use of hospice services for persons with dementia would require adapting hospice methods to the needs of cognitively impaired people and greater knowledge of the physical, emotional, and social aspects of patient functioning in the late stages of dementia. Since inpatient hospice units seldom serve dementia patients at present, they are not discussed in this chapter.

THE CURRENT ROLE OF THE FEDERAL GOVERNMENT IN LONG-TERM CARE

The United States has no national long-term care policy, but the Federal Government is extensively involved in providing, funding, and regulating a wide range of long-term care services. At least 80 Federal programs provide or fund such services, either directly or indirectly. The five programs described in table 6-2 are the major sources of Federal funding for long-term care (88). Their role in funding services for dementia patients is discussed briefly here and at greater length in chapters 11 and 12.

The programs listed in table 6-2 pay for a substantial proportion of all long-term care in this country. In 1983, Medicaid paid about $12.4 billion for nursing home care, which represented 43 percent of all public and private spending for such services. Medicare paid $500 million, or about

Table 6-2.—Major Federal Programs That Fund Long-Term Care Services

Medicare/Title XVIII of the Social Security Act

Medicare is the Federal insurance program intended to provide medical care for elderly people. Generally those who are 65 or older are eligible, and about 95 percent of these Americans are enrolled in Medicare. People under 65 who have been receiving social security disability payments for at least 2 years are also eligible. Medicare provides reimbursement for hospital and physician services and limited benefits for skilled nursing home care, home health care, and hospice. By law, Medicare does not cover custodial care.

Medicaid/Title XIX of the Social Security Act

Medicaid is the joint Federal/State program intended to provide medical and health-related services for low-income individuals. Medicaid regulations are established by each State within Federal guidelines; eligibility requirements and the long-term care services that are covered vary significantly among the States. In general, however, Medicaid pays for nursing home and home health care for individuals who meet financial and medical eligibility requirements. In some States Medicaid also covers adult day care and in-home services such as personal care and homemaker services.

Social Services Block Grant/Title XX of the Social Security Act

The Social Services Block Grant provides Federal funding to States for social services for elderly and disabled people, among others. There are no Federal requirements for specific services that must be provided, but many States use a portion of their Social Services Block Grant funds for board and care, adult day care, home health aide, homemaker, and chore services. States determine the eligibility requirements for these services and may require means tests.

Title III of the Older Americans Act

Title III of the Older Americans Act provides Federal funding to States for social services for people over 60. The specific services that are provided are determined by each State and local Area Agencies on Aging, but Title III funds are often used for home health aide, homemaker, and chore services; telephone reassurance; adult day care; respite care; case management; and congregate and home-delivered meals. Means tests are not used to determine eligibility, but Title III services are supposed to be targeted to elderly people with social or economic need.

Supplemental Security Income (SSI)

SSI is the Federal income support program that provides monthly payments to aged, disabled, and blind people with incomes below a minimum standard ($336 for individuals and $504 for couples in 1986) and assets below $1,700 for individuals and $2,550 for couples. States may supplement the Federal benefit for all SSI recipients in the State or for specified groups, such as those living in board and care facilities. Some States also provide SSI supplements for home health care and homemaker services.

SOURCE: U.S. Congress, Office of Technology Assessment, *Technology and Aging in America*, OTA-BA-264 (Washington, DC: U.S. Government Printing Office, June 1985); U.S. Congress, Congressional Research Service, "Financing and Delivery of Long-Term Care Services for the Elderly," Oct. 17, 1985.

2 percent of all spending for nursing home care (88). Both programs require eligible individuals to contribute their own resources to pay for part of the cost of their care. For example, individuals who are covered by Medicaid in a nursing home and who receive a social security check or any other income are required to pay almost all of it to the nursing home.

As a result, the 45 percent of total nursing home spending covered by Medicare and Medicaid actually represented a much larger proportion of all nursing home residents, perhaps as high as 65 to 75 percent nationally (37,114) and 85 to 90 percent in some States (21). This somewhat complicated point is important for understanding the extent of government involvement in nursing home care: that is, although Medicaid and Medicare pay less than half the total cost of nursing home care, anyone who receives any Medicaid or Medicare funding—whether it is $1 or $1,000—for nursing home care (i.e., 65 to 90 percent of all residents) is a "Medicaid or Medicare patient" for purposes of regulatory requirements discussed below.

The proportion of home care paid for by the programs listed in table 6-2 is not known, but experts estimate that Medicare and Medicaid pay for one-third to one-half of all home care (18,72). In 1983, Medicare spent about $1.5 billion for home health care, and Medicaid about $600 million. Social Services Block Grant funds for in-home services for recipients of all ages amounted to some $555 million in 1983. Expenditures for in-home services under Title III of the Older Americans Act are not known, but the fiscal year 1985 appropriation for all Title III services (except congregate and home-delivered meals) amounted to $256 million (88).

Little is known about the total cost of board and care or adult day care or the proportion of those costs that is covered by publicly funded programs. However, about 43 percent of all residents of board and care facilities receive Supplemental Security Income (SSI) (58), and Social Services Block Grant funds are used for board and care in some states. Likewise, Medicaid, Social Services Block

Grant, and Title III funds are used for adult day care in some States (15).

Because government programs pay for such a large portion of long-term care services, government regulations play a significant role in defining and structuring the entire care system. Legislation and program regulations that define which long-term care services are covered determine to a great extent what services are available at all. Thus, for example, Medicare and Medicaid legislation and regulations that restrict coverage to medical and physical care services have resulted in these services becoming predominant over social and mental health services in the long-term care system as a whole. (The impact of Medicare and Medicaid coverage policies on the availability of appropriate services for persons with dementia is discussed in ch. 11.)

Similarly, legislation and regulations that define eligibility requirements determine which individuals receive any publicly funded services. For instance, Medicare legislation and regulations define eligibility in terms of the medical and skilled nursing care needs of the patient; as a result, individuals who need only personal care and supervision are ineligible. Long-term care is costly, especially when services are needed for prolonged periods, as is often the case for someone with dementia. Since relatively few individuals or families have sufficient income or assets to pay privately for services for an extended amount of time, the eligibility requirements for publicly funded services determine to a great extent who receives services, at least for extended periods. Some individuals, however, are given wrong diagnoses or diagnoses that are not directly related to their care needs in order to meet the eligibility requirements. (The impact of Medicare and Medicaid eligibility requirements on access to long-term care for dementia patients is discussed in ch. 11. Alternate methods for determining eligibility are discussed in ch. 8.)

Legislation and program regulations also define which facilities and agencies may provide covered services. Federal regulations determine which nursing homes and home health care agencies are certified to provide Medicare-funded services. Federal, State, and local government regulations determine which facilities and agencies are certified to provide services funded by Medicaid, the Social Services Block Grant, Title III of the Older Americans Act, and SSI.

Certification and licensing requirements regulate aspects of each facility's physical plant, services that must be provided, and the number and type of health care and social service professionals and others who must be available in each facility. For example, regulations specify overall staff-to-resident ratios for nursing homes that care for Medicare and Medicaid recipients; the number of required physician visits per year; and the minimum level of involvement of dietitians, social workers, physical therapists, occupational therapists, pharmacists, and other professionals. Although some nursing homes have a physical plant, services, and staffing levels that exceed Medicare and Medicaid requirements, many barely meet the minimum requirements (37). (Licensing and certification procedures and the role of government in regulating quality of care in long-term care facilities and agencies are discussed in ch. 10.)

The Federal Government's significant role in funding long-term care is well known. Less well recognized is the extent to which Federal legislation and regulations and State legislation and regulations developed within those Federal guidelines determine what services are available, who receives them, and who provides them. Moreover, since Medicaid pays for such a large proportion of all nursing home care, the program's reimbursement rates also have a significant impact on the prevailing charges for nursing home care (38). In many localities, Medicaid rates function as a floor for nursing home charges.

Even the long-term care services available to individuals who pay privately are determined in large part by Federal and State program regulations and reimbursement rates. This is because these individuals are often treated in facilities and by agencies that also serve Medicare and Medicaid patients and are, therefore, subject to those programs' requirements for physical plant, services, and staffing.

A final component of the Federal Government's role in this area is the Veterans Administration (VA), the largest, single provider of long-term care services in the country. As of 1983, VA operated 99 nursing homes, with an average daily census of 8,849 residents, and 16 large board and care facilities (called domiciliary care facilities) with an average daily census of 6,852. VA also paid for nursing home care in non-VA facilities for a daily average of 10,212 veterans, for board and care in private homes for a daily average of 11,195 veterans, and for nursing home and board and care in 45 State veterans' homes in 33 States, with a daily average of about 11,000 veterans. Home care services were provided through 30 of the 172 VA Medical Centers for more than 7,000 veterans.

Adult day care was provided at 5 VA Medical Centers and respite care at 12 (111).

The pervasive role of the Federal Government in providing, funding, and regulating long-term care underlines the importance of national legislation and regulations in determining access, quality, and cost of care. Although Federal policies affect the availability of services for anyone in need of long-term care, they particularly affect those who require services for extended periods, including many persons with dementia.

CONCEPTUAL ISSUES IN LONG-TERM CARE OF PERSONS WITH DEMENTIA

Several basic conceptual issues arise repeatedly in discussions about long-term care for persons with dementia and underlie policy-related questions about eligibility, personnel and training, quality assurance, and financing. These issues are summarized below; their policy-related implications are introduced here and discussed at greater length in relevant chapters.

- ***What are or should be the relative roles of families and formal long-term care services in the care of persons with dementia?***

This question (also discussed in ch. 4) is answered in different ways by different people. Some people believe that formal long-term care services completely replace services once provided by the family. Thus they believe that when a family is overcome by the burden of care and gives up, long-term care facilities and agencies should take over. Other people believe that formal long-term care facilities and agencies provide specific services that families cannot provide, such as skilled nursing care, occupational or physical therapy, or, on a simpler level, assisting an elderly caregiver with bathing a patient he or she is unable to lift. Thus, they believe that when such services are provided in the home, they forestall nursing home placement, allow individuals to remain at home longer, save public dollars, and mitigate the burden of care for families, without taking over tasks family members are able to perform.

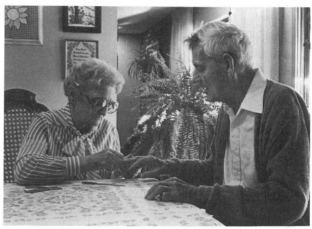

Photo credit: ADRDA and Peter Carrol, PhotoSynthesis Productions, Inc.

Families and paid caregivers may be equally capable of providing some long-term care services for persons with dementia.

Still others believe that families and formal long-term care facilities and agencies are equally capable of providing needed services and that formal services should be used on an intermittent basis to provide relief for a family. This model of care—the respite care model—appears to be evolving concurrently with the growing recognition of the care needs of persons with dementia and may, in fact, be developing in response to their care needs. Specifically, respite care would be a uniquely appropriate model of care if those with dementia are seen to require supervision and assistance with activities of daily living (services that many families *can* provide) more frequently than others receiving long-term care, and to require skilled nursing care, occupational therapy, and physical therapy (services that families ordinarily *cannot* provide) less frequently.

It is unclear whether one of these models is most appropriate for everyone with dementia or whether the appropriate model depends on patient characteristics, family characteristics, stage of illness, or all three. Obviously, the question of responsibility for the care of persons with dementia involves both providing provision of services and paying for them. Theoretical and practical considerations in deciding who should pay for long-term care for persons with dementia are discussed in chapter 12.

● *How does the concept of respite care relate to the underlying rationale for existing long-term care services?*

Long-term care services funded by Medicare and Medicaid are intended to address medical and health-related needs, while services funded by the Social Services Block Grant and Title III of the Older Americans Act are meant to meet specific social service needs. In contrast, respite care aims to temporarily relieve families of caregiving responsibilities. It can involve any services that fulfill that purpose and often consists primarily of patient supervision during the absence of a family caregiver.

In general, using long-term care services funded by Medicare and Medicaid for respite care is inconsistent with the current intent of the programs, and regulations often restrict such use. (Medicare and Medicaid waiver programs discussed in this chapter and ch. 11 do sometimes allow respite care.) Similarly, the intent and regulations of programs that fund specific social services must be stretched when the need is not necessarily for these services but rather for a temporary caretaker. Thus, the concept of respite care and the underlying rationale for existing long-term care services are mismatched: existing services are intended to address specific needs, while respite care does not imply specific services. Further, the emphasis in existing services is on a patient and his or her needs; respite care, although required because of an individual's condition, responds primarily to family needs.

These conceptual differences raise questions about the kinds of services that should be included in respite care programs and how they can be defined in legislation and regulations. The difference in focus on the needs of recipients versus those of families raises questions about how to determine eligibility for publicly funded respite care services and whether it should be based on individual needs, family needs, or some combination. (The difficulty of defining and measuring family needs for the purpose of eligibility determination is discussed in ch. 8.)

● *What is the appropriate role of mental health services and settings in the care of people with dementia?*

Primarily for historical reasons, most individuals with dementia receive long-term care services from facilities and agencies that focus on medical and physical care needs. Relatively few are cared for in State mental hospitals or other psychiatric facilities or receive services from outpatient mental health centers. Moreover, mental health professionals, such as psychiatrists, clinical psychologists, psychiatric social workers, and psychiatric nurses, are seldom employed in nursing homes or other facilities and agencies that provide long-term care for those with dementia (9,92). Although experts agree that dementia is an organic condition and not a mental illness per se, the emotional and behavioral problems often associated with it suggest that the expertise of mental health professionals may be particularly relevant to the care of persons with dementia (34,69,70).

In nursing homes and in board and care facilities, residents with dementia and those with chronic mental illnesses, such as schizophrenia, are sometimes considered to have similar care needs. However, the emotional and behavioral problems of nursing home residents are seldom identified or evaluated (123). As a result, it is not clear whether the problems and long-term care needs of these two groups are similar. It is also unclear whether either or both groups could be better cared for in mental health settings. It is interesting to note that in some countries a significant portion of long-term care services for elderly people is called "psychogeriatric care." In the United States, although many State mental hospitals have psychogeriatric units and VA maintains some psychogeriatric wards (12 in 1981) (111), the concept of psychogeriatric care is not widely recognized, nor are long-term care services usually provided in this model.

For Federal policy purposes, the question of the role of mental health services and settings in the care of persons with dementia has implications for personnel and quality assurance regulations and requirements for funding for mental health services in nursing homes and board and care facilities. For example, Medicare and Medicaid do not require nursing homes to provide mental health services for residents (9,34). If such services are believed to be important for individuals with dementia, changes in these regulations may be needed. A related issue is whether government should promote long-term care for persons with dementia in mental health facilities.

- *Can the long-term care needs of persons with dementia who are under 65 be adequately met within the existing system?*

Individuals with dementia usually receive long-term care services in facilities and agencies that primarily serve elderly people. It is unclear whether the long-term care needs of younger people differ significantly from those of older ones and whether the needs of both groups are equally well (or poorly) met in these settings. In addition, eligibility requirements for some long-term care services exclude those who are under 60 or 65, and the process of establishing eligibility for other programs, such as Medicare, is considerably more difficult for those under 65 (see ch. 11). Whether and how long-term care services should be adapted to the needs of younger persons with dementia and whether public funding programs should be restructured to include all everyone with dementia on the same basis is an important policy issue.

- *What is the role of the Veterans Administration in providing long-term care services for dementia patients, and how are VA services related to non-VA services?*

Although VA provides and funds long-term care services for many veterans, providing services for those with dementia is problematic for two reasons. First, VA services are provided on a priority basis to veterans with service-connected disabilities. Since dementia is seldom service-connected, veterans with dementia are accorded a lower priority than those with a service-connected disability. About 70 percent of those receiving VA services do not have service-connected disabilities (89), but an OTA survey of family caregivers found that 45 percent of persons with dementia who applied for VA long-term care services were refused, most often because of lack of a service-connected disability (122). A second problem is that VA services have traditionally focused on the veteran and not the family. Providing respite care would require a change in this traditional focus (112).

Despite these problems, VA is providing services for many veterans with dementia. In fiscal year 1983, VA hospitals and nursing homes treated 11,200 veterans with a primary diagnosis of a dementing disorder and about 9,000 others who had dementia as a secondary diagnosis. VA has developed several special care units for persons with dementia (112), and the agency is currently surveying all its facilities to determine service availability and gaps for such persons (19).

Over the next 15 years, the number of veterans in older age groups—and therefore at greater risk for dementia—will increase dramatically. In 1980, some 3 million veterans were over 65, but by 2000 that number will increase to 9 million, representing 63 percent of all males over 65 (111). In view of this very large population base, VA could build more facilities, purchase care for veterans in non-VA facilities, restrict eligibility for no-cost services, or limit the services it covers. Legislation passed by Congress in 1986 limits eligibility for veterans with non-service-connected disabilities to those who have incomes of $15,000 or less for a single veteran, $18,000 or less for a veteran with one dependent, with $1,000 added for each additional dependent. Veterans with non-service-connected disabilities and income above these levels may receive VA services if the services are available and if the veteran contributes to the cost of care (106).

Although VA has traditionally limited care for veterans with non-service-connected disabilities, such as dementia, the families of these individuals often expect VA to provide care and sometimes complain to their Representative or Senator when it is denied. Several bills have been introduced in Congress to require VA services for veterans with dementia. For example, HR 1102 would have required VA to allocate 10 percent of its long-term care beds to dementia patients. This bill was not enacted.

As the number of elderly veterans increases, Federal policies that provide long-term care in VA facilities for veterans with dementia would relieve non-VA facilities of the burden of caring for them but would simultaneously increase VA expenditures. Policies that allow the agency to purchase care from non-VA facilities would also increase VA expenditures but eliminate the need to build more VA facilities. Policies that deny VA services and coverage of services in non-VA facilities would shift the burden and cost of caring for veterans with dementia to non-VA facilities and to Medicare and Medicaid. Thus, VA eligibility and funding policies affect the need for non-VA facilities and services and Medicare and Medicaid expenditures for long-term care. Although the problem of integrating VA and non-VA long-term care services has received considerable attention in general (96,105,110,111,120), the relationship of the two in providing services for persons with dementia has received little attention.

- *What long-term care services can and should be provided for persons with dementia in rural areas?*

Many rural areas lack long-term care facilities, and lengthy travel times may make services such as adult day care impractical. Long distances and insufficiently trained personnel can also interfere with delivery of home care services. In some cases, lack of home care and adult day care may result in early placement of individuals with dementia in long-term facilities far from their homes. In other cases, lack of services intensifies the burden for families who care for them at home. Analysis of long-term care policy options should include consideration of their effect on persons with dementia in rural as well as suburban and urban areas.

- *How do the long-term care needs of minority group members with dementia differ from those of nonminority group members?*

Little is known about the care of minority group members with dementia. Although epidemiologic research indicates no difference in the prevalence of most dementing conditions among minority groups (see ch. 1), differences in attitudes, beliefs, and other characteristics among such groups may affect the way persons with dementia are regarded by their families and the larger community—for example, whether they are seen as physically ill, mentally ill, or simply old. Ethnic and cultural factors affect patterns of informal caregiving and the use of medical, mental health, and social services. They also determine the most effective methods of informing patients and their families of available services (54). Differences in minority group characteristics affect the validity of assessment procedures used to determine eligibility for services (see ch. 8), and they have important implications for staffing requirements and quality assurance regulations for long-term care facilities and agencies.

Because minority group status is frequently associated with low income, minority group members are more likely than others to depend on publicly funded programs that are means-tested. For example, 22 percent of black elderly and 25 percent of Hispanic elderly received SSI in 1981, compared with only 5 percent of the elderly population in general (57). Thus SSI policies can be expected to have a greater impact on access to long-term care services for minority group members than for the general population. Similarly, a higher proportion of blacks and Hispanics use VA as their sole source of health care (111). Therefore, VA policies may affect long-term care for minority groups disproportionately.

Different minority groups vary greatly on a wide range of characteristics, and no generalizations can be made about how all or even the majority of these groups react to and care for persons with dementia. Examples from minority groups are used throughout this and the following chapters to point out variations in patient care needs, informal caregiving patterns, and formal service utilization that are relevant to the development of public policy. At the same time, OTA recognizes the considerable differences in attitudes, beliefs, and characteristics within and between minority groups, and no stereotypes are intended.

- ● *What is the appropriate balance of institutional and noninstitutional long-term care services for persons with dementia?*

Some publicly funded programs, notably Medicaid and the VA, have encouraged institutional long-term care over home care in general (81,88, 111). Long-term care experts agree, however, that services for all kinds of patients should be provided in the home whenever possible and that program regulations should be changed to promote home care and services such as adult day care for those living at home. This approach is generally accepted for those with dementia, and as a result, families, health care and social service providers, and others are asking for increased services for individuals with dementia who are living at home.

The bias in favor of home care is strong, and nursing homes and other such institutions are often perceived negatively. At the same time, the OTA survey of family caregivers found that 80 percent agree that "a patient with a severe case of Alzheimer's disease should be living in a nursing home" (122). Similarly, the Massachusetts Governor's Committee on Alzheimer's Disease found that "because all patients with Alzheimer's Disease who survive long enough eventually require total care, the majority end up in institutions" (27). Thus institutional care is seen as unavoidable for many individuals in late stages of dementing illnesses.

For several reasons, institutional care may also be appropriate for some patients in earlier stages of the illnesses:

- ● Because of decreased cognitive ability and judgment, most individuals with dementia require 24-hour supervision. Those who do not have a family member or other person willing and able to provide that supervision may need institutional care, regardless of their other care needs, because the cost of 24-hour supervision at home is usually prohibitive.
- ● For family caregivers, behavioral disorders of some persons with dementia may be emo-

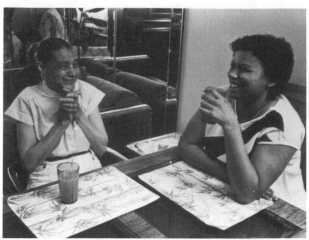

Photo credit: ADRDA and Peter Carrol, PhotoSynthesis Productions, Inc.

Families and health care and social service providers agree that home care is the first choice of persons with dementia.

tionally intolerable. In addition, some family caregivers who are smaller than the patient or who have sensory impairments may be physically at risk from some behavioral disorders. Such disorders may be more likely in the early or middle rather than the late stages of the illnesses.
- ● Although the home is often said to be the least restrictive setting for long-term care, individuals who wander and whose behavior is socially unacceptable may actually require fewer restrictions in institutional settings that allow such behaviors.
- ● Some environmental adaptations believed to facilitate improved functioning are feasible in institutional settings and adult day care centers but less so in the home. Social stimulation is also easier to provide in a group setting.
- ● In situations where the relationship between the patient and caregiver is poor, institutional placement may be necessary to avoid possible neglect or abuse at home.

For these reasons, institutional care may be the most appropriate long-term care option for some individuals with dementia even if they are not in the late stages of the illness, when total nursing care is needed, and even if formal home care services are available. The prevailing negative attitudes about nursing homes and other institutional settings increase the guilt of family members who decide that institutional placement is the best course. Such attitudes also discourage the use of nursing homes for respite care and may discourage some family members from remaining involved with their relative after placement.

* ***Do persons with dementia require special long-term care services?***

Perhaps the most important conceptual issue in long-term care for persons with dementia is whether they constitute a definable group with distinct care needs. The related policy issue is whether the Federal Government should create incentives for developing special long-term care services for them. Although most people agree that the long-term care system needs improvement, in general, some argue that the needs of this group are different and that special services and settings are needed. Others believe that everyone who requires long-term care has special care needs, and that making the existing system more responsive to the needs of each individual is a better approach than singling out one group for special care.

These two points of view raise important theoretical questions that have received little attention despite the growing interest in special services for persons with dementia. One overriding question is whether the category "dementia patients" is conceptually clear. Who is included? Only those with Alzheimer's disease or other primary degenerative dementias? What about individuals with multi-infarct dementia or Huntington's disease, or elderly persons with physical conditions that have dementia as a side effect of the disease or its treatment? If a category can be delineated, what are the long-term care needs of that group? Are their needs sufficiently similar—and sufficiently different from those of other patients—to warrant a separate care system?

The corresponding practical questions are whether persons with dementia can be accurately distinguished from other long-term care patients, which services they need, who can best provide them, and how much they should cost. Thus far, these questions have been answered in different ways by the many different individuals, groups, and agencies that have developed special services for persons with dementia. At the point when Federal, State, or local government begins to provide or fund special services for persons with dementia, these questions require answers that can be translated into eligibility requirements, staffing and quality assurance regulations, and reimbursement guidelines.

LONG-TERM CARE SETTINGS AND SERVICES

The following sections describe six settings that provide long-term care services for persons with dementia and other persons. Each section discusses the nature of those who are served, the quality of care, and access to the services for persons with dementia and their families.

Three distinct systems provide long-term care services:

1. the medical or physical care system, which includes nursing homes and home health care agencies and is funded primarily by Medicare and Medicaid;
2. the aging services system, which includes Area Agencies on Aging and homemaker and home nutrition providers and is funded by Title III, the Social Services Block Grant, and State and local funds; and

3. the mental health system, which includes State mental hospitals and community mental health centers and is funded by Medicaid, a Federal block grant, and State and local funds.

Persons with dementia are seldom differentiated from others who receive services in each of these systems. Thus individuals with dementia who receive services in the medical or physical care system are grouped conceptually with physically impaired elderly people, and increasingly both groups are described in terms of limitations in their self-care abilities or activities of daily living (ADLs). Those with dementia who receive services through the aging services system are grouped with physically impaired elderly people, and both groups are described under the rubric "frail elderly."

Finally, persons with dementia who receive services through the mental health system are grouped with those who have chronic mental illnesses, and both sets of patients are described as "mentally ill."

Individuals with dementia are seldom identified as a discrete group in long-term care research, and as a result, there are few studies comparing them with others who receive long-term care in terms of their characteristics, care needs, or experiences with facilities and agencies. Failure to identify them as a discrete group occurs partly because interest in these patients as a group has developed only recently, partly because of conceptual and practical difficulties in defining the group, and partly because aspects of the existing long-term care system, including eligibility, certification, and reimbursement regulations, tend to discourage their identification as a group.

Information in the following sections is largely from research in which the study populations include an unknown number of individuals with dementia. Although the population of elderly State mental hospital patients with a diagnosis of organic brain syndrome clearly includes many persons with dementia, it is more difficult for example to identify such persons in the three categories that have been used in research on board and care facilities: aged, mentally ill, and mentally retarded residents. Thus the accuracy of available information about the number of people with dementia in each setting varies. Moreover, for most settings, no comparisons are available of the characteristics and care needs of persons with and without dementia, or of the services most frequently provided for each group.

The following sections draw on the OTA survey of family caregivers (122) described in more detail in chapter 4. In addition, in the past few years, several State-sponsored committees and task forces have studied services for persons with dementia, and their reports specifically address the needs of these persons. Some of their findings are cited here; in general, they are based on anecdotal reports and should be interpreted as such.

The six long-term care settings described below are:

1. State mental hospitals,
2. nursing homes,
3. board and care facilities,
4. home care,
5. adult day care centers, and
6. community mental health centers.

State Mental Hospitals

State mental hospitals are usually large psychiatric facilities that provide acute and long-term care for mentally ill people. They are seldom included in reviews of long-term care settings, but until 30 to 40 years ago, they were the formal long-term care setting used most frequently for persons with dementia. Since then, factors largely unrelated to the care needs of such persons have resulted in decreased use of State mental hospitals for institutional care of persons with dementia and increased use of nursing homes and, to a lesser extent, board and care facilities.

During the 1700s and early 1800s, people who could not live independently because of acute or chronic physical or mental impairments and who had no source of informal care lived in locally supported almshouses. It is not known how many individuals with dementia lived in almshouses because the category "dementia patients" was unknown at that time; many of the diseases that cause dementia were not understood, and confusion was seen as a natural concomitant of old age. Some portion of those in almshouses undoubtedly had a dementing disorder, however.

Beginning in the mid-1800s, mentally ill people who would previously have been placed in almshouses were instead cared for in State-supported mental hospitals, called asylums. At first, these facilities admitted only patients with acute mental illnesses. Over the next century, however, and particularly after 1900, State mental hospitals provided care for an increasing number of chronically mentally ill and senile people (29,60). By 1946, some 44 percent of all first admissions to State and county mental hospitals had a diagnosis of organic brain syndrome (not including drug- or alcohol-induced organic brain syndrome) (102), and 30 percent of the residents of State mental hospitals were over 65 (48). Even though the term dementia was not used to describe the ailments of these individuals, it is clear that many and perhaps most of them had dementing illnesses.

In the late 1940s and 1950s, several developments combined to create a new direction in treatment of those with mental illness—the community mental health movement. This movement grew in part from the recognition that large State mental hospitals had become primarily custodial facilities where little treatment was provided, and in part from the development of psychotropic drugs and brief therapy methods that made outpatient care feasible for many patients. The movement, with its primary tenet that mental health services should be provided in the community whenever possible, led to the process of deinstitutionalization. As a result, between 1955 and 1980, the overall population of State mental hospitals decreased by 75 percent (44,60). Likewise, between 1946 and 1972, the proportion of first admissions to State mental hospitals with a diagnosis of organic brain syndrome dropped from 44 to 10 percent (102).

For elderly people, deinstitutionalization resulted primarily in reduced use of State mental hospitals and increased use of nursing homes and related care facilities. Table 6-3 documents the magnitude of this change.

Increased use of nursing homes was spurred by the enactment of Medicaid in 1965, which for the first time provided public funding for nursing home care on a national basis. With the introduction of Supplemental Security Income (SSI) in 1972, a federally guaranteed minimum income for elderly and disabled people was available for the first time. Moreover, some States provided additional funds for SSI residents in board and care facilities. The availability of SSI and State SSI supplements encouraged the discharge of persons with dementia (and of other State hospital residents) to board and care facilities (48).

Table 6-3.—Residents of Mental Hospitals and Homes for the Aged Who Were 65 or Older: 1950, 1960, 1970, and 1980

Type of institution	Rate per 100,000 persons 65 or older			
	1950	1960	1970	1980
Mental hospitals	1,150	1,074	563	200
Homes for the aged/dependent	1,769	2,342	3,966	4,835

SOURCE: Based on P. Lerman, ''Deinstitutionalization and Welfare Policies in the Welfare State in America: Trends and Prospects,'' *American Academy of Political and Social Sciences-1985 Annals* 479:132-155, 1985.

Historically, changes in the primary locus of institutional care for persons with dementia—from almshouses to State mental hospitals, and from there to nursing homes and board and care facilities—have occurred primarily in response to financial incentives. Placing these persons in State mental hospitals instead of almshouses transferred the cost of their care from local to State government (29). Similarly, placing them in nursing homes and board and care facilities instead of State mental hospitals transferred part of the costs to the Federal Government through Medicaid and SSI (48,60). There is no evidence that these changes occurred in response to the care needs of individuals with dementia, or that their care needs and the effect on them of changes in the locus of care were even considered.

The number of persons with dementia in State mental hospitals is not known. The 1980 census counted 51,000 elderly people in all mental hospitals (48), and some observers suggest that many of them have dementia even though their diagnoses may indicate mental illness (6). The National Association of State Mental Health Commissioners recently appointed a Task Force on Alzheimer's Disease that will develop estimates of the number of persons with dementia in such facilities (49).

Current admission practices in many State mental hospitals discourage admission of persons with dementia who can be managed in other settings (64,68), but clearly some, and perhaps many, are admitted. The Rhode Island Legislative Commission on Dementias Related to Aging described why persons with dementia might be transferred from nursing homes to State mental hospitals:

> If . . . the patient becomes aggressive, combative or in some manner endangers himself, other patients, or members of the nursing home staff, and such behavior cannot be controlled adequately through the use of physician-ordered pharmacological or physical restraints, the nursing home facility will then arrange for his transfer to one of the state . . . hospitals. Transfer may also be initiated if the patient wanders continually and cannot be restrained or monitored effectively (68).

In some cases, State mental hospitals are able to adjust medications to bring the behavior of these persons under control so that they can return to the nursing home.

Persons with dementia who are living in the community are sometimes brought to State mental hospitals because of behavior that is considered dangerous to themselves or others, and some are brought in by the police on an emergency basis when they are picked up wandering in the streets (27). How often such situations occur is not known, however.

Although State mental hospitals have been criticized for providing only custodial care, some persons with dementia receive excellent treatment in these facilities, as the Massachusetts Governor's Committee on Alzheimer's Disease heard:

> To my surprise and relief our experience with (the) State Hospital turned out to be a positive one during most of my father's 18-month stay there. He was taken off all medication immediately. The doctors, nurses, and attendants we met there were kind and competent. Within six weeks my father's behavior had adjusted to the point where it was thought that he could function in a nursing home. On the recommendation of the hospital social worker my father was placed in a particular nursing home. She brought him there on a Friday. We decided to give him a few days to adjust to his new surroundings. On Sunday afternoon my mother, brother, and I walked into my father's room to find him tied to a chair, naked, drugged, and in a pool of urine. I called up the social worker at (the hospital) and told her what we had found. She said she would investigate. The next day she found my father in the same condition and returned him to (the) State Hospital where he stayed until he died 18 months later (27).

Although little consideration has been given to providing long-term care for persons with dementia in State mental hospitals, at least one State task force has proposed developing a demonstration special care unit in one facility (68). Such a unit could provide a model of care based on a mental health rather than medical or physical care principles. One problem with this approach is that care in State mental hospitals can cost considerably more than in nursing homes. Since Medicaid funding is available for elderly patients in mental hospitals, the cost of care for Medicaid-eligible elderly people is shared by the Federal and State govern-ment. Medicaid does not cover those under 65 in mental institutions, and there is variation among States in how these patients are paid for. Generally, however, the cost is borne by State and local government.

Nursing Homes

Nursing homes are health care facilities that provide 24-hour supervision, skilled nursing services, and personal care. They are now the most frequently used institutional setting for persons with dementia. Care is provided primarily by nurses and by nurse's aides under their supervision. Although both Medicare and Medicaid regulations emphasize the nursing component of nursing home care, many persons with dementia do not need skilled nursing services, and for them the most important components of nursing home care may be 24-hour supervision and personal care.

At present, there are 14,000 to 15,000 nursing homes in the United States, with about 1.5 million beds (37,77). (Both the National Master Facility Inventory (NMFI) and the National Nursing Home Survey include a large number of facilities (about 11,000 in the 1982 NMFI) that do not employ any nurses or provide nursing services. These are discussed in the section on board and care facilities in this chapter.) About 75 percent of nursing homes are for-profit facilities, 20 percent are non-profit, and 5 percent are government-owned (101).

In 1982, some 7,000 nursing homes were certified to provide Medicare and/or Medicaid skilled nursing care and are called skilled nursing facilities (SNFs). About 5,500 others were certified to provide Medicaid intermediate level care (101) and are called intermediate care facilities (ICFs). Many nursing homes have some beds certified at the SNF level and some at the ICF level. Another 1,500 nursing homes, although they provided nursing care, were not certified by either Medicare or Medicaid (77).

The main difference between skilled nursing facilities and intermediate care facilities is that Federal regulations require SNFs to provide 24-hour services by licensed practical nurses (LPNs) and to employ at least one registered nurse on the day shift, 7 days a week. ICFs must have at least one LPN on duty during the day shift 7 days a week. State Medicaid regulations that define SNFs and ICFs vary greatly, and the proportion of nursing homes in each category also varies. For example, all or almost all nursing homes in Arizona and Connecticut are certified as SNFs, while almost all those in Iowa and the District of Columbia are certified as ICFs. Few differences have been found in the kinds of individuals cared for in SNFs and ICFs in different States, and the Institute of Medicine's Committee on Nursing Home Regulation recently recommended that the distinction between them should be dropped (37). The impact of such a change on access to nursing homes by persons with dementia requires further analysis.

Nursing home bed supply varies widely, from a low of 22 beds per 1,000 elderly residents in Florida to a high of 94 in Wisconsin (94). Total bed supply increased steadily from 1963 to 1977, but the rate of increase has slowed since then, partly in response to State efforts to limit bed supply in order to contain Medicaid expenditures. Since 1977 the supply has grown at a rate slower than the growth in the population age 75 or older, thus limiting access to nursing home care in general (94,114).

Residents With Dementia in Nursing Homes

Until recently, scant information was available about the number of persons with dementia in nursing homes. The 1977 National Nursing Home Survey found that 7 percent of residents had a primary diagnosis of chronic brain syndrome, and 2 percent had a primary diagnosis of senility without psychosis (97). No information was obtained about other diagnoses associated with dementia. However, nurses were asked about each resident's chronic conditions. According to the nurses, about 25 percent of all residents had chronic brain syndrome and 32 percent were senile, with prevalence increasing with age (see figure 6-1) (97).

The difference between the small proportion of nursing home residents with a primary diagnosis of chronic brain syndrome or senility and the much higher proportions identified by the nurses is partly explained by diagnostic practices

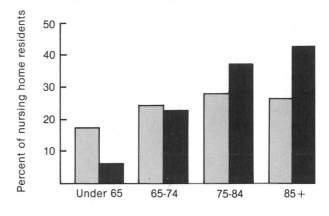

Figure 6-1.—Nursing Home Residents With Chronic Brain Syndrome or Senility as Assessed by Nurse Respondents, by Age, United States, 1977

☐ Chronic brain syndrome

■ Senility

SOURCE: U.S. Department of Health and Human Services, Public Health Service, National Center for Health Statistics, *Characteristics of Nursing Home Residents, Health Status, and Care Received: National Nursing Home Survey, United States, May-December 1977*, series 13, No. 51, DHHS Pub. No. (PHS) 81-1712, Hyattsville, MD, 1981.

that resulted in underdiagnosis of dementia, as discussed in chapters 1 and 3. In addition, Medicare and Medicaid policies that define eligibility in terms of medical and nursing care needs discourage the use of diagnoses that suggest the need for personal care and supervision instead. (See also the discussion of the "50 percent rule" in ch. 11.)

Since 1977, diagnostic practices have changed considerably, and higher proportions of nursing home residents now have a primary or secondary diagnosis of dementing disorders, at least in some States. A 1985 survey of Texas nursing homes found that 45 percent of the residents had a diagnosis of Alzheimer's disease and an additional 21 percent had diagnoses of other dementing disorders (86). A 1984 survey of New York nursing homes found that 41 percent of residents had a diagnosis of a dementing disorder (22).

Although some observers believe that dementia, and particularly Alzheimer's disease, is now being overdiagnosed for nursing home residents, research based on assessments of cognitive status rather than diagnoses suggests that at least

40 percent have a dementing disorder, and in some facilities the proportion is even higher. A 1983 study in Rhode Island using a cognitive rating scale to assess mental status found that 40 percent of those under 80 and 50 percent of those older had dementia (68). Another study found that 56 percent of the residents of a Maryland nursing home had a primary degenerative dementia, another 18 percent had multi-infarct dementia, and 4 percent had dementia associated with Parkinson's disease—a total of 78 percent with dementing disorders (70).

In addition to residents with cognitive impairment caused by the dementing disorders that are the subject of this OTA assessment, nursing homes serve people with cognitive impairments caused by acute and chronic diseases, by drugs taken to treat those diseases, by pain or terminal illness, and by mental retardation. They also serve people who appear to be cognitively impaired because of hearing and speech impairments or emotional withdrawal associated with depression. Nurses, nurse's aides, and other staff often do not distinguish between cognitive impairments caused by dementing disorders and those due to these other factors. (Some of the difficulties involved in making such distinctions are discussed in ch. 8.)

Little research has been done on the characteristics and care needs of persons with dementia in nursing homes. One study (70) found that many of these persons have coexisting psychiatric disorders (e.g., delusions, hallucinations, or depression) and behavioral disorders (e.g., restlessness, agitation, wandering). The length of stay of nursing home residents varies greatly, and several studies indicate that residents with mental disorders, including chronic brain syndrome and senility, tend to be among those who stay longest and, therefore, may be more likely than other residents to become eligible for Medicaid (42,53).

Many nursing home administrators and employees believe that persons with dementia are more difficult to care for and require more staff time than other residents. A study of Maryland nursing home residents found that those with behavioral disorders required 35 percent more staff time than those without behavioral disorders; however, the residents were not identified by diagnosis or cognitive status (2). To investigate this question, OTA contracted with Rensellear Polytechnic Institute for a retrospective analysis of data collected in the development of a new reimbursement system for New York State nursing homes, called RUG-II. Initial findings showed that nursing home residents with a diagnosis of dementia varied greatly in terms of limitations on activities of daily living, behavioral disorders, and care needs (22).

The New York State data included no measure of cognitive status, so the severity of dementia could not be determined. Nevertheless, an attempt was made to develop a rough index of severity by combining data on five survey items that may be related to cognitive status—resident's learning ability, motivation, refusal to care for self, expressive communication, and receptive communication/comprehension. (The wording of these items and the resident descriptors used to develop the index of severity are presented in app. A.) Analysis of the New York State data using resident diagnosis and the index of severity showed that persons with dementia were in general more impaired than other residents in activities of daily living and behavior, and that their level of impairment became greater with increasing severity of the dementia. For example, a greater number of those with dementia required continuous supervision with eating or had to be fed by hand; 61 percent of those in the high severity group required assistance compared with about 6 percent in the low severity group. Similar results were obtained for dressing, bathing, toileting, bowel and bladder control, and personal hygiene.

The data also showed that residents with a diagnosis of dementia were more likely than others to be wanderers, but that wandering was most frequent among those in the low and middle severity groups and decreased in the high severity group. Other behavioral disorders, including verbal abuse, physical aggression, and regressive or inappropriate behavior also occurred more frequently among residents with dementia (22) (see app. A).

These findings suggest that although many nursing home residents who do not have dementia require substantial assistance with activities of daily living, on average those with dementia require more aid. Because they are also more likely to have behavioral disorders, residents with dementia generally require more staff time. Thus, as nursing home administrators and employees maintain, persons with dementia are frequently "heavy care patients." The more severe the dementia, the more assistance is needed, although behavioral disorders appear to lessen at the highest level of severity. It should be noted, however, that these data were collected almost entirely in facilities that do not provide special services for persons with dementia. As discussed in chapter 7, some nursing homes with special services for these persons report decreased limitations in activities of daily living and behavioral disorders among their residents.

Quality of Care for Residents With Dementia

Nursing homes have been criticized for a long list of deficiencies that affect all residents, regardless of cognitive status. The criticisms range from widespread complaints about inadequate attention to residents' emotional and social needs and need for privacy to less frequent but serious complaints about dangerous medication errors and resident abuse and neglect (37,105). This assessment does not discuss these general problems in nursing homes except to note that some deficiencies are related to low levels of reimbursement for Medicaid patients and to Medicare and Medicaid regulations that focus on physical and nursing care needs to the exclusion of emotional and social ones.

In addition to problems that affect all nursing home residents, some care practices even in "good" nursing homes are inappropriate for persons with dementia:

- Cognitive status is not routinely assessed. As a result, the primary reason the person with dementia needs nursing home care is not identified or evaluated. Although some residents with dementia need nursing home care because of other physical problems, failure to identify cognitive deficits affects the quality of their care overall.
- Most nursing home personnel are not trained to care for people with dementia and are not

aware of management techniques that could lessen functional disability and behavioral disorders.
- Medications that could reduce agitation and other behavioral problems associated with dementia are frequently not used, sometimes because the physician is not aware of the behavioral problems but more commonly because he or she does not know which drugs to use or in what dosage. In some cases, individuals with dementia are given the wrong drug or excessive doses of drugs that increase their confusion and may cause extreme drowsiness and falls.
- Most nursing homes are designed to accommodate residents who are relatively immobile, and there is seldom enough space for those with dementia who may be physically active until the late stages of their illness. Restraints are frequently used to keep them from wandering or restless pacing, and some develop physical disabilites associated with forced immobility. Since exercise is seldom part of the daily routine, residents with dementia who are capable of physical activity often become increasingly agitated.
- The regular practice of rotating staff from one unit to another is a problem for persons with dementia who may be able to remember staff they see every day but cannot remember over longer periods of time and may become agitated when repeatedly confronted with caregivers they do not recognize.
- Increased noise and activity associated with shift changes, fire drills, or even activities that are pleasant for other residents, such as a parade through the nursing home of schoolchildren in Halloween costumes, can be agitating for people with dementia. The disembodied voice heard over an intercom can also be confusing.

Staff-to-resident ratios in most nursing homes may be inadequate for residents with moderate to severe dementia. It is possible, however, that in nursing home units designed specifically for persons with dementia, good care can be provided without higher staff-to-resident ratios (see ch. 7).

Residents from minority groups may have particular difficulty adjusting to nursing home care because of differences in attitudes, expectations, and typical behavior patterns. Those with dementing disorders may have even more difficulty because they often cannot understand or adapt to these differences. And those who are non-English speaking are most severely affected for they cannot communicate with staff or other residents at all.

In many areas of the country, nurse's aides are primarily from minority groups, and some are recent immigrants. When the residents of the home are predominantly of the majority culture, misunderstandings and tension can develop between the staff and the residents. Residents with dementia may be particularly unable to understand and adjust to staff from minority groups or from other countries. By the same token, however, such staff members are able to communicate with and relate to residents from the same minority group or country who might otherwise be isolated in the facility. The care of non-English speaking residents with language deficits associated with dementia is greatly facilitated if someone on staff speaks the residents' original language.

Residents with dementia not only experience problems in nursing homes but also create them. Due to deficits of memory and judgment, they may touch, move, or take other residents' possessions. In addition, their agitation, restlessness, noisiness, and occasional physical or verbal aggressiveness can upset other residents. Some nursing homes place cognitively impaired and cognitively normal residents in the same room, sometimes because they fail to consider cognitive differences but more often because they believe that the cognitively normal resident can help orient the cognitively impaired one. Although the efficacy of this approach has not been tested, other providers believe it is generally unfair to nondemented residents to be placed in a 24-hour living situation with someone with dementia and that residents with similar cognitive abilities should be roommates (1,13,121). Research on the effects of pairing residents with and without cognitive impairment is needed.

Despite the many problems of nursing home residents with dementia, the OTA survey of family caregivers found that 55 percent of those who had experience with a family member living in a nursing home reported that the care was excellent or good, and that only 16 percent reported that it was poor or very poor. Comparing these findings with the answers to other questions on the survey indicates that families who had experience with nursing homes had more positive attitudes about them than families who had no such experience (122). It is possible, however, that these attitudes mask a feeling of guilt about having placed a family member in a nursing home.

Few examples of positive experiences of dementia patients in nursing homes are found in the literature, but anecdotal evidence suggests that some people benefit from placement:

Mrs. P, suffering from Alzheimer's disease, had been living with her daughter, a tense woman who had difficulty tolerating Mrs. P's repetitious questions and seemingly aimless "fussing around the house." Over a period of months, the daughter became increasingly irritated and often spoke sharply to Mrs. P, who grew more and more agitated in response. Finally, when Mrs. P began to have occasional episodes of incontinence, her daughter could tolerate the situation no longer and placed her in a nursing home.

Mrs. P had a pleasant personality, and despite her increasing confusion, she was well liked by the staff. She did not receive any special services, but she enjoyed weekly activities, such as bingo and sing-alongs, and was obviously content to sit near the nurses' station much of the day, talking to staff and other patients and watching the goings on around the unit. Since staff expectations for her were not high, she felt more comfortable with herself than she had in her daughter's home. The daughter also felt calmer and was able to express genuine affection for her mother during her frequent visits.

Over a period of 5 years Mrs. P's disease progressed to the point where she was bedridden, and it was no longer possible to communicate with her. However, it was clear that her life in the nursing home had been better than it would have been at her daughter's home.

Evaluating the experience with nursing home care of a dementia patient and of his or her family is difficult partly because the patient is often unable to formulate or express feelings and thoughts. Some familes may be relieved that they no longer have to provide 24-hour care, although many feel intense guilt about the placement. Research indicates that quality of life for caregivers who place a relative with dementia in a nursing home improves in some ways and not in others (16). These mixed findings and the difficulty of distinguishing between the debilitating effects of progressive dementias and the effects of poor care may preclude valid generalizations about the individual and family experiences.

Access to Nursing Home Care

It is clear from the large number of residents with dementia in nursing homes that such individuals are regularly admitted. At the same time, several problems continue to restrict access for some people with dementia:

- Nursing homes are reluctant to admit someone they believe will be difficult to care for or require disproportionate amounts of staff time.
- In States where Medicaid reimbursement levels are exceptionally low, nursing homes are reluctant to admit individuals who are likely to stay long enough to deplete their private funds and become eligible for Medicaid.
- Nursing homes are especially reluctant to admit Medicaid recipients who they believe will be difficult to care for and for whom the Medicaid reimbursement rate is low. (Case mix reimbursement systems that may reverse this disincentive are discussed in chs. 8 and 12.)
- In some States, Medicaid policies restrict eligibility for publicly funded nursing home care for persons with dementia. (These problems are discussed in detail in ch. 11.)

The limited supply of nursing home beds in many States restricts access for all types of people and is a particularly severe problem in rural areas. When bed supply is limited, access to nursing home care for individuals with dementia may be restricted disproportionately for the reasons above.

In general, the proportion of minority group residents in nursing homes is lower than would be expected from their proportion in the population as a whole. That may reflect barriers to access (e.g., lack of information, discrimination, cost, and geographic location of the facilities), personal choice, greater availability of informal home care,

or a combination of all three (10,54,61,80). No information is available about the proportion of minority individuals with dementia in nursing homes.

Short-term nursing home placement to provide respite for family caregivers is an important service but one that is frequently not available (28,68). Nursing homes may be reluctant to provide short-term respite care because the costs of staff time and administrative procedures associated with admission and discharge are not adequately reimbursed at the prevailing daily rates. In addition, beds used for respite care may be vacant more frequently than other beds (46). Anecdotal evidence suggests that persons with dementia are often disoriented, agitated, and difficult to care for when first moved to any new setting. They may also be more likely to wander off during the first days after admission to a nursing home than they would be if they were accustomed to the facility. Such behaviors upset more permanent residents, particularly if they detract from staff attention to the "old timers" (32). For these reasons, nursing homes may be more reluctant to admit someone with dementia for short-term respite care than other types of patients. Research is needed to evaluate the frequency of these problems and to develop potential solutions.

Board and Care Facilities

Board and care facilities are nonmedical residences that provide room and board and 24-hour supervision. Some also provide personal care and a variety of other services. They differ from nursing homes in that they generally do not provide nursing care. They differ from boarding homes and congregate housing facilities because they generally provide 24-hour supervision. However, there are no clear-cut boundaries, and some facilities might be classified differently by different observers. Some large facilities provide board and care in some sections and nursing home care in others (59).

Board and care facilities vary in size from adult foster care homes for one or two individuals, to personal care homes and group homes that may serve 3 to 10 or more, retirement homes and homes for the aged that serve up to 100 or more, and large domiciliary care facilities that serve several hundred residents. The number and type of board and care facilities vary greatly in different States. In addition, one study identified more than 20 different names used for these facilities around the country (67).

Board and care facilities also vary in the type of care they provide. In adult foster care homes, for example, one or several residents may be cared for by one person who shops and cooks for them and assists with bathing and dressing. Care is informal, and the atmosphere may be homelike. In contrast, residents of large domiciliary care facilities are cared for by a staff with a formal daily schedule and structured activities. Between these extremes, tremendous variety exists in patterns of care.

Board and care is sometimes referred to as "residential care" or "community care," while nursing home care is called "institutional care." The first two terms have positive connotations in contrast to the last one, but the positive image they convey may not apply to all board and care facilities. Although many small board and care facilities and some larger ones are homelike or residential, larger facilities are often just as institutional as any nursing home. Furthermore, some nursing homes are closely involved with their communities, while some board and care facilities are isolated. Thus the distinction between "residential" or "community care" in board and care facilities and "institutional care" in nursing homes can camouflage real differences in atmosphere and patterns of care in specific facilities. These terms are not used to differentiate board and care facilities from nursing homes in this report.

Little is known about the services provided in board and care facilities. One study of small facilities (up to 13 residents) in Pennsylvania showed the following services were provided: laundry (97 percent); personal shopping (83 percent); cleaning a resident's room (80 percent); transportation to social activities (77 percent); handling money (65 percent); supervising or administering medications (65 percent); assistance in bathing (37 percent); and assistance in dressing (26 percent) (75). Similar services are required by State programs that regulate some types of board and care facilities (67).

No Federal Government agency has responsibility for collecting data on board and care facilities, and the definitions of these facilities used by different researchers vary significantly. Accurate national figures are therefore not available. Several sources estimate that there are at least 30,000 board and care facilities in this country, providing beds for 350,000 or more people (67,98). Other sources estimate that if facilities that serve only one or two residents are included, there may be 100,000 or more (73). Still others believe that both these estimates are low and that, in fact, we have no idea how many such facilities there are (84).

State and Federal programs pay for a significant portion of board and care. Although neither Medicare nor Medicaid covers these services, many board and care residents receive Federal SSI benefits. In 1983, 34 States and the District of Columbia provided supplemental payments for SSI recipients who lived in board and care facilities (100). VA provides board and care in 16 large domiciliary care facilities and pays for board and care in State Veterans Homes and small group homes. In addition, some States (20 in fiscal year 1984) use a portion of their Social Services Block Grant funds for adult foster care. Total spending for this purpose is not known because States are no longer required to report how they spend Block Grant Funds. In 1980, however, before Title XX funding was converted to the Social Services Block grant, Title XX funds constituted about 4 percent of all public funding for board and care, while SSI accounted for 73 percent and VA accounted for 23 percent (15).

Residents With Dementia in Board and Care Facilities

Much less is known about residents of board and care facilities than about residents of nursing homes, and no research has been reported on those with dementia. Studies have generally identified three groups of residents: the aged, mentally ill, and mentally retarded residents. One survey found that among 230,000 board and care residents for whom information was available, about 45 percent were elderly, 37 percent were mentally ill, 15 percent were mentally retarded, and the remainder were substance abusers or persons placed by the courts (67). The groups overlap, however, and some of the mentally ill and mentally retarded residents are elderly, and vice versa.

Among the mentally ill and elderly residents are an unknown number of persons with dementia. One study of applicants for Pennsylvania facilities found that 36 percent of the mentally ill group and 38 percent of the elderly group needed supervision due to disorientation or memory impairment (74). Another study of board and care residents in seven states found that about one-third were disoriented or exhibited some memory impairment (17). However, no diagnoses are available to determine the cause of these conditions.

Many residents of board and care facilities have psychiatric diagnoses or a history of psychiatric hospitalization. For example, 27 percent of those in board and care facilities in five States were found to have a history of psychiatric hospitalization (58). Among residents of VA board and care facilities, 55 percent of those in the large domiciliary care facilities and more than 70 percent of those in smaller homes had a primary diagnosis of psychiatric disorder (15). It is not known how many of the residents with psychiatric diagnoses or a history of psychiatric hospitalization actually have a dementing disorder.

Quality of Care for Residents With Dementia

Board and care facilities may be particularly appropriate care settings for many individuals with dementia because they provide protective supervision but are often less restrictive than nursing homes. Moreover, board and care usually costs one-third to one-half as much as nursing home care. However, many of these facilities provide inadequate care (17,85,90), and residents with dementia are particularly unlikely to be able to report or resist poor care. Among board and care facilities identified in one national survey, about 85 percent were licensed by the States, but licensing requirements often focus on physical plant and fire and safety code regulations rather than quality of care. Furthermore, few States regularly inspect these facilities (67). (Quality assurance standards and inspection procedures for board and care facilities are discussed in ch. 10.)

Although no research has been done on board and care specifically for those with dementia, there are reports of good care in some facilities that serve individuals with dementia along with others. For example, one study (108) described an adult foster care program in Hawaii that serves elderly clients, 38 percent of whom were significantly disoriented and 40 percent were incontinent of bowel and bladder. The study reported positive relationships between the foster families and the residents and improvements in self-care abilities and continence over time.

In contrast, anecdotal evidence suggests that there are instances of very poor care:

> Mrs. N, an 89-year-old black woman with no family, was brought to the hospital emergency room in a state of severe malnutrition and dehydration. She was confused on admission and remained confused even after her nutritional status had improved with treatment. Investigation by the local Adult Protective Services Unit revealed that Mrs. N and two other elderly woman with dementia had been living for an unknown period in a filthy apartment, cared for by a man who took their SSI checks every month, visited them daily during the week and brought them food, but apparently left them entirely alone on weekends. None of the women had relatives who visited them, and while little specific information could be obtained about their care, their physical condition suggested that they had received little care and little to eat.

It is not known how often such situations occur.

When board and care is provided by one person, changes in that individual's physical or mental health can jeopardize the safety and continuity of care for residents, just as changes in a family caregiver's physical or mental health can jeopardize the care of a person with dementia at home. For many board and care facilities, there is no established procedure for notifying a relative of the resident or another responsible person when such problems arise.

Access to Board and Care Facilities

Access to board and care facilities for all kinds of people is limited by lack of information about them. Although some facilities, especially large retirement homes and VA domiciliary care facilities, are well known in their communities, others are largely unknown, even to health care and social service providers. The OTA survey of family caregivers found that 55 percent did not know whether board and care was available in their area—a larger proportion than those who did not know about the availability of other long-term care services (122). Some States have case management programs that place people in board and care facilities, and some continue to monitor resident adjustment after placement (59). However, these programs are often limited to certain types of facilities and certain types of people, particularly mentally retarded individuals and those who receive public funding.

The cost of board and care may also limit access for all kinds of people, including those with dementia. Although board and care is considerably less expensive than nursing home care, it often costs more than the individual's social security or SSI benefit and any State SSI supplement (83).

In some localities, there are no board and care facilities. For example, one survey of six States identified several rural counties without any such facilities (76). Lack of SSI supplements for board and care in some States and extremely low SSI supplements in other States discourage the development of these facilities, thus limiting access to this form of care for all types of people (67,85).

For someone with dementia, access may be restricted because providers sometimes refuse to accept residents with behavioral problems or incontinence. The six-State survey cited above found that 35 percent of board and care operators refused to admit people with behavioral problems, night wanderers, and people with bowel or bladder problems (31).

Little is known about minority group access to or use of board and care facilities. Some research suggests that minorities may be excluded from specific kinds of facilities. For example, few black people live in homes for the aged (12). In contrast, many board and care providers, especially in small facilities, are black, at least in some localities. In the Pennsylvania domiciliary care program, 30 percent of the providers but only 13 percent of the residents were black (76). No information is available about access to or use of board and care facilities by Hispanic elderly or other minorities.

Home Care

Home care services include medical, social, and supportive services provided in someone's home. They range from complex, technologically sophisticated interventions, such as the administration of intravenous antibiotics and nutritional support, to relatively simple interventions, such as home-delivered meals. Between these extremes are services such as skilled nursing care, physical therapy, speech therapy, occupational therapy, home health aide, personal care, homemaker, paid home companion, and chore services. (These services were defined earlier in table 6-1.)

Family caregivers who responded to the 1985 OTA survey said that each home care service they were asked about was important for their family member with dementia:

- 96 percent said that a paid companion who can come to the home a few hours each week to give caregivers a rest is essential, very important, or important;
- 94 percent said that home health aide services—that is, a person paid to provide personal care such as bathing, dressing, or feeding—are essential, very important, or important;
- 93 percent said that a paid companion who can come to the home and provide overnight care is essential, very important, or important; and
- 87 percent said that visiting nurse services—a registered nurse to provide nursing care—are essential, very important, or important (122).

Unfortunately for persons with dementia and their families, some of these services do not correspond to the services usually funded or provided by public programs. Although some families can pay privately for home care services, the long duration of dementing illnesses and thus the long period during which services are needed mean that families must often turn to publicly funded services or do without.

Federal funding for home care is provided by Medicare, Medicaid, the Social Services Block Grant, Title III of the Older Americans Act, and VA. Medicare is the largest payer for home care, and Medicare expenditures for home care have grown rapidly during the past 10 years. However, in 1983 they still constituted only 2.7 percent of Medicare spending (88). Medicare is a medical insurance program, and its coverage of home care is limited to the following medically related services:

- part-time or intermittent skilled nursing care;
- physical therapy, speech therapy, and occupational therapy;
- medical social services provided under the direction of a physician;
- medical supplies and equipment (other than medicines); and
- part-time or intermittent home health aide services.

Medicare services must be prescribed by a physician and provided by an agency certified to participate in the program, of which there were 5,237 in 1985 (35).

Federal regulations do not restrict the number of home health care visits that can be covered and the period of time over which they may be received, but because of the requirement that Medicare-covered home health care services must be "intermittent," daily visits for more than 2 to 3 weeks require additional documentation by a physician. Home care providers complain that some Medicare intermediaries who handle reimbursement routinely deny payment for daily visits that extend for more than 2 to 3 weeks and that the intermediaries are erratic in their reimbursement decisions. Testifying before the Subcommittee on Health of the Senate Finance Committee, the director of a home health care agency stated:

A visiting nurse association in the Southwest was denied all visits to an 80-year-old Alzheimer's disease victim for March and April after being reimbursed for daily visits in previous months. Then the intermediary turned around after denying these two months, and paid for two additional months of daily visits . . . there is no consistency at all in those types of decisions.

The patient had [decubitus] ulcers. I have the pictures here . . . I would like to enter these pictures in with our testimony in the record. [Ten pictures of severe decubitus ulcers are submitted.] You cannot look at these photos and not see that this man had the need for the daily visits; and the . . . intermediary looked at the pictures and denied the visits anyway (103).

For many persons with dementia, home health aide services are the most useful Medicare-covered home care service. Covered services include assistance with medications and exercise; personal care, such as bathing, dressing, and feeding; and homemaker services when these can be shown to prevent or postpone placement in a nursing home or other institutional setting. To be eligible, however, the patient must also need skilled nursing care, physical therapy, or speech therapy—a condition that many with dementia do not meet. Using a home health aide as a paid companion—one of the services considered essential by many family caregivers—is not legitimately covered by Medicare.

Studies by the General Accounting Office and the Health Care Financing Administration indicate that Medicare reimbursement for one-fourth to one-third of all home health care claims was or should have been denied—sometimes because the individual was not eligible for such services, according to program regulations, but more often because the person received too many visits (91,109). It is not known how many individuals with dementia actually receive any Medicare-covered home health care services or how many receive services for which reimbursement is later denied.

Statistical analysis of the characteristics of a national sample of people receiving Medicare-covered home health care services indicates that six clinically distinct groups can be identified (56). Four of the groups generally do not include cognitively impaired people:

1. people with acute medical problems such as cancer;
2. people with hip or other fractures;
3. people with acute and chronic medical problems and limitations in self-care abilities; and
4. people with severe circulatory and respiratory problems.

The other two groups, which do include cognitively impaired people, are:

5. people who have many chronic medical conditions, including senility and stroke, but few acute or severe conditions and few limitations in self-care abilities; and

6. people with severe neurological impairments, including senility and stroke, and significant difficulty in self-care abilities.

Among all six groups, group 5 received the lowest amount of Medicare reimbursement for home health care services, while group 6 received the highest amount—an average of six times as much. The primary differences between the two groups are the absence or presence of acute medical care problems and limitations in self-care abilities. These findings suggest that persons with dementia and with acute medical problems and severe limitations in self-care abilities may receive substantial Medicare reimbursement for home health care services, and that those with fewer acute medical problems and fewer limitations in self-care abilities probably receive much less. The latter group may be among home care recipients for whom reimbursement is frequently denied.

Medicaid also covers home health care services, although in 1983 they accounted for less than 2 percent of all spending in the program (88). Within Federal guidelines, States determine what services their Medicaid programs cover, and tremendous variation exists. Although some States have legislative, regulatory, and administrative policies that make a range of services available to Medicaid-eligible people, others do not (14). Federal regulations require State Medicaid programs to cover skilled nursing care and home health aide services. Personal care is optional; as of 1983, only 25 States and the District of Columbia covered it (95). Even so, three-quarters of Medicaid home care expenditures were for personal care (18). All Medicaid-covered home care services must be ordered by a physician, and home health aide and personal care services must be supervised by a licensed nurse.

In many States, home health care services covered by Medicaid match the needs of someone with dementia more closely than those covered by Medicare; however, only people who meet Medicaid financial eligibility criteria can receive Medicaid-covered services. The criteria include limits on income and assets that vary among States but are low everywhere and extremely low in some States. As a result, even where Medicaid covers the home care services for a person with dementia, the allowable income and asset levels are so low that it is difficult to support the person in the community. When a spouse is involved, he or she must also live at these low income and asset levels (see ch. 11 for further discussion of this problem).

In 1981, Congress authorized the Medicaid 2176 waiver program to allow States increased flexibility in the home care services they provide. Under this program, States may provide home health aide, homemaker, personal care, and respite services as long as these services are said to prevent nursing home placement. States may target the expanded services to specific areas and to certain groups of people instead of making them available statewide and to all Medicaid-eligible individuals.

As of April 1985, 95 waiver applications had been approved: 50 include services for the aged and disabled and 4 including services for the mentally ill. Among waiver programs for the aged and disabled, 11 included home health aide services, 26 included homemaker services, 18 provided personal care, and 24 provided respite care (87). The number of persons with dementia who receive services through these programs is not known. Since recipients must meet Medicaid financial eligibility requirements, however, services are generally available only to those with low income and assets. In some States, individuals with income up to three times the SSI level in the community are eligible for 2176 waiver benefits, but they must have medical expenses higher than the difference between their income and the SSI benefit level (see ch. 11 for a description of the 2176 waiver program).

Funding for home care services through the Social Services Block Grant and Title III of the Older Americans Act is administered at the State and local levels, and little information is available about services provided and the financial or other factors used to determine eligibility. Although many

States use these funds to provide personal care, homemaker, and chore services not covered by Medicare or Medicaid, they are generally insufficient to meet demonstrated need (27,28,88). Again, the number of persons with dementia who receive home care services through these funding sources is not known.

VA provides relatively little home care compared with the amount of hospital, nursing home, and board and care services it provides. Only 30 of 172 VA Medical Centers provide home care services, and veterans who live far from these centers do not have access to VA home care. Estimates for fiscal year 1985 indicated that about 15,000 veterans would receive home care, but the need for these services is much greater. For example, VA figures indicate that 460,000 veterans will need home care services by 1990 (111). No breakdown of these figures for veterans with dementia is available.

Persons With Dementia Receiving Home Care Services

As indicated, the number of persons with dementia who receive federally funded home care services is not known, and OTA is unaware of any national or State data on the number who receive any publicly or privately funded home care services. The eligibility criteria for relevant Federal programs discourage identification of this group by focusing on different types of needs: medical, skilled nursing, and health-related needs (Medicare, Medicaid, VA); social service needs (Social Services Block Grant); or age-related needs (Title III of the Older Americans Act). Although several national, State, and community surveys include measures of cognitive status and information about service utilization (52), these data have not yet been analyzed to determine the number or proportion of persons with dementia who receive home care services or, conversely, the proportion of all home care recipients who have a dementing disorder.

Despite this lack of information, it is clear that individuals with dementia constitute a significant proportion of home care recipients, at least in some programs. For example, one study of 50 people who received home care services following hospitalization in Little Rock, Arkansas, found that

48 percent had mild or moderate cognitive impairments, and 10 percent were severely impaired (24).

A person's mental status may affect the efficacy and chance for success of formal home care services. National data indicate that mental status is one of the most important predictors of nursing home placement. For example, analysis of data from the 1977 Health Interview Survey and the 1977 National Nursing Home Survey showed that 66 percent of elderly persons with diagnoses of mental illness (including cognitive impairments and functional mental illnesses) are in nursing homes. By contrast, only 22 percent of those with cancer, digestive, metabolic, or blood diseases and a smaller proportion of those with other diagnoses are in nursing homes (119). Similarly, hospital data suggest that cognitively impaired persons are much more likely than other patients to be discharged to nursing homes (20,71). These findings imply that persons with dementia are more difficult to maintain at home than others who need long-term care. They also raise questions about whether formal home care services can be effective in keeping someone with dementia at home and whether it is more difficult to arrange home care services for such a person. OTA is not aware of research that addresses these questions.

One characteristic that limits the usefulness of home care services for some persons with dementia is their need for 24-hour supervision. Although not unique to this group, this need is probably universal among persons with dementia. While some families can provide 24-hour supervision, persons with dementia who have no family cannot be safely maintained at home without 24-hour formal care—a service that is seldom available.

One home health aide who works for a Medicare-certified home health care agency has 11 elderly clients, most of whom live alone. She visits six of them daily and the others on alternate days, to help with bathing and dressing, and—for those who live alone—shopping, cooking, and other housekeeping chores.

Agency policy is that the home health aides do not visit clients who live in rural areas on days when the county schools are closed because of snow. The aides have been told that their services are intended to be "part-time and intermittent," as required by Medicare regulations and

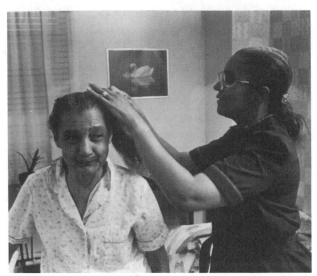

Photo credit: ADRDA and Peter Carrol, PhotoSynthesis Productions, Inc.

Some families are able to provide 24-hour care for a relative with dementia.

that their clients are not supposed to need 24-hour care.

On this "snow day," however, the aide decides to visit one of her clients anyway. The client is confused, and the aide is always worried about how she will manage between the aide's daily visits. In good conscience, the aide cannot imagine failing to check in on the woman. It is not the aide's decision whether or when the woman should be placed in a nursing home, and in fact her instructions do not mention the woman's increasing confusion—only her need for assistance with bathing, dressing, shopping, and cooking.

Data from the 1979 Home Care Supplement to the National Health Interview Survey indicate that individuals who need supervision plus assistance in activities of daily living and medical care use formal home care services more often than those who need only assistance in activities of daily living and medical care (79). Further, some 56 percent of those 65 or older who needed home care also needed supervision all or most of the time (78). However, it is now known how many of these people had a dementing disorder. Analysis of these data in terms of the cognitive status of home care recipients might clarify the relationship between dementia, the need for 24-hour supervision, and the use of formal home care services.

For many years it has been believed that home care services can help people who need long-term care remain in their homes and avoid nursing home placement, thus reducing expenditures for nursing home care. Many studies have tested this hypothesis, and although some are methodologically flawed, analysis of the findings indicates that home care services do not, in general, substitute for nursing home care. Nor are home care services generally less expensive than nursing home care, although they often improve the quality of life for those who remain at home (36,93,117).

Analysis of the reasons for these unexpected results is beyond the scope of this assessment. However, it appears that none of the studies considered the effect of the individual's cognitive status on whether home care services prevent institutionalization. One recent study indicated that caregiver characteristics and caregiver well-being are more important predictors of placing someone with dementia in a nursing home than any characteristic of the person (16). However, the person's cognitive status could affect caregiver well-being or, alternatively, the emotional or behavioral characteristics associated with dementia could be intervening variables that affect caregiver well-being and thus decisions about placement. Further research is needed on the factors that predict institutionalization of persons with dementia and therefore the potential impact of home care services on such decisions.

Quality of Home Care Services for Persons With Dementia

Several problems limit the quality of home care services for persons with dementia:

- The services most needed—paid companion, homemaker, personal care, and 24-hour supervision—are frequently not available. Home care services that can be used for respite care are particularly difficult to find (28,40,68).
- Many of the people who provide home care services are not trained to work with individuals with dementia (68), and they may create more problems for the patient and the primary caregiver than they solve.

- There are few standards or procedures for monitoring quality of home care services for anyone, particularly someone with dementia.

In addition, different expectations about the role of the family and the role of the paid home care worker can cause problems. Although there may be little disagreement about the role and responsibilities of a nurse, physical therapist, occupational therapist, or speech therapist who provides home health care, the responsibilities of a home health aide who provides personal care and homemaker services may be difficult to distinguish from those of the family. This lack of clear roles and responsibilities can lead to tension. Home care workers sent out to provide home health care may become upset by a family's requests or demands for services that do not match the worker's job description. Likewise, family caregivers may become upset when services they want are not provided (41). Families and home care workers can also disagree about how much help the patient needs (32).

Close supervision of home care workers by the agency is virtually impossible, and families complain that some of these employees do not do their jobs. For example, one woman told the Massachusetts Governor's Committee on Alzheimer's Disease about a home health aide who seldom showed up on time, and when she finally arrived did little more than watch the woman care for her mother (27). Anecdotal reports indicate that some home care workers do not show up at all or merely sit and watch television. Theft, neglect, and exploitation of cognitively impaired people by home care workers have also been reported. Although it is not known how often such problems occur, they are clearly a cause of concern, especially for families who live a considerable distance from the person receiving the care (47).

Access to Home Care Services

In many areas, access to formal home care services by persons with dementia can be limited by lack of any home care services, lack of appropriate services, lack of funding, and fragmentation of the service delivery system. Home care services of all kinds are particularly difficult to obtain in rural areas. National data indicate that elderly people who need home care services do without them more frequently in farm areas than in urban, suburban, or rural, nonfarm areas. At the level of ADL impairment at which informal caregiving is usually augmented by formal home care services, almost twice as many people do without formal services in farm areas than in all other geographic locations (79). These findings are not specific for persons with dementia, but the Kansas Alzheimer's and Related Diseases Task Force has documented the difficulty of finding home care services for such persons in rural areas of the state (40).

Problems in obtaining appropriate home care services have been discussed throughout this section. One overriding problem is the emphasis on medical and skilled nursing services in Medicare, Medicaid, and VA home health care programs, as opposed to the personal care, supervision, and social services most often needed by persons with dementia. A second problem that has received almost no attention concerns home care services for different ethnic, cultural, and socioeconomic groups. When services are provided in the home, differences among groups and individuals in lifestyle, expectations, attitudes, and patterns of interpersonal behavior are particularly salient and can affect acceptance of the services, the level of trust and cooperation that can be achieved between the paid home care worker and the patient and family, and the overall efficacy of the service. Adaptations of home care services for different ethnic, cultural, and socioeconomic groups are needed.

The cost of services can also limit access, and many home care services are expensive. One woman told the Kansas Alzheimer's and Related Diseases Task Force:

> I was told that I might be able to get someone in for an hour a day—that might be long enough to bathe and dress my husband. When I asked how much I was told it would cost $40 an hour from the minute they left their office until they returned (40).

Some agencies provide home care services on a sliding fee basis, but the client's share of the cost may still be high (64). As a result, some families hire maids to provide home care services. One study showed that 41 percent of caregivers of persons with Alzheimer's disease hired private maids or sitters because it was cheaper than paying for home care services from a home health care agency. Most of the other caregivers did not use any home care services (25).

A final and serious problem that affects access to home care services is the complexity and fragmentation of the service delivery system. Although in some localities there are no agencies to provide home care services, in other areas there are many such agencies, each providing a variety of services with differing eligibility requirements and reimbursement procedures (114).

The complexity of Federal regulations on what home care services are covered, who can receive them, and who can provide them is compounded by interpretations of Federal Medicare regulations by Medicare intermediaries; State legislation, regulations, and administrative policies that determine Medicaid coverage and eligibility requirements; and State and local regulatory and administrative decisions about the use of Social Service Block Grant and Title III funds. In addition, some services are available through State and local programs unrelated to Federal funding sources, or through private nonprofit groups, each of which has its own eligibility, coverage, and reimbursement guidelines.

Several States have created programs to pool and administer funds that are available for home care. Examples are the Massachusetts Home Care Corporations and the Maryland Gateway II program. Both provide home health aide, personal care, and homemaker services using more liberal and flexible eligibility criteria than are applied elsewhere. The primary problem they face is inadequate funding to meet the home care needs they identify (27,28). Thus even these programs are frequently unable to provide appropriate home care services for persons with dementia.

Adult Day Care Centers

Adult day care centers provide a range of health, mental health, and social services for physically, emotionally, and cognitively impaired and socially isolated people. The centers all provide some common services, but they differ in their emphasis and the clients they serve. Several types have been identified in the literature (33,118). Some emphasize medical and rehabilitative services, such as physical, occupational, and speech therapy, and serve people who are recovering from physical illnesses such as stroke. Other centers emphasize personal care, supervision, socialization, and activities, and serve mentally retarded and developmentally disabled adults or frail elderly persons and those with dementia. A third type emphasizes mental health services, supervision, socialization, and recreation, and serves primarily mentally ill people, some of whom have been discharged from public and private mental hospitals. The three types overlap, and some analysts have questioned how closely this typology reflects real differences between existing centers (8).

Before 1972, there were fewer than 10 nonpsychiatric adult day care centers in the United States. By 1977, that number had grown to 300, and by 1982-83, there were between 700 and 1,000 centers serving 15,000 to 20,000 people (33,55,65). A 1985-86 survey sponsored by the National Institute of Adult Daycare (NIAD) received responses from 847 centers, and the report suggests that 1,200 is a conservative estimate of the number of existing centers (8).

Unlike nursing homes and home health care agencies, adult day care centers have developed largely without Federal regulation. As a result, they vary greatly in physical setting, clientele, staffing, mode of operation, and services provided. To some extent, this diversity reflects local needs and resources (7).

Adult day care centers may be located in buildings used solely by the center or in hospitals, nursing homes, senior centers, churches, schools, community centers, clinics, housing for the elderly, private homes, or life care communities. A few are open 7 days a week, but most are open 5 days a week (7). Many clients do not attend every day, however; one study of four centers found that the average days of attendance ranged from 48 to 114 days per person per year (82). Although the services provided in different centers vary, as mentioned earlier, many centers have similar goals—to avoid premature or inappropriate institutional placement, to maximize client functioning, to provide respite for family caregivers, and to provide supportive services in the community (8).

According to the NIAD survey, the average cost of adult day care is $27 to $31 a day (8). However, some programs cost significantly more (65). Medicare does not cover adult day care per se, but may cover medical or skilled nursing care and physical and speech therapy provided for adult day care clients. Adult day care is an optional service under Medicaid, and some states cover it either as a separate service or as part of clinic or outpatient services (15). Coverage is usually limited to centers that provide medical and rehabilitative services as opposed to those that emphasize personal care, supervision, and activities (45). Financial eligibility criteria further limit Medicaid-covered adult day care to persons with low income and assets.

Nevertheless, the NIAD survey found that Medicaid and participant fees were the two main sources of funding for adult day care centers (8). Adult day care is an allowable service under the Medicaid 2176 waiver program, and as of April 1985 it was a part of 42 of the 95 approved 2176 waiver proposals—26 for the aged and disabled, 14 for the mentally retarded and developmentally disabled, and 2 for the mentally ill (87).

Some States (29 in fiscal year 1984) use Social Service Block Grant funds to support clients in adult day care (104), and some use funds allocated under Title III of the Older Americans Act. Other state and local funds and contributions from United Way organizations, churches, synagogues, service clubs, and other charity groups also support these centers (45).

As of 1985, the VA provided adult day care at five medical centers. Veterans with service-connected disabilities are eligible for adult day care for an indefinite period, but those with non-service-connected disabilities are limited to 6 months of this care (43).

Persons With Dementia in Adult Day Care Centers

A 1984 survey of adult day care centers found that about 45 percent served persons with dementia (55). The recent NIAD survey did not ask specifi-

cially about dementia, but it did ask about characteristics of clients that may be related to dementia, such as supervision needs and incontinence. The survey found that about 45 percent of clients require supervision, and about 20 percent require constant supervision. In addition, about 8 percent are incontinent to the degree that they require changing during the attendance day (8). Many individuals in each of these categories may have dementing disorders.

Although the majority of adult day care centers continue to serve a mixed population, an increasing number are specializing in services for specific client groups (65). Specialization may evolve as providers encounter problems in serving clients with differing needs and capabilities or may occur in response to community needs (23). Adult day care centers designed specifically for persons with dementia are discussed in chapter 7.

The Alzheimer's Disease and Related Disorders Association (ADRDA), families, and many health care and social service providers are enthusiastic about the role of adult day care in the treatment of persons with dementia because they believe it can do three things: improve quality of life for these persons; provide respite for family caregivers; and perhaps postpone the need for nursing home care in some cases. The efficacy of adult day care in attaining these objectives for persons with dementia is discussed in chapter 7.

Research not specifically focused on persons with dementia indicates that adult day care programs can and do serve quite severely debilitated persons. For example, one study compared clients in an adult day care center and residents of a nursing home and found that the adult day care clients were more impaired in physical and mental health and self-care abilities than the nursing home residents, but the latter had more limited social and financial resources (166).

Although these findings indicate that severely debilitated clients can be maintained in adult day care centers, it is unclear whether adult day care is a substitute for nursing home care. Analysis of seven studies that addressed this question indicates that these centers were generally serving a different group of people than those who enter nursing homes, that the cost of adult day care was not less than the cost of nursing home care, but that like home care clients, people in adult day care had higher morale than those in nursing homes (33).

Access to Adult Day Care

Lack of a stable funding source for adult day care is a pervasive problem that limits access for individual clients and discourages the development of new centers (27,33). As discussed, many public programs and private groups provide some funding for adult day care. Still, among all long-term care services, adult day care is one of the two most commonly associated with client fees for service (the other is homemaker services) (15). At $27 to $31 a day, adult day care is clearly too expensive for most clients and families to afford on a regular basis.

Lack of centers also restricts access. Rural areas are particularly unlikely to have such centers because of low population density and lengthy travel time for clients. Innovative models of service delivery based on the satellite site concept have been developed (30), but OTA is not aware of any research that evaluates their effectiveness for persons with dementia.

NIAD survey data indicate that about half the centers that responded serve some black clients, and in these centers an average of 15 percent of all clients are black. About one-fourth of all centers said they serve some Hispanics, and in those centers 2 to 3 percent of the clients are Hispanic. Ten percent of centers said they serve some Native Americans, and 12 percent said they serve some Asians and Pacific Islanders (8). No information is available about why some centers serve no minority group clients.

A final factor that restricts access to adult day care is the admission and discharge policies of some centers. The NIAD survey found that many centers determine eligibility on a case-by-case basis. However, a minority reported that they deny admission to people who are incontinent, disruptive, combative, psychotic, too confused, or in need of constant supervision (8). Clearly, many persons with dementia would not be admitted to these centers.

Community Mental Health Centers

Community mental health centers (CMHCs) are agencies that provide a range of mental health services to persons of all ages, primarily on an outpatient basis, although some also provide short-term inpatient care. CMHCs are not usually included in discussions of long-term care services. They are included here because they are local sites of mental health expertise—an element clearly lacking in the care provided by most long-term care facilities and agencies serving persons with dementia. Elderly people, the group that includes the vast majority of persons with dementia, have generally been underserved by CMHCs. However, some CMHC services regularly provided to other age groups and patient types, such as assessment, counseling, and support groups for patients and families, are needed by persons with dementia and not available in many communities.

Outpatient mental health centers have existed in this country for a long time, but the Federal program that created CMHCs was initiated in 1963 with passage of the Community Mental Health Services Act and subsequent authorization of Federal funding for the centers. Special services for elderly people were not required in the original act, and few such services were provided. However, amendments to the act passed in 1975 and 1978 mandated increased services for that group. In 1980, legislation was passed to provide additional funding for CMHCs with special programs for the elderly, but that legislation was never implemented because direct Federal funding for CMHCs and other programs was replaced by the Alcohol and Drug Abuse and Mental Health Services Block Grant, to be administered by the states. Federal funding for the block grant in its first year was 25 percent lower than combined Federal funding for CMHCs and substance abuse programs in the previous year (3,62,92).

No information is available about the number or proportion of persons with dementia served by CMHCs. The proportion of elderly persons among all clients served by these agencies increased from 3.4 percent in 1971 to 6 percent in 1982—still far below the proportion of elderly people in the population as a whole. The proportion of elderly people served by CMHCs did not change from 1981 to 1984, but many CMHCs report a decrease in special programs for elderly people since 1981 (3,5).

Not all CMHCs that provide special services for elderly people also have special services for persons with dementia, but one study indicates that the two are often associated (51). The study found that CMHCs with special services for elderly people are five times more likely than other CHMCs to provide services for individuals with Alzheimer's disease and their families. Those that also had staff trained to provide services for persons with dementia were more than 8 times as likely to provide such services. And they were also more likely to provide services in satellite sites, such as nursing homes, senior centers, community residential facilities, or in the patient's home. Thus reported cutbacks in special CMHC programs for elderly people since 1981 could indicate that services for persons with dementia have also been cut back and that they are less frequently available in settings where such persons are usually seen and treated. Interestingly, CMHCs responding to the study cited above (51) reported that their most important need was for information about memory and cognitive problems in elderly people (50).

The change to block grant funding and the decrease in Federal funding for CMHCs resulted in reduced staff and increased caseloads in many centers, a decrease in the number of psychiatrists employed in CMHCs, and an increase in client fees (39,62). These changes may have affected the availability and quality of services for persons with dementia.

Outpatient mental health services for persons with dementia could be provided by mental health professionals who are in private practice, including psychiatrists, clinical psychologists, psychiatric social workers, and psychiatric nurses, but research indicates that such services are seldom used by these patients. For example, the Epidemiologic Catchment Area survey in Baltimore found that no one with cognitive impairment who was over 65 had seen any mental health specialist in the preceding 6 months (26). A 1978 study found that fewer than 3 percent of the patients of mental health professionals in private practice were over 65 (107), and although this proportion has probably increased in recent years, relatively few such professionals treat elderly persons with dementia.

The original intent of the Federal legislation that created CHMCs was that those centers would provide mental health services and also would work with other community agencies and private practitioners to create a coordinated system of mental health care at the local level. This latter aspect has been particularly affected by decreases in funding, with the result that in many localities mental health services for all kinds of people are now more fragmented (39).

Despite funding cutbacks, some CMHCs do provide comprehensive mental health services for persons with dementia and their families and outreach to facilities and agencies in the community where such persons are cared for (4,63). Analysis of how these services are organized and funded could provide a model of service delivery that might be duplicated in other CMHCs.

SERVICE DELIVERY SYSTEMS

Service delivery systems are methods for matching the needs of an individual with appropriate services. Some are relatively simple, such as providing the person or family with a list of community agencies that they can use to select the services they need. Others involve comprehensive assessment of an individual's needs, counseling with the person and family to evaluate different care options, and followup to monitor the individual's adjustment and ensure that services are provided regularly. Still others are based on agreement among community agencies to designate a single agency as the entry point for long-term care services or to use a common assessment instrument to evaluate client needs. Another type of service delivery system is the Social/Health Maintenance Organization (see ch. 12) and similar systems that provide a range of long-term care services through a single agency or program.

Each of these methods and many others are being used for persons with dementia and others who need long-term care. Although some have been analyzed extensively in terms of their effect on access, appropriateness, and cost of long-term care services for all kinds of people, OTA is not aware of any research that compares alternate methods of service delivery for persons with dementia.

The need for a service delivery system arises in part from the fragmentation of long-term care services at the community level and the complexity of Federal, State, and local programs that provide and fund such services. The three systems that provide services for persons with dementia—the medical or physical care system, the aging services system, and the mental health system—are generally disconnected. Gaps and overlapping services within each and between systems are common, and providers in one system are often unaware of services in the other two.

In addition to these problems, some individuals and families need assistance in evaluating their needs before they can select appropriate services. Others need counseling and emotional support to work through feelings of sadness, anger, and guilt associated with the patient's condition and care needs before they can evaluate long-term care options rationally or follow through on decisions about institutional placement or continued care at home.

Although the same problems affect everyone who needs long-term care, several characteristics may intensify the problems for persons with dementia and their families:

- persons with dementia frequently do not understand their condition and care needs and may refuse services they need;
- persons with dementia frequently lack the ability to evaluate care options, and family members or others must make important decisions for them (nursing home placement, sale of a home, etc.);
- there is no generally accepted assessment instrument to measure their care needs;

- there is no generally accepted method of evaluating their capacity to make decisions; and
- they often come to the attention of health care and social service providers and community agencies only when their need for services is desperate, and the assessment/referral/decisionmaking process frequently takes place in an atmosphere of crisis.

The need for improving in the service delivery system for persons with dementia is evident from the responses to the OTA survey of family caregivers. Many respondents did not know whether home care, board and care, respite, adult day care, or nursing home services were available. Likewise, almost half reported that they had difficulty finding a doctor who could adequately care for the person with dementia. When asked about the most important services, families identified the need for assistance in locating people or organizations that provide care and for help in applying for Medicaid, Social Security Disability benefits, SSI, and so on as the second and third most essential (following only the need for a paid companion to give caregivers a rest) (122).

The reports of several State Alzheimer's disease task forces stress the need for good information and referral systems (27,28,40). The experience of the Massachusetts Governor's Committee on Alzheimer's Disease is instructive:

At the beginning of our examination of available community services, one member was assigned the task of calling facilities on a random list and asking if they had specialized services for Alzheimer's patients. Without exception, the caller was told that such specialized services existed. When questioned more specificially, most facilities failed to demonstrate any special capability to assist the Alzheimer's client. In fact, in some cases, facilities which initially stated that they had "specialized units or services" were ill-prepared to assist an Alzheimer's patient or family member (27).

Many different agencies and community service providers are involved in matching the needs of persons with dementia to available services. Hospitals play a major role in service delivery, sometimes because no other agency has been available to serve this function. Anecdotal evidence indicates that persons with dementia are frequently admitted to a hospital when family caregivers are no longer able to manage them, or when their ability to function independently has deteriorated to such a low level that neighbors or others insist that something must be done. In such situations, the person may or may not have an acute medical condition, but the primary (although sometimes unspoken) reason for hospitalization is the need for a long-term care plan.

Hospital discharge planning units, often staffed by social workers, are primarily responsible for developing a plan of care for patients who need long-term institutional care or formal services at home. This process—which may involve assessment of the patient's physical, emotional, and cognitive status and social supports; consultation with the patient, the family, the doctor, nurses, and others; and location of appropriate services and funding—can be time-consuming. In the past, patients sometimes remained in the hospital for prolonged periods while a discharge plan was developed. Now, however, the Medicare Prospective Payment System and other public and private programs that create incentives for shorter stays are reducing the time available for discharge planning in hospitals. Analysis of the impact of these changes on discharge planning for persons with dementia is needed.

Physicians, other health care providers, staff in agencies that serve elderly and disabled people, and many others are also involved in referring persons with dementia to long-term care services. Staff in adult day care centers that serve persons with dementia and ADRDA staff and support groups frequently provide information about available services and assistance with decisionmaking for families of these patients.

Evaluation of alternate methods of service delivery for persons with dementia is beyond the scope of this OTA assessment. Some of the questions that need to be answered are:

- Which methods of service delivery are most effective?
- Are they are best served by a delivery system that focuses on persons with dementia or by a system that serves all persons who need long-term care?
- What are the appropriate roles of families, voluntary caregiver support groups, and public and private agencies in the service delivery system?

Some answers may be found on analysis of data collected for the National Channelling Demonstration project—a large-scale study of two models of service delivery funded by the U.S. Department of Health and Human Services—and other studies of service delivery systems (52). Other answers must await the outcome of new studies and demonstration projects.

CHAPTER 6 REFERENCES

1. Ablowitz, M., "Pairing Rational and Demented Patients in Long-Term Care Facilities" (letter to the editor), *Journal of the American Geriatrics Society* 31:627, 1983.
2. Abt Associates, Inc., "Analysis of the Maryland Patient Assessment System With Emphasis on the Needs of Behavior Problem Residents," Washington, DC, Jan. 11, 1985.
3. Action Committee To Implement the Mental Health Recommendations of the 1981 White House Conference on Aging, *Mental Health Services for the Elderly: Report on a Survey of Community Mental Health Centers, Vol. I*, Washington, DC, 1984.
4. Action Committee To Implement the Mental Health Recommendations of the 1981 White House Conference on Aging, *Mental Health Services for the Elderly: Report on a Survey of Community Mental Health Centers, Vol. II*, Washington, DC, 1984.
5. Action Committee To Implement the Mental Health Recommendations of the 1981 White House Conference on Aging, *Mental Health Services for the Elderly: Report on a Survey of Community Mental Health Centers, Vol. III*, Washington, DC, 1986.
6. Baldwin, B., RN, consultant, Crofton, MD, personal communication, May 18, 1986.
7. Behren, R.V., "Adult Day Care: Progress, Problems, and Promise," *Perspective on Aging* 14(6):5-39, 1985.
8. Behren, R.V., "Adult Day Care in America: Preliminary Report of the Results of the National In-

stitute of Adult Daycare/National Council on Aging Survey, 1985-86," Washington, DC, July 1986.

9. Brody, E.M., "The Social Aspects of Nursing Home Care," *The Teaching Nursing Home*, E.L. Schneider, C.J. Wendland, A.W. Zimmer, et al. (eds.) (New York, NY: Raven Press, 1985).

10. Brody, J.A., and Foley, D.J., "Epidemiologic Considerations," *The Teaching Nursing Home*, E.L. Schneider, C.J. Wendland, A.W. Zimmer, et al. (eds.) (New York, NY: Raven Press, 1985).

11. Brody, S.J., and Magel, J.S., "DRG: The Second Revolution in Health Care for the Elderly," *Journal of the American Geriatrics Society* 32:676-679, 1984.

12. Butler, R.N., and Lewis, M.I., *Aging and Mental Health* (St. Louis, MO: C.V. Mosby Co., 1982).

13. Cameli, S., "Pairing Rational and Demented Patients in Long-Term Care Facilities, Continued" (letter to the editor), *Journal of the American Geriatrics Society* 32:409, 1984.

14. Chavkin, D., "Interstate Variability in Medicaid Eligibility and Reimbursement for Dementia Patients," contract report prepared for the Office of Technology Assessment, U.S. Congress, Washington, DC, 1986.

15. Cohen, J., "Public Programs Financing Long-Term Care," The Urban Institute, Washington, DC, draft (revised), January 1983.

16. Colerick, E.J., and George, L.K., "Predictors of Institutionalization Among Caregivers of Patients With Alzheimer's Disease," *Journal of the American Geriatrics Society* 34:493-498, 1986.

17. Dittmar, N.D., and Smith, G.P., "Evaluation of Board and Care Homes: Summary of Survey Procedures and Findings," Denver Research Institute, University of Denver, CO, Feb. 22, 1983.

18. Doty, P., Liu, K., and Weiner, J., "An Overview of Long-Term Care," *Health Care Financing Review* 6(3):69-78, 1985.

19. Fago, D., Veterans Administration, personal communication, June 9, 1986.

20. Fields, S.D., MacKenzie, C.R., Charlson, M.E., et al., "Cognitive Impairment, Can It Predict the Course of Hospitalized Patients?" *Journal of the American Geriatrics Society* 34(8):579-585, 1986.

21. Foley, W.J., assistant professor, Industrial and Management Engineering Department Rensselaer Polytechnic Institute, Troy, NY, personal communication, May 6, 1986.

22. Foley, W.J., "Dementia Among Nursing Home Patients: Defining the Condition, Characteristics of the Demented, and Dementia on the RUG-II Classification System," contract report prepared for

the Office of Technology Assessment, U.S. Congress, Washington, DC, 1986.

23. Frankel, E.R., Sherman, S.R., Newman, E.S., et al., "The Continuum of Care Within Psychogeriatric Day Programming: A Study of Program Evolution," *Gerontological Social Work in Home Health Care*, R. Dobrof (ed.) (New York, NY: Haworth Press, 1984).

24. Garner, J.D., "From Hospital to Home Health Care: Who Goes There? A Descriptive Study of Elderly Users of Home Health Care Services Post Hospitalization," *Gerontological Social Work In Home Health Care*, R. Dobrof (ed.) (New York, NY: Haworth Press, 1984).

25. George, L.K.,"The Dynamics of Caregiver Burden," final report to the American Association of Retired Persons, Washington, DC, December 1984.

26. German, P.S., Shapiro, S., and Skinner, E.A., "Mental Health of the Elderly: Use of Health and Mental Health Services," *Journal of the American Geriatrics Society* 33:246-252, 1985.

27. Governor's Committee on Alzheimer's Disease, "Final Report," The Commonwealth of Massachusetts, Boston, 1985.

28. Governor's Task Force on Alzheimer's Disease and Related Disorders, "The Maryland Report on Alzheimer's Disease and Related Disorders," Annapolis, MD, 1985.

29. Grob, G.N., "The Transformation of the Mental Hospital in the United States," *American Behavioral Scientist* 28:639-654, 1985.

30. Gunter, P.L., "Rural Adult Day Care Means Nontraditional Delivery," *Perspective on Aging* 14(6):8,9,18, 1985.

31. Gutkin, C.E., and Morris, S.A., "A Description of Facility and Program Characteristics in Nine Domiciliary Care Programs," *Domiciliary Care Clients and the Facilities in Which They Reside*, S. Sherwood, V. Mor, and C.E. Gutkin (eds.) (Boston, MA: Hebrew Rehabilitation Center for the Aged, 1981).

32. Gwyther, L., director, Center for the Study of Aging and Human Development, Duke University Medical Center, Durham, NC, personal communication, June 16, 1986.

33. Harder, W.P., Gornick, J.C., and Burt, M.R., "Adult Day Care: Supplement or Substitute," The Urban Institute, Washington, DC, draft, 1983.

34. Harper, M.S., "Introduction," *Mental Illness in Nursing Homes: Agenda for Research*, M. Harper and B. Lebowitz (eds.) (Rockville, MD: National Institute of Mental Health, 1986).

35. "Health Facilities Participating in Health Care

Financing Administration Programs, 1985," *Health Care Financing Review* 6(4):143, 1985.

36. Hedrick, S.C., and Inui, T.S., "The Effectiveness and Cost of Home Care: An Information Synthesis," *Health Services Research* 20:851-880, 1986.

37. Institute of Medicine, *Improving the Quality of Care in Nursing Homes* (Washington, DC: National Academy Press, 1986).

38. Intergovernmental Health Policy Project, "Nursing Home Reimbursement Under Medicaid," *Focus On*, February 1986, p. 8.

39. Jerrell, J.M., and Larsen, J.K., "How Community Mental Health Centers Deal With Cutbacks and Competition," *Hospital and Community Psychiatry* 36:1169-1174, 1985.

40. Kansas Alzheimer's and Related Diseases Task Force, *Final Report to the Kansas Department on Aging*, Topeka, KS, 1986.

41. Kaye, L.W., "Home Care for the Aged: A Fragile Partnership," *Social Work* 30:312-317, 1985.

42. Keeler, E.B., Kane, R.L., and Solomon, D.H., "Short- and Long-Term Residents of Nursing Homes," *Medical Care* 19:363-369, 1981.

43. Kelly, J., "Veterans Administration Embarks on Day Care Program," *Perspective on Aging* 14(6):23, 1985.

44. Kramer, M., "Trends of Institutionalization and Prevalence of Mental Disorders in Nursing Homes," *Mental Illness in Nursing Homes: Agenda for Research*, M.S. Harper and B. Lebowitz (eds.) (Rockville, MD: National Institute of Mental Health, 1986).

45. Kurland, C.H., "Constituency Speaks Out," *Perspective on Aging* 14(6):29,34, 1985.

46. Lane, L., Director for Special Programs, American Health Care Association, Statement to the OTA Workshop on Financing Long-Term Care for Patients With Dementia, Washington, DC, May 19, 1986.

47. Larson, E.B., Associate Professor of Medicine, University of Washington, Seattle, letter to OTA, Sept. 11, 1986.

48. Lerman, P., "Deinstitutionalization and Welfare Policies in the Welfare State in America: Trends and Prospects," *American Academy of Political and Social Science Annals—1985* 479:132-155, 1985.

49. Light, E., National Institute of Mental Health, Rockville, MD, personal communication, May 6, 1986.

50. Light, E., National Institute of Mental Health, Rockville, MD, personal communication, Sept. 2, 1986.

51. Light, E., Lebowitz, B., and Bailey, F., "CMHCs [Community Mental Health Centers] and Elderly Services: An Analysis of Direct and Indirect Services and Services Delivery Sites," *Community Mental Health Journal*, 22(4):294-302, 1986.

52. Liu, K., "Analysis of Data Bases for Health Services Research on Dementia," contract report prepared for the Office of Technology Assessment, U.S. Congress, Washington, DC, 1986.

53. Liu, K., and Manton, K.G., "The Characteristics and Utilization Pattern of an Admission Cohort of Nursing Home Patients," *The Gerontologist* 23:92-96, 1983.

54. Lockery, S.A., "Impact of Dementia Within Minority Groups," contract report prepared for the Office of Technology Assessment, U.S. Congress, Washington, DC, 1986.

55. Mace, N.L., and Rabins, P.V., "A Survey of Day Care for the Demented Adult in the United States," National Council on the Aging, Washington, DC, 1984.

56. Manton, K.G., and Hausner, T., "Prospective Reimbursement Systems for LTC: An Illustration of a Case Mix Methodology for Home Health Services," Duke University, Durham, NC, draft, March 1986.

57. Manuel, R.C., and Berk, M.L., "A Look at Similarities and Differences in Older Minority Populations," *Aging* 339:21-29, 1983.

58. Mor, V., Sherwood, S., and Gutkin, C.E., "Psychiatric History as a Barrier to Residential Care," *Hospital and Community Psychiatry* 35:368-372, 1984.

59. Mor, V., Gutkin, C.E., and Sherwood, S., "The Cost of Residential Care Homes Serving Elderly Adults," *Journal of Gerontology* 40(2):164-171, 1985.

60. Morrissey, J.P., and Goldman, H.H., "Cycles of Reform in the Care of the Chronically Mentally Ill," *Hospital and Community Psychiatry* 35:785-793, 1984.

61. Moss, F., and Halamandaris, V., *Too Old, Too Sick, Too Bad: Nursing Homes in America* (Germantown, MD: Aspen Systems Co., 1977).

62. Okin, R.L., "How Community Mental Health Centers Are Coping," *Hospital and Community Psychiatry* 35:1118-1125, 1984.

63. Orr, N., director, Hillhaven Corp. Special Care Units, statement to the OTA Advisory Panel on Disorders Causing Dementia, Washington, DC, June 16, 1986.

64. Petty, D., executive director, Family Survival Project, San Francisco, CA, personal communication, June 16, 1986.

65. Ransom, B., and Kelly, W., "Rising to the Challenge," *Perspective on Aging* 14(6):13,14, 1985.

66. Rathbone-McCuan, E., and Elliott, M., "Geriatric Day Care in Theory and Practice," *Social Work in Health Care* 2(2):153-177, 1976-77.

67. Reichstein, K.J., and Bergofsky, L., "Summary and Report of the National Survey of State Administered Domiciliary Care Programs in the Fifty States and the District of Columbia," Horizon House Institute, Boston, MA, December 1980.

68. Rhode Island Legislative Commission on Dementias Related to Aging, "Final Report," May 1, 1984.

69. Rovner, B.W., and Rabins, P.V., "Mental Illness Among Nursing Home Patients," *Hospital and Community Psychiatry* 36:119-128, 1985.

70. Rovner, B.W., Kalanek, S., Filipp, L., et al., "Prevalence of Mental Illness in a Community Nursing Home," *American Journal of Psychiatry* 143:1446-1449, 1986.

71. Rubenstein, L.Z., Josephson, K.R., Wieland, G.D., et al., "Differential Prognosis and Utilization Patterns Among Clinical Subgroups of Hospitalized Geriatric Patients," *Health Services Research* 20:881-895, 1986.

72. Samuel, F., Health Industry Manufacturers Association, Washington, DC, personal communication, Feb. 14, 1984.

73. Sherwood, C.C., and Seltzer, M.M., *Task III Report: Board and Care Literature Review*, Boston University School of Social Work (Boston, MA: Hebrew Rehabilitation Center for the Aged, 1981).

74. Sherwood, S., and Gruenberg, L., "A Descriptive Study of Functionally Eligible Applicants to the Domiciliary Program: Commonwealth of Pennsylvania" (Boston, MA: Hebrew Rehabilitation Center for the Aged, 1978).

75. Sherwood, S., and Morris, J.N., "The Pennsylvania Domiciliary Care Experiment: #1, Impact on Quality of Life," *American Journal of Public Health* 73:646-653, 1983.

76. Sherwood, S., Mor, V., and Gutlin, C.E., "Domiciliary Care Clients and the Facilities in Which They Reside," contract report prepared for the Department of Health and Human Services, Administration on Aging, December 1981.

77. Sirrocco, A., National Center for Health Statistics, Division of Health Care Statistics, Rockville, MD, personal communication, May 9, 1986.

78. Soldo, B.J., "In-Home Services for the Dependent Elderly: Determinants of Current Use and Implications for Future Demand," working paper, The Urban Institute, Washington, DC, May 1983.

79. Soldo, B.J., "The Elderly Home Care Population: National Prevalence Rates, Select Characteristics, and Alternative Sources of Assistance," working paper, The Urban Institute, Washington, DC, May 1983.

80. Solomon, B., "Ethnic Minority Elderly and Long-Term Care: A Historical Perspective," *Minority Aging and Long-Term Care*, E.P. Stanford and S.A. Lockery (eds.) (San Diego, CA: University Center on Aging, San Diego State University, 1982).

81. Somers, A.R., "Long-Term Care for the Elderly: Policy and Economic Issues," *The Teaching Nursing Home*, E.L. Schneider, C.J. Wendland, A.W. Zimmer, et al. (eds.) (New York, NY: Raven Press, 1985).

82. Stassen, M., and Holahan, J., "Long-Term Care Demonstration Projects: A Review of Recent Evaluations," The Urban Institute, Washington, DC, February 1981.

83. Stone, R., National Center for Health Services Research, personal communication, May 19, 1986.

84. Stone, R., National Center for Health Services Research, personal communication, Sept. 18, 1986.

85. Stone, R., and Newcomer, R., "The State Role in Board and Care Housing," *Long-Term Care of the Elderly: Public Policy Issues*, C. Harrington, R.J. Newcomer, C. Estes, et al. (eds.) (Beverly Hills, CA: Sage Publications, 1985).

86. Texas Department of Health, *Alzheimer's Disease Initiative Nursing Home Study* (Austin, TX, 1985).

87. U.S. Congress, Congressional Research Service, Library of Congress, O'Shaughnessy, C., and Price, R., "Medicaid 2176 Waivers for Home and Community Based Care," Pub. No. 85-817 EPW, June 21, 1985.

88. U.S. Congress, Congressional Research Service, Library of Congress, O'Shaughnessy, C., Price, R., and Griffith, J., "Financing and Delivery of Long-Term Care Services for the Elderly," Pub. No. 85-1033 EPW, Oct. 17, 1985.

89. U.S. Congress, Congressional Research Service, Library of Congress, McClure, B., "Medical Care Programs of the Veterans Administration," Pub. No. 86-41 EPW, Jan. 31, 1986.

90. U.S. Congress, General Accounting Office, "Identifying Boarding Homes Housing the Needy Aged, Blind, and Disabled: A Major Step Toward Resolving a National Problem," Washington, DC, 1979.

91. U.S. Congress, General Accounting Office, "Medicare Home Health Services: A Difficult Program to Control," GAO Pub. No. HRD 81-155, Washington, DC, Sept. 25, 1981.

92. U.S. Congress, General Accounting Office, "The Elderly Remain in Need of Mental Health Services," GAO Pub. No. HRD-82-112, Washington, DC, Sept. 16, 1982.

93. U.S. Congress, General Accounting Office, "The Elderly Should Benefit From Expanded Home Health Care But Increasing These Services Will Not Insure Cost Reductions," GAO Pub. No. IPE-44-1, Washington, DC, Dec. 7, 1982.

94. U.S. Congress, General Accounting Office, "Medicaid and Nursing Home Care: Cost Increases and The Need for Services Are Creating Problems for the States and the Elderly," GAO Pub. No. IPE-84-1, Washington, DC, Oct. 21, 1983.

95. U.S. Congress, General Accounting Office, "Constraining National Health Care Expenditures: Achieving Quality Care at an Affordable Cost," GAO Pub. No. HRD-85-105, Sept. 30, 1985.

96. U.S. Congress, General Accounting Office, "VA Health Care: Issues and Concerns for VA Nursing Home Programs," GAO Pub. No. HRD-86-111BR, Washington, DC, August 1986.

97. U.S. Department of Health and Human Services, Public Health Service, National Center for Health Statistics, *Characteristics of Nursing Home Residents, Health Status, and Care Received: National Nursing Home Survey, United States, May-December, 1977*, series 13, No. 51, DHHS Pub. No. PHS81-1712 (Hyattsville, MD, 1981).

98. U.S. Department of Health and Human Services, Office of the Inspector General, *Board and Care Homes* (Washington, DC, 1982).

99. U.S. Department of Health and Human Services, Social Security Administration, Office of Operational Policy and Procedures, Office of Assistance Programs, "Supplemental Security Income for the Aged, Blind and Disabled—Summary of State Payment Levels, State Supplementation, and Medicaid Decisions," Jan. 1, 1983.

100. U.S. Department of Health and Human Services, Health Care Financing Administration, Office of Research and Demonstrations, "The Medicare and Medicaid Data Book, 1983," D. Sawyer, M. Ruther, A. Pagan-Berlucchi, et al., HCFA Pub. No. 03156 (Baltimore, MD, 1983).

101. U.S. Department of Health and Human Services, Public Health Service, National Center for Health Statistics, *Advancedata*, No. 111, Sept. 20, 1985.

102. U.S. Department of Health, Education, and Welfare, Public Health Service, National Institute of Mental Health, Kramer, M., *Psychiatric Services and the Changing Institutional Scene*, DHEW Pub. No. ADM77-433 (Bethesda, MD, 1977).

103. U.S. Senate, Subcommittee on Health of the Committee on Finance, "Medicare Home Health Benefit," hearing held June 22, 1984.

104. U.S. Senate, Special Committee on Aging, *Developments in Aging, 1984*, vol. 2 (Washington, DC: U.S. Government Printing Office, February 1985).

105. U.S. Senate, Special Committee on Aging, "Nursing Home Care: The Unfinished Agenda," No. 99-J, May 1986 (Washington, DC: U.S. Government Printing Office, 1986).

106. U.S. Senate, Committee on Veterans Affairs, *Title XIX of the Consolidated Omnibus Budget Reconciliation Act of 1985 (Public Law 99-272; April 7, 1986) Veterans Health-Care Amendments of 1986*, committee print (Washington, DC: U.S. Government Printing Office, 1986).

107. VandenBos, G.R., Stapp, J., and Kilberg, R.R., "Health Service Providers in Psychology: Results of the 1978 APA Human Resources Survey," *American Psychologist* 36:1395-1418, 1981.

108. Vandivort, R., Kurran, G.M., and Braun, K., "Foster Family Care for Frail Elderly: A Cost Effective Quality Care Alternative," *Gerontological Social Work in Home Health Care*, R. Dobrof (ed.) (New York, NY: Haworth Press, 1984).

109. Van Gelder, S., General Accounting Office, U.S. Congress, personal communication, May 22, 1986.

110. Veterans Administration, Harvard Conference on VA/Community Resources and the Older Veteran, Boston, MA, 1983.

111. Veterans Administration, *Caring for the Older Veteran* (Washington, DC, July 1984).

112. Veterans Administration, Department of Medicine and Surgery, *Guidelines for Diagnosis and Treatment*, IB 18-3 (Washington, DC, Oct. 10, 1985).

113. Vladeck, B.C., *Unloving Care: The Nursing Home Tragedy* (New York, NY: Basic Books, 1980).

114. Vladeck, B.C., "The Static Dynamics of Long-Term Care Policy," *The Health Policy Agenda: Some Critical Questions*, M.E. Lewin (ed.) (Washington, DC: American Enterprise Institute for Public Policy Research, 1985).

115. Volicer, L., "Need for Hospice Approach to Treatment of Patients With Advance Progressive Dementia," *Journal of the American Geriatric Society* 34(9):655-658, 1986.

116. Weiler, P., director, Center for Aging and Health, School of Medicine, University of California, Davis, statement to the OTA Advisory Panel on Disorders Causing Dementia, Washington, DC, June 16, 1986.

117. Weissert, W.G., "Seven Reasons Why It Is So Difficult To Make Community-Based Long-Term Care Cost-Effective," *Health Services Research* 20:423-433, 1985.

118. Weissert, W.G., "Two Models of Geriatric Day Care: Findings From a Comparative Study," *The Gerontologist* 16:420-427, 1976.

119. Weissert, W.G., and Scanlon, W., "Determinants of Institutionalization of the Aged," working pa-

per, The Urban Institute, Washington, DC, July 1983.

120. Wetle, T., and Rowe, J.W., *Older Veterans: Linking VA and Community Resources* (Cambridge, MA: Harvard University Press, 1984).

121. Wolfson, S., "The Policy of Pairing Patients With Different Cognitive Skills in the Same Room of a Nursing Home" (letter to the editor), *Journal of the American Geriatric Society* 31:246, 1983.

122. Yankelovich, Skelly, and White, "Caregivers of Patients With Dementia," contract report prepared for the Office of Technology Assessment, U.S. Congress, 1986.

123. Zimmer, J.G., Watson, N., and Treat, A., "Behavioral Problems Among Patients in Skilled Nursing Facilities," *American Journal of Public Health* 74:1118-1121, 1984.

Programs and Services That Specialize in the Care of Persons With Dementia

CONTENTS

Programs and Services That Specialize in the Care of Persons With Dementia*

The increasing recognition of the needs of those with dementing illnesses has led to the development of programs and services—day care, home care, short-term residential care programs, and nursing home programs—that specialize in caring for those persons. This interest in special services arises in part from recognition of the potential market, in part from the demand of family members and voluntary associations, and in part from the hope that special resources and skills may improve the care of these people.

Although there are now only a handful of these specialized programs, the growing number of them raises important policy questions: What standards should these programs meet? how should they be reimbursed? and is it in the individuals' best interests to be segregated? Some answers depend on understanding whether the care needs of these people are different from those of other chronically ill elderly individuals. Since many of them have been served all along by long-term care programs, particularly nursing homes, what is "new" about special dementia care? Indeed, some of the changes advocated for specialized dementia care are improvements that would benefit many other long-term care recipients.

This is the first generation of such special care programs. Although a few nursing homes have had specialized units for more than a decade, most such programs are less than 5 years old, and the total number of persons receiving special care is small. It cannot be assumed that services that have been found to be beneficial to a few people will be of value to over a million others. Nevertheless, enough information is available to consider some questions:

- Who is served in special units?
- What are the advantages and disadvantages of specialization?
- What kinds of services and programs do patients and families need?
- What kinds of services and programs are appropriate in specialized care?
- What specialized care is currently being provided?

Although an extensive body of literature exists on nursing home care (93) and on respite care for the elderly (91), there is limited information on special dementia care programs; what there is represents the opinions and experiences of clinicians rather than reports of controlled studies. Although there is some research on interventions with the elderly mentally ill and with nursing home residents, much is poorly designed and most does not discriminate between persons with and without dementing disorders (100). Thus this chapter must rely on anecdotal material and "best guesses" of experienced clinicians. Policymakers cannot assume that these represent the best ultimate approaches to care. Additional research is urgently needed.

Seven providers of special services were asked to document their experiences for OTA (18,25,32, 42,67,74,84). One contractor had previously surveyed other special care programs (95). Another reviewed in detail the management of incontinence (96). In addition, OTA reviewed reports of specialized nursing home programs, and OTA contractors and staff attended conferences, visited facilities, and consulted with providers in the industry and the nonprofit sector. A few of those providers have worked for many years with chronically mentally ill elderly individuals (a term that includes many persons with dementia). This chapter also draws on the studies of elderly mentally ill persons in State mental hospitals prior to deinstitutionalism (efforts to move people out of such facilities) (20,30,35,36,51,55).

OTA found variations in services and no consensus about what constitutes ideal or cost-efficient care. But OTA did observe a clear move-

---

*This chapter is a contract report by Nancy Mace, consultant in Gerontology, Towson, MD.

ment toward providing specialty care for persons with dementia and agreement among leading clinicians about the principles of such care.

Specialized care for individuals with dementia can be delivered in any setting and can provide most services noted in chapter 6, including respite for families or long-term residential care. The options for care should be a part of a network of resources for families and those with dementia, who will need different resources as the person's health and the family status change through the course of the illness, and who may need to move back and forth between formal and informal care (100). Ideally, resource clearinghouses, information and referral systems, and case management services would be available to assist patients in locating specialized care programs and in moving easily from one setting to another. In fact, resources are fragmented, funding is discontinuous, and information is often not available.

Patients and families also need allied resources such as legal advice from attorneys familiar with dementia. Legal issues are described in chapters 5 and 11 and will not be dealt with here. This chapter will be limited to a discussion of special respite and long-term care programs which specialize in care of persons with dementia. However, such services must be thought of as links in a broader spectrum of care needs.

THE RECENT INTEREST IN SPECIAL CARE

What Is New About Special Programs?

Persons with dementia are not entirely new to formal care providers. Until the movement toward deinstitutionalization, persons with dementia whose families could not care for them were housed in State mental hospitals along with individuals suffering from a range of mental disorders. State mental institutions therefore had a history of caring for persons with dementia, and a few institutions developed special care programs for them. Deinstitutionalization resulted in the transfer of public care for those with dementia from State mental hospitals to nursing homes (13). More than half the current residents of nursing homes apparently suffer from dementing illnesses (see ch. 1).

The number of persons with dementia and in need of care is increasing (see ch. 1), and there is a growing concern that the nursing home system—facilities, funding sources, and regulating agencies—does not serve such individuals well. With the increasing public interest in these illnesses has come a parallel interest in both care outside of nursing homes or mental hospitals and in different approaches to care within such facilities.

Who Is Served by Special Units?

The kind of care offered by the few existing special programs is not considered appropriate for everyone with a dementing illness. In nursing homes that have established a special care unit, most individuals with dementia still reside on mixed units. Many nursing home residents are frail and suffer from multiple, severe illnesses. Their mental confusion may result from Alzheimer's disease or from delirium brought about by their illness. These people need more nursing care than the special programs offer. Thus most people with dementia are now cared for in programs designed to serve all frail or ill elderly individuals. Programs that specialize in dementia care address the needs of those who are most difficult to care for or whose care needs have been overlooked.

No generally accepted criteria defining who will be served in special programs have been established. The criteria followed by many programs can be summarized as:

- **Presence of irreversible dementia:** Most programs serve only adults with a clear history of intellectual decline, excluding persons with mental retardation and those with treatable causes of mental impairment.

- **Presence of disruptive behaviors:** In contrast to programs that historically have excluded persons who are incontinent, agitated, combative, prone to wandering, etc., these programs focus on the behaviorally disabled whom they see as most in need of services.
- **Ability to benefit from the program:** This vague criterion is used to describe persons in the midstages of an illness, when behavior problems are most likely to be present, and when the individuals can be observed to respond to social activities. Later in the illness these programs may discharge or transfer persons who need extensive nursing care, who are not ambulatory, who are too ill to show disruptive behaviors, or who are less responsive to group social activities. (Programs that serve people individually in their homes may serve persons who are more seriously impaired than those in group programs.)

Opinions differ on the ideal diagnostic mix of persons who should be served in specialized programs. Some families of individuals with Alzheimer's disease advocate programs that serve only that group. Some programs, notably the Family Survival Project in San Francisco (27), serve all brain-damaged adults, including those suffering from stroke, trauma, Parkinson's disease, Huntington's disease, normal pressure hydrocephalus, and Alzheimer's disease. These programs strongly advocate a noncategorical program for all brain-injured adults.

The argument centers on whether persons with Alzheimer's disease are more or differently impaired and require different care than other brain-damaged adults. In practice, most programs serve mainly persons with Alzheimer's disease and a sprinkling of persons with various other conditions, reflecting the mix in the community as a whole.

While people with Alzheimer's disease do have characteristic symptoms that distinguish them from those with related disorders, providers report that the behaviors and care needs of most persons with dementia are based as much on the stage of the illness or on individual characteristics as on diagnosis. No service provider reported to OTA that problems were caused by serving individuals with other diagnoses, although a person with any disorder, including Alzheimer's disease, can prove unsuitable for a given program. Several reported that a diagnostic mix was beneficial.

Designing programs for these active and difficult persons who can benefit from such efforts has one major drawback: It could result in choosing only the most responsive individuals, leaving the more difficult or withdrawn to receive less care.

ADVANTAGES AND DISADVANTAGES OF SPECIALIZATION

Table 7-1 summarizes some of the arguments for and against special units for persons with dementia. Few solid data support either side. But care providers seem increasingly convinced that these persons have unique limitations best met by specialized care. The results of the programs discussed in this chapter support that belief. In addition, enthusiasm for special care programs has probably been influenced by a common frustration that long-term care has failed this group.

It should be noted that, although these arguments are most often raised in discussion of nursing home special units, similar concerns confront day care or respite providers. Also, these arguments assume that special care is targeted toward those with dementia alone. Different issues are raised by the care of persons who are both cognitively impaired and have serious physical illness. Finally, the trend toward specialized care challenges the long-held assumptions of therapeutic nihilism—that there is nothing that can be done for people who are old and "senile" (60).

In weighing the advantages and disadvantages of special care, the effect of widespread adoption of programs must be considered. The few existing programs have enthusiastic staff and are the focus of community interest. Those qualities may not carry over to large-scale programs and may need to be supplemented or enhanced by staffing requirements or formal quality assurance mechanisms.

Table 7-1.—Arguments For and Against Special Programs/Units for Persons With Dementia

Arguments for	Arguments against
The needs of individuals with dementia are not the same. Trained staff in a special environment can produce measurable evidence of benefit in persons with dementia.	People need much the same care. Most nursing home residents suffer multiple illnesses, of which mental impairment is only one. They need regular nursing care.
Quality care should be available to all nursing home residents, but even in the best possible setting the needs of the cognitively impaired are different from those of the cognitively intact.	Provision of special units is unfair to other people who would also benefit from many of the environmental changes that help people with dementia. Instead of segregating people, the quality of all care should be upgraded.
Being around people whose mental functioning is higher can be stressful for persons with dementia, who must constantly struggle to process even simple information. This may be one cause of behavior problems.	Placing persons with dementia with cognitively well persons helps the person with dementia stay alert by providing role models. Isolation in all-dementia units may lead to greater deterioration.
Special units permit special interior design, fire safety equipment, trained staff, and marketing efforts to attract private pay clients. The demand for quality ensures that beds in good facilities will fill quickly.	Special units must hold a bed open until a person with dementia needs it. This is more expensive than quickly filling beds with the next available client.
Cognitively well elderly persons have made it clear in several informal surveys that they do not want to spend their lives with persons who act "crazy" or are disruptive. The lucid client is vulnerable to loss of privacy, loss of personal property, interrupted sleep, and fear of harm by the agitated person. Efforts to protect the lucid client may result in overmedication and restraints, which have negative effects on persons with dementia. There are ethical issues involved in using persons who are paying for their own care as supervisors of other patients.	In mixed units, cognitively well individuals can help "look after" the person with dementia, which allows lower staffing levels and gives the well client something to do.
The current demand for specialized units is such that people will transport family members long distances for residential care.	In areas with a low population density, there will not be enough persons with dementia to support special units, particularly day care.
An all-dementia unit allows staff to develop expertise in care for clients. This benefits residents and is rewarding to staff. Experience has shown that staff do not necessarily "burn out."	Staff will quickly "burn out" on a dementia unit. The issue of burnout and staff satisfaction is not unique to dementia care, but reflects pervasive problems in long-term care.
Patients' rights laws, ombudsmen, and quality assurance regulations assure oversight of persons who are not competent. The new focus on dementia reduces the risk that individuals would be poorly served.	A program serving persons with dementia would create a ghetto in which no one would be able to report abuses or be a legally capable witness. Ombudsmen rarely serve board and care facilities. Persons with dementia often outlive the family members who advocate for them.
Dementia is a medical specialty long overdue for recognition. Specialty programs would attract physicians and nurses interested in this field.	Dementia is not a medical specialty, deserving of separate designation and specialization, because the needs of these individuals are primarily psychological and social.

SOURCES: M. Ablowitz, "Pairing Rational and Demented Patients in Long-Term Care Facilities," *Journal of the American Geriatrics Society* 31:627-628, 1983; J. Bergman, "Mentally Ill in Nursing Homes? Yes, if . . . .," *Geriatric Nursing* 3:98-100, 1983; R. Cook-Deegan and N. Mace, "Care of Patients With Dementia," Testimony, California Task Force on Alzheimer's Disease, 1986; D. Coons, "A Residential Care Unit for Persons With Dementia," contract report prepared for the Office of Technology Assessment, U.S. Congress, 1986; G. Hall, V. Kirshling, and S. Todd, "Sheltered Freedom: The Creation of an Alzheimer's Unit in an Intermediate Care Facility," unpublished paper, 1985; Hebrew Home for the Aged at Riverdale, "Institutional Approaches to the Care of Individuals With Dementia," contract report prepared for the Office of Technology Assessment, U.S. Congress, 1986; N. L. Mace, "Home and Community Services for Alzheimer's Disease: A National Conference for Families," U.S. Department of Health and Human Services and Alzheimer's Disease and Related Disorders Association, May 2, 1985; J. Pynoos and C.A. Stacey, "Specialized Facilities for Senile Dementia Patients," *The Dementias: Policy and Management* M.L.M. Gilhooly, S. Zarit, and J.E. Birren (eds.) (Englewood Cliffs, NJ: Prentice Hall, 1986).

SERVICES AND PROGRAMS NEEDED BY THOSE WITH DEMENTIA AND THEIR FAMILIES

Chapter 2 describes the characteristics of individuals with dementia, and chapter 4 documents the needs of family caregivers. Ideally, these needs will define the shape of special care programs.

In addition, services should be tailored to surmount the problems of service delivery in rural areas and to meet the needs of varied ethnic groups. For example, since people with dementia

Table 7-2.—OTA Survey: Availability and Use of Services for Persons With Dementia

100%→	Available				Used[a]		
	Yes %	No %	Don't know %	No answer %	Yes[b] %	No, never used %	No answer %
Visiting nurse...................................	51	10	31	7	44	53	4
Paid companion/home health aide	48	16	29	8	59	38	3
Temporary, round the clock respite care.........	21	24	47	8	13	61	27
Special dementia unit nursing home care........	21	33	37	9	44	50	7
Adult day care	29	24	39	8	31	66	3
Domiciliary/boarding care....................	14	26	51	9	33	61	6

NOTE: Percentages rounded to the nearest whole number.
[a]Base = those who knew service was available.
[b]Current and past used combined.

SOURCE: Yankelovich, Skelly, & White, Inc., "Caregivers of Patients With Dementia and Their Families," contract report prepared for the Office of Technology Assessment, U.S. Congress, 1986.

have problems in learning, persons from other cultures may have great difficulty adapting to "mainstream" programs.

Needs of Families

Although families report high levels of need for services, an OTA survey of caregivers of individuals with dementia found that services were not available for many (99) (see ch. 4; the study is referred to in this chapter as the OTA survey or study). Table 7-2 shows that many families know services are available, yet families do not always use available services. Of the families surveyed who knew a service was available, 38 percent did not use a home health aide and between 50 and 66 percent did not use other services. Many families are noticeably reluctant to turn any care over to others.

The OTA survey and others (33) have identified several characteristics of care provided by families that could affect the use of specialized services. Care must be affordable. Some resources are available but beyond the reach of families. Although they are concerned that their resources not be exhausted, families prefer to share with the formal system, rather than completely turn over, the costs and tasks of caregiving whenever possible. Current funding sources, notably Medicaid, impoverish the family before providing assistance, and the emphasis on nursing home placement reduces the caregiver's continued participation in care.

Evidence from respite programs (37,74) indicates that families can remain in control of the care

process by paying a portion of respite care costs, by using voucher systems that allow a family to select the provider, by participating in caregiving, and by helping paid providers develop care plans.

Needs of Individuals With Dementia

Arguments for and against specialized care turn, in part, on different views about medical v. social needs, about the potential of these individuals for treatment, and about the benefits of treating the person v. treating the environment.

First, the handicaps of people with dementia, and therefore their needs, differ from those of the physically ill. Since the symptoms are behavioral and the difficulties mental, for much of their illness individuals need physical less care than supervision and support of their remaining mental capacities. That difference makes one of the strongest arguments for specialized care. As these diseases progress, however, the need for physical care increases and the effectiveness of existing special units appears to lessen. More medical and nursing care will be needed. The existence of these shifting needs over time fuels the debate over a social rather than medical model of care. Each model tends to explain the individual behaviors on the basis of its own tenets, despite the fact that the distressing behaviors of dementing illnesses are explained in part by organic illnesses and in part by the social environment (see ch. 2).

Dementia has been described as a "bio-psycho-social phenomenon." Although the biological aspects are not currently treatable, the psychological and social aspects may be amenable to intervention (52). But the shape of future programs will be heavily influenced by policy and funding, which until now have focused on either a strict medical model (Medicare and Medicaid) or a primarily social one (Older Americans Act). Many persons with dementing illnesses have psychiatric symptoms that may be amenable to treatment (see ch. 2). Services need to include psychiatric skills or access to a psychiatric consultant for help in decreasing such symptoms and maximizing function.

A second unknown is how much can be done for persons with dementia. Current funding policy assumes that people with dementia do not have rehabilitative potential and therefore are eligible only for custodial services at rates that discourage efforts to search for treatable aspects of the individual's illness. Funding does not support the employment of persons skilled in dementia care.

Function may be improved in some individuals by treating "excess disability" (52) (see ch. 2). The term refers to impairments in everyday functioning that are worse than expected considering the underlying biological deficits. Little is known about the prevalence of excess disability among persons with dementia, or about the capacity of persons to respond to treatment. Estimates of the number of those persons in nursing homes and acute care institutions with untreated conditions are high (53). Some but not all will improve significantly if treated. Much of the "improvement" documented among demented nursing home residents (discussed later in this chapter) may actually be elimination of excess disability.

A third disagreement is whether treatment should be directed at the individual or the environment. Federal policy is generally limited to funding interventions that treat the person. Reimbursement of caregiver supports or construction of facilities with special modifications for the purpose of treating someone with dementia would require a change in funding policy. Some techniques, such as reality orientation (29,30,76), behavior modification, remotivation therapy (64), fantasy and validation therapy (28), use of drugs to control behavior, and the potential use of drugs to enhance memory, are intended to effect change

in a person by acting directly on that person. Studies to date have not shown that these techniques consistently improve the functioning of persons with dementia (100). In contrast, some observers (19,60,63) argue that the individual benefits from the creation of a physical and psychosocial environment that supports function and that, conversely, inappropriate environments can result in unnecessary impairment in persons with dementia.

It may be that the environment can be modified (both physically and interpersonally) to support greater function for persons with dementia (48,56,60). The percent of individuals who would respond to an improved physical and psychosocial environment is unknown, but of the special nursing home units reviewed by OTA, all that attended to some type of excess disability or made changes in environment reported improvements in the residents with dementia. One researcher maintains that:

> . . . there is now good evidence that even elderly demented patients are capable of showing a beneficial response to environmental manipulation. However, unlike physical therapy or similar treatments, maintenance of behavior change is dependent on the continuation of the intervention (63).

Evidence that environmental changes may be beneficial if they are continued raises another problem of policy. In general, the intent of Federal programs (such as Medicare) has been to support rehabilitative, short-term care that will enable a person to return to more normal functions, rather than interventions that must remain in place to support improvement.

Many of the people now in nursing homes and included in the estimates of the number of those with dementia, suffer from multiple, severe illnesses. Their cognitive impairment is often due both to delirium and to dementia. They are too ill to benefit from the kinds of programs described in this chapter. Even the best medical care can do little to alter their overall condition. Programs designed to improve the quality of life for people with dementia probably will have little effect on this group. However, there are also an unknown number of people who would respond to interventions but have been consigned to the "hopeless" category. Questions about the size of the group that could be helped raise another issue of policy: Since not all cognitively impaired people will benefit from special programs, how should those who would benefit be identified? There is a need for physicians trained in geriatrics to be available for those in nursing homes and similar settings.

SERVICES THAT CAN BE TAILORED TO PERSONS WITH DEMENTIA

In its survey, OTA asked why families did not use a service if it were available (see table 7-3). Only a few reported that the service would not accept a person with a diagnosis of dementia but, depending on the service, 5 to 18 percent reported that staff was not sufficiently knowledgeable about dementia. The most common reasons for not using or no longer using respite services, among those who knew that such services were available, were that the person entered a nursing home, the service was too expensive, the ill person died, or the service was not needed. Thus, some individuals apparently used appropriate respite services until their condition worsened, leading to placement in a nursing home or to death. This conclusion also indicates that respite care is a temporary solution and does not necessarily replace nursing home care (75).

Several different alternative services are being tried by chapters of the Alzheimer's Disease and Related Disorders Association (ADRDA), individual entrepreneurs, family service organizations, and the health care industry. The search for appropriate care is international (65,81). At this point in the development of dementia care options, the programs are highly individualized. Providers are trying different interventions and exploring innovative ways to reach clients and hold down costs. Special programs apparently are still rare, however. There is no listing of existing services, but the special units in nursing homes and respite programs are estimated to be serving between 1 and 2 percent of persons with dementia. (This figure is based on programs known to American Association of Homes for the Aged (AAHA), American Health Care Association, ADRDA, New York State

Table 7-3.—OTA Survey: Reasons for Not Using Available Support Services[a]

Reasons	Base[b]	Paid companion/ health aide	Visiting nurse	Respite care	Adult day care	Domiciliary/ boarding care	Special dementia nursing home care
		36%	42%	17%	24%	10%	13%
The patient entered a nursing home ...		46	43	40	35	40	24
The service is too expensive..........		31	23	24	11	16	19
The patient got worse or died.........		21	21	15	17	9	20
The service is not needed		19	27	25	19	26	27
The people available to provide this service are not sufficiently knowledgeable about dementia		16	11	5	5	9	4
The patient refused to accept the service.........................		15	10	10	25	13	5
Lack of knowledge about how to arrange for this service		9	2	6	4	6	10
The waiting list is too long		4	1	3	2	2	7
The service would not accept the patient because of the patient's diagnosis		1	3	4	6	6	5
Other reasons		12	6	13	11	11	14
No answer		6	9	9	8	15	11

[a]Question was asked of respondents who said respective service was available but was not used.
[b]Percent of total surveyed. Totals more than 100% because of multiple responses.

SOURCE: Yankelovich, Skelly, & White, Inc., "Caregivers of Patients With Dementia and Their Families," contract report prepared for the Office of Technology Assessment, U.S. Congress, 1986.

Department of Health, Hebrew Home for the Aged at Riverdale, Hillhaven Corp., National Council on Aging, and OTA.)

Companion Care, Home Health Aides, and Visiting Nurses

Families report that part-time help at home is the form of respite they need most (37,99). In programs providing such care, a nonprofessional person with special training spends a few hours a week with the individuals with dementia so that the caregiver can leave the home or rest. Fifty-nine percent of the respondents in the OTA study had used an aide in the home and 44 percent had used a visiting nurse. Families often used a home health care agency or made private arrangements, thus the number of these providers who had special training is not known. Some specialized programs use volunteers, others use "paid volunteers," and some pay a salary.

Several ADRDA chapters offer help at home, and others are allied with respite providers. The three programs described in boxes 7-A, 7-B, and 7-C found that a half-day per week, or less than 6 hours weekly, was what families most often needed. Relief was requested most often during regular business hours.

Although programs affiliated with ADRDA or with universities attempt to ensure the quality of in-home providers, there is little or no mandated monitoring of the quality of home care. Home care aides generally are not required to have special training or to be bonded. There is often no requirement for background checks of persons going into the homes of vulnerable persons. Possibilities exist, therefore, that individuals with dementia and their families might be exploited. Some families have refused to use in-home care for these reasons.

Adult Day Care

Adult day care has developed as an option of care for frail elderly persons mainly in the past 15 years. It has served primarily individuals who were cognitively intact, but many day care centers have always served a few confused persons. Over the past 5 years, with the increasing interest in

---

Box 7-A.—Senior Respite Care Program

The Senior Respite Care Program in Portland, OR, is a nonprofit project begun in 1983 by a group of concerned citizens. Persons interested in part-time work are given 2 days training in providing respite in the home. The program has produced a manual for staff training. A trained staff person supervises the providers, talks with families, and does some informal case management. Fees are on a sliding scale. Clients tend to be ambulatory but have behavioral problems, are continent but need reminders, are in need of constant supervision, and have sleep disturbances. Families are urged to leave the home during respite provision. The director of the program visits families before the service begins and follows up carefully after the provider visit. She reports that the same person should consistently provide care. The person with dementia gradually learns to accept the care provider, family trust is gained, and the provider learns how to manage the individual. The program also notes that caregivers tend to wait too long and to seek respite care "after the caregiver is already broken, and no matter how much relief is provided, the health and commitment is gone" (24).

---

dementia, several day care centers have been established solely for individuals with dementia.

Adult day care contrasts with geriatric day hospitals that have been developed in England. A day hospital offers many of the same services as a regular hospital, except that patients live at home. The emphasis is on medical treatment and rehabilitation (7). Clients have a potential for improvement and the staff includes rehabilitation therapists. There are few day hospitals in the United States, where the focus has been on adult day care.

Day care differs from day hospitals in services offered (less medical, psychiatric, and rehabilitative care), client population (more chronically impaired), the expected outcomes (less client improvement), and staffing pattern (68). Some States (e.g., California) further distinguished between adult day care and adult day health care. Although it offers social programming, day health care places greater emphasis on nursing needs of clients. This distinction is often difficult to make

Box 7-B.—Duke University/American Association of Retired Persons (AARP) Project

The Duke University/American Association of Retired Persons (AARP) project is a research study that is following caregivers who receive in-home respite for 2 years. The study is examining changes in the caregiver's well-being, changes in the employability of the respite care provider, effect on the person with dementia, and impact on the provider agency. Providers are aides who are employed by a home health agency and a non-profit nursing home. Both agencies have a nursing supervisor for supervision, monitoring, and case coordination. Duke has provided the additional training. The home health agency is skilled in negotiating and coordinating other services the family also needs.

This project has a cap on the amount of service available; families can purchase additional time or use the same providers through other funding sources. Duke/AARP's clients include more minority, low-income families than those originally surveyed in a study of caregiver burden. The clients are sicker than expected; many are not ambulatory and most are occasionally incontinent. Caregivers do not have to leave the home during the visit; some go to bed to rest and some are ill. Some are employed and manage care by coordinating the help of other family members, neighbors, and the respite service. Since family reluctance to use a respite service is common, the Duke/AARP project provides case management, gaining the family member's trust as well as helping families locate other needed programs.

One site in the Duke/AARP project offers overnight companion care, providing someone to stay in a client's home for one or more nights so the caregiver can get away. The OTA study found that 53 percent of families listed overnight care as a most important option. Many informal arrangements include overnight respite, and some home care facilities offer this service. Duke/AARP reports that few families have requested overnight care. Neither Medicaid nor Medicare will cover such a program (37).

Box 7-C.—Atlanta Area Chapter of ADRDA

The Atlanta area chapter of ADRDA provides both day care and in-home respite through its community service program. The staff reports that in-home clients are more impaired than their day care clients. This chapter has been exceptionally successful in generating both a full census and adequate funding through a series of small local grants. It recently received funds from the State.

As with most centers, the Atlanta program has guidelines for what in-home workers can and cannot do. The approved duties of the in-home worker include assisting with personal care; bathing patient; helping with brushing teeth, eating, toileting; assisting with exercise or recreation; assisting in transfer to and from bed; accompanying the ill person to doctor; and changing bed linens. Providers do not do housework or prepare meals.

in practice and can serve to exclude persons with dementia, who characteristically need nursing care, socialization, and social services.

Despite enthusiastic reports of the positive effect of day care on persons with dementing illnesses, questions remain about the role of day care and its effect on individuals and families (34,61). One problem is the number of different expectations people have about day care. It has been seen as a treatment, assessment, and rehabilitation program; as a form of support for families; as a means of providing stimulation; and as a vehicle for promoting and maintaining quality of life. Such diverse goals make attempts to study day care's effectiveness difficult. However, care is clearly not appropriate for some individuals and families (e.g., people who have no caregiver or those who are too ill to benefit from the social experience).

A 1984 survey of adult day care programs in the United States estimated that some 2,200 to 2,400 persons with dementia were being served (61). The majority of centers served a mixture of confused and alert clients, but 17 centers (5 percent) specialized in care of persons with dementia. Although still relatively rare, the number of programs focusing on dementia is increasing.

Three special adult day care centers—Atlanta Community Services Program, Family Respite Center in Falls Church, VA, and Harbor Area Adult Day Care in Costa Mesa, CA—reported to OTA on their programs (see boxes 7-D, 7-E, and 7-F). OTA staff visited the latter two programs, as well

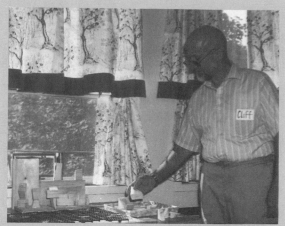

Photo credit: Gretchen Kolsrud

At the Family Respite Center, one client sands wood blocks and glues them together to make wood sculptures.

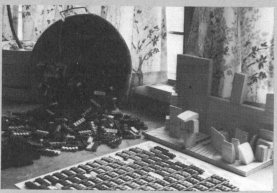

Photo credit: Gretchen Kolsrud

The same client makes designs with colored plastic blocks. The art therapist has noted that his choice of colors changes with major changes in his mood.

Box 7-D.—Atlanta Community Services Program

The Atlanta Community Services Program provides both home care and day care. The program observed that its day care clients become less withdrawn, enjoy peer contacts, and show decreased agitation and "appear happier." This program was developed by the Atlanta ADRDA and has been enthusiastically used by caregivers (also see box 7-C) (32).

Box 7-E.—Family Respite Center

At the Family Respite Center in Virginia, staff members work to improve the individual's self-image and community living skills. They reported that:

. . . as [clients] are integrated into a group and function within it their physical and social adjustment improves. In many cases their personality returns toward their premorbid state.

Of the 53 clients admitted, 22 required help moving around and 9 were not ambulatory. Twenty-six needed help with meals and two needed help with all activities. Forty-two required assistance in the bathroom and 13 had lost control of their bladders and/or bowels. On the Folstein Mini-Mental Status Exam (see ch. 8), with a possible high score of 30, no client scored higher than 9, indicating significant impairment. Thirteen had been discharged from other programs due to behavior disorders. Eighteen exhibited either wandering or hitting behavior.

Quite interestingly, visitors to the Center are astonished to learn of participants previous behavior problems or level of dementia because they function so well in this setting.

The program employs an art therapist (67).

Box 7-F.—Harbor Area Adult Day Care

At the Harbor Area Adult Day Care Program, in Costa Mesa, CA, which provides both boarding care and day care, clients appear brighter, happier, less panicked, and more alert than comparable individuals in other settings. They initiate conversation and exhibit a sense of humor. It is speculated that these people respond to and benefit from the social environment. Although no studies have documented these changes or their causes, this pattern has been observed repeatedly in other day care centers specializing in care of people with dementia (61,84).

as the Alzheimer's Family Center in San Diego (see box 7-G). All were started with the assistance of community groups. All have succeeded in providing care to people who need one-to-one help with meals, who are ambulatory and prone to wander, who need assistance with toileting, and who have behavioral outbursts. All report significant benefits to clients and families. Most programs provide some nursing management to clients and some social services to caregivers.

Day care is consistently reported to be beneficial to clients, in addition to providing respite to families. In the national survey, 84 percent of the centers said their clients with dementia made friends with others, 79 percent thought that clients enjoyed day care, 67 percent reported that pacing and wandering decreased, and 71 percent reported that clients had fewer emotional outbursts (61).

The 1984 survey of day care reported a mean charge per day of $20 (61). It did not determine costs. The ADRDA estimates a current average daily cost of $25 to $30 (5), and the National Institute on Adult Day Care reports an average cost, with subsidies, of $31 per day (78). The survey reported ratios of one staff person to four or five clients. Some programs are open from early morning to late evening weekdays in order to accommodate working caregivers. These centers were also found to be providing considerable informal support to families through teaching, case coordination, and short-term counseling. Centers supplement staff with volunteers (61).

These findings indicate that, as with other forms of respite, day care probably does not replace nursing homes, but serves instead as a vital support to families in the period before nursing home placement is needed (see also ch. 4). And they show that not all individuals or families can use day care. Other physical illnesses; a greater need for help with walking, toileting, and eating than the center can manage; and inability to adjust to a new environment prevent some people from using day care. About one client in five dropped out because of inability to adjust to the setting (61). To date there is no way to identify these people in advance. The OTA study found that among families who had access to adult day care, 25 percent reported that the person with dementia rejected the service (i.e., could not adjust to day care or was unable to function in a group).

The most common reasons for discharge from day care, according to the national survey, were (in descending order) client's transfer to a nursing home, client's death, and client's inability to adjust to the program. The OTA study findings were similar. Transportation problems and client moves from one household to another are other reasons for discharge.

Transportation is a serious problem both in the United States (61) and in Great Britain, where day care has been used much longer (3). Elderly caregivers may not be able to drive, and confused, disoriented individuals cannot tolerate a long bus ride—necessary unless the clients live in an area with a high population density. They may be unwilling to board the bus or may wander away when they are dropped off. Some programs have a staff person on the bus to assist clients in and out of the home and the transport vehicle.

Regardless of problems associated with day care, the social responsiveness of those with dementia confirms that it is one way to improve the quality of life for these individuals as well as provide respite for caregivers. Multiple factors of both client and caregiver determine who will successfully use this resource. As with child day care, adult day care may prove to be an excellent employee benefit for adult children caring for a parent.

Unlike some other methods of providing special care, most day care programs are providing substantially the same services and have had enough experience with clients to establish guidelines on what these services should be (54,71,72,

Box 7-G.—Alzheimer's Family Center, Inc.

The Alzheimer's Family Center in San Diego is able to care for clients until close to their death, and reports that some never enter a nursing home. This program is affiliated with the University of California at San Diego—one of the federally funded Alzheimer's Research Centers. The program has opened a second day care center and has received a grant from American Express to train in-home respite workers (2).

85,101). The National Council on the Aging has published a bibliography of sources (87). Night care has also been proposed for people who could live with family but whose nighttime activities seriously stress the caregiver.

Short-Term Residential Care

Short-term residential care provides stays of days or weeks in a residential setting, usually a nursing home. Only 13 percent of caregivers responding to the OTA survey used short-term residential care, perhaps because it is rarely available. Forty-three percent, however, ranked it as "most important."

These programs have several problems, however. Because the stay is too brief for residents to adjust to the surroundings, they may be more restless and agitated than participants in other programs. Short-term programs may therefore need additional staff. Care may be more difficult if individuals are placed on units with residents who are not confused. And nursing homes report that regulations and paperwork for a short-term admission are so cumbersome that short stays are not cost-effective.

In the past, the urgent need for short-term respite has led to acute hospital admissions for persons whose caregiver must have medical care or rest. Used that way, this is an extraordinarily ex-

---

Box 7-H.—Veterans Administration Residential Respite Programs

The Veterans Administration (VA) has 12 short-term residential respite programs. OTA staff visited the VA hospital and respite program in Palo Alto, CA, which allows patients to stay for 1 or 2 weeks, scheduled in advance (23). Families may use the service year after year. Some of these patients are in the advanced stages of their illness or may also have other impairments. Other VA hospitals, a few nursing homes, retirement communities, and retirement homes offer short-term stays, usually with the restriction that the person is continent and does not wander (1). The Southern Baptist Hospital in New Orleans, for example, offers a weekend respite program to patients who are not violent (also see ref. 75).

---

pensive resource; it has been proposed, however, that empty hospital beds could be used for respite.

Some programs have found that families are reluctant to take the ill persons with dementia back at the end of the respite period. These are probably families who actually needed to have the person placed in a nursing home but who tried to compromise by using respite. For some caregivers, short-term admission helps them realize how ill the individual is or that the person does not know where he or she is or who is providing care. The presence of nursing staff may confirm for the family that the person really needs more care than they can provide (37,43). These things all make it easier for reluctant caregivers to accept nursing home placement.

Multi-Service Programs

Programs are being developed that offer a wide range of services to the family and the person with dementia. These multi-service programs have the advantage of coordinating care and facilitating referral from one program to another, and allowing staff members to get to know individual clients and families. In addition, the staff at such programs has access to a broad database for research.

California recently authorized a 4-year demonstration project for three Alzheimer's disease institutes that would provide a continuum of traditional and innovative services including diagnosis and assessment, day care, home care, hospice care, and skilled nursing care (Assembly Bill 999).

Other Settings

Other forms of care being considered or tried include vacation programs that serve both the ill person and the caregiver (1), sitter programs in a group site (75), client recreation and therapy while families are being provided group therapy (57), medical teams that do an in-home evaluation, and family-run cooperatives (1,75). Publications on these various programs are slowly becoming available (15,21,38,77,79,101).

Although the family is clearly the most common provider of care, little attention has been given to training family members—the primary caregiver and members of the extended family—in the

Box 7-I.—Family Survival Project

The Family Survival Project is a freestanding program in San Francisco that provides information, advice and referral; case coordination; legal counseling; and in-home supportive services to brain-damaged adults. The program attributes its success to its decision to include adults with any form of brain damage: dementia, trauma, vascular accidents, etc. It also sought to form a partnership with the public sector and to identify the family, as well as the patient, as the target population. It did not include income criteria in its model programs and has avoided becoming yet another categorically based service.

The program has been remarkably successful in serving caregivers in a previously unserved segment and in generating government support for its programs, which have been called a "good buy" (74). The Family Survival Project has contracted with the Institute for Health and Aging at the University of California, San Francisco to conduct a study concerning the costs of formal and informal care provided to brain-impaired adults (74).

Box 7-J.—Comprehensive Services on Aging Institute

The COPSA (Comprehensive Services on Aging) Institute for Alzheimer's Disease and Related Disorders in New Jersey is a statewide program funded by the State for persons with dementia, their families, and the professionals who care for them.

A resource center provides information and referral to families and professionals, ongoing phone consultations, family education and counseling, and liaison with family support groups and professionals. A diagnostic clinic provides diagnostic workups for the memory-impaired and confused, second opinions, and coordination of followup recommendations. A day hospital provides rehabilitation and treatment for persons with dementia, education and support for families, and it is also a training site for health professionals. The consultation and education program provides training and seminars for professionals and technical assistance for the development of dementia programs (22).

techniques of care. Some ADRDA chapters have launched programs that train family members or lay persons in the community to care for persons with dementia. Caregivers might learn to care with less stress to themselves. Other members of the extended family may not provide support or give respite to the caregiver because they feel helpless and do not know what to do. In such situations, a family member can learn to be a respite care provider.

Family training is often done informally by professionals who observe the need. A nurse visiting in the home to treat a person with dementia offers extensive bedside training for the caregiver, for example. Although such services are not covered by Medicare or other sources, they may be of significant value in keeping the individual with dementia in good health and in sustaining the caregiver.

Hospice

Programs and services similar to hospice, which assist individuals and families at the end of the person's life, may be needed. OTA found no such programs except for the excellent care of families and patients provided by major research institutions. The needs of a dying person with dementia and his or her family have needs that differ in some ways from those of other dying individuals. The person may be terminally ill for many months or years, and approaching death can be difficult to predict. Unlike patients dying with cancer, for example, people with dementia are often unable to communicate with family or express their wishes. They may be mute and immobile. Because of the long, slow, deteriorating progress of the illness, the family may have been grieving for a long time, and some families have already begun to emotionally separate from their relative.

A major concern of many families is providing appropriate, but not aggressive, medical care for a person with dementia who is nearing the end of life. Nursing homes may have unwritten policies that are not discussed with families. These policies may include transferring a dying patient to an acute hospital against family wishes, or "not calling the ambulance until morning"—in effect, letting the person die (see ch. 5) (9). Facilities with such unwritten policies do not take into consideration the wishes of the family.

RESIDENTIAL SPECIAL CARE

At some point in a dementing illness, many individuals and families need long-term residential (institutional) care. Such care is most often provided by intermediate and skilled nursing homes. In what ways should these offer persons with dementia special services or specialized care? and in what ways is their care the same as that for other persons with chronic illnesses? Although these facilities have always cared for persons with dementia, some are now developing special units or offering special services.

Foster Homes, Domiciliary Care, and Boarding Homes

Few residential facilities other than nursing homes specialize in the care of persons with dementia (see boxes 7-K and 7-L for descriptions of

> **Box 7-L.—Valenti Alzheimer's Care Center**
>
> The Valenti Alzheimer's Care Centers in southeastern Pennsylvania operate under that State's personal care license. Their advertisement accurately describes the program:
>
> **Care**—In comfortable, home-life settings, we provide round-the-clock care in areas where residents can no longer cope, lots of encouragement, and a positive outlook.
>
> **Therapy**—A specially oriented staff administers a varied program of daily exercises, music therapy, and participation in simple projects and familiar chores to help clients retain confidence and self-worth (94).

> **Box 7-K.—Suncoast Institute for Applied Gerontology**
>
> The Suncoast Institute for Applied Gerontology in Costa Mesa, CA has combined adult day care and boarding home care. It reports that the use of a boarding home exclusively to care for persons with Alzheimer's disease has increased its capacity to tolerate deviant behavior. The program uses a registered nurse who consults at both the day care center and the boarding homes. She helps the staff manage client medications, incontinence, impactions, sleep disorders, nutrition needs, and behavior problems. She also acts as an intermediary between the facility and the client's physicians.
>
> The philosophy of this program includes supporting clients' dignity, sense of control, and opportunity for choices. Clients have frequent outings, which are cited as important in reducing their agitation. Most of the clients in this program are ambulatory and partially continent. Many have had severe behavior problems. Average monthly costs per client are $2,021 and $1,330. Residents in the higher cost unit are more infirm and need a nurse, and the facility also carries a mortgage. The reported monthly costs are lower than the $2,200 average nursing home cost in the area (84).

two such programs). Those that do cite limited regulation as one reason they are able to devise creative programs at costs competitive with nursing homes, although as discussed below, that absence of regulation can be exploited by less scrupulous programs.

The Johns Hopkins Hospital in Baltimore operates an adult foster care program that accepts some persons with dementia (69). In Michigan, two foster care homes accept persons with dementia. Illinois reports that a small group home there accepts persons with dementia for short stays (1).

Facilities such as these can offer clients individual attention, a day filled with activities, a sense of safety and security, and a life much closer to normal than that in a larger facility. Although residents in both the Suncoast Institute and the Valenti centers are visibly impaired, the behavioral problems commonly seen in boarding houses and nursing homes—apathy, drowsiness, pacing, screaming, aggression, absence of initiative, and lack of humor—are not evident (although both report that these occasionally occur).

These programs report that quality boarding home care for persons in the middle stages of their illness is possible. However, such homes are extremely rare. The norm, unfortunately, is substandard facilities that offer no special services and only minimal services that are not appropriate for clients with dementia. Boarding homes rarely employ a nurse (although the two profiled programs do), nor do they provide activities or adequate supervision.

Special facilities can provide a level of supervision and care that is higher than that of most other boarding homes. Although they can provide excellent care for a portion of a person's illness, however, they are neither safe nor appropriate for very ill individuals.

California recently passed legislation addressing quality assurance in board and care (Senate Bill 185). It calls for the development of three levels of care: basic care and supervision, nonmedical personal care, and health-related assistance. The legislation provides for standards and supervision designed to ensure the facility's ability to serve clients at each level of care they intend to offer.

As noted, the same absence of regulation that allows creative programming by dedicated staff can also allow unscrupulous operators to take advantage of individuals with dementia. Although family members are urging the expansion of boarding facilities, many State regulations governing these facilities are lax or absent. If such care is not to be funded by the State, or costs less than nursing home care, some States may overlook the potential for abuse.

Even dedicated providers can make mistakes. One operator is known to have established a "step down" unit for more severely impaired individuals. These residents appeared to be receiving excellent care, and their families were reportedly satisfied. Although the facility had smoke alarms and exterior fire escapes, however, the residents could not assist in their own evacuation in the event of fire and therefore were in an unsafe situation.

Another problem with boarding homes is cost: The profiled facilities are competing successfully with private pay nursing home care and offering excellent programming and professional care, yet no evidence indicates that this kind of care can be provided at rates for boarding homes paid for by Supplemental Security Income (SSI) or the Veterans Administration (VA).

Finally, good quality boarding care is so rare that many families may not be aware of it. Five percent of the respondents in the OTA study had used boarding home care and only 25 percent identified it as "most important." Both the California facility and the one in Pennsylvania were at or near capacity, suggesting that there may be an unmet demand.

Special Units in Nursing Homes

A rapidly growing and controversial program is the development in nursing homes of long-term care units that specialize in the care of persons with dementia. Both the for-profit and the non-profit sectors are hiring experts, establishing planning committees, holding conferences (66), and opening "special" units. Some are drafting "national" guidelines or local standards (14). Some have developed policy and procedures documents (50). Others have not segregated the residents, but offer them special programs in regular units (86).

Special nursing home units are being developed largely in response to the belief that they foster better care and, conversely, that nursing home residents who do not have a dementing illness prefer separate living space. But these reasons do not fully account for the rapid development of special units. Some people in the nursing home industry see separate units as good marketing strategy, and some argue that individuals with dementia are easier to care for in a special setting where they are all together.

There are many persons with dementia in nursing homes (92), but traditional forms of care have failed to successfully treat behavioral problems. One survey of 42 skilled nursing facilities (1,139 patients) found that 64 percent of residents had significant behavioral problems (102). Some specialized programs report successful reduction of these behaviors (16,18).

Major differences have been noted in the amount and type of changes facilities have made for residents with dementia. Some units appear no different from the other units of a facility; others have significant changes in structure or decor, in staffing and staff training, in the amount and type of services offered, in admission procedures, and in the appearance of residents. Most notable is the variation in what experts perceive these individuals need. For example, some propose that the units be painted in bright primary colors, but others suggest all white, and still others propose pastels. Arguments are buttressed with theories of cognition. Less trivial differences of opinion involve philosophy, staff-to-patient ratios, floor plans, and the number of persons on a unit. Decisions about these factors can represent significant investments for the facilities. Rigorous comparative study is needed to resolve such controversies.

Availability and Costs

The number of special nursing home units open or planned is unknown; OTA found 110 facilities. Specialists in the field report that they frequently hear of new units being developed (5,37,70). Based on this information, and on the opinions of those in the industry, it can be estimated that fewer than 500 special units are developed or close to completion, although more are being planned.

A major for-profit chain, Hillhaven Corp., has a full-time employee to set up special units. The corporation has opened 49 units, and one facility is devoted entirely to persons with dementia. Nonprofit organizations are also involved in developing special programs. The Hebrew Home for the Aged at Riverdale (Riverdale, NY) surveyed 38 homes that provide special services or have a special unit (95). AAHA is developing resources for facilities that are opening special units.

Despite the growing movement to create such units, they serve only a small portion of the large number of persons with dementia who live in nursing homes; an estimated 60 to 74 percent of nursing home residents in traditional mixed units have dementia (8,83). Even when a facility has a special unit for some residents, a majority of other residents in the facility also have dementia. Some home health agencies and nursing homes offering special care accept only those who can pay for care privately, excluding those whose care is covered by Medicaid. These programs report that they cannot provide quality care for persons with dementia at Medicaid's low payment rates.

Little information is available on the costs of special care. Because changes in cost are partially tied to changes in the physical plant, extent of programming, and staffing, they can vary according to the facility's perception of what constitutes a special unit. Care approaches vary so widely that costs for individual programs cannot be assumed to be representative, but most units report costs of $5 to $10 per day higher than for standard care, although some excellent programs report no difference, and in fact, cost significantly less than other special units. Some programs, both for-profit and not-for-profit, have cost information that is not publicly available.

In a report on the special residential unit, Wesley Hall in Michigan, an OTA contractor wrote:

> . . . residents have consistently scored on the Mental Status Questionnaire by Kehn, et al. (1960), in the range of 0-2, placing them in the category of the severely impaired.

> At the time of the completion of the project [12/85], daily costs to residents of the old age home unit were $29.70; Wesley Hall residents paid $42.65 a day; and the nursing home section cost $60.00 per day (18).

The consensus is that good care in special units requires more staffing and better-trained staff, and probably more square feet per patient than required by Medicare, Medicaid, or State standards. Some clinicians argue that residents of special units exhibit fewer disturbed behaviors and therefore will use less nursing time than in mixed facilities, and that changes in staffing patterns and task assignment will increase efficiency (26). But it is unlikely that good care can be provided to these difficult individuals with staff-to-resident ratios lower than current minimums. Good studies of cost are urgently needed, but must await a determination of what components are necessary or ideal in a special unit.

Architectural Design

The architectural design of special units is controversial. The most common nursing home design is a long corridor with double rooms opening onto it. There is often a small room for visitors. Meals are eaten in a large communal dining hall and activities are conducted in a separate area. Each unit has a nurses' station similar to those in hospitals. This design is thought to be detrimental to the functioning of persons with dementia. It discourages social functioning, it is disorienting and noisy, and the communal dining room overstresses people with dementia (17,18).

A "racetrack" design has been proposed for persons with dementia (65). The building's corridor is circular, encouraging the resident with dementia to wander in safety. But the design probably discourages social functioning and orientation. The Philadelphia Geriatric Center has a large central room with residents' rooms opening onto it (55). That arrangement encouraged social interaction and simplified supervision.

Some of the programs observed by OTA were small—from 8 to 15 residents (6,18). Residents had small single rooms. There were one or two small sitting rooms that also served as dining areas and activity spaces. It is easier for residents to orient themselves and to interact with others on small units. Small dining rooms are quieter and less confusing. This type of setting helps people relax so that they can regain old skills or make friends. The industry reports that this design is expensive, although it is not yet clear that variations, such as groups of clusters, would be significantly costlier than traditional units.

Many facilities emphasize the importance of access to a secure outside area where residents may walk, keep a pet, grow flowers, or enjoy the sun. Outside exercise is thought to contribute to the restoration of normal sleep cycles.

Most nursing homes planning a special dementia unit are restricted by the design of the existing building. Some convert a resident room into a sitting room or locate the unit at the end of a corridor where it can be cut off from traffic through the facility. The resulting loss of bed space increases costs.

Interior Decor

Successful programs have encouraged residents and families to furnish rooms extensively with the resident's own possessions. That appears to help them to accept that they live there. Administra-

tors in some facilities argue that personal possessions will be stolen, although small special units report that this has not been a problem. The smaller units and higher staff ratio probably prevent that problem.

Controlling resident egress is a significant concern for institutions caring for wandering individuals. Locked doors may be forbidden by fire codes. While some facilities use buzzers that sound when doors are opened, others report that this system caused staff to check doors constantly. Several electronic sensing devices are now available. Facilities can be secured without locks, however, and successful units have disguised exits or located them so that residents must pass several staff persons before reaching the outside.

There are several schools of thought on decor. (Although many facilities, however, decorate according to their expectation of the family's taste, not the resident's needs.) Low stimulus decorating means reducing visual stimuli—color, decorations, clutter—as much as possible. A pastel decor is a variation of that school of thought. In contrast, Wesley Hall at the University of Michigan uses bright, high-contrast colors (yellow, red, and kelly green with white) to provide visual stimulus and to help those residents who have visual problems (18). The aging eye is better able to see these colors and the contrasts help residents distinguish the boundaries between toilet and floor, or between floor and wall. The lighting level in the unit was increased and glare was reduced, again to assist the aging eye. Wesley Hall has a small kitchen where residents prepare snacks and clean up after meals. The staff uses a desk in the kitchen. There is no nurses' station. These unusual components help to restore normal roles to the residents—for example, getting oneself a glass of milk or helping to dry dishes. The absence of a nurses' station helps to make the relationship of staff to residents more therapeutic.

Furnishings in the most successful units visited by OTA were more "home-like" than in most nursing homes or hospitals. Many of the special units have no paging system, and extraneous, distracting noises such as those of the main kitchen, hallway traffic, or meal carts are reduced or eliminated. Pianos and record players are used often (18).

There is a substantial amount of literature on the characteristics of architecture and environment that benefit the aging person (18,46,47,48, 49,55,88,89). Environmental changes must consider the visual, hearing, and gait impairments of this age group and analyze each aspect of the environment for its tendency to confuse or disorient (101). For the doubly impaired elderly person with a dementia, these factors are even more important but are frequently ignored.

Step Down Units

Special dementia units in nursing homes usually serve residents in the middle stages of their illnesses. As the cognitive abilities of these individuals gradually deteriorates, however, they eventually need a level of care different from that originally established by the unit. Some nursing homes transfer these residents to regular skilled nursing units; others have established "step down units" where these more impaired persons can still be given special sensory stimulation, passive exercise, nutrition support, and be kept as alert and physically active as possible.

Characteristics of Special Programs

Many of the characteristics of special programs in nursing homes and board and care homes are similar to those in day care and respite care.

Characteristics of Residents

The special programs reviewed by OTA were fairly consistent specifying the type of client they serve: those who were ambulatory, exhibited problem behaviors, and, in some cases, were incontinent. In general, these are people in the middle stages of a dementing illness. These individuals are capable of participating in activities and in helping to care for themselves. Some programs report that it is preferable to group residents homogeneously by severity of mental impairment. Others point out that a workable resident mix, staffing, and programming vary with the stage of the illness. Thus existing programs vary in their practices, and most focus on subgroups of these with dementia.

Benefits to Residents

The crucial issue of special services—for family members as well as the government—is whether they are significantly better for people with dementia than other forms of care. Until recently it was assumed that little could be done for persons with dementia beyond providing for their physical needs. The recent interest in dementing disorders has focused clinicians' attention on the quality of life of these persons. Some now assert that people with dementia are capable of considerable improvement in behavior, social function, and life satisfaction or happiness (6,13,16,18,60).

A few programs claim that their clients improve in some respects when given special care. This idea is by no means universally accepted, however, and few practitioners are willing to accept the extent of change claimed by some of these programs. It is agreed that a person's underlying dementia cannot now be reversed, and that individuals with dementia will move toward more severe illness and eventual death. Some programs report an initial improvement in participants, followed by a gradual, but less precipitous decline.

Among the changes reported are:

1. decrease in wandering (18,86);
2. decrease in episodes of agitation (18,39);
3. no screaming or a decrease in screaming (42);
4. few or no drugs needed to control behavior (18,39,90);
5. improved orientation (18,90);
6. decrease in socially unacceptable behaviors (masturbation, rummaging in other patients' rooms, etc.) (18,90);
7. weight gains or improved eating (18,39,90);
8. decrease in depression (18);
9. greater ability to sleep through the night (18,39);
10. a sense of humor (18);
11. a happy, relaxed appearance (18,39);
12. the formation of friendships (18,39,61);
13. reduction or elimination of incontinence (18,96);
14. the initiation of interpersonal exchanges (18); and
15. decrease in hallucinations (39).

It is noteworthy that these changes reflect either decreases in extreme disturbed behavior or increases in socially appropriate behavior. No program reports that residents consistently improved in language skills, motor skills, or memory—problems that are likely evidence of the disease itself, rather than responses to the environment.

The surprising finding that some participants can improve in certain kinds of function may have several explanations. In most experiments, the focus on the intervention and increased staff enthusiasm lead to some improvement. Second, people who are severely impaired may be even more responsive to slight improvements in the environment (55). Third, this finding may also reflect the extent to which inappropriate forms of care add to resident impairment.

All three factors probably contribute to the changes seen. Most clinicians agree that some of the changes listed (often the first seven) can be achieved in some individuals by maintaining them in good health—that is, by eliminating excess disability (see ch. 2). Almost all the residential programs reviewed by OTA that made some environmental changes when they created special units report improvements in their residents. Many day care centers report the same changes in some clients (61), and observation and unpublished reports from other nursing homes suggest similar results. OTA found no appropriately designed and controlled study of participant change. Anecdotal reports of partial improvement are encouraging, however, and fail to support the common position of therapeutic nihilism. OTA found no study seeking to improve psychosocial function in individuals with dementia living at home (and not in day care).

The remaining eight changes were reported by fewer programs, which have served a total of only about 200 individuals. It is not known whether these results can be replicated and, if so, which patients are most likely to respond, and over how much time. The techniques for this special care are only now being developed and have not been tested. Yet the initial reports are encouraging.

It is also important to note, as mentioned, that behavioral gains made by individuals receiving special care will not carry over if the special care is stopped. In some States, when individuals improve in functioning levels, they are reclassified from skilled to intermediate care and can no longer stay in the special units; they therefore will not maintain any gains. Day care clients in programs that have a rehabilitative mandate may be discharged when clients improve, setting up a "revolving door" pattern, with improvement under special care followed by discharge and worsening symptoms and subsequent readmission.

Overall Approach to Care

Since special programs and reported change vary considerably, it is premature to describe the characteristics of special programs in a final form, or to establish standards or criteria for these programs. Indeed, guidelines or standards could freeze into place approaches that may later prove less than optimal, or could block experimentation with other interventions. Further clinical experience and the replication of the most successful programs are needed.

But that does not mean that nothing can be done. A considerable body of knowledge exists on the nature of dementia (53) that can be applied to techniques of care. And a good deal is known about similar patients—geriatric patients in State hospitals (20,35,36,51) and nursing home residents in general (many of whom are demented). Finally, the overall approach to patient care is widely agreed upon (4,10,11,41,62,98). These findings permit some general observations on the approach of special units. The most successful programs (in residential and day care) resemble each other in key factors and strive toward common goals:

- to prevent excess disability due to other health problems or medication;
- to use as few psychoactive medications as possible, and use few if any, physical restraints;
- to maximize an individual's ability to hear and see;
- to enhance remaining function rather than to restore function lost through the disease process;
- to reduce long hours of idleness;
- to use activities and a caregiving style that enhance resident comprehension of appropriate roles as friend, parent, or volunteer,

and that reinforce a sense of personhood and dignity;

- to create a "homey" environment in which residents are dressed and well groomed;
- to use a mixture of flexibility, creativity, and both structured and nonstructured approaches of activities;
- to emphasize the importance of respect for residents and to individualize approaches;
- to recognize the importance of environmental accommodation and the significance of a benign, nonstressful, supportive environment; and
- to support the family in a continuing relationship with the resident.

One observer of special unit residents reports:

. . . spontaneous interaction between and among residents, staff, and visitors . . . joy or the manifestations of joy—smiling, laughter (13).

The director of Wesley Hall reports residents who appear happy, exhibit spontaneous laughter, and initiate communication with staff and other residents. This unit also has successfully experimented with clowning and focused on the role of humor (17).

Staff

The way a facility's staff relates to resident's clearly affects behavior (38). For much of their illness, persons with Alzheimer's disease seem to retain the capacity to read nonverbal communication correctly (26). That has important clinical implications: Staff members who are hurried or irritable, or who belittle a person, may trigger behavioral outbursts. Programs in which staff members "talk down" to participants tend to produce patients who either become stubborn or behaviorally regressed. Staff approaches should be cheerful and calm, allowing patients to make what decisions they are able to.

Changing staff behavior toward residents raises several problems often reported in connection with nursing homes: the need for a motivated, concerned administration; for adequate staff salaries commensurate with the tasks required; and for a stable, adequately trained staff (see ch. 9) (26). The existing special units have attracted professionals and nurse's aides who wanted a psychological and emotional challenge, who want to be able to give to others (80), and who enjoy the rewards of community interest and the administration's enthusiasm.

Initial training and strong, ongoing support appear to be necessary for staff to work successfully on these units. Several training packages are being prepared or planned (13,17,26,38,45,79,101). The philosophy, techniques, and objectives of these training materials differ, but most emphasize the need for all staff members to be trained—administrators, nurse's aides, therapists, and even housekeeping, dietary, and janitorial personnel. (Housekeeping staff, for example, spend significant amounts of time with residents and therefore affect behavior (44)). A team approach with communication among staff members and across shifts is emphasized (26).

Some programs report that staff members can work on a dementia unit regularly, rather than rotate on and off, if given adequate support. Contrary to the prediction that the staff on all dementia units would "burn out," some programs have found lower turnover among the staff of special units. Other programs, however, report problems with staff burnout. Consistent staffing seems to be reassuring to the residents. Staff members develop expertise, and they learn the habits of individuals (26).

Persons with dementia usually have a mixture of social and medical needs. The emphasis on social v. medical needs is influenced by the severity of the resident's medical problems. Successful programs have staff members with differing expertise who work together as a team. The delivery of a person's care is provided by nonprofessional nurse's aides just as in traditional nursing homes. With training and ongoing support, aides have provided excellent care in special units. One recent book gives instructions and guidance for this group of caregivers (38), and a second addresses nursing staff (26).

The optimal ratio of staff to residents has not been established. Needed levels probably will vary with severity of participant impairment. Wesley Hall reports a day shift staff-to-resident ratio of 1 to 4.4 (18). Green Hills Center reports a day shift ratio of 1 to 5.8 (90). The ratio in programs examined by OTA varied considerably, but most reported a ratio of no more than 1 to 10, better than the minimum ratio required for licensure in most States. In addition, some programs augment the effective ratio by using trained volunteers to accompany wanderers, or to give one-to-one attention to some individuals during exercises, meals, or activities.

The cognitive difficulties of persons with dementia become a factor when staff members are suspected of robbing or abusing someone. An employee cannot be fired on the basis of a charge by a person who is not mentally competent. Yet retaining such a person may jeopardize residents who cannot complain. At the same time, persons with dementia can erroneously charge that they have been robbed or abused (see ch. 2). In special facilities where all the potential witnesses are cognitively impaired, steps will be needed to ensure the quality of employees and to protect both employees and residents.

Activities

Some believe there is a relationship between the number of hours of completely unstructured idle time and some behavioral problems such as wandering and perservation (59). Because persons with dementia are unable to initiate and plan independently, most new programs reduce the number of hours that the client is idle. Programs are developing varied philosophies about activities, but all agree that activities are a key part of success. Activities cannot be limited to games offered by a nonprofessional for a few hours a week if they are to benefit individuals with a dementing disorder. Some programs fill a good part of the day with structured tasks. There is also evidence, though, that structured programming should allow flexibility and spontaneity (18,101).

People with dementia live from moment to moment—a truly existential life. Therefore, programming for them should be designed to be enjoyable at the moment, possibly leaving some good feeling retained, rather than being designed to produce a worthwhile product or provide later satisfaction (26). Some programs use projects that allow their clients to work as volunteers or for

pay: stuffing envelopes, assembling garnishes for the main kitchen, etc. One program reports that trips and outings reduce agitation (84).

Activities must be meaningful to the client, must be voluntary, and must offer the client a reasonable chance for success (58). They must address the client's personal and psychosocial needs, and their purpose must be obvious to the person with dementia (101). In Wesley Hall, activities that enable residents to assume old roles—such as homemaker, friend, or volunteer—are emphasized. Exercise, music, personal grooming, housekeeping, preparation of snacks, repetitive, rhythmic activities, visits from children or pets, and simple volunteer tasks have been recommended (18,61,101).

Reality orientation is offered in most programs for persons with dementia, although its usefulness is debated. The term has been applied to several different techniques, some of which are more beneficial than others (26). In general, it is agreed that persons with irreversible dementia will not relearn information but do benefit from a program that gives frequent multiple cues for orientation.

Meals

Persons with dementing illnesses may fail to eat or may eat only one kind of food. They need good nutritional planning, food that enhances sensory information, and a supportive environment. Several programs report that midmorning, midafternoon, and bedtime snacks are helpful.

Behavior Management

Techniques for managing the inappropriate behaviors of special unit residents are as varied as the models of the physical plant (12,18,26,31,40, 42). What is most striking is that many units have successfully reduced problem behaviors, but even the most successful programs report that these behaviors still occur occasionally. At Wesley Hall, in addition to planned activities and changes in the physical environment, several staff techniques are used: first, to divert the individual; when unsuccessful, to withdraw and try later; to use touch and a sympathetic approach; to reinterpret the behavior as normal (e.g., if a staff member acts in an authoritarian way, it is normal for the client to resist); and to use humor and a lighthearted approach (18).

Others point out that "responses to problematic behaviors cannot be set out in a formula basis. Flexibility and variety are essential qualities which staff must maintain in caring for the [dementia] patient" (13). Problem behaviors are greatly reduced when the environment orients participants and when meaningful activities fill their time. The quality of the interpersonal relationships between staff and participants may be at least as important as techniques of behavior management.

Management of Incontinence

Incontinence is often assumed to be a symptom of dementia. It has been reported as 3.5 times more common in persons with dementia than in persons without dementia; the causes of this dysfunction have not been reported and are rarely evaluated. The problem can lead to further withdrawal and isolation, skin breakdown, and infections (96). Traditional nursing home care has focused on containment, not reversal of the problem.

Many things other than a person's dementia can prevent that person from being continent: medications, too little fluid, diuretics such as coffee in the diet, inability to get to a toilet in time, chair design (causing problems getting up out of it), lack of a well-lighted and visible path to the toilet, loss of eyeglasses, inaccessibility of a walker or cane, insufficient visual contrast to distinguish the toilet, fecal impaction, and urinary tract infections. In addition, cognitively impaired elderly individuals have the same causes of urinary problems as other elderly persons, and may also respond to social cues of appropriate behavior (96). People who still have problems are successfully managed in many day care programs by being taken

to the toilet every 2 hours or on individualized toilet schedules. Many of the unacceptable behaviors that accompany incontinence result from the person's confusion or from inappropriate care that can be easily avoided.

Four of the eleven residents in Wesley Hall had been incontinent before admission, but after several months in the unit this was no longer a problem (18). A best-guess clinical estimate is that at least 50 percent of cognitively impaired elderly individuals with loss of urine control could regain control (96).

Application of Technologies to Care

Little has been done to identify ways in which technologies developed for other uses could be applied to the care of persons with dementia. The application of technologies to care does not necessarily imply that there will be less compassionate or less humane care to these individuals. It may free caregivers from routine tasks and allow them to provide more supportive activities or social experiences. Research Triangle Institute, for example, assessed the feasibility of a wandering notification system, sponsored by the Administration on Aging, National Aeronautics and Space Administration, National Institute on Aging, the National Institute for Handicapped Research, and the Veterans Administration (82). Families would also benefit from more efficient methods for managing human wastes in persons who are incontinent. Devices to prevent a person with dementia from turning on a stove, technologies that would enable a caregiver to locate the person who had wandered away, more efficient equipment to enable a frail caregiver to lift, turn, or bathe a person, and safer bathroom facilities—all would be greatly beneficial to both ill persons and their caregivers (93).

THE EFFECT OF REGULATIONS ON THE DEVELOPMENT OF SPECIAL CARE

Nursing homes are subject to numerous State and Federal quality assurance standards that they say impede quality care of persons with demen-

tia. Other service delivery settings (day care, in-home respite) are subject to so few quality assurance standards that experts express concern over the lack of protection for persons in these settings who cannot protect themselves. The problems of quality assurance are discussed in chapter 10. This section briefly reviews some of the ways standards may directly interfere with patient care on special units.

Some problems arise from local interpretation of regulations and lack of understanding about the needs of persons with dementia. For example, for sanitary reasons, some facilities are required to use plastic dishes and utensils. Yet people with dementia can be confused because these do not have the familiar color and weight of crockery and silverware. Individuals who are easily distracted do better with one item of food on their plate at a time, but one facility reported that the inspector did not allow this. Food too hot to eat should not be served to confused persons, but one facility reported that serving cooler food violated health standards. Freshly waxed floors create glare, but are required by some inspectors as an indication of a clean facility. Reports of such episodes are scattered and seem to represent a lack of information on the part of State inspection agencies or the need for revision of regulations.

A more general problem is the emphasis of standards on physical evidence of quality—shining floors and sparkling bathrooms, beds perfectly made, and everything put away. Staff members are discouraged from letting residents make their own beds, even if sloppily, or talking with residents instead of tidying up. The pervasive tone of regulations, more than specific incidents, shapes patient care. The focus on the physical plant, combined with financial pressure for efficiency, has resulted in an atmosphere that more resembles a hospital than a home. Long corridors, lack of personal items, glare from waxed floors, and a paging system are disorienting to persons with dementia, who respond to a more homelike environment (18,46,47,49).

Quality assurance regulation depends heavily on paper documentation. Nursing homes report that nurses cannot spend time getting to know their patients or training aides to care for persons with dementia because their time is filled with the required paperwork (97).

The emphasis of regulations on the physical plant and on recordkeeping, in combination with low reimbursement rates for patient care, has resulted in efforts to increase efficiency. For example, an assembly line approach to resident care may be taken: one aide gets the person up, another toilets the person, a third gives out suppositories, and a fourth feeds the residents as a group. This is dehumanizing to all residents and stressful to those who are cognitively impaired (26). There are many examples of such problems. However, facilities have demonstrated that they can improve care within the framework of existing standards. Some have done so without increasing costs. Staffing patterns can be improved without a loss of efficiency (26) and physical plants can be improved (18,70).

Fire and safety regulations in domiciliary homes and respite settings present more difficult problems. Persons with dementia may not respond to a fire alarm; they move slowly, and when they become frightened they are likely to become stubborn and uncooperative. They may not be able to negotiate stairs and cannot follow instructions. They may wander off as soon as they are evacuated or may try to reenter a building. Fire safety standards in some areas do not address these special problems. For example, some day care centers have been approved by fire marshals under a code that was established to set requirements for a public meeting hall or office; such standards do not consider the special needs of those who use day care centers.

Fire safety regulations can also present obstacles. One design for a specialized unit proposes a large communal room surrounded by residents' rooms (55), but is not acceptable to fire safety experts in some cities. Locked exits, which protect residents from wandering and therefore reduce staff stress, are often not allowed because of safety hazards in case of fire. Some devices that confine an agitated person to his or her room in order for the person to relax (screen doors, half doors, or a bar across the door) are approved by fire marshals in some communities but not in others. Fire safety guidelines that take into consideration the care needs and special limitations of persons with dementia are urgently needed.

Persons with dementing illnesses can be so frail that any intervention may place them at greater risk of injury. For example, if a facility permits a frail person to continue walking, that person is at risk of falling and breaking a hip—a serious injury. If restrained from walking, the individual may lose the ability to walk or may develop pressure sores. When number of falls is used as a criterion of quality, facilities will restrict frail persons from walking. Research is needed to identify ways in which care can be provided while allowing marginal freedom. The risks of various interventions are not well known. A better understanding of which risk is greater—e.g., walking or restraint—would help programs and families make wiser choices.

Standards for domiciliary care and respite care programs (day care, short stay respite, in-home care) are limited or nonexistent in some States. Even where standards exist they are often poorly enforced or are not designed to protect persons with intellectual impairments. Persons with dementing illnesses are unable to act in their own behalf in unsafe situations. These individuals may not be able to report abuse to their families. Yet severely impaired individuals reside in domiciliary care facilities with minimal standards or in facilities that are consistently out of compliance; OTA found no information on the number of domiciliary care, day care, or in-home respite programs with inadequate safeguards. Recent attention to the problems of dementia and the eagerness of some families to locate special care may attract unscrupulous or incompetent providers to the business.

ISSUES AND OPTIONS

This discussion of services for persons with dementia has identified a number of concerns:

- the fragmented service system;
- inadequate funding of services;
- inadequate staff and poor staff training;
- lack of programs that assist family caregivers; and
- service designs that emphasize acute medical care and cost efficiency at the expense of humane care, quality of life, and patient dignity.

The need for changes that respond to these concerns affect not only persons with dementia but all recipients of long-term care. Given the scope of this assessment, the options discussed here are limited to service that address the needs of persons with dementia.

Would services for persons with dementia replace existing, more costly services? Would establishment of services such as respite reduce the need for nursing home care? These issues are raised repeatedly throughout this report. Although it is tempting for model programs to see themselves as more economical than other programs, it is unlikely that the provision of respite services and specialized dementia care will reduce costs. These programs are often not direct substitutes for nursing home care and therefore will almost certainly result in greater overall expenditures.

Concern over costs means that planners and taxpayers must ultimately make value judgments about the care of the individuals with dementia. Quality of life for the cognitively impaired person must be balanced against cost, individual safety must be balanced against personal autonomy, the maintenance of those who are chronically ill must be balanced against expenditures to seek a cure, and support of family caregivers must be balanced against the more traditional patient-only treatment.

ISSUE 1: Should the Federal Government support the development of special care for persons with dementia?

Option 1: Implement programs of care for persons with dementia.

Option 2: Offer incentives to develop specialized care.

Option 3: Support health services research into special respite and residential programs for persons with dementia.

Policymakers face a dilemma: Identifying the best kind of care for persons with dementing disorders awaits a better understanding of how much can be done for them. Standards and the establishment of appropriate funding levels must await more information about the kind of care that can be achieved.

The specific changes needed in facilities that serve persons with dementia seem to be controversial. But a body of knowledge already exists about compensating for sensory deficits late in life. Experience was gained in treatment of persons with dementia in some State mental hospitals. Milieu therapy (modifying the social and physical environment to support function) has been generally endorsed as the preferred approach to such individuals. There is also a body of literature on family needs. Finally, there is some generally accepted literature on the style of care and approach to persons with dementia. Thus the general principles that special units need to follow are known. The finding that residents improve somewhat in most special settings is encouraging because it indicates that some benefit can be achieved in the absence of precise knowledge about optimal care.

There is an obvious need for formal care for a large segment of those with dementia, either on a short-term, respite basis or—for some—on a residential basis. Caregivers and voluntary associations are pressing for such care, and it may be that providing it will have significant benefits in caregiver health and employment status.

However, a large Federal investment in special care at this point (option 1) might result in the development of inappropriate services or the replication of existing models that do not serve persons with dementia well. Improving some "special services" on top of existing inappropriate models of care may cost more than developing new care models that better suit the needs of people with dementia.

Use of incentives (option 2) would expedite the development of much-needed services. It would also rely on market forces to determine the nature of quality care. Although this appears to be an excellent option, the generally pervasive belief that little or nothing can be done for persons with dementia may lead to a situation in which consumers, professionals, and providers have lower than appropriate expectations for care.

Health service research would test underlying principles and the various hypotheses proposed by individual project. It would identify the amount of change possible in people with dementia, the people who are likely to benefit, the points at which they should enter and leave programs, and the impact of specific services on family caregivers. Table 7-4 identifies major questions which such research would answer.

Federal support of research (option 3) helps ensure the quality of research. The Federal Government can provide a focal point or a coordinating task force for health service delivery research that would ensure the coordination of research. A national scope would expedite coordination of State and private sector endeavors as well (also see issue 2, option 3 below).

Federal support of a group of care models with a strong health service research component, although it would leave many people unserved, would be seen by caregivers as a major step forward and would give better information regarding the design and cost of services. In addition, the costs of an experimental program are controlled and predictable. The private sector is moving forward with programs for persons with dementia, holding promise of possible collaboration with the government.

Health service delivery research often establishes model programs that are set up, run, and studied with specific objectives in mind. Such programs would be welcomed by caregivers who are eager to encourage the development of better care. Yet demonstration projects tend to drop their clients after their funding ends. That would be particularly difficult for the frail, confused, elderly person who may take weeks or months to adjust to a new setting. In some areas there may be no other respite programs for families after the model program is completed, thus placing serious stresses on caregivers or precipitate nursing home placement. If such model programs are funded, plans for client care after their completion could be required, or programs could be planned with gradual funding phase-out.

Table 7-4.—Issues in Health Service Research

Patient outcomes:
Which of the patient benefits that have been reported actually occur?
How can these be measured?
Which patients benefit?
How can they be identified?

Family caregiver outcomes:
What are the benefits to caregivers of the various services?
Do they reduce symptoms of stress, enable caregivers to remain employed, or extend the time people with dementia can remain at home?
Which caregivers will benefit from which services?
Can family members of persons in special residential units continue to provide some of the individualized care the residents need?

Settings:
How much does care cost in each of the settings—residential, day care, or home?
Which setting is right for which patient/family?
Are stage of illness, family situation, or other factors the critical elements in determining which setting is used?

Services:
Which services are essential and which optional for people with dementia? (full-day programming, special activities, special diet or meals, behavior management, continence management, medical care, nursing care, social services, occupational therapy, physical therapy, outdoor recreation, exercise, memory retraining, etc.)
How can delivery of the various service be evaluated?
Which elements of the physical plant (e.g., architecture, interior design) are essential and which are optional for people with dementia?
How much does each of these items of service and physical plant cost?
What technologies can make patient care easier or more humane?

Staff:
What kind of staff are needed for which patient/settings (geriatricians, neurologists, psychiatrists, nurses, social workers, occupational and physical therapists, nonprofessional staff, etc.)?
How can professionals best be trained to care for people with dementia?
Do existing training methods work?
What staff-patient ratios are necessary for which patients/settings?
What is the role of volunteers? How should they be selected and trained?

Admission/discharge criteria:
What admission/discharge criteria are used?
Where do patients come from?
Where are they discharged to?
What stage, functional level, or behavioral problems do different programs accept? Why?
Is special care beneficial to the patient/family? Cost effective?

Cost structures:
Who should pay for which kinds of care (the patient, the family, the government, the private sector)?
What is the impact of payment adjusted for case mix?
Does special care cost more per patient?

Quality assurance policy:
How can safe and humane care be ensured for people with dementia?
How can existing standards and regulations be modified to benefit people with dementia?
Should Federal regulation be extended to adult day care, board and care, and other programs not now regulated by the Federal Government?
How can quality assurance standards be designed that ensure quality of life?

SOURCE: Office of Technology Assessment, 1987.

ISSUE 2: Should the Federal Government set standards for special residential care, respite care, or both, for persons with dementing illnesses?

Option 1: *Keep existing Federal standards as they are and leave standards for special units and respite care to the States.*

Option 2: *Develop guidelines to be met in all federally supported programs and in programs in which care is purchased with Federal funds. Encourage adoption of these standards by the States.*

Option 3: *Support research that will generate information needed to develop care standards for programs serving people with dementia.*

Option 4: *Require that persons purchasing care with Federal funds receive care appropriate to their level of impairment.*

Option 5: *Enforce existing standards.*

In the past, the Federal Government has not set standards for facilities and services that do not fall under Medicare or Medicaid. (An entirely separate issue is whether the Federal Government should now become involved on behalf of impaired persons.) The Federal Government could leave standards-setting to the States (option 1). Several States have set or are considering guidelines for care of persons with dementia (14; California Senate Bill 195), but many States are unlikely to do so and the degree of protection varies widely.

Basic standards for protection and fire safety are needed for all settings. The Federal Government could develop guidelines to be met in federally supported programs or when care is purchased with Federal funds (including SSI and VA pensions), and could encourage States to adopt them (option 2). Basic guidelines would provide some protection quickly to individuals who may be in jeopardy and would relieve the States of the expense of separately investigating this issue.

Better enforcement of existing standards (option 5) and requirements that these individuals be cared for in facilities offering an appropriate level of care (option 4) would provide some protection without developing additional standards.

Should quality assurance standards be developed for special dementia programs—either respite, day care, or nursing homes? Existing standards sometimes get in the way of service provision, some programs have no standards to ensure basic safety, and standards do not always result in the desired outcome—quality care (see ch. 10). In addition, limited knowledge of the characteristics and costs of special programs makes it difficult to set standards. Standards for nursing or social work time, staff-to-client ratios, or services provided could freeze certain programs in place and prevent innovation and development of more creative ones. Research into models of care is a necessary preparation for establishing standards of care. The Federal Government could support the research (option 3) needed to identify expected participant outcomes in special programs, to discriminate between severity of dementia and the presence of excess disabilities, and to identify the required inputs that result in optimal recipient function.

CHAPTER 7 REFERENCES

1. Alzheimer's Disease and Related Disorders Association, *Respite Care Manual* (Chicago, IL: 1986).
2. Alzheimer's Family Center, Inc., *1985 Annual Report* (San Diego, CA: 1986).
3. Arie, T., "Day Care and Geriatric Psychiatry," *Geriatric Clinics* 17:31-391, 1975.
4. Bartol, M.A., "Nonverbal Communication in Patients With Alzheimer's Disease," *Journal of Geriatric Nursing* 5(4):21-31, 1979.
5. Billington, R., Alzheimer's Disease and Related Disorders Association, New York, NY, personal communication, May 1986.
6. Bowsher, M., "A Unique and Successful Approach to Care for Moderate Stage Alzheimer's Victims," Green Hills Center, West Liberty, OH (no date).
7. Brocklehurst, J.C., "The British Experience With Day Care and Day Hospital," *Day Care for Older Adults: A Conference Report*, E. Pfeiffer (ed.) (Durham, NC: Center for the Study of Aging and Human Development, Duke University, 1976).
8. Brody, E., "The Formal Support Network: Congregate Treatment Settings for Residents With Senescent Brain Dysfunction," *Clinical Aspects of Alzheimer's Disease and Senile Dementia, Aging, Vol. 15*, N.E. Miller and G.D. Cohen (eds.) (New York, NY: Raven Press, 1981).
9. Buchanan, A., Brock, D., and Gilfix, M., "Surrogate Decisionmaking for Elderly Individuals Who Are Incompetent or of Questionable Competence," contract report prepared for the Office of Technology Assessment, U.S. Congress, 1986, forthcoming in *Milbank Memorial Fund Quarterly*.
10. Burnside, I.M., "Alzheimer's Disease: An Overview," *Journal of Geriatric Nursing* 5:(4):14-20, 1979.
11. Burnside, I.M., "Care of the Alzheimer's Patient in an Institution," *Generations* 7:1, 1982.
12. Clarke, T., "A Special Nursing Home Unit for Ambulatory Demented Patients," *Generations* 7:1, 1982.
13. Cohen, E., "NIMH SBIR Phase II Proposal," Community Services, Inc., Narberth, PA, 1986.
14. Commonwealth of Massachusetts, Final Rough Draft of Guidelines on Special Projects, Boston, MA, Jan. 10, 1986.
15. Coons, D., "Alive and Well at Wesley Hall," *Quarterly, A Journal of Long-Term Care*, Ontario Association of Homes for the Aged, 21(2), July 1985.
16. Coons, D., "Wesley Hall: A Special Life," Institute of Gerontology, University of Michigan, Ann Arbor, MI (no date).
17. Coons, D.H., Institute of Gerontology, University of Michigan, Ann Arbor, MI, personal communication, 1985.
18. Coons, D.H., "A Residential Care Unit for Persons With Dementia," contract report prepared for the Office of Technology Assessment, U.S. Congress, 1986.
19. Coons, D.H., "The Therapeutic Milieu: Social and Psychological Aspects of Treatment," *Clinical Aspects of Aging*, 2d ed., W. Reichel (ed.) (Baltimore, MD: Williams & Wilkins, 1983).
20. Coons, D.H., and Spencer, B., "The Older Person's Response to Therapy," *Psychiatric Quarterly, In-Hospital Therapeutic Community* 55(2&3): summer/fall 1983.
21. Coons, D.H., Metzelaar, L., Robinson, A., et al., *A Better Life: Helping Family Members, Volunteers and Staff Improve the Quality of Life of Nursing Home Residents Suffering From Alzheimer's*

Disease and Related Disorders (Columbus, OH: Source for Nursing Home Literature, 1986).

22. COPSA (Comprehensive Services on Aging) Institute for Alzheimer's Disease and Related Disorders, brochure, University of Medicine and Dentistry of New Jersey, Community Health Center at Piscataway, Piscataway, NJ.

23. Delaney, N., and Platt, K., "Nuts and Bolts in Patient Respite Program," Veterans Administration Medical Center, Palo Alto, CA, 1983.

24. Dunn, L., "Senior Respite Care Training Manual," Portland, OR, 1986.

25. Dunn, L., "The Senior Respite Care Program," contract report prepared for the Office of Technology Assessment, U.S. Congress, 1986.

26. Edelson, J.S., and Lyons, W.H., *Institutional Care of the Elderly Mentally Impaired Elderly* (New York, NY: Van Nostrand Reinhold, 1985).

27. Family Survival Project, *Annual Report, July 1, 1984—July 1, 1985*, San Francisco, CA, 1985.

28. Feil, N., "The More We Get Together," videotape, Feil Productions, Cleveland, OH (no date).

29. Folsom, J.C., "Intensive Hospital Therapy of Geriatric Patients," *Current Psychiatric Therapies* 7:209-215, 1967.

30. Folsom, J.C., "Reality Orientation for the Elderly Mental Patient," *Journal of Geriatric Psychiatry* 1:291-307, 1968.

31. Frazier, C., Hellman, L., and Seaman, J.D., "A Model for Developing a Geriatric Behavioral Treatment Unit," paper presented at Caracas, Venezuela, International Congress of Psychology, July 1985.

32. French, C.J., "Experiences in the Development and Management of the Community Services Program of the Atlanta Area Chapter of the Alzheimer's Disease and Related Disorders Association, Inc.," contract report prepared for the Office of Technology Assessment, U.S. Congress, 1986.

33. George, L.K., "The Dynamics of Caregiver Burden," final report, submitted to American Association of Retired Persons, Andrus Foundation, Washington, DC, 1984.

34. Gilleard, C.J., "Predicting the Outcome of Psychogeriatric Day Care," *The Gerontologist* 25:280-285, June 1985.

35. Gottesman, L., "Organizing Rehabilitation Services for the Elderly," *The Gerontologist* 10:287-293, 1970.

36. Gottesman, L., "Resocialization of the Geriatric Mental Patient," *American Journal of Public Health* 55:1964-1970, 1965.

37. Gwyther, L., director, Family Support Program, Center for the Study of Aging and Human Development, Duke University, personal communication, Mar. 7, 1986.

38. Gwyther, L.P., *Care of Alzheimer's Patients: A Manual for Nursing Home Staff* (Washington, DC: Alzheimer's Disease and Related Disorder Association and American Health Care Association, 1985).

39. Hall, G., Kirschling, V., and Todd, S., "Sheltered Freedom: The Creation of an Alzheimer's Unit in an Intermediate Care Facility," 1985.

40. Hanczaryk, D.P., and Batzka, D.L., Taylor Care Center, Adventure Program, Jacksonville, FL, 1986.

41. Hayter, J., "Patients Who Have Alzheimer's Disease," *American Journal of Nursing* 74(8):1460-1463, 1974.

42. Hebrew Home for the Aged at Riverdale, "Institutional Approaches to the Care of Individuals With Dementia," contract report prepared for the Office of Technology Assessment, U.S. Congress, 1986.

43. Hegeman, C., letter to the editor, *The Gerontologist* 26:325, 1986.

44. Henderson, J.N., "Nursing Home Housekeepers: Ingenious Agents of Psychosocial Support," *Human Organization* 40(4):300-305, 1981.

45. Henderson, J.N., and Pfeiffer, E., "Mental Health and Aging: A Curriculum Guide for Nursing Home Caregivers," Suncoast Gerontology Center, University of South Florida, 1984.

46. Hiatt, L.G., "Disorientation Is More Than A State of Mind," *Nursing Homes* 29(4):30-36, 1980.

47. Hiatt, L.G., "Environmental Design and Mental Impaired Older People," *Mentally Impaired Aging, Bridging the Gap*, H. McBride (ed.) (American Association of Homes for the Aging, 1982).

48. Hiatt, L.G., "Understanding the Physical Environment," *Pride Institute Journal of Long-Term Home Health Care* 4(2):12-22, 1985.

49. Hiatt, L.G., "Wandering Behavior of Older People (doctoral dissertation, Graduate Center, City University of New York), *Dissertation Abstracts International* 46 (University Microfilms No. 86-01, 653) 1985.

50. Hillhaven Corp., "Special Care Unit Pre-Admission Interviewer's Guide," Tacoma, WA (no date).

51. Institute of Gerontology, *Workbook for the Workshop on Principles of Milieu Practice* (Ann Arbor, MI: University of Michigan, 1980).

52. Kahn, R.L., "The Mental Health System and the Future Aged," *The Gerontologist*, 24-31, 1975.

53. Katzman, R., Lasker, B., and Bernstein, N., "Accuracy of Diagnosis and Consequences of Misdiagnosis of Disorders Causing Dementia," contract

report prepared for the Office of Technology Assessment, U.S. Congress, 1986.

54. Keys, B., and Szpak, G., "Day Care for Alzheimer's Disease, Profile of One Program," *Postgraduate Medicine* 73:245-248, 1983.

55. Lawton, M.P., "Sensory Deprivation and the Effect of the Environment on Management of the Patient With Senile Dementia," *Aspects of Alzheimer's Disease and Senile Dementia*, N. Miller and G.D. Cohen (eds.) (New York, NY: Raven Press, 1981).

56. Lawton, M.P., Fulcomer, M., and Kleban, M., "Architecture for the Mentally Impaired Elderly," *Environment and Behavior* 16(6):730-757, 1984.

57. Libkowitz, R., "Research Builds Esteem: A Model Patient/Family Group Program," *Generations* 7(1), 1982.

58. Mace, N.L., "Activities for the Cognitively Impaired," *Physical and Occupational Therapy in Geriatrics*, in press.

59. Mace, N.L., "Adult Day Care," paper presented at New York State Health Department conference, Innovations in the Care of the Memory Impaired Elderly, New York, NY, June 12, 1986.

60. Mace, N.L., "Home and Community Services for Alzheimer's Disease: A National Conference for Families," U.S. Department of Health and Human Services and ADRDA, May 2, 1985.

61. Mace, N.L., and Rabins, P.V., "A Survey of Day Care for the Demented Adult in the United States," National Council on Aging, Washington, DC, 1984

62. Mace, N.L., and Rabins, P.V., *The 36-Hour Day: A Family Guide to Caring for Persons With Alzheimer's Disease, Related Dementing Illnesses, and Memory Loss in Later Life* (Baltimore, MD: The Johns Hopkins University Press, 1981).

63. Miller, E., "The Management of Dementia: A Review of Some Possibilities," *British Journal of Social Clinical Psychology* 16:77-83, 1977.

64. Miller, M.A., "Remotivation Therapy: A Way To Reach the Confused Elderly Patient," *Journal of Gerontological Nursing* 1(2):28-31, 1975.

65. Moss, B., "Nursing Home Care for the Senile Dementia Sufferer," paper presented at the 13th International Congress of Gerontology, New York, NY, July 1985.

66. New York State Department of Health, "Innovations in the Care of the Memory Impaired Elderly," conference, June 12, 1986.

67. Noyes, L., and Wittenborn, R., "The Family Respite Center: Day Care for the Demented," contract report prepared for the Office of Technology Assessment, U.S. Congress, 1986.

68. O'Brien, C.L., *Adult Day Care: A Practical Guide* (Monterey, CA: Health Sciences, 1982).

69. Octay, J.S., and Volland, P.J., "Community Care Program for the Elderly," *Health and Social Work* 41-47, 1981.

70. Orr, N., director, Hillhaven Corporation Special Care Units, personal communication, 1986.

71. Pannella, J., Jr., and McDowell, F., "Day Care for Dementia: A Manual to Instruction for Developing a Program," The Burke Rehabilitation Center Auxiliary, Burke Rehabilitation Center, White Plains, NY, 1983.

72. Pannella, J., Jr., Lilliston, B.A., et al., "Day Care for Dementia Patients: An Analysis of a Four-Year Program," *Journal of the American Geriatrics Society* 32:883-886, 1984.

73. Petty, D., director, Family Survival Project, San Francisco, CA, personal communication, 1986.

74. Petty, D., "Family Survival Project," contract report prepared for the Office of Technology Assessment, U.S. Congress, 1986.

75. Petty, D., "Respite Care, A Growing National Alternative," *The Coordinator* 34-36, October 1984.

76. Powell-Proctor, L., and Miller, E., "Reality Orientation: A Critical Appraisal," *British Journal of Psychiatry* 140:457-463, 1982.

77. Pride Institute, *Journal of Long-Term Home Health Care* 3(4), fall 1986.

78. Ransom, B., coordinator, National Institute on Adult Daycare, and National Center on Rural Aging, National Council on the Aging, personal communication, 1986.

79. Reifler, B., and Orr, N., *Alzheimer's Disease in the Nursing Home: A Staff Training Manual* (Tacoma, WA: Westprint Division of Hillhaven Corp., 1985).

80. Ronch, J., Minutes, 1986 Planning Meeting for Training Program for Nursing Home Staff, Community Services, Inc., Narberth, PA.

81. Roth, M., and Mountjoy, C.Q., "Mental Health Services for the Elderly Living in the Community: A United Kingdom Perspective," *International Journal of Mental Health* 8(3-4):6-35, 1979.

82. Rouse, D.J., Griffith, J.D., Trachtman, L.H., et al., "Aid for Memory Impaired Older Persons: Wandering Notification," Research Triangle Institute, Research Triangle Park, NC, 1986.

83. Rovner, B.W., Kafanek, S., Philipp, L., et al., "Prevalence of Mental Illness in a Community Nursing Home," in press.

84. Sands, D., and Belman, J., "Evaluation of a 24-Hour Care System for Alzheimer's and Related Disorders," contract report prepared for the Office of Technology Assessment, U.S. Congress, 1986.

85. Sands D., and Suzuki, T., "Adult Day Care for Alzheimer's Patients and Their Families," *The Gerontologist* 23:21-23, 1983.

86. Sawyer, J.C., and Mendlovitz, A.A., "A Manage-

ment Program for Ambulatory Institutionalized Patients With Alzheimer's Disease and Related Disorders," paper presented at the annual conference of the Gerontological Society of America, Nov. 21, 1982.

87. Shepherd, B., and Howley, D., "Adult Day Care: Annotated Bibliography," National Institute on Adult Day Care, Washington, DC, 1983.

88. Snyder, L.H., "Living Environments, Geriatric Wheelchairs and Older Persons Rehabilitation," *Human Ecology Forum* 3(2):17-20, fall 1972.

89. Snyder, L.H., Rupprecht, P., Pyrek, J., et al., "Wandering," *The Gerontologist* 18:272-280, 1978.

90. Sommers, C., administrator, Green Hills Center, West Liberty, OH, personal communication, Nov. 22, 1985.

91. Stone, R., "Recent Developments in Respite Care Services for Caregivers of the Impaired Elderly," Aging Health Policy Center, 1985.

92. U.S. Congress, General Accounting Office, "Medicaid and Nursing Home Care: Cost Increases and the Need for Services Are Creating Problems for the States and the Elderly," Washington, DC, Oct. 21, 1983.

93. U.S. Congress, Office of Technology Assessment, *Technology and Aging in America*, OTA-BA-264 (Washington, DC: U.S. Government Printing Office, June 1985).

94. Valenti's Alzheimer's Care Centers, Lancaster and Columbia, PA, advertisement (no date).

95. Weiner, A.S., "Confronting Alzheimer's Disease, Strategies for the Long-Term Care Provider, Programming To Meet the Special Needs of the Alzheimer's Patient," Hebrew Home for the Aged, Riverdale, NY, 1985.

96. Wells, T.J., "Urinary Incontinence in Alzheimer's Disease," contract report prepared for the Office of Technology Assessment, U.S. Congress, 1986.

97. Willging, P., American Health Care Association, press release, Washington, DC, May 21, 1986.

98. Winograd, C.H., and Jarvik, L.F., "Physician Management of the Demented Patient," *Journal of the American Geriatrics Society* 34:295-308, 1986.

99. Yankelovich, Skelley, & White, Inc., "Caregivers of Patients With Dementia," contract report prepared for the Office of Technology Assessment, U.S. Congress, 1986.

100. Zarit, S.H., and Anthony, C.R., "Interventions With Dementia Patients and Their Families," *The Dementias: Policy and Management*, M.L.M. Gilhooly, S.H. Zarit, and J.E. Birren (eds.) (Englewood Cliffs, NJ: Prentice-Hall, 1986).

101. Zgola, Y., *Doing Things, A Guide to Programming Activities for Persons With Alzheimer's Disease and Related Disorders* (Baltimore, MD: The Johns Hopkins University Press, in press).

102. Zimmer, J.G., Watson, N., and Treat, A., "Behavioral Problems Among Patients in Skilled Nursing Facilities," *American Journal of Public Health* 74: 1118-1121, 1984.

Chapter 8
Patient Assessment and Eligibility for Services

CONTENTS

Patient Assessment and Eligibility for Services

In the context of dementia research and treatment of persons with dementia, assessment is the process of identifying, describing, and evaluating individual characteristics associated with the dementing illness. Assessment can focus on cognitive deficits, changes in self-care abilities, behavioral problems, or all three. It can also focus on the impact of the person's functioning on the caregiver.

Diagnosis and assessment are related, but distinct. Since dementia is defined as the decline of memory and other cognitive abilities in an individual with no disturbance in consciousness (see ch. 2), assessment of cognitive abilities is a prerequisite for the diagnosis of dementia and diseases that cause dementia. However, diagnosis and assessment also differ in several ways. Diagnosis results in the identification of a specific disease, while assessment results in a description of the impact of the disease on the patient. A diagnosis of Alzheimer's or of another disease that causes dementia does not provide information about the severity of the condition, and individuals with such diagnoses vary greatly in their cognitive and self-care abilities and behavior, and therefore in their care needs. Assessment provides information about a person's current functioning and care needs but generally does not distinguish among the diseases that can cause dementia. This distinction is important because some dementias (an estimated 2 to 3 percent) are reversible with treat-

ment, and diagnosis is essential for identifying these conditions. Both diagnosis and assessment are necessary for good patient care, and neither is sufficient by itself (18,74,179).

Assessment of persons with dementia is often an unstructured process in which a physician or another health care or social service professional evaluates the person based on conversations with the person, the family, and other caregivers and on informal observations of the person's behavior. Structured assessment procedures and instruments have been developed to assist in this process. They include questions to be asked of the person, performance tasks to measure cognitive and self-care abilities, and lists of cognitive and self-care abilities and behaviors that can be used to rate the person.

This chapter discusses the role of assessment in the study of dementia and treatment of persons with a dementing illness; the kinds of assessment procedures and instruments that are used to evaluate cognitive, self-care, and behavioral deficits and caregiver burden; and problems that affect the accuracy of these procedures and instruments. The primary focus of the chapter is the potential use of such procedures and instruments in identifying long-term care needs and in establishing eligibility for publicly funded long-term care services.

USES OF STRUCTURED ASSESSMENT PROCEDURES AND INSTRUMENTS

Clinicians, researchers, and caregivers agree in theory that cognitive abilities are diminished or lost in individuals with a dementing illness, that self-care abilities such as bathing, dressing, eating, and continence are frequently lessened, and that many caregivers have difficulty managing these individuals. When these concepts are ap-

plied to specific individuals and their caregivers, however, agreement often ends. In practice, clinicians, researchers, and caregivers may disagree about answers to the following questions:

- Does this individual have a dementing illness?
- How severe is the dementia?

- Which cognitive abilities have been diminished or lost?
- How does the cognitive deficit affect the individual's ability to care for himself or herself?
- Which self-care functions does the person need help with?
- How much help does he or she need?
- How burdensome are these care requirements for family members or others who take care of the person?

Structured assessment procedures and instruments are intended to provide objective answers to these questions.

One reason for disagreement about the answers is that many of the terms used in the questions are vague and have different meanings to different people. With no definitive physiological markers for dementia and no precise physical methods for measuring the severity of cognitive, behavioral, or self-care deficits, it is difficult for clinicians, researchers, and caregivers to communicate clearly with each other about the condition and its impact. Thus, several individuals observing the same person can disagree about whether to call his or her cognitive or self-care deficits mild, moderate, or severe. Structured assessment procedures and instruments provide a common methodology for evaluating deficits and a common language for communication among those who study, diagnose, treat, and care for persons with dementia. In the absence of precise physical markers, these measures provide the only operational definitions of the terms "dementia," "cognitive impairment," "behavioral and self-care deficits," and "caregiver burden."

Structured assessment procedures and instruments can be used for a variety of purposes, and the purpose of the assessment determines which procedure or instrument should be used and the extent and type of errors that are acceptable (75,172). For some applications, it is necessary to identify only those individuals who certainly have a dementing illness; false positives are unacceptable. Appropriate instruments in these situations may miss some mild or borderline cases. Other applications require identification of all individuals with any possible dementia; false negatives are unacceptable. The appropriate procedures and instruments in this case will sometimes classify cognitively normal individuals as having dementia.

Research, Clinical, and Legal Applications

Almost all formal research on dementia uses structured assessment procedures and instruments to identify and classify research subjects. In fact, many available instruments were developed for research projects. Measures of cognitive abilities are used in survey research to identify individuals with dementia; they are used in clinical research to identify symptoms of diseases that cause dementia, to describe the course of the diseases, and to study the relationship between cognitive abilities and physiological findings, such as the results of brain imaging tests.

The measures are also used to evaluate outcome in research on experimental treatments, such as drug therapies and behavioral interventions. In long-term care research, findings based on assessment of cognitive and self-care abilities, behavioral problems, and caregiver burden are compared with information about service use to determine why, for example, some persons with dementia are placed in nursing homes while others can be maintained at home. For each of these research applications, accurate and reliable assessment procedures are important, because the research findings can only be as good as the measurement procedures that have been used (21,93).

Clinical applications for these assessment procedures and instruments are numerous and diverse. Measures of cognitive abilities can be used to screen for dementia and to assist in its diagnosis. Behavioral measures can be used to identify disturbing behaviors that can be treated and controlled even if the underlying cause of dementia is not treatable, thus allowing some families to maintain patients at home. Physicians and case managers who assist families with decisions about long-term care can use measures of cognitive and self-care abilities to determine whether the person should continue to live independently and what long-term care services are needed (127,166,187). In nursing homes, adult day care centers, and home care agencies, these instruments can be used to plan appropriate services, to determine the number and type of staff needed to provide them, and to monitor patient progress. Finally, measures of caregiver burden, which have thus far been used almost exclusively for research, might help to identify supportive services needed by families and other caregivers.

In geriatric assessment centers and specialized health care settings, such as teaching nursing homes and some teaching hospitals, structured assessment procedures and instruments are part of a comprehensive multidisciplinary evaluation of persons with probable dementias. In most cases, such an evaluation results in accurate identification of deficits associated with dementia, and frequently the cause of dementia can also be specified (45,78,138,185).

Yet, most persons with probable dementias are not seen in these specialized settings. In community hospitals, nursing homes, adult day care centers, home care agencies, and the offices of general practitioners—the settings where persons with probable dementias are most often seen and treated—comprehensive multidisciplinary evaluation is usually not available, and structured assessment procedures and instruments are seldom used. Instead, health care and social service providers in these settings often make intuitive judgments about an individual's abilities based on informal observations. Many experts believe that structured assessments could increase the accuracy of these judgments, facilitate communication among caregivers, and assist health care and social service providers in identifying an individual's long-term care needs (6,73,74,187).

Assessment procedures that are acceptable for research applications may be unsatisfactory for clinical applications, where errors or inaccuracy could have serious implications for the health care, safety, and quality of life of patients. In a research study, the failure of an assessment instrument to correctly identify a few individuals with dementia among a large number of subjects or, conversely, the incorrect classification of a few cognitively normal individuals as having dementia may have negligible statistical impact. In clinical settings, however, the same errors can cause serious problems, including inappropriate treatment and the failure to provide needed services and supervision. Since available assessment instruments are sometimes inaccurate, many experts advocate their use for initial screening only, to be followed by a comprehensive clinical evaluation of the individual (3,34,39,169,187).

In the future, structured assessment procedures and instruments may be used for legal purposes. For example, current procedures for determining competence to make legally binding decisions have been criticized for lack of objectivity. Particularly troublesome is the observation that the competence of individuals who agree with the decisions of their caregivers is rarely questioned, whereas individuals who do not agree with caregivers' recommendations are more frequently judged incompetent (see ch. 5) (116,146). Assessment instruments could provide a more objective measure of cognitive abilities.

Assessment instruments are rarely used for legal purposes at present, although assessing cognitive and self-care abilities as a basis for decisions about guardianship has been suggested (116). Since assessment focuses on the individual in relation to his or her physical and social environment, that suggestion would appear to fit well conceptually with the growing enthusiasm among legal and health care experts for the idea of "decision-specific competence"—i.e., competence for a specific decision rather than as a general attribute of a person (see ch. 5 and ref. 15).

The questions raised about the reliability and validity of assessment instruments for research and clinical applications are also relevant to legal applications. Careful testing of the reliability and validity of any instrument to be used for legal purposes is essential, since errors in the assessment could wrongfully deprive individuals of the right to make their own decisions, on the one hand, or wrongfully deny them protective services, such as guardianship, on the other hand.

Public Policy Applications

Public policy applications for structured assessment procedures and instruments include:

- establishing eligibility for publicly funded services,

- determining level of reimbursement for publicly funded services,
- measuring patient outcome for quality assurance programs, and
- identifying persons with dementia in health services research—the results of which are used by government agencies and others to plan and evaluate long-term care services.

Establishing Eligibility for Services

Eligibility for most publicly funded long-term care services is based on medical and nursing care needs. As described in chapter 6, eligibility for Medicare reimbursement for long-term care services depends on medical diagnosis, prognosis, and physician certification that the individual needs the services. Eligibility for Medicaid long-term care services varies from State to State, but generally depends on a need for medical and health-related services (in addition to income, assets, and other criteria discussed in ch. 11). Some States provide Medicaid funding for intermediate-level nursing home care based on an individual's need for personal care services supervised by a nurse. Although the need for personal care is clearly related to the self-care deficits of the patient, most States do not use an assessment of these abilities to determine eligibility. For Veterans Administration (VA) long-term care services, eligibility depends on medical and health care needs, age, income, whether the individual has a service-connected disability, and whether a bed is available in a VA facility.

The focus on medical and health care needs in Medicare, Medicaid, and VA eligibility requirements means that some persons with dementia do not receive the long-term care services they need. Others receive these services only because they have been given another diagnosis or certified by a physician to have medical, skilled nursing, or health care needs that make them eligible. Distorting the person's diagnosis and care needs, however, interferes with appropriate treatment.

Concern in Congress about Medicare, Medicaid, and VA eligibility requirements that may exclude persons with dementia from long-term care services has led to the introduction of several bills to make the necessary services available. Similar

legislation is expected to be introduced in future sessions. The framers of this legislation face the difficult task of defining which individuals and groups will be eligible for services. Some of the proposed bills describe an eligible individual as:

- one who "suffers from Alzheimer's disease (or a related organic brain disorder) and is physically or mentally incapable of caring for himself, as determined by a physician";
- one "who is diagnosed as having Alzheimer's disease or a related disorder (including dementia)";
- one who is "diagnosed by a physician as having senile dementia of the Alzheimer type"; and
- one who is a victim "of Alzheimer's disease or a related memory disorder."

If these or other bills are enacted, Federal agencies will be responsible for formulating regulations to implement them, based primarily on the intent of Congress as expressed in debate prior to enactment. These regulations will further define how eligibility will be determined and whether structured assessment procedures and instruments will be used in the process. **The terms used to describe eligible individuals in Federal legislation and the methods of determining eligibility established by Federal regulations have serious implications for the numbers and kinds of individuals who are eligible and, therefore, the public cost of any such programs.**

One approach to defining eligibility is to identify specific diseases as a criterion. For example, each description just cited identifies individuals with Alzheimer's disease as eligible. This theoretically simple approach would correct biases against such persons in existing Federal programs, but it might also introduce new problems. At present, many middle-aged and elderly individuals who cannot care for themselves independently because of a variety of physical, mental, or emotional problems do not meet the eligibility requirements for publicly funded long-term care services. As indicated in chapter 3, the diagnosis of Alzheimer's disease is often an uncertain one. Given that uncertainty and the commitment of most physicians to the welfare of their patients, legislation that provided services specifically for individuals with Alzheimer's disease would create strong incentives for physicians to diagnose their patients who need these services as having that disease.

With no physiological marker for Alzheimer's disease, there would be no definitive method for disputing the diagnosis, and many individuals who do not have Alzheimer's disease would be mislabeled. That would have serious implications for the kinds of health care these "Alzheimer's disease patients" would receive. Long-term care facilities would be filled with "Alzheimer's disease patients," and systematic errors would be introduced into research findings about the prevalence of this illness. In addition, the number of individuals eligible for services and the public cost would be higher than anticipated based on current prevalence estimates.

A second approach, as indicated, is to identify more general conditions such as "related disorder (including dementia)," "organic brain disorder," or "related memory disorder" as criteria for eligibility. That approach would eliminate incentives for the overdiagnosis of Alzheimer's disease. Yet diagnosis of these general conditions may be more susceptible to error and misinterpretation and more difficult to verify than the diagnosis of Alzheimer's disease. Thus, estimates of the number of individuals eligible for services based on these criteria and predictions about the public cost of services would be subject to significant errors. Terms such as "related memory disorder" raise additional questions because memory disorders can be due to many conditions, including Korsakoff's syndrome, depression, chronic schizophrenia, chronic alcoholism, and, to a lesser extent, normal aging. Legislation that created eligibility for services based on memory disorders could mandate services for individuals with any of these conditions.

Basing eligibility on either specific diseases or general conditions, such as dementia, creates another problem because these criteria do not account for the severity of a person's condition or for his or her need for services. One proposal just cited incorporates a measure of severity and need for services by requiring a physician's determination that the person is "physically or mentally

incapable of caring for himself." These terms are vague, however, and permit wide possible interpretation. An alternative is to use assessment instruments that measure cognitive and self-care deficits to establish eligibility.

Although it is possible that no legislation to provide expanded services for persons with dementia will be passed soon, the pressure on Congress to enact legislation to improve services for such persons will continue. Being aware of the implications of defining eligibility in one way or another and understanding the kinds of assessment procedures and instruments that might be used for this purpose could result in legislation that accurately reflects the intent of congressional sponsors and that avoids potential problems in implementation.

Determining Reimbursement for Services

Availability of publicly funded services for persons with dementia is affected not only by eligibility requirements but also by regulations that set the reimbursement levels for these services. Most States reimburse nursing homes for the care of Medicaid patients at flat rates that do not reflect differences in the cost of caring for individuals with different needs. That reimbursement policy creates a strong incentive for nursing homes to admit individuals who require relatively little care and refuse those who require a lot of care, many of whom are persons with dementia. An alternative that has been adopted by at least five States (Illinois, Maryland, New York, Ohio, and West Virginia) is to adjust Medicaid reimbursement for different patient characteristics and care needs (42,165).

Several methods have been developed for grouping persons with similar characteristics and care needs (42,103,165). Known as "case mix formulas," these methods can focus on medical care indicators, such as diagnosis and prognosis; patient characteristics, such as cognitive, self-care, and behavioral deficits; or specific treatment needs, such as oxygen therapy or intravenous feeding. Case mix formulas based entirely or in part on patient characteristics use the assessment procedures discussed in this chapter. The specific characteris-

at are included can encourage or discourage admission of persons with dementia to nursing homes. For example, formulas that assess cognitive status could encourage admission of persons with dementia, assuming that the level of reimbursement is high enough to meet the cost of caring for them. Similarly, formulas based on self-care abilities or behavioral problems and tied to adequate reimbursement rates could encourage admission of such persons.

The Health Care Financing Administration is currently developing a case mix formula for Medicare reimbursement to nursing homes. It may be based primarily on medical care indicators and thus biased against Medicare reimbursement for nursing home care for persons with dementia. If a measure of patient characteristics is included, however, Medicare reimbursement for nursing home care might become available for some persons with dementing illnesses.

Measuring Patient Outcome for Quality Assurance Programs

Government programs that regulate quality of care in nursing homes have focused on inputs—physical aspects of the facility, staffing, and caregiving procedures. An alternative is to focus on patient outcome as an indicator of quality of care. With this approach, changes in patients' physical condition and cognitive, self-care, and behavioral characteristics are monitored to determine quality of care. Aspects of this approach have been incorporated in the new survey instrument now being used in facilities that serve Medicare and Medicaid patients (see ch. 10). However, many nursing home administrators and others fear that the inspectors who use the new survey instrument will make subjective judgments about patient characteristics. Use of assessment procedures and instruments that have been shown to be reliable and valid could increase their confidence in the objectivity of the survey process.

Government quality assurance programs have legal status because they are based on Federal, State, and local law and because they can impose legally binding financial and administrative penalties on facilities and service providers that are out of compliance with regulations. Likewise, govern-

ment regulations that mandate eligibility requirements and level of reimbursement for services have legal status because they define the rights of individuals to receive services and the contractual obligation of government to pay for the services. The legal status of government programs and regulations suggests the need for highly precise and reliable assessment procedures.

The available procedures generally lack that high degree of accuracy, as discussed in this chapter. Yet they have been proposed and are being used in some instances to replace less satisfactory methods of establishing eligibility for services, determining level of reimbursement, and monitoring quality of care. Although the existing methods are generally precise and relatively easy to use, they do not measure the aspects of patient functioning that are most relevant to the need for long-term care and quality of care received. For example, measuring quality of care in terms of the hot water temperature in a nursing home or the number of square feet per patient in an adult day care center is easier and more precise than measuring quality of care in terms of patient outcome in either setting. Precision and ease of measurement are not the only important considerations, however, and public policy must balance these concerns with the need for assessment procedures that reflect the true intent of government programs.

Identifying Dementia Patients in Health Services Research

Information about the prevalence of specific diseases, the characteristics of affected persons, their care needs, patterns of service utilization, and cost of care is derived primarily from large-scale surveys and smaller studies of specific population groups and care settings. Almost all this research is sponsored by agencies of the Department of Health and Human Services (e.g., the National Center for Health Statistics, the National Center for Health Services Research, the National Institutes of Health, the National Institute of Mental Health, the Office of the Assistant Secretary for Planning and Evaluation, the Office of Human Development Services, and the Health Care Financing Administration) and by VA. Research findings are used to plan and evaluate services.

In general, persons with dementia have not been identified as a distinct group in health services research (100). Information about patient diagnosis is routinely obtained in many studies but is often unreliable. That is partly because of the difficulty of differential diagnosis in dementia but more often because the individual's diagnosis is obtained either from family members or other informants who do not know or may report it incorrectly, or from hospital or nursing home medical records that may be out of date or unreliable for other reasons. Furthermore, as indicated, diagnosis alone is not a good indicator of care needs.

Relatively few studies have used cognitive assessment instruments, and in some studies where these instruments were included, they were not administered to the subjects who were most likely to be cognitively impaired—i.e., those for whom a proxy was interviewed. As a result, although it is clear that persons with dementia constitute some proportion of the subjects in many studies of elderly and long-term care populations, their identity can only be inferred by combining information about diagnosis, self-care deficits, behavioral problems, and excessive caregiver burden (100). More accurate procedures for identifying these individuals are essential for government policy analysis and program planning and evaluation.

The remainder of this chapter discusses assessment of cognitive abilities, self-care abilities, behavior, and caregiver burden. Multidimensional assessment instruments that measure a wide range of patient and family characteristics are also discussed. Each section describes some of the available procedures and instruments, their reliability and validity, their capacity to differentiate between different patient groups, and their potential usefulness for public policy applications.

Some researchers and clinicians use the term "functional abilities" to refer to some or all of the cognitive and self-care abilities and behaviors discussed in this chapter, and some refer to the process of identifying and evaluating such abilities and behaviors as "functional assessment." Their use of the word "functional" emphasizes the concept that these patient characteristics are more closely related to the individual's ability to care for himself or herself independently and to the individual's need for long-term care services than factors such as diagnosis and medical care needs. While recognizing the validity of that concept, OTA finds that the term functional is used by different people to mean different patient characteristics and different combinations of characteristics. For that reason, it is not used in this chapter, and its use in legislation would create problems in implementation.

ASSESSMENT OF COGNITIVE ABILITIES

Cognitive impairment is the central feature of dementia and the primary cause of self-care and behavioral problems associated with it. The cognitive abilities that can be diminished or lost in dementia include memory, intelligence, learning ability, calculation, problem solving, judgment, comprehension, recognition, orientation, and attention. Many structured assessment procedures and instruments measure some or all of these.

The most commonly used method for evaluating cognitive abilities in persons with possible dementia is the clinical mental status exam in which a physician evaluates the person, based on verbal responses and behavior during an interview. Most clinicians ask questions to determine orientation—i.e., whether the individual knows who he or she is, who others are, where he or she is, and the date or day of the week. Mathematical questions and proverb interpretation are often used to measure higher cognitive functions. Yet there is considerable variation in the specific questions included and the cognitive functions evaluated (74,85,108). The result of a mental status exam is a judgment by the clinician, based on observations, experience, and intuition, about the person's cognitive abilities. Although that judgment may be accurate in many cases, lack of uniformity in questions asked and in cognitive abilities evaluated by different clinicians leads to uncertainty about the results.

In some cases, no mental status evaluation is done, and the cognitive impairments of patients are not identified. One study in a hospital medical ward found that ward physicians and nurses failed to identify cognitive impairments in 37 and 55 percent, respectively, of the affected patients (84). Other studies have noted the same problem in a rehabilitation hospital (46), in a medical inpatient service (109,144), in a neurology inpatient service (28), in a geriatric inpatient service (118), and for elderly persons in the community (190). The researchers suggest that routine use of assessment instruments could improve identification of patients with cognitive deficits.

Results of one study that tested that approach do not support their contention, however. The study involved the use of a brief cognitive assessment instrument, the Short Portable Mental Status Questionnaire (SPMSQ), to assess patients in a general internal medicine practice. Its use resulted in increased recording of patients' mental status: cognitive status was recorded in 35 percent of patient charts before the study began and 65 percent of the charts when the SPMSQ was used. Yet, routine use of the SPMSQ did not raise the proportion who were found to have cognitive deficits (about 9 percent in both periods) (193). Replication of the study is needed in other settings and using other cognitive assessment instruments.

Instruments To Measure Cognitive Abilities

Some instruments used to measure cognitive abilities in persons with dementia are derived from tests first used by psychologists and educators to measure intelligence quotient (IQ) in young people. An example is the Wechsler Adult Intelligence Scale (WAIS), developed in 1955 and used widely today to assess healthy and cognitively impaired adults (12,89). The WAIS includes subtests that can be used separately or combined into verbal and performance IQ scores.

Other instruments focus primarily on memory. The Wechsler Memory Scale (WMS), the most widely used of these, includes subtests that measure orientation; ability to recite the alphabet and count by threes; and ability to remember words, numbers, and geometric designs (132). Another such instrument is the Object Memory Evaluation (OME), in which an individual is presented with 10 easily recognized objects; the objects are then removed, and the person is asked to name them (44).

A third type of cognitive assessment instrument is derived from the clinical mental status exam described above. Examples (see tables 8-1, 8-2, 8-3, and 8-4) include the Information-Memory-Concentration Test (9); the Mental Status Questionnaire (MSQ) (73); the Short Portable Mental Status Questionnaire (127); and the Mini-Mental State Exam

Table 8-1.—Information-Memory-Concentration Test

Information test:
Name
Age
Time (hour)
Time of day
Day of week
Date
Month
Season
Year
Street
Town
Type of place (e.g., home, hospital, etc.)
Recognition of persons (cleaner, doctor, nurse, patient, relative; any two available)

Memory:
1. *Personal*
    Date of birth
    Place of birth
    School attended
    Occupation
    Name of siblings or name of wife
    Name of any town where patient had worked
    Name of employers
2. *Nonpersonal*
    Date of World War I
    Date of World War II
    Monarch
    Prime Minister
3. *Name and address (5-minute recall)*
    Mr. John Brown
    42 West Street
    Gateshead

Concentration:
Months of year backwards
Counting 1-20
Counting 20-1

SOURCE: G. Blessed, B.E. Tomlinson, and M. Roth, ''The Association Between Quantitative Measures of Dementia and of Senile Change in the Cerebral Grey Matter of Elderly Subjects,'' *British Journal of Psychiatry* 114:797-811, 1968.

Table 8-2.—Mental Status Questionnaire (MSQ)

1. What is this place?
2. Where is this place located?
3. What day in the month is it today?
4. What day of the week is it?
5. What year is it?
6. How old are you?
7. When is your birthday?
8. In what year were you born?
9. What is the name of the president?
10. Who was president before this one?

SOURCE: R.L. Kahn, A.I. Goldfarb, M. Pollack, et al., "Brief Objective Measures for the Determination of Mental Status in the Aged," *American Journal of Psychiatry* 117:326-328, 1963.

Table 8-3.—Mini-Mental State Examination (MMSE)

Orientation:
What is the (year) (season) (date) (day) (month)?
Where are we (State) (hospital) (floor)?

Registration:
Name three objects: One second to say each. Then ask patient all three after you have said them. Repeat them until he learns all three. (Count trials.)

Attention and calculation:
Begin with 100 and count backwards by 7 (stop after five answers). Alternatively, spell "world" backwards.

Recall:
Repeat the three objects above.

Language:
Show a pencil and a watch and ask subject to name them.
Repeat the following; "No 'ifs' 'ands' or 'buts.' "
A three-stage command, "Take a paper in your right hand; fold it in half and put it on the floor."
Read and obey the following: (Show subject the written item).
CLOSE YOUR EYES
Write a sentence.
Copy a design (complex polygon as in Bender-Gestalt).

SOURCE: M.R. Folstein, S. Folstein, and P.R. McHugh, "Mini-Mental State: A Practical Method for Grading the Cognitive State of Patients for the Clinician," *Journal of Psychiatric Research* 12:189-98, 1975.

Table 8-4.—Short Portable Mental Status Questionnaire (SPMSQ)

1. What is the date of today? (month) (day) (year)?
2. What day of the week is it?
3. What is the name of this place?
4. What is your telephone number?
4a. What is your street address? (Ask only if patient does not have a telephone.)
5. How old are you?
6. When were you born?
7. Who is the President of the United States now?
8. Who was the president just before him?
9. What was your mother's maiden name?
10. Subtract 3 from 20 and keep subtracting 3 from each new number, all the way down.

SOURCE: E. Pfeiffer, "A Short Portable Mental Status Questionnaire for the Assessment of Organic Brain Deficits in Elderly Patients, *Journal of the American Geriatrics Society* 23:433-441, 1975.

have been used extensively in research and clinical settings.

A fourth type of assessment instrument uses neurological tests to differentiate between cognitively normal individuals and those with organic dementias. An example is the Face-Hand Test (FHT) in which the person is touched simultaneously on the face and the hand, first with his eyes open and then with eyes closed. Persons with organic dementias frequently report only one of the two stimuli (36).

Many other cognitive assessment instruments have been developed for research and clinical applications. This chapter focuses on the instruments just described because they are used most often in the United States.

Reliability and Validity of Cognitive Assessment Instruments

The accuracy of assessment instruments in identifying individuals with cognitive deficits depends on two factors—reliability and validity. Reliability is the capacity to produce the same results when used by two different raters (interrater reliability) or at different times (test-retest reliability). Interrater reliability has not been reported for all the assessment instruments just mentioned, but it has been shown to be high for those that have been tested. Although raters are usually trained to use the instrument beforehand, some instruments, such as the MMSE, are designed for use by untrained raters, and these too have demonstrated

(MMSE) (39). Designed specifically for evaluating individuals with probable dementia, these instruments are shorter than the WAIS and WMS because such individuals frequently cannot tolerate lengthy assessment procedures. Test items are generally simpler than items on the WAIS.

All four of these instruments measure orientation and memory. Both the MMSE and SPMSQ measure ability to subtract a number from 100 and continue subtracting serially. In fact, many items on the four tests are similar and can be combined with slight rewording into a single test with fewer than 40 questions (78). All four measures high interrater reliability (3). Test-retest reliability has not been reported for all the instruments but has been high when reported (38,127,169).

Validity is the capacity of an instrument to measure cognitive abilities accurately and to distinguish between individuals who are cognitively impaired and those who are not. Experience with the four types of assessment instruments described indicates that they usually distinguish correctly between cognitively normal individuals and those with moderate or severe cognitive impairments; they are less accurate, however, in identifying individuals with mild cognitive impairments. In addition, some persons with obvious cognitive impairments do well on these tests, and some persons who are cognitively normal do poorly (3,36,39,89,125).

Validity of these instruments is usually tested by comparing the results of one test with another or with the judgment of a clinician who evaluates the same person in an unstructured or semistructured interview. Often the subjects in these studies have been previously identified as either cognitively impaired or cognitively normal; individuals with questionable cognitive status or characteristics that might complicate cognitive assessment are not included. When tested in this way, the instruments are generally effective in differentiating between those who are cognitively impaired and those who are not (3,36,80,166).

When the same instruments are used with subjects who have not been previously screened, however, their ability to correctly identify individuals with cognitive deficits is significantly reduced. For example, when the MMSE was used recently for a large survey in Baltimore, a significant proportion of individuals were incorrectly identified as cognitively impaired (14 to 33 percent, depending on which cutoff score was used) (38).

Similarly, when the MMSE was used to evaluate hospital patients on a general medical ward, 33 of the 97 subjects were identified as cognitively impaired on the basis of the test, but only 20 were so judged on the basis of a comprehensive clinical evaluation by a psychiatrist. That is a false positive rate of 39 percent. Eleven of the 13 false positives had an eighth grade education or less, and level of education was not known for the other

two. In contrast, there were no false positives among those who had more than an eighth grade education. More false positives were also noted for those aged 60 and over than for those under 60 (3). Thus, educational background and age appear to affect the validity of the MMSE.

The use of cognitive assessment measures for long-term care decisionmaking, as eligibility criteria, or in survey research requires evaluation of individuals with a wide range of cognitive functioning who have not been previously screened for such cognitive impairments. Many are over 60, and many have less than an eighth grade education. Thus, there may be serious drawbacks to using the MMSE or similar assessment instruments alone for these purposes. The authors of the MMSE have not suggested such use and emphasize that it is a screening instrument and should be followed by clinical evaluation of the patient (39). It is considered here only as a prototype of the kind of instrument that might have public policy applications.

Research indicates that cognitive test items differ in their tendency to produce false positive or false negative findings (83). Orientation items often produce false negatives—that is, some persons with dementia answer these questions correctly. Conversely, cognitively normal individuals seldom miss these questions. Other test items, such as spelling a word backwards or remembering three items after five minutes, tend to result in false positives—that is, some cognitively normal individuals miss these items. Conversely, dementia patients seldom get them right. These findings suggest the possibility of varying the mix of test items for different applications depending on the acceptability of each kind of error.

Problems That Complicate the Assessment of Cognitive Abilities

A variety of problems affect performance on cognitive tests and, therefore, complicate the assessment process. Many are related to the fact that most individuals with possible dementia are elderly and have physical, psychological, and sociodemographic characteristics that can reduce test performance even when there is no real cognitive impairment. Just as prevalence of dementia increases with increasing age, so does the prevalence of problems that interfere with accurate assessment.

One overriding problem is that the diagnosis of dementia requires a decline in cognitive function. Individuals of all ages, but especially the elderly, vary widely in cognitive ability (89), and a given level of performance on a cognitive test may be normal for one individual but indicate serious cognitive loss for another. Thus, poor test performance can indicate either a low level of intelligence that has been characteristic of an individual throughout life or a decline in cognitive abilities associated with dementia. Similarly, an average score can indicate either normal cognitive status or a significant decline in an individual who once had high intellectual ability.

Few elderly people have taken these tests earlier in life, and test results are seldom available for those who have; thus, there is no personal standard against which to measure change. Furthermore, age-related norms have not been developed for most instruments (110). Since verbal skills change less in old age than other cognitive functions, some experts have suggested that measures of such skills may reflect an individual's previous cognitive abilities (74,89,147). These findings have not been sufficiently documented, however, to form a basis for long-term care decisionmaking or for establishing eligibility for services.

Many experts recommend interviewing a relative or friend of the person to determine the person's previous cognitive abilities (147,163). Sometimes, however, no well-informed relative or friend is available. Even when information is available, it is often difficult to evaluate since relatives and friends may have a different frame of reference from the clinician for judging cognitive abilities.

The difficulty of determining whether there has been a decline in cognitive abilities is a serious problem in the assessment of patients with dementia (40,172). For research applications, averaging of data may minimize the effect of this problem, but for long-term care decisionmaking or eligibility determination, errors in classification of individuals due to lack of information about previous intellectual ability cannot be averaged out.

Physical Conditions

Visual impairments, hearing loss, speech impairments, acute and chronic diseases, and the effects of various medications can reduce cognitive test performance and complicate the assessment of cognitive abilities. Although individuals with these conditions are often excluded from studies that test the validity of assessment instruments, they are part of the population that must be assessed for long-term care decisionmaking, eligibility determination, and other public policy purposes.

About 14 percent of those over 65 have visual impairments (173), and prevalence increases in successively older age groups. On cognitive tests that involve visual stimuli, individuals with visual impairments perform poorly despite normal cognitive abilities (25). If this problem is recognized, test items can be modified. But in some testing situations, especially when assessment instruments are used by untrained persons or for large-scale screening, visual impairments that affect test performance may not be noticed.

Hearing impairments are also very common among the elderly and can interfere with performance on tests that involve verbal instructions or a verbal response (53). As with visual impairments, assessment procedures can be modified if the hearing loss is recognized; however, many people are unaware of or try to hide such impairments. If they answer questions they have not heard clearly, it is extremely difficult to determine whether errors are caused by failure to hear the question or by cognitive impairments. A comprehensive multidisciplinary evaluation conducted by a trained professional lessens the chance of mistaking hearing loss for cognitive impairment, but when less well trained observers conduct the assessment and a single instrument involving verbal stimuli is used, there is a much greater probability of error.

Some individuals have both hearing loss and cognitive impairment. Among those over 65, at least 28 percent have moderate to severe hearing loss, and coexistence of hearing loss and dementia is not uncommon (171,174). Among nursing home residents and those over 80, prevalence of both conditions is higher, and many of these individuals are both hearing impaired and cognitively impaired. In such cases, identification of cognitive deficits and measurement of their severity is particularly difficult.

Speech impairments also affect cognitive test performance when verbal responses are required. In some cases, inability to communicate verbally is a symptom of dementia, resulting directly from the disease or other condition that causes the dementia. (Certain kinds of speech impairment are associated with specific diseases that cause dementia, and careful evaluation of an individual's speech impairment may facilitate differential diagnosis.) In other cases, inability to communicate verbally is unrelated to cognitive ability; yet it is often perceived by laypersons and many health care and social service providers as a sign of cognitive impairment (174). For a patient who can write, assessment procedures can be adapted, but for those who can neither write nor speak clearly, accurate assessment is difficult, whether done in a structured or unstructured clinical interview, and with or without an assessment instrument.

Acute and chronic diseases that are common among the elderly affect cognitive test performance. Because of the sensitivity of the aged brain to any changes in physical condition, almost all diseases can affect cognitive ability. Infections, cardiovascular disease, dehydration, electrolyte disturbances, nutritional deficiencies, and many other conditions can lessen cognitive functioning (174). Pain or fatigue associated with acute or chronic disease can also take a toll. Furthermore, fluctuations in cognitive functioning associated with pain, fatigue, or episodes of acute disease can result in different evaluations of a person's cognitive abilities by observers who see the person at different times.

For research purposes and some clinical applications, assessment can be postponed until acute conditions have been treated and cognitive functioning has returned to normal; however, long-term care decisions and eligibility determination often cannot be postponed. Elderly individuals with diminished cognitive abilities frequently live independently until a medical crisis brings them to a hospital, where discharge plans based at least in part on an assessment of cognitive abilities are often made before they are entirely well. Indeed, the Medicare Prospective Payment System and other government and private initiatives that encourage early discharge of hospital patients are now increasing the pressure on hospital staffs to formulate discharge plans, including plans for nursing home placement, while patients are still acutely ill. For example:

> Mrs. C., a 75-year-old woman who had been living alone, was admitted to the hospital after a friend called an ambulance because Mrs. C. had become weak, confused, and incontinent. In the hospital, an infection was diagnosed and treatment begun. Mrs. C. was definitely confused in the hospital. Informal evaluation by the physician indicated poor orientation to time and place, memory loss, and poor judgment. The doctor and the hospital social worker had to decide quickly whether it was safe for Mrs. C. to go home alone or whether she should be placed in a nursing home. This decision depended primarily on whether her confusion would lessen as the infection subsided. They both knew that the infection could be causing the confusion; there was no way to accurately assess her cognitive abilities while it continued. They both also knew that if she was placed in a nursing home now, discharge to home would be unlikely at a later time.

In this hypothetical case that represents an increasingly common occurrence in hospitals, most physicians and social workers would rely on a history of the patient's illness and prior functioning to make a tentative judgment about her underlying cognitive abilities. Structured assessment procedures and instruments would not provide accurate information about her long-term cognitive functioning.

Eligibility for long-term care services, such as Medicaid funding for nursing home care, is often determined at times when a person is acutely ill and accurate measurement of cognitive abilities is difficult. Eligibility determinations based on cognitive test performance would be subject to frequent errors at these times.

Many medications affect cognitive functioning, particularly in the elderly (78,170,174). Even if reversible, such cognitive deficits are real and affect both test performance and the results of informal patient evaluation (36). Some clinicians may not be aware of the effect of drugs on cognitive functioning (66), but even those who are aware have no way to evaluate a person's cognitive abilities in a drug-free condition without stopping the drugs, which is dangerous for some patients. As with acute illness, a history of the patient's functioning prior to the use of medications may help determine underlying cognitive abilities. Use of structured assessment procedures and instruments usually cannot differentiate between patients with medication-induced cognitive deficits and those with primary degenerative dementias.

Emotional and Psychological Conditions

Depression and other emotional and psychological conditions common among elderly people can complicate assessment of cognitive abilities. Severe depression, particularly in the elderly, can cause cognitive deficits that are the same or similar to those associated with multi-infarct disease, Alzheimer's disease, and other degenerative brain diseases. Less severe depression causes some elderly individuals to doubt their own cognitive abilities and exaggerate the importance of minor memory lapses. Their complaints about memory loss seldom reflect real cognitive deficits (25,41, 110,133), but they can complicate the assessment process.

Other psychological and emotional characteristics common among elderly people can affect test performance even for those with no cognitive deficits. Elderly people are more cautious than younger people on cognitive tests and tend to be less confident about their answers (10,25,89). They may respond more slowly and omit items they are unsure of, resulting in lower test scores. Such behavior is especially a problem on timed tests (120,25).

Cognitive testing is a familiar experience for many young people today but is often something new for elderly people, and anxiety related to an unfamiliar test situation can reduce test performance. Any actual errors on the test can also increase anxiety (25,36). Research indicates that success on one test item increases the probability of success on the next item (4), and some experts advise that testing should at least begin with items that allow a high rate of success in order to alleviate anxiety and increase the validity of the results.

That is an important consideration in test design and administration for persons with Alzheimer's disease who may have very limited cognitive abilities and limited tolerance for stress and may become so agitated by failures that they have a catastrophic reaction and are unable to complete the assessment (36,190).

The validity of cognitive tests depends on the assumption that the individual is attentive (89), but research indicates that some cognitively normal elderly people do not concentrate on tests that have no meaning to them. Lack of attention can reduce performance on simple tests, such as the Face-Hand Test (FHT) (31), and on tests of rote memory, such as recalling random numbers. Inability to concentrate, however, can be an integral part of dementia, affecting both cognitive test performance and the individual's ability to function independently. Distinguishing between poor test performance due to lack of attention and poor test performance due to dementia may be easy when the clinician knows the person and several tests are used. In large-scale screening, when the clinician does not know the person or when only one measure is used, that distinction can be difficult.

Sociodemographic Characteristics

Educational level attained, ethnic and cultural background, and language barriers all affect cognitive test performance (172). The relationship between educational background and cognitive test performance has been noted frequently (3,38,67, 70,89,127). Test items that are especially difficult for individuals with limited formal education include orientation to time (3,113) and serial subtraction tests in which the individual is asked to subtract a number from 100 and continue subtracting repeatedly (3,65,89).

The FHT has been recommended for cognitive assessment because it uses an unlearned perceptual task that is not affected by educational background (73,89). Alternatively, some experts have recommended adjusting the scoring of cognitive tests, depending on the educational level of the individual (82,127). Others have suggested that new test items should be devised that are less affected by educational background (3). In a recent survey, subjects who could not complete the serial subtraction test were offered an alternative—spelling the word "world" backwards. All those with an eighth grade education or less had to resort to this alternative, and some who were not cognitively impaired were, nevertheless, unable to complete the item correctly (3).

In a related area, some studies of hospital or nursing home patients have replaced test items such as the name of the President with more personally relevant information, such as the name of a head nurse or a neighbor. Surprisingly, at least one study has indicated that these items were more difficult for subjects (31). It has been suggested that the new items may tap different cognitive functions than the original items (78).

Ethnic and cultural background also affect cognitive test performance, but little research has been done on this issue. Some test items may have little meaning or a different meaning for subjects from different ethnic backgrounds (89). For example, research indicates that Hispanics in Los Angeles had more difficulty with the MMSE items "state," "season," and "country" than non-Hispanics, possibly because many had recently immigrated from Mexico or other Latin American countries where these concepts are seldom used (33). Similarly, anecdotal evidence indicates that time orientation may be different for some minority group individuals (175). Some ethnic and cultural minority groups have negative attitudes about psychological testing and mental health professionals that can distort cognitive test performance. In addition, clinicians may have problems evaluating background information about clients from ethnic or cultural minority groups different from their own.

To compensate for language barriers, test instruments can be translated, but some items, such as proverb interpretation, lose their meaning in translation. When the test is in English, those for whom English is a second language may have particular difficulty with items such as vocabulary. Some will switch back and forth between English and their native language during the interview, and it can be difficult for the clinician to tell whether that behavior indicates regression associated with dementia, resistance to the test situation, or the person's normal behavior (23).

Ethnic minority groups of color (black Americans, Native Americans, and Asian Americans) constitute about 10 percent of the elderly population, and an additional 3 percent of the elderly are of Spanish origin (97). These percentages will increase as life expectancy rises for ethnic minority groups. In addition to these groups, many other elderly individuals immigrated to this country and retain cultural and language characteristics that reflect their countries of origin. Assessment procedures that can be adapted for these individuals are needed for research and clinical applications, for accurate evaluation of cognitive abilities related to long-term care decisionmaking, and for potential use in eligibility determination and other public policy applications.

Cognitive Assessment and Differential Diagnosis

Federal legislation that defines eligibility in terms of specific diseases or general conditions would require a method for differentiating among cognitive deficits associated with normal aging, depression, and organic brain diseases such as Alzheimer's, Pick's, and Huntington's diseases. Although physiological markers and lab tests can help identify some conditions, there are no definitive markers or tests for others. While diagnosis of these diseases and conditions is often accomplished in an unstructured or semistructured clinical evaluation, assessment procedures and instruments are sometimes used.

Age-Related Cognitive Decrements

Extensive psychological research indicates that cognitive functions such as response speed and short-term memory are often diminished in elderly people (110,172,176). Experts disagree, however, about the extent and inevitability of cognitive loss associated with aging. Some studies show that average cognitive test scores for elderly subjects are 30 percent below those of younger subjects (195). Yet it appears that up to one-third of the elderly show no age-related cognitive loss (110).

Age-related cognitive decrements differ from dementia in that they usually do not progress to the point of interfering with independent functioning. At any one time, however, it can be difficult to distinguish between age-related cognitive decrements and those that signal early stages of dementia (24,110).

The assessment instruments used most often for this purpose are subtests of the WAIS, the WMS, the OME, and similar measures (11,91,111, 121). For example, one study differentiated with 98 percent accuracy between cognitively normal elderly persons and those with mild dementia using four tests (WMS logical memory, Trailmaking A, word fluency, and WMS mental control) (168). Another study identified a battery of three tests (Visual Retention Test, Controlled Oral Word Association Test, and Temporal Orientation) that correctly classified 87 percent of the subjects (34).

A third study showed that individuals with age-related cognitive loss could be differentiated from those with dementia on the basis of short-term (3-minute) memory and from younger controls on the basis of longer (24-hour) memory (119). Finally, one group of researchers found that scores on two measures (the WAIS digit symbol test[1] and an aphasia battery) were the best predictors of whether individuals with mild cognitive deficits would progress to moderate or severe dementia over a 1-year period (5).

Some researchers and clinicians have used the term "benign senescent forgetfulness" to describe significant memory loss that does not interfere with the individual's functioning and is not expected to progress (87,86). Research suggests, however, that such memory loss may not be benign in some people:

> In a prospective study of 488 volunteers, age 75 to 85 years, who were nondemented on initial examination, approximately 50 developed an unequivocal dementia over a 3-year period. Extensive neuropsychological tests had been carried out annually: the best predictor of dementia was the score on the Blessed mental status test. Subjects who initially made zero to two errors (out of 33 possible errors) on this mental status examination

developed dementia at a rate of less than 1 percent per year; those who made five to eight errors developed dementia at a rate over 10 percent per year. But only one-third of those who made five to eight errors have developed dementia as yet. The latter subset of subjects may be best described as an "at risk" group (78).

Even a comprehensive clinical evaluation using the best neuropsychological tests cannot predict which of the individuals with mild cognitive loss will develop progressive dementias (78).

Cognitive Deficits Caused by Depression

As noted earlier, depression can cause significant cognitive impairment, especially in the elderly, and much of the research on cognitive assessment for dementia has focused on methods of differentiating between depression-induced dementia and primary degenerative dementias.[2] The impetus behind research on cognitive assessment for dementia is that the cognitive deficits caused by depression are sometimes reversible if the depression is treated (60,129,135,156,194).

Several clinical features are said to distinguish depression-induced dementia from primary degenerative dementia (see table 8-5). Inconsistent performance on cognitive assessment tests is one such feature, but several researchers have been unable to confirm its validity (81,130). Likewise, "I don't know" responses have been identified as characteristic of depression-induced dementia, but several studies have found no significant differences in the number of these responses given by the two groups of patients (107,196). One study (180) found that depressed individuals have more difficulty remembering random than nonrandom words, while individuals with dementia have equal difficulty with random and nonrandom words.

An individual's history, behavior, and mood can provide clues for differentiating between the two conditions (48,184), and a multidimensional assessment instrument (discussed later in this chapter)

---

[1]The digit symbol test involves showing the subject a sheet on which the digits 1-9 are paired with 9 geometric figures. The subject is then asked to draw the appropriate geometric figure after each digit on a test sheet. He or she is allowed to look back at the originial sheet on which the digits and figures are paired (Berg, et al., 1984b).

[2]A review of instruments to assess depression is beyond the scope of this report. In the context of differential diagnosis, however, it is important to note that some researchers and clinicians believe that many of the commonly used instruments do not assess the symptoms of depression most common in elderly people (Weiss, et al., 1986) and are of little value in evaluating them (Garcia, et al., 1981; Katzman, et al., 1986).

Table 8-5.—Major Clinical Features Differentiating Depression-Induced and Primary Degenerative Dementia

Depression-induced dementia	Primary degenerative dementia
Clinical course and history	
Family always aware of dysfunction and its severity	Family often unaware of dysfunction and its severity
Onset can be dated with some precision	Onset can be dated only within broad limits
Symptoms of short duration before medical help is sought	Symptoms usually of long duration before medical help is sought
Rapid progression of symptoms after onset	Slow progression of symptoms throughout course
History of previous psychiatric dysfunction common	History of previous psychiatric dysfunction unusual
Complaints and clinical behavior	
Patients usually complain much of cognitive loss	Patients usually complain little of cognitive loss
Patients' complaints of cognitive dysfunction usually detailed	Patients' complaints of cognitive dysfunction usually vague
Patients emphasize disability	Patients conceal disability
Patients highlight failures	Patients delight in accomplishments, however trivial
Patients make little effort to perform even simple tasks	Patients struggle to perform tasks
Patients do not try to keep up	Patients rely on notes, calendars, etc., to keep up
Patients usually communicate strong sense of distress	Patients often appear unconcerned
Affective change often pervasive	Affect labile and shallow
Loss of social skills often early and prominent	Social skills often retained
Behavior often incongruent with severity of cognitive dysfunction	Behavior usually compatible with severity of cognitive dysfunction
Nocturnal accentuation of dysfunction uncommon	Nocturnal accentuation of dysfunctions common
Clinical features related to memory, cognitive, and intellectual dysfunctions	
Attention and concentration often well preserved	Attention and concentration usually faulty
"Don't know" answers typical	Near-miss answers frequent
On tests of orientation, patients often give "don't know" answers	On tests of orientation, patients often mistake unusual for usual
Memory loss for recent and remote events usually equally severe	Memory loss for recent events usually more severe than for remote
Memory gaps for specific periods or events common	Memory gaps for specific periods unusual[a]
Marked variability in performance on tasks of similar difficulty	Consistently poor performance on tasks of similar difficulty

[a]Except when due to delirium, trauma, seizures, etc.

SOURCE: C.E. Wells, "Pseudodementia," *American Journal of Psychiatry* 136:895-900, 1979.

has been developed for this purpose (59). In addition, some have recommended a trial with antidepressant medications or electroconvulsive therapy for cases that are otherwise impossible to diagnose accurately (107,110).

The relationship between depression-induced and primary degenerative dementia may be considerably more complex than indicated by this discussion. Research indicates that the two conditions coexist in as many as one-fourth of cognitively impaired elderly persons (139). Differentiating persons with coexisting conditions from those with only depression is extremely difficult. Furthermore, several studies have shown that some persons who were originally identified as having depression-induced dementia go on to develop primary degenerative dementia (87,107,137). It has been suggested that depression and primary degenerative dementia may be biologically related in some as yet unexplained fashion (78,102).

Given the difficulty of distinguishing between depression-induced dementia and primary degenerative dementia, programs designed to serve persons with Alzheimer's and other organic dementias will probably also serve those with dementia caused by depression and those with coexisting depression and primary degenerative dementia. Federal legislation and regulations that restrict eligibility to those with primary degenerative dementias would create incentives for physicians to diagnose individuals with depression-induced dementia as having organic dementias. Conversely, legislation and regulations that extend eligibility to individuals with depression-induced dementias would encourage correct diagnosis and appropriate treatment for these individuals but might also result in overdiagnosis of depression.

Diseases That Cause Dementia

Diagnosis of the specific diseases that cause dementia is often made on the basis of factors such as age of onset, course of the disease, associated motor disorders, and other physical findings (see ch. 3). Differences in typical cognitive functioning in each of the diseases have been noted, however (50,60), and some researchers have tested the ability of cognitive assessment instruments to differentiate among these diseases. For example, one study used six WAIS subtests to assess cognitive impairment in patients with multi-infarct dementia or Alzheimer's disease: 74 percent of the patients were correctly classified (123). Another used cognitive tests to compare test performance in patients with Alzheimer's and Pick's diseases and multi-infarct dementia (72).

In an attempt to differentiate Alzheimer's from other diseases that cause dementia, researchers have developed an assessment procedure based on the concept that Alzheimer patients with obvious cognitive deficits retain normal motor functions longer than patients with other diseases (26). In a retrospective study of 50 patients, that assessment procedure, which involves rating patients on five cognitive functions and five motor functions (speech, psychomotor speed, posture, gait, and involuntary motor disturbances), successfully classified all Alzheimer patients and all but two of the non-Alzheimer patients (one with Pick's disease and one with post-traumatic dementia). The researchers point out that the procedure is least useful in the earliest stage of dementia when cognitive deficits are mild and in the latest stage when motor functions have deteriorated, and that it may misclassify Alzheimer patients with atypical presentations. Further validation of this assessment procedure is needed.

Differential diagnosis is complicated by the coexistence in some patients of diseases that cause dementia. For example, some patients have both Parkinson's and Alzheimer's diseases (14,94). Similarly, autopsy research indicates that 12 to 25 percent of patients with dementia show physiological signs of both multi-infarct dementia and Alzheimer's disease. Coexistence of these conditions is particularly common in the very old (16,43).

Assessment instruments have been used for differential diagnosis primarily in the context of comprehensive multidisciplinary evaluations that include physical examination, lab tests, a patient history, and neurological, psychiatric, and social work evaluation. Even with such a comprehensive assessment, differential diagnosis is often difficult, and some individuals are misclassified (7,162,172). For legislative purposes, it is important to recognize the difficulty of differential diagnosis when considering proposed legislation that would provide eligibility for individuals with specific illnesses, such as Alzheimer's disease, while excluding those with others that cause dementia.

Cognitive Rating Scales

Some assessment instruments have been used not only to identify and describe cognitive impairments but also to rate them from mild to severe. Most such instruments combine measures of cognitive, self-care, and behavioral deficits; these multidimensional scales are discussed later in this chapter. One instrument that focuses only on cognitive abilities is the Dementia Rating Scale (DRS), which is based on a series of tests that measure attention, memory, and other cognitive abilities (106). DRS has shown high test-retest reliability over a 1 week interval and significant correlation with a measure of self-care deficits. However, one study suggests that the cutoff point between normal cognitive functioning and mild dementia is set too high because cognitively normal persons are sometimes classified by the test as having a mild dementia (177).

Most of the other cognitive assessment instruments discussed earlier also result in numerical scores that have been used to differentiate mild, moderate, and severe dementia. Although such scores convey an impression of precise measurement, it should be remembered that selected cutoff points in this process are somewhat arbitrary, and that individuals found to have mild, moderate, or severe dementia on the basis of one test may be classified differently on the basis of another test. Any cognitive rating scale to be used for eligibility determination or in other public policy applications would require extensive validation of its cutoff scores.

Public Policy Applications

Establishing Eligibility for Services

As discussed earlier, eligibility for most publicly funded long-term care services is based on medical and health care needs, with the result that some persons with dementia are ineligible for services they need. An alternative—determining eligibility on the basis of structured assessment procedures and instruments—could benefit such persons if the assessment focused on areas of disability that are common among them. The obvious choice is a measure of cognitive deficits. Yet the research cited earlier points to many problems that limit the reliability and validity of cognitive assessment procedures. These include:

- visual, hearing, and speech impairments;
- acute and chronic diseases, pain, and medications that affect cognitive abilities;
- anxiety, depression, or lack of attention that affect cognitive test performance;
- limited educational background, ethnic and cultural minority group status, and language barriers; and
- the difficulty of differentiating between cognitive deficits caused by normal aging and those caused by dementia.

These problems suggest that despite the recognized ability of individual practitioners and specialized assessment centers to correctly identify dementia, with or without the use of structured assessment procedures and instruments, no available procedure or instrument is sufficiently reliable and valid to be used alone as a basis for eligibility. This finding does not dispute the value of these procedures and instruments for research and clinical applications. Nor does it mean that cognitive measures cannot be used along with diagnosis and other measures of patient care needs to establish eligibility. However, it does indicate a need for continued research to refine and validate cognitive assessment procedures for the diverse population served by publicly funded long-term care services.

Determining Reimbursement for Services

An evaluation of the patient's cognitive status is included in the case mix formulas used to determine the level of Medicaid reimbursement for nursing home care in Illinois and West Virginia (165) but not elsewhere. New York has recently instituted a reimbursement system based on research that compared a large number of patient descriptors (including diagnosis, prognosis, medical and skilled nursing care needs, cognitive and self-care abilities, and behavioral problems) with the amount of staff time required to care for nursing home residents with those characteristics.

Results of one phase of this research showed that differences among patients in mental status were less effective than other patient characteristics (such as self-care abilities and behavioral problems) in explaining differences in the amount of staff time spent caring for them. The cognitive measure used in this research was a judgment by the rater about the person's "mental status," with six choices for ratings: clear, minimal confusion, moderate confusion, severe confusion, comatose, or not determined (42). The research also showed that diagnoses indicating dementia, such as "senile dementia," "presenile dementia," and "Alzheimer's disease," were not helpful in explaining differences in the amount of staff time spent caring for patients (159).

In a second phase of the research in New York, other, less direct measures of cognitive status were used (see table 8-6). Together these items accounted for 12 to 15 percent of the differences in staff time required to care for residents. They were highly correlated with measures of self-care abilities, and the self-care items were more effective in explaining differences in staff time needed to care for individual residents. The cognitive items were not included in the final assessment instrument because they did not add to the accuracy of the instrument in accounting for staff time once the other factors in the assessment—primarily self-care items—were accounted for. In addition, the researchers concluded that the cognitive items were less reliable, more difficult to define, and more difficult for auditors to review than self-care items (114,158).

Since most long-term care providers agree that the care of persons with dementia is difficult and time-consuming, it is significant that the New York State research did not show a stronger and more direct relationship between cognitive status and staff time required to care for patients. One possible explanation is that the providers are incorrect. Alternatively, the measures of cognitive status that were used may not be valid indicators of the cognitive deficits that are most closely re-

Table 8-6.—Items Related to Cognitive Status: New York State Patient Assessment Instrument

Learning ability—*Process of understanding and retaining concepts or instructions.*
1. Listens, retains, and comprehends directions or teaching instructions. Knows what to do and when.
2. Difficulties retaining or comprehending instructions. Needs clues or continuous reminding.
3. Cannot comprehend and retain instructions. Must be shown every time.
4. Cannot comprehend and retain instructions. No instructions given.
5. Cannot determine.

Motivation—*Process of stimulating one's self to perform activities without external influence.*
1. High—Initiates activity, keeps appointments, willing to tolerate discomfort/pain to achieve goals.
2. Moderate—Will work toward goals but needs external support and urging.
3. Minimal—Passive, participates in activities when told or when it is required. Activities may be performed in a slow, mediocre or inaccurate fashion.
4. Poor—Resists activity, feels someone else should do everything.
5. None—Due to organic causes.
6. Cannot determine.

Refusal to care for one's self—*Physically capable but mentally unwilling to perform routine activities.*
(This is not due to physical limitations.)
1. Performs routine activities (e.g., Activities of Daily Living (ADLs)) to the extent physically capable.
2. Performs routine activities (e.g., ADLs) but not to the extent physically capable. Activities are performed incompletely or of mediocre quality.
3. Resists assistance by others in performing routine activities (e.g., ADLs), though needs assistance from others.
4. Refuses to perform routine activities (e.g., ADLs) of which physically capable. Staff must perform the activities.
5. Unable mentally to perform routine activities (e.g., ADLs), regardless of willingness.

SOURCE: New York State Department of Health and Rensselear Polytechnic Institute, New York State Patient Assessment Instrument, Albany, NY, March 1984.

lated to care needs. Another possibility is that severity of cognitive deficits is not accurately reflected in the response categories used. Since wide variations among patients in severity of cognitive deficits are manifested in wide variations in care needs, accurate measures of severity and careful analysis of the data in terms of severity would be needed to test the view of providers that dementia patients are particularly difficult to care for. Retrospective analysis of the New York State data for OTA showed that within each category of patients defined by self-care and behavioral measures and by nursing care needs, dementia patients were more impaired and required more

care than patients who did not have dementia (37) (see also ch. 6). Further research is needed to define the cognitive deficits and severity measures that are most closely associated with care needs.

Measuring Patient Outcome for Quality Assurance Programs

Government quality assurance programs primarily affect nursing homes at present. Since all the physical conditions that complicate cognitive assessment are common among nursing home residents, using the available instruments to measure changes in residents' cognitive status as an indicator of quality of care is premature. Analysis of the relationship between cognitive status and quality of care and a better understanding of how cognitive abilities can be expected to change over time in persons with dementia are both needed before cognitive assessment instruments are used as an outcome measure in quality assurance programs.

Identifying Dementia Patients in Health Services Research

Measures of cognitive status have been used with varying degrees of success in health services research. The MMSE was used in the Epidemiologic Catchment Area (ECA) Survey in 1981 and was successfully administered to 869 of the 923 respondents; 54 respondents were not or could not be tested (40). (Questions that arose in the ECA about the validity of MMSE for elderly respondents and those with less than an eighth grade education were discussed earlier.)

The 1982 to 1984 Long-Term Care Survey, a nationally representative survey of the Medicare population over 65, also incorporated a measure of cognitive status, the Short Portable Mental Status Questionnaire. However, the SPMSQ was not administered to many of the respondents with diagnoses suggesting dementia because a proxy answered the questionnaire for them (100). As a result, information cannot be derived from the survey about the relationship between cognitive status, self-care abilities, caregiver burden, and service utilization.

Finally, the pretest for the 1985 National Nursing Home Survey included a special study of mental status and mental health problems. However, the response rate for the special study was somewhat lower than for the other sections of the survey, and it was eliminated after the pretest (100). Thus, potentially valuable information about the relationship between the individual's mental status and other aspects of his or her functioning and care needs cannot be derived from the survey results. The pretest data, however, provide a source of pertinent information for the study of dementia among nursing home residents (100).

Supplementing Current Procedures

Although available cognitive assessment procedures frequently lack the accuracy needed for public policy applications, their use in conjunction with other measures would help to focus the attention of the long-term care system on the needs of persons with dementia. **Just as current procedures for establishing eligibility, determining reimbursement, monitoring quality of care, and identifying patients in health services research emphasize medical and health care needs, new procedures that require assessment of cognitive status would emphasize the role of cognitive impairment in long-term care and ensure at a minimum that the cognitive deficits of patients would be identified**. That beneficial side effect is an important consideration in public policy decisions about the use of cognitive assessment procedures and instruments.

ASSESSMENT OF SELF-CARE ABILITIES

Self-care abilities include those related to personal care (such as bathing, dressing, eating, and using the toilet) commonly referred to as activities of daily living (ADLs) and abilities related to independent living, commonly referred to as instrumental activities of daily living (IADLs). IADLs include handling money, using the telephone, shopping, cleaning, and preparing meals.

Although cognitive deficits are the most basic and universal feature of dementia, it is the deterioration in patients' self-care abilities that most often necessitates long-term care. Assessment of such abilities can help to identify activities an individual needs help with and the services he or she needs. Patient response to various treatment approaches can also be monitored in terms of changes in self-care abilities (151). Since decline in self-care abilities results from cognitive loss, assessment of self-care abilities is sometimes used in research as an indicator of the severity of the cognitive loss. Finally, measures of self-care abilities are less affected by ethnic, cultural, or educational background than measures of cognitive abilities, and may therefore be a more valid indicator of an individual's condition and care needs than cognitive test performance.

Research indicates that self-care deficits are more closely correlated with institutional placement than either diagnosis or the need for specific medical or skilled nursing care services (183). As a result, some experts have suggested that measures of self-care abilities should be used to determine eligibility for nursing home care. Although that approach has not yet been tried, some States are using these measures to determine level of Medicaid reimbursement for nursing home residents (as discussed later in this section).

Instruments To Measure Self-Care Abilities

Most assessment instruments to measure self-care abilities were developed for physically impaired individuals. The Index of Independence in Activities of Daily Living, the most widely used measure of ADLs, was developed for evaluation of patients with hip fractures (77). Also known as the Katz ADL Scale, it assesses six abilities: bathing, dressing, going to the toilet, transferring from bed or chair, continence, and feeding (see figure 8-1). Other ADL instruments include these personal care abilities plus others, such as grooming. Items related to mobility, such as walking, using a wheelchair, climbing stairs, and going outside, are included in some ADL scales but are considered as a distinct area of functioning in other assessment batteries (74,76).

Figure 8-1.—Index of Independence in Activities of Daily Living

Independence means without supervision, direction, or active personal assistance, except as specifically noted below. This is based on actual status and not on ability. A patient who refuses to perform a function is considered as not performing the function, even though he or she is deemed able.

Bathing (sponge, shower, or tub):
Independent: assistance in bathing a single part (as back or disabled extremity) or bathes self completely.
Dependent: assistance in bathing more than one part of body; assistance in getting in or out of tub or does not bathe self.

Dressing:
Independent: gets clothes from closets and drawers; puts on clothes, outer garments, braces; manages fasteners; act of tying shoes is excluded.
Dependent: does not dress self or remains partly undressed.

Going to toilet:
Independent: gets to toilet; gets on and off toilet; arranges clothes, cleans organs of excretion (may manage own bedpan used at night only and may or may not be using mechanical supports).
Dependent: uses bedpan or commode or receives assistance in getting to and using toilet.

Transfer:
Independent: moves in and out of bed independently and moves in and out of chair independently (may or may not be using mechanical supports).
Dependent: assistance in moving in or out of bed and/or chair; does not perform one or more transfers.

Continence:
Independent: urination and defecation entirely self-controlled.
Dependent: partial or total incontinence in urination or defecation, partial or total control by enemas, catheters, or regulated use of urinals or bedpans.

Feeding:
Independent: gets food from plate or its equivalent into mouth (precutting of meat and preparation of food, as buttering bread, are excluded from evaluation).
Dependent: assistance in act of feeding (see above); does not eat at all or parenteral feeding.

For each area of functioning listed below, check description that applies. (The word "assistance" means supervision, direction of personal assistance.)

Bathing—either sponge bath, tub bath, or shower:

☐	☐	☐
Receives no assistance (gets in and out of tub by self if tub is usual means of bathing)	Receives assistance in bathing only one part of body (such as back or a leg)	Receives assistance in bathing more than one part of body (or not bathed)

Dressing—Gets clothes from closets and drawers—including underclothes, outer garments, and using fasteners (including braces, if worn):

☐	☐	☐
Gets clothes and gets completely dressed without assistance	Gets clothes and gets dressed without assistance except for assistance in tying shoes	Receives assistance in getting clothes or in getting dressed, or stays partly or completely undressed.

Toileting—Going to the "toilet room" for bowel and urine elimination; cleaning self after elimination and arranging clothes:

☐	☐	☐
Goes to "toilet room," cleans self, and arranges clothes without assistance (may use object for support, such as cane, walker, or wheelchair and may manage night bedpan or commode, emptying same in morning	Receives assistance in going to "toilet room" or in cleaning self or in arranging clothes after elimination or in use of night bedpan or commode	Does not go to room termed "toilet" for the elimination process

Transfer:

☐	☐	☐
Moves in and out of bed as well as in and out of chair without assistance (may be using object for support such as cane or walker)	Moves in or out of bed or chair with assistance	Does not get out of bed

Continence:

☐	☐	☐
Controls urination and bowel movement completely by self	Has occasional "accidents"	Supervision helps keep urine or bowel control; catheter is used or is incontinent

Feeding:

☐	☐	☐
Feeds self without assistance	Feeds self except for getting assistance in cutting meat or buttering bread	Receives assistance in feeding or is fed partly or completely by using tubes or intravenous fluids

SOURCE: S. Katz, A.B. Ford, R.W. Moskowitz, et al., "Studies of Illness in the Aged. The Index of ADL: A Standardized Measure of Biological and Psychosocial Function," *Journal of the American Medical Association* 185:914-919, 1963.

IADL scales measure a wider range of activities. For example, the Philadelphia Geriatric Center Instrumental Activities of Daily Living Scale assesses patient ability to use the telephone, use public transportation, take medications, handle finances, prepare meals, and do housework and laundry (92). The OARS Instrumental ADL Scale measures most of these items plus shopping (30). The Performance Activities of Daily Living Scale includes telling time, signing one's name, locking the door, and turning faucets and lights on and off (90).

Although some consensus has developed about the most important ADL items to measure, there is less agreement about IADL items because of uncertainty about which activities are necessary for independent functioning (74). Since IADL items are primarily used to assess individuals who are living in the community, differences in lifestyle and living arrangements affect which test items are relevant. For persons who live alone, all the IADL items just listed may be relevant, while those who have someone to live with may not need to perform any of them. The sex and role responsibilities of the person also affect which IADL items are relevant (74,79,92). Thus, inability to cook and shop may not be considered a serious self-care deficit for a married man because it is assumed that his wife will perform these tasks (at least among the current cohort of older Americans). Yet the same deficits are regarded as a serious problem for a married woman who has always performed these tasks for her family.

Some instruments to measure self-care abilities are designed for self-rating, but most are designed to be completed by a caregiver, such as a nurse, nurse's aide, relative, or friend. Some instruct the observer to ask the individual to perform some of the ADL functions being rated (77,79).

Reliability and Validity of ADL and IADL Instruments

At first glance, the determination of whether someone can bathe, dress, and feed himself or herself would seem to be relatively simple and straightforward. Certainly ADLs can be more easily measured than some aspects of cognitive functioning, and when ADL measures have been tested using trained observers, standardized definitions of each item, and standardized assessment procedures, interrater reliability has been high. Interrater reliability may be higher for some ADL items than for others (122), but little research has been reported on this question. Interrater reliability is lower for IADL than ADL measures, but it is still acceptable (76,189). Observers can and sometimes do disagree about how to rate a given patient on these scales for several reasons.

First, there can be disagreement about how to rate a patient who is physically capable of performing a certain activity but does not perform it. As it is the individual's actual behavior rather than latent capabilities that determines that person's need for services, researchers and clinicians generally agree that self-care ratings should be based on whether the individual does perform a certain activity rather than whether he or she is capable of it (74,157,167). That approach seems appropriate for persons with dementia because little is known on a theoretical level about how cognitive deficits affect their capabilities.

A second problem is how to rate individuals who do not have an opportunity to perform certain activities. For example, patients in hospitals and nursing homes are seldom allowed to bathe without supervision. Yet they may be quite able to bathe themselves independently at home. Reliable measurement requires agreement about how to score activities an individual has no opportunity to perform (74).

A third problem is how to rate individuals who are neither completely independent nor completely dependent in certain activities—that is, those who need some assistance or who perform activities very slowly or in an unsatisfactory manner. The Katz ADL scale offers the rater three choices for each activity—complete independence, partial dependence, or complete dependence—but in the final rating, partial and complete dependence are combined, giving a dichotomous scale (77). Other ADL instruments use rating scales that include more options for categorizing the patient, but there is disagreement about the effect on reliability of the number and type of rating points. Some researchers assert that multiple rating points increase agreement between observers

(79) and that raters can be trained to correctly use scales with up to seven points. Others disagree.

The Functional Life Scale (157) has a complex system that involves rating the individual on 44 activities on the basis of overall efficiency in performing the activity, speed, frequency, and self initiation (see figure 8-2). For each category, individuals are scored on a five-point scale, from 0 ("does not perform the activity at all") to 4 ("normal"). This scale has been criticized for being too complex to be either reliable or useful (74). Initial testing indicated high interrater reliability for the points at each end of the scale, but lower reliability for the three intermediate points (157).

Assessment instruments with many rating points are inappropriate for certain settings because the amount of detail included is greater than the distinctions that can be made accurately. The appropriate amount of detail should be determined by the time available for assessment, the background and expertise of the raters, and the purpose for which the assessment will be used (74,186). When complex rating scales are used in nursing homes with limited staff and few professionally trained nurses to complete the assessment, reliability may suffer. In contrast, the same instruments may have high interrater and test-retest reliability in research or specialized care settings, where highly trained raters have time to carefully consider fine line distinctions between levels of self-care functioning.

The reliability of ADL and IADL instruments is also affected by raters' biases. One study that compared ratings by patients, their nurses, and a relative or friend on three ADL and IADL scales showed that patients generally rated themselves higher than their nurses did (154). Family members and friends rated the patients lower than the nurses did, and spouses tended to rate patients lower than other relatives or friends did. The researchers suggested that patients may rate themselves high because they deny their disabilities, while family members and friends may exaggerate patients' disabilities in order to emphasize their caregiving role and the burden of caring for the patient. Others have found that staff of an adult day care center rated patients much higher on self-care abilities than their families did (192).

Another study looked at ADL and IADL ratings of the same individuals by trained observers using an assessment questionnaire and by physicians and "health visitors" who had known the individuals over a period of time (179). The three rating sources agreed about ADL ratings in most cases but agreed less often about IADLs. Physicians' ADL ratings tended to match the ADL ratings based on the questionnaire, while health visitors' IADL ratings agreed more often with the IADL ratings based on the questionnaire. These findings suggest that self-care ratings derived from different sources may not be directly comparable (79,154).

Validity of ADL and IADL instruments has been evaluated by comparing findings from different tests or by comparing findings with patient outcome or clinical judgment (74). In general, however, ADL instruments have been assumed to be valid—that is, a rating of an individual's ability to get dressed is assumed to be a valid indicator of his or her ability to get dressed, and ability to dress oneself is assumed to be an essential aspect of independent functioning. Thus, the rating of ability to dress oneself is assumed to be a valid indicator of self-care ability. IADL items are also assumed to be valid measures of the activities they measure, but their validity as indicators of self-care ability is less certain because of the difficulty of determining which IADL items are relevant for various individuals.

More importantly in the context of this OTA report, ADL and IADL instruments are assumed to be valid indicators of self-care abilities for cognitively impaired people even though most such instruments were developed to measure self-care abilities in physically impaired people. There has been little analysis or formal testing of reliability and validity of these instruments for people with dementia, thus raising several theoretical and practical questions about their use with these individuals.

- **How do fluctuations in self-care abilities of persons with dementia affect the reliability and validity of self-care measures?**

For reasons that are only partially understood, fluctuations in self-care abilities are quite common in people with dementia and may be more

Figure 8-2.—The Functional Life Scale

	Self-initiation	Frequency	Speed	Overall efficiency	Total
Cognition:					
1. Is oriented for time (e.g., hour, day, week)					
2. Uses "yes" and "no" appropriately					
3. Understands speech (e.g., simple commands, directions, television)					
4. Calculates change (money)					
5. Does higher calculation (balance checkbook, etc.)					
6. Uses appropriate gestures in lieu of speech (not applicable for patients without speech impairment)					
7. Uses speech for communication					
8. Reads (e.g., street signs, ability to follow written instructions, books)					
9. Writes (e.g., signs name, writes or types letters) (include motor disability)					
10. Social behavior is appropriate					
11. Able to shift from one task to another with relative ease and speed					
12. Aware of self (e.g., of mistakes, inappropriate behavior, poor judgment, etc.)					
13. Attempts to correct own errors (e.g., of judgment, mistakes)					
14. Has good memory (e.g., names of people, recent events)					
Activities of daily living:					
15. Able to get about (with or without brace, wheelchair, etc.)					
16. Does transfers					
17. Feeds self					
18. Uses toilet					
19. Grooms self (e.g., wash, brush teeth, shave)					
20. Dresses self					
21. Bathes self (including getting in and out of tub or stall)					
Home activities:					
22. Prepares simple food or drink (e.g., snacks, light breakfast)					
23. Performs light housekeeping chores (e.g., meals, dishes, dusting)					
24. Performs heavy housekeeping chores (e.g., floor or window washing)					
25. Performs odd jobs in or around house (e.g., gardening, electrical, auto, mending, sewing)					
26. Engages in solo pleasure activities (e.g., puzzles, painting, reading, stamps)					
27. Uses telephone (e.g., dialing, handling. Do not rate speech proficiency)					
28. Uses television set (e.g., changing channel)					
29. Uses record player or tape recorder					
Outside activities:					
30. Engages in simple pleasure activities (e.g., walk, car rides)					
31. Goes shopping for food					
32. Does general shopping (e.g., clothes, gifts)					
33. Performs errands (e.g., post-office, cleaner, bank, pick up newspaper)					
34. Attends spectator events (e.g., theatre, concert, sports, movies)					
35. Uses public transportation accompanied (mass transportation)					
36. Uses public transportation alone (rate NA if item 35 is 0)					
37. Takes longer trips accompanied (plane, train, boat, car)					
38. Takes longer trips alone (rate NA if item 37 is 0)					
Social interaction:					
39. Participates in games with other people (e.g., cards, chess, checkers)					
40. Participates in home social activities (e.g., family gathering, party, dancing)					
41. Attends social functions outside of home (e.g., home of friend, dining at restaurant, dance)					
42. Participates in organizational activities (e.g., religious, union, service club, professional)					
43. Goes to work or school at comparable premorbid level (not housekeeping at home) (*Do not rate if item 44 is to be rated*)					
44. Goes to work or school at lower than premorbid level (*Do not rate if item 43 has been rated*) (Multiply item 43 or 44 by 2)					

SOURCE: J.E. Sarno, M.T. Sarno, and E. Levita, "The Functional Life Scale," *Archives of Physical Medicine and Rehabilitation* 54:214-220, 1973.

frequent and more extreme than in people with physical impairments. For example, some Alzheimer patients become more confused and agitated in the late afternoon, probably as a result of fatigue and the cumulative impact of overstimulation throughout the day. Self-care abilities may be markedly reduced at this time (called the "sundowning" period) than in the morning when they are well rested. Extreme fluctuations also occur at night, when persons with dementia frequently become much more confused. For example, some persons with dementia who are continent in the day become incontinent at night.

Because of fluctuations in self-care abilities, assessments for one individual completed by day, evening, and night staff in nursing homes can look like they observed three different people. Although some of these differences may reflect the way patients are handled by the three shifts and differences in opportunity (e.g., at night patients who need to go to the bathroom may be unable to get assistance or to get out of bed over the bed rails), others indicate real changes in self-care abilities. On a theoretical level, research is needed on how fluctuations in self-care abilities are related to cognitive deficits. On a practical level, research is needed to determine how fluctuations in self-care abilities affect the reliability and validity of ADL and IADL measures for persons with dementia.

- **How does environment affect the reliability and validity of ADL and IADL measures for persons with dementia?**

For physically impaired people, self-care abilities primarily depend on individual characteristics that remain constant from one setting to another, although the availability of assistive devices and the lack of environmental barriers affect self-care functioning to some extent. For persons with dementia, however, environment seems to affect self-care abilities in a more pervasive and fundamental way. Anecdotal evidence suggests that persons with dementia test better at home (101). They become more confused in an unfamiliar setting, and therefore less able to perform ADLs and IADLs. Yet little is known about the aspects of setting that are most important. Better understanding of the relationship between self-

care abilities and setting is a necessary prerequisite for evaluating the validity of ADL and IADL measures for these patients.

- **Do ADL and IADL instruments measure the aspects of independent functioning that are most often affected in dementia?**

The activities usually included in ADL and IADL instruments and the rating choices provided may not encompass the aspects of functioning that are most often affected in dementia. For example, while persons with physical impairments that cause weakness or restrict movement can be relatively easily rated as independent, partially dependent, or completely dependent in dressing, persons with dementia are more difficult to rate because they are often physically capable of getting dressed but lack judgment about when to do so and what to put on. Similarly, dependence in eating is easier to assess for physically impaired persons who cannot feed themselves due to weakness or limitations in use of their arms and hands than for those with dementia who sometimes feed themselves independently but other times wander away from the table without eating, take food off the trays of other patients, or attempt to eat things that are not edible.

When ADL and IADL instruments are used to project care needs, the differences between self-care deficits of the physically impaired and dementia patients become evident. For example, physically impaired individuals may be unable to shop because of weakness, poor vision, inability to walk, or inability to carry their purchases; they need someone to shop for them. In contrast, persons with dementia may be unable to shop because they cannot find the store or remember what to buy, but they can remember that it is necessary to shop; thus, they need someone to shop for them *and* someone to stop them from wandering off to "go shopping." **The tendency of a person with dementia to try to perform certain activities he or she is no longer capable of performing safely or effectively is not included on most ADL or IADL instruments. Yet it is an important aspect of the individual's functioning and has important implications for the kind of care the person needs.** In fact, that tendency often results in the need for 24-

hour supervision—a need that distinguishes persons with dementia from many physically impaired people.

To the extent that ADL and IADL instruments do not measure aspects of functioning that are often affected in dementia, they lack validity for these individuals. ADL and IADL instruments designed specifically for persons with dementia include two sections of the Dementia Scale (9) and the Functional Activities Questionnaire (126) (see tables 8-7 and 8-8). Both instruments use items that are particularly relevant for individuals with

Table 8-7.—Dementia Scale

Changes in performance of everyday activities
1. Inability to perform household tasks
2. Inability to cope with small sums of money
3. Inability to remember short list of items, e.g., in shopping
4. Inability to find way about indoors
5. Inability to find way about familiar streets
6. Inability to interpret surrounds (e.g., to recognize whether in hospital, or at home, to discriminate between patients, doctors and nurses, relatives and hospital staff, etc.)
7. Inability to recall events (e.g. recent outings, visits of relatives or friends to hospital, etc.)
8. Tendency to dwell in past

Changes in habits
9. Eating:
    Cleanly with proper utensils
    Messily with spoon only
    Simple solids, e.g., biscuits
    Has to be fed
10. Dressing:
    Unaided
    Occasionally misplaced buttons, etc.
    Wrong sequence, commonly forgetting items
    Unable to dress
11. Complete sphincter control
    Occasional wet beds
    Frequent wet beds
    Doubly incontinent

Changes in personality, interests, drive
    No change
12. Increased rigidity
13. Increased egocentricity
14. Impairment of regard for feelings of others
15. Coarsening of affect
16. Impairment of emotional control, e.g. increased petulance and irritability
17. Hilarity in inappropriate situations
18. Diminished emotional responsiveness
19. Sexual misdemeanour (appearing *de novo* in old age)
    Interests retained
20. Hobbies relinquished
21. Diminished initiative or growing apathy
22. Purposeless hyperactivity

SOURCE: G. Blessed, B.E. Tomlinson, and M. Roth, "The Associations Between Quantitative Measures of Dementia and of Senile Change in the Cerebral Grey Matter of Elderly Subjects," *British Journal of Psychiatry* 114:797-811, 1968.

Table 8-8.—Functional Activities Questionnaire

Writing checks, paying bills, balancing checkbook
Assembling tax records, business affairs, or papers
Shopping alone for clothes, household necessities, and groceries
Playing a game of skill, working on a hobby
Heat water, make a cup of coffee, turn off stove
Prepare a balanced meal
Keep track of current events
Pay attention to, understand, discuss TV, book, magazine
Remember appointments, family occasions, holidays, medications
Travel out of neighborhood, driving, arranging to take buses

SOURCE: R.I. Pfeffer, T.T. Kurosaki, C.H. Harrah, et al., "Measurement of Functional Activities in Older Adults in the Community," *Journal of Gerontology* 37:323-329, 1982.

dementia—for example, self-care items defined in terms of memory and attention deficits that are characteristic of dementia patients.

The ability to give and receive information and to interact verbally with others is an important aspect of independent functioning. One study found, for instance, that receptive and expressive communication were highly correlated with the amount of staff time required to care for nursing home residents (42). Language difficulties are common in persons with dementia. Yet ability to communicate is not part of most commonly used ADL instruments (76).

In many research and clinical settings, assessments are conducted by health care professionals trained to notice and evaluate communication problems. For public policy purposes, however, assessment instruments may be used by individuals who are not trained to assess communication problems. If communication difficulties are not incorporated into the assessment instrument, deficits relevant to an individual's safety and ability to function independently will not be noted.

- **What effect does the medical care emphasis in many agencies and facilities that serve individuals with dementia have on the validity of self-care assessment?**

Medicare and Medicaid regulations focus on medical and physical care needs, and facilities and agencies that serve Medicare and Medicaid patients tend to adopt this focus—to provide primarily physical care, to perceive their patients as needing medical and physical care, and to use assessment procedures and instruments that measure medical and physical care needs. Within this context, it may be difficult for nurses and nurse's aides, who are often responsible for assessment in long-term care agencies and facilities, to recognize other characteristics and care needs of dementia patients. This is especially true since the background and training of nurses and nurse's aides are usually in physical care. Moreover, when the assessment instrument that is used includes only two rating choices, dependent and independent, nurses and nurse's aides may have difficulty rating as dependent both a person with dementia who is physically able to bathe, dress, or feed himself or herself but needs supervision and reminders and a person with terminal cancer who is often too weak to bathe or get dressed.

Public Policy Applications

Establishing Eligibility for Services

Use of self-care measures to determine eligibility for federally funded health care and social services would increase access for persons with dementia because they frequently have self-care deficits but often do not have the medical and health-related needs currently used to establish eligibility. Clearly, the specific self-care items chosen as eligibility criteria would affect the number of such persons who would be eligible. Other variables that would affect which individuals would be eligible include the training given to staff members who perform the self-care ratings and administrative decisions about how to rate fluctuations in patient abilities at different times and in different settings and about how to define the selected self-care items.

Using self-care measures to determine eligibility would also make services available to many people without dementia who have other physical, emotional, and psychiatric conditions that cause self-care deficits. The public cost of services for these individuals would be considerably higher than that for dementia patients alone, and some people may oppose using self-care measures to determine eligibility for this reason.

Determining Reimbursement for Services

Several States include self-care measures in the case mix formulas they use to determine Medicaid reimbursement for nursing home care. Since 1983, for example, Maryland has used an assessment instrument that measures five ADLs (mobility, bathing, dressing, continence, and eating) to determine reimbursement levels. New York State uses four ADLs (eating, mobility, transfer, and toileting) in addition to other items concerned with medical care needs and patient behavior (32).

The impact on persons with dementia of using ADL items in case mix formulas depends partly on the relative reimbursement provided for groups with high ADL needs compared with other patient groups. It also depends on the specific ADL items and rating choices included. The Maryland system requires a rating of either independent or dependent on each item, so the problems in rating persons with dementia as completely independent or dependent apply to this system. The New York system offers rating choices that more adequately describe the problems dementia patients have with ADL functions (see table 8-9).

Measuring Patient Outcome for Quality Assurance Programs

Measures of self-care abilities provide a patient-oriented index of quality of care to replace the facility- and resource-oriented standards that have been used. However, validation of these measures for dementia patients is needed.

Relationship Between Cognitive Deficits and Self-Care Abilities

Cognitive loss associated with dementia is known to lessen self-care abilities, but little is known about the specific relationship between the two (13,63,178). It is often assumed that the cognitive deficits measured by commonly used assessment instruments are directly related to self-care deficits. Yet researchers and clinicians report that

Table 8-9.—Activities for Daily Living (ADLs) from the New York State Patient Review Instrument

Eating: process of getting food by any means from the receptacle into the body (for example, plate, cup, tube).

1. Feeds self without supervisions or physical assistance. May use adaptive equipment.
2. Requires *intermittent* supervision (i.e., verbal encouragement/guidance) and/or minimal physical assistance with minor parts of eating, such as cutting food, buttering bread or opening milk carton.

3. Requires continual help (encouragement/teaching/physical assistance) with eating or meal will not be completed.
4. Totally fed by hand; patient does not manually participate. (Include syringe feeding.)
5. Tube or parenteral feeding for primary intake of dood. (*Not* just for supplemental nourishments.)

Mobility: how the patient moves about.

1. Walks with no supervision or human assistance. May require mechanical device (e.g., a walker), but not a wheelchair.
2. Walks with intermittent supervision (that is, verbal cueing and observation). May require human assistance for difficult parts of walking (e.g., stairs, ramps).
3. Walks with *constant* one-to-one supervision and/or constant physical assistance.

4. *Wheels* with *no* supervision or assistance, except for difficult maneuvers (e.g., elevators, ramps). May actually be able to walk, but generally does not move.
5. Is *wheeled*, chairfast or bedfast. Relies on someone else to move about, if at all.

Transfer: process of moving between positions, to/from bed, chair, standing, (exclude transfers to/from bath and toilet).

1. Requires not supervision or physical assistance to complete necessary transfers. May use equipment, such as railings, trapeze.
2. Requires *intermittent* supervision (i.e., verbal cueing, guidance) and/or physical assistance for difficult maneuvers only.
3. Requires *one* person to provide constant guidance, steadiness and/or physical assistance. Patient participates in transfer.

4. Requires *two* people to provide constant supervision and/or physically lift. May need lifting equipment.
5. Cannot and is not gotten out of bed.

Toileting: process of getting to and from a toilet (or use of other toileting equipment, e.g., bedpan), transferring on and off toilet, cleansing self after elimination, and adjusting clothes.

1. Requires no supervision or physical assistance. May require special equipment, such as a raised toilet or grab bars.
2. Requires *intermittent* supervision for safety or encouragement; or *minor* physical assistance (e.g., clothes adjustment or washing hands).
3. Continent of bowel *and* bladder. Requires constant supervision and/or physical assistance with major or all parts of the task or task will not be completed.

4. Incontinent of bowel *and/or* bladder and is not taken to a toilet.
5. Incontinent of bowel *and/or* bladder, but is taken to a toilet every 2 to 4 hours during the day and as needed at night.

SOURCE: D. El-Ani, D. Schneider, and M. Desmond, *The New York State Patient Review Instrument* (Albany, NY: New York State Department of Health, 1985).

some patients who do poorly on cognitive tests are nevertheless able to function independently (46,181,189,191).

The correlations between individual scores on cognitive and self-care measures are far from perfect (12,31,192,194). For example, one researcher compared the scores of nursing home residents on the Short Portable Mental Status Questionnaire (SPMSQ) and on three self-care items—dressing, eating, and ambulation (191). Not surprisingly, among patients with normal or only slightly impaired cognitive abilities, none had impaired self-care abilities due to cognitive impairment.

Among those with moderate or severe cognitive impairment, however, half were completely independent in self-care abilities or required assis-

tance only because of physical impairments, while another one-third of the subjects required assistance only with dressing. Thus, most individuals who scored low on the measure of cognitive abilities were able to care for themselves, and the statistical correlation between the SPMSQ and self-care abilities was small (37). A stronger correlation (47) was found between the results of a semistructured clinical evaluation of the person and the assessment of self-care abilities. The researcher concluded that some aspects of functioning evaluated in the clinical interview, such as ability to respond sensibly to questions, may be more directly related to self-care abilities than the cognitive functions assessed by the SPMSQ.

Others assessed persons with Alzheimer's disease living in the community by using items from the Mini-Mental State Exam and the Dementia Rating Scale to measure five cognitive abilities: attention, calculations, recognition memory, recall, and orientation. ADLs and IADLs were also measured. The results indicated that measures of attention and the ability to recognize a design were associated with ability to perform ADLs, while other test items, such as ability to follow a three-step command, orientation to time, math score, and design recognition, were related to ability to perform IADLs (178).

These findings suggest that at least some commonly used cognitive test items may not be directly related to ability to function independently. In some cases, the test item may not be a valid indicator of the cognitive ability it is intended to measure (124,198). In other cases, the cognitive ability measured may be irrelevant to self-care abilities. Although assessment of such cognitive abilities may be valuable for research and clinical applications, it is less helpful in determining a person's need for long-term care or establishing eligibility for services. Further research on the relationship between cognitive and self-care abilities could identify measures of cognitive function that are closely correlated with the need for services.

Many researchers and clinicians have suggested that some persons with dementia have areas of

cognitive functioning that are relatively unaffected by the illness or have personality characteristics that should be seen as strengths in assessing the person's overall functioning (22,63,75,191). These patient strengths may explain some of the lack of correlation between cognitive and self-care deficits. Methods of measuring patient strengths have not received much attention, and research is needed on this issue.

Because of the apparent complexity of the relationship between cognitive and self-care deficits, measures of self-care abilities may be more reliable and valid than even the best cognitive measures for public policy applications such as establishing eligibility and determining reimbursement for long-term care services. Still, many persons with self-care deficits do not have cognitive impairment. Thus measures of self-care abilities are clearly not valid indicators of cognitive status. Likewise, they are inadequate for planning clinical and long-term care for persons with and without cognitive impairment. For these purposes, knowledge of the individual's cognitive status and the relationship between his or her cognitive abilities and self-care deficits is essential.

ASSESSMENT OF BEHAVIOR

Behavioral problems of persons with dementia can include wandering and getting lost; agitation; pacing; emotional outbursts; suspiciousness and angry accusations; physical aggression; combativeness; cursing; socially unacceptable sexual behavior; chronic screaming or noisiness; repetition of meaningless words, phrases, or actions; withdrawal and apathy; hoarding; and sleep disruption that results in nighttime wakefulness (see ch. 2). Obviously, not all persons with dementia exhibit these behaviors, but many go through stages in which they exhibit some of them.

Some researchers and clinicians refer to some of these problem behaviors as "mood disturbances." Although that term may accurately describe the problems from the patient's point of

view, the focus here is on behaviors that are problems for caregivers. "Mood disturbances" are therefore included only when they are manifested as behaviors that affect caregivers.

Cognitive deficits are the most basic and universal effects of dementia, and impaired self-care abilities usually cause the need for informal and formal long-term care services, but behavioral problems are often the most burdensome aspect of dementia for caregivers (see ch. 4). For family members and other caregivers, these behaviors can cause anxiety, embarrassment, fear, anger, exhaustion, and in some cases the decision to place the patient in a nursing home. In nursing homes, the same behaviors upset other residents and are disruptive and time-consuming for staff.

Some behavioral problems of persons with dementia are treatable even if the underlying disease is not (8,61,64,134). Yet in many settings these problems are not systematically identified. One study of nursing homes in upstate New York found that 23 percent of all residents had behavioral problems that were considered serious by the researchers (see table 8-10) (199). Attending physicians for these residents had noted problem behaviors in fewer than 10 percent of the cases. Nurses were much more likely to have documented the problems in the resident's chart. Since such problems are often treatable, methodical and thorough procedures for identifying them are essential for good patient care.

Table 8-10.—Serious Behavioral Problems Among Nursing Home Residents

Types of problem behaviors	Percent exhibiting the behavior
Endangering others:	
Physically agressive (deliberate striking, biting, etc.)	8.3
Indirectly endangering (unfastening others' restraints, dangerous smoking habits, etc.)	0.4
Endangering self:	
Physical self-abuse (scratching, banging head, removing catheter, etc.)	4.3
Dangerous ambulation (into unsafe areas, escaping restraints, etc.)	5.4
Physically resistive to care (spitting out medication, refusing to eat, etc.)	11.4
Other possibly endangering (verbal suicidal expression, severe agitation, etc.)	4.2
Disturbing to others:	
Verbally (noisy, abusive, etc.)	12.6
Inappropriate ambulation (into others' rooms, beds, etc.)	3.8
Physically disruptive (throwing food and objects, lying on floor, etc.)	2.5
Taking others' belongings and food	1.1
Inappropriate urination/defecation (urinating in waste baskets, smearing feces, etc.)	1.0
Sexually disturbing (exposing self, masturbating publicly, etc.)	0.4
Other bothersome behaviors	1.6
Nonendangering or disturbing to others but of concern to staff:	
Reclusive (refusing to leave room, socialize, etc.)	5.0
Hoarding (food, clothes, etc.)	0.6
Other	2.8

SOURCE: Adapted from J.G. Zimmer, N. Watson, and A. Treat, "Behavioral Problems Among Patients in Skilled Nursing Facilities," *American Journal of Public Health* 74:1118-1121, 1984.

Instruments To Measure Behavioral Problems

All assessment instruments that measure behavioral problems of persons with dementia are based on ratings by caregivers. Dementia rating scales are designed to measure the severity of dementia, and many of these instruments include some questions about patient behavior. For example, the Dementia Scale (9) includes questions about impairment of emotional control, diminished initiative, and purposeless hyperactivity. Other rating scales that assess patient behavior are the Alzheimer's Disease Assessment Scale (145), the Global Deterioration Scale (141), the Haycox Behavioral Scale (62), and the Clinical Dementia Rating Scale (69). Although these are useful in identifying some behavioral problems, none includes the full range of behavioral problems common among persons with dementia.

Assessment instruments developed for use by nurses and aides in evaluating psychiatric patients are sometimes used to assess behavior in persons with dementia. Examples are the Psychogeriatric Dependency Rating Scale (PGDRS) (186) (see figure 8-3); the Nurses' Observation Scale for Inpatient Evaluation (NOSIE) (68,164), and the Physical and Mental Impairment of Function Evaluation (PAMIE) (55). The Sandoz Clinical Assessment Geriatric Scale (SCAG) (161) and the Brief Psychiatric Rating Scale (BPRS) (121) were designed to measure treatment effects, including response to drug treatments. Although all these instruments include many of the behavioral problems seen in dementia patients, they were developed for psychiatric patients and do not include all the problem behaviors common among persons with dementing illnesses.

One behavioral instrument designed specifically for dementia patients living in the community (54) is illustrated in table 8-11. Relatives are asked to rate the frequency and severity of each item on a five-point scale. A companion instrument measures the impact on the caregiver of the patient's behavioral and mood disturbances (see table 8-12). One study that used these instruments found that passive and withdrawn behavior was much more distressing to caregivers than cognitive deficits, self-care deficits, or actively disturbed behavior

Figure 8-3.—Behavior Scale: Psychogeriatric Dependency Rating Scale

N	O	F	
☐	☐	☐	Disruptive
☐	☐	☐	Manipulating
☐	☐	☐	Wandering
☐	☐	☐	Socially objectionable
☐	☐	☐	Demanding interaction
☐	☐	☐	Communication difficulties
☐	☐	☐	Noisy
☐	☐	☐	Active aggression
☐	☐	☐	Passive aggression
☐	☐	☐	Verbal aggression
☐	☐	☐	Restless
☐	☐	☐	Destructive (self)
☐	☐	☐	Destructive (property)
☐	☐	☐	Affect—elated
☐	☐	☐	Delusions/hallucinations
☐	☐	☐	Speech content

N = Never.
O = Occasionally = 2 to 5 days or less.
F = Frequently = 3 to 5 days or more.

SOURCE: I.A. Wilkinson and J. Graham-White, "Phychogeriatric Dependency Rating Scales (PGDRS): A Method of Assessment for Use by Nurses," *British Journal of Psychiatry* 137:558-565, 1980.

(54). Another assessment instrument includes 52 questions about patient behaviors and problems the family experiences in caring for the individual (134). Researchers using this instrument found that violent behaviors, memory disturbance, and incontinence were the most disturbing behaviors for family caregivers. Using a third behavioral instrument, researchers found that no cognitive, self-care, or behavioral variables were related to the caregiver's perception of burden (197). Analysis of the differences among the three assessment instruments could explain these divergent findings and indicate changes that are needed in the behavioral measures.

Reliability and Validity of Behavioral Measures

Since most of the instruments described here include questions about a variety of patient characteristics, reliability and validity figures for the instruments as a whole do not provide information about the reliability and validity of the behavioral items. Several studies indicate, however, that reliability is lower for behavioral than for self-care items (122,145,186). One reason is that the terms used for behavioral problems have different meanings for different people. A second reason is that behavior is profoundly affected by

Table 8-11.—Behavioral and Mood Disturbance Scale

1. Does not take part in family conversations
2. Does not read newspapers, magazines, etc.
3. Sits around doing nothing
4. Does not show an interest in news about friends and relations
5. Does not start and maintain a sensible conversation
6. Does not respond sensibly when spoken to
7. Does not understand what is said to him/her
8. Does not watch and follow television
9. Does not keep him/herself busy doing useful things
10. Fails to recognize familiar people
11. Gets mixed up about where he/she is
12. Gets mixed up about the day, year, etc.
13. Has to be prevented from wandering outside the house
14. Hoards useless things
15. Talks nonsense
16. Appears restless and agitated
17. Gets lost in the house
18. Wanders outside the house at night
19. Wanders outside the house and gets lost
20. Endangers him/herself
21. Paces up and down wringing his/her hands
22. Wanders off the subject
23. Talks aloud to him/herself
24. Seems lost in a world of his/her own
25. Mood changes for no apparent reason
26. Becomes irritable and easily upset
27. Goes on and on about certain things
28. Accuses people of things
29. Becomes angry and threatening
30. Appears unhappy and depressed
31. Talks all the time
32. Cries for no obvious reason
33. Looks frightened and anxious
34. Gets up unusually early in the morning

SOURCE: J.G. Greene, R. Smith, M. Gardiner, et al., "Measuring Behavioural Disturbance of Elderly Demented Patients in the Community and Its Effects on Relatives: A Factor Analytic Study," *Age and Aging* 11(2): 121-126, 1982.

Table 8-12.—Relatives' Stress Scale

1. Do you ever feel you can no longer cope with the situation?
2. Do you ever feel that you need a break?
3. Do you ever get depressed by the situation?
4. Has your own health suffered at all?
5. Do you worry about accidents happening to ......?
6. Do you ever feel that there will be no end to the problem?
7. Do you find it difficult to get away on holiday?
8. How much has your social life been affected?
9. How much has the household routine been upset?
10. Is your sleep interrupted by ......?
11. Has your standard of living been reduced?
12. Do you ever feel embarassed by ......?
13. Are you at all prevented from having visitors?
14. Do you ever get cross and angry with ......?
15. Do you ever feel frustrated at times with ......?

SOURCE: J.G. Greene, R. Smith, M. Gardiner, et al., "Measuring Behavioural Disturbance of Elderly Demented Patients in the Community and Its Effects on Relatives: A Factor Analytic Study," *Age and Aging* 11(2): 121-126, 1982.

many factors, including the person's physical condition, the time of day, the presence of different staff and family caregivers, and environmental factors such as noise and commotion. The fact that patient behavior changes in response to all these factors reinforces the importance of identifying problem behaviors; it also means that test-retest reliability ratings may be low.

Public Policy Applications

Although it is clear that assessment of problem behaviors is essential for good patient care, it is unclear whether behavioral measures are appropriate for public policy applications. At present, these measures are not being used for eligibility determination, but they are included in some case mix formulas to determine the level of Medicaid reimbursement for nursing home residents. Behavioral items are used, for example, in the New York State assessment instrument (see table 8-13).

In contrast, the assessment instrument used in Maryland does not include behavioral problems. Nursing home administrators in that State have argued that behavioral problems should be assessed and that reimbursement should be higher for residents with behavioral problems because these individuals require significantly more staff time than other residents. A study to evaluate these assertions found that behavioral problems, such as wandering and abusive, disruptive, and inappropriate behavior, do significantly increase the amount of staff time needed to care for these residents. However, no change was made in the assessment instrument or the reimbursement system. The State argued that residents with and without behavioral problems had been included in the original research that measured staff time requirements, so that the reimbursement level derived from that research covers the cost of caring for all residents (1).

In response, Maryland nursing home administrators have pointed out that the current reim-

Table 8-13.—Behaviors: New York State Patient Review Instrument

Verbal disruption: by yelling, baiting, threatening, etc.

1. None during the past 4 weeks. (May have verbal outbursts which are not disruptive.)
2. Verbal disruption one to three times during the past 4 weeks.
3. Short-lived disruption at least once per week during the past 4 weeks or *predictable* disruption regardless of frequency (e.g., during specific care routines, such as bathing).
4. Unpredictable, recurring verbal disruption *at least once per week* for no foretold reason.
5. Patient is at level #4 above, but does not fulfill the active treatment and psychiatric assessment qualifiers (in the instructions).

Physical aggression: assertive or combative to self or others with **intent for injury**. (For example, hits self, throws objects, punches, dangerous maneuvers with wheelchair).

1. None during the past 4 weeks.
2. Unpredictable aggression during the past 4 weeks (whether mild or extreme), *but not at least once per week*.
3. Predictable aggression during specific care routines or as a reaction to normal stimuli (e.g., bumped into), regardless of frequency. May strike or fight.
4. Unpredictable, recurring aggression at least once per week during the past 4 weeks for no apparent or foretold reason (i.e., not just during specific care routines or as a reaction to normal stimuli).
5. Patient is at level #4 above, but does not fulfill the active treatment and psychiatric assessment qualifiers (in the instructions).

Disruptive, infantile or socially inappropriate behavior: childish, repetitive or antisocial **physical** behavior which creates *disruption with others* (e.g., constantly undressing self, stealing, smearing feces, sexually displaying oneself to others), exclude verbal actions. Read the instructions for other exclusions.

1. No infantile or socially inappropriate behavior, whether or not disruptive, during the past 4 weeks.
2. Displays this behavior, but is not disruptive to others (e.g., rocking in place).
3. Disruptive behavior during the past 4 weeks, but *not* at least once per week.
4. Disruptive behavior at least *once per week* during the past 4 weeks.
5. Patients is at level #4 above, but does not fulfill the active treatment and psychiatric assessment qualifiers (in instructions).

Hallucinations: experienced at least once per week during the past 4 weeks, visual, auditory or tactile perceptions that have no basis in external reality.

1. Yes
2. No
3. Yes, but does not fulfill the active treatment and psychiatric assessment qualifiers (in the instructions).

SOURCE: D. El-Ani, D. Schneider, and M. Desmond, *The New York State Patient Review Instrument* (Albany, NY: New York State Department of Health, 1985).

bursement level is fair only if the mix of patients with and without behavioral problems is the same in all nursing homes and at all times, which it clearly is not. Consultants hired by the State have suggested that nursing homes should be reimbursed separately for programs and services designed to resolve behavior problems. The consultants remain convinced, however, that behavioral problems are too changeable to be used to determine level of reimbursement (1).

The use of behavioral measures for quality assurance programs is also problematic. The prevalence of behavioral problems and an unexpected deterioration in patient behavior may be useful indicators of quality of care. However, questions about the reliability and validity of behavioral measures and the lack of well-documented information about the relationship between treatment methods and patient behavior limits the current utility of this approach.

Relationship Between Cognitive Deficits and Behavioral Problems

Although many persons with dementia exhibit behavioral problems at times during the course of their illness, some may never exhibit such problems. Conversely, many people with behavioral problems do not have dementia. Data from the Epidemiologic Catchment Area (ECA) survey in Baltimore show that persons with dementia make up about 9 percent of the population over 65, but they account for 15 percent of persons over 65 with behavioral disorders. Thus, persons with dementia are more likely to have behavioral disorders than those without dementia. At the same time, among all persons with dementia aged 65 to 74, one-fourth had no behavioral disorders. Among persons with dementia aged 75 to 84, more than a third had no behavioral problems. Finally, among persons with dementia who were over 85, about one-fifth had no behavioral problems. Conversely, almost one-fifth of persons who were not demented had behavioral problems (136).

These findings indicate that the relationship between cognitive deficits and behavioral problems is neither simple nor straightforward. In retrospective analysis of data from studies that did not collect information about the cognitive abilities of subjects, some analysts have used findings about behavioral problems along with other indices, such as self-care deficits, to try to identify subjects with probable dementia. In fact, several OTA contractors have used this procedure, which, while necessary for analyzing studies that did not include a measure of cognitive abilities, is far from ideal. Assessment of behavioral problems is clearly not a valid substitute for cognitive assessment for most purposes. Such studies in the future should include a measure of cognitive abilities.

MULTIDIMENSIONAL ASSESSMENT INSTRUMENTS

Multidimensional assessment instruments focus on some or all of the following: diagnosis, physical condition, cognitive status, self-care abilities, emotional and behavioral characteristics, family and social supports, financial status, and health and social service utilization patterns. Thus, they combine many of the elements of assessment instruments already discussed in this chapter.

Some multidimensional instruments are designed for evaluation of all elderly individuals. Others are designed specifically for persons with dementia and are referred to as dementia rating scales. Assessments using multidimensional instruments are recommended for elderly individuals because the physical, mental, emotional, and social aspects of their functioning are closely related, and information gathered about one area is frequently relevant to others as well (48,59,74,120). For persons with dementia, these instruments are valuable because dementia is manifested differently in each area of functioning in different individuals (29), and treatment planning requires evaluation of all aspects of functioning.

General Multidimensional Instruments

Many multidimensional assessment instruments have been developed for general use with elderly individuals. Each of the four described here has been used in research and, to a lesser extent, for clinical purposes and long-term care planning.

The Older American's Research and Service Center Instrument (OARS) (30) is a 105-item questionnaire that assesses physical and mental health, self-care abilities, social and financial resources, and patterns of formal and informal service utilization. No measure of behavioral problems is included. The Short Portable Mental Status Questionnaire is used to measure cognitive status. Once the questionnaire has been completed, a trained interviewer rates the individual based on the questionnaire results (74). These ratings are potentially unreliable because they involve raters' subjective judgments, and a computerized rating procedure has been developed to replace them for some applications (48).

The Functional Assessment Inventory (FAI) (128) is a shortened version of OARS that takes about 30 minutes to complete, compared with about an hour for OARS. Like OARS, FAI uses the SPMSQ to assess cognitive status and also measures physical and mental health, self-care abilities, social and financial resources, and service utilization. A trained interviewer rates the subject based on responses to the questionnaire. FAI has fewer response categories for each item than OARS and a somewhat different coding scheme (17,128).

The Comprehensive Assessment and Referral Evaluation (CARE) (58) is a lengthy multidimensional instrument developed to compare health and social problems of community dwelling elderly in New York and London (see table 8-14 for the topic areas covered). The Mental Status Questionnaire and Face-Hand Test are used along with other items to evaluate cognitive status, and some items from OARS are also included. As with OARS and FAI, the subject is rated by the interviewer based on responses to the questionnaire. While CARE evaluates many of the same patient characteristics as OARS and FAI, it has a stronger emphasis on assessment of medical and psychiatric problems (59).

SHORTCARE is an abbreviated version of CARE that includes 143 items to assess dementia, depression, subjective memory impairment, sleep

Table 8-14.—Topic Areas in the Comprehensive Assessment and Referral Evaluation (CARE)

Identifying data/Dementia I: census type data/country of origin/race/length of time spoken English

Dementia II: Error in length of residence/telephone number
General enquiries about main problems
Worry/depression/suicide/self-depreciation
Elation
Anxiety/fear of going out/infrequency of excursions
Referential and paranoid ideas
Household arrangement/loneliness
Family and friendly relationships/present and past isolation index/closeness
Emergency assistance
Anger/family burden on subject
Obsessions/thought reading
Weight/appetite/digestion/difficulties in shopping and preparing food/dietary intake/alcohol intake
Sleep disturbance
Depersonalization

Dementia III: subjective and objective difficulty with memory/tests of recall
Fits and faints/autonomic functions/bowel and bladder
Slowness and anergia/restlessness
Self-rating of health
Fractures and operations/medical and nonmedical attention/examinations/medicines or drugs/drug addiction
Arthritis/aches and pains
Breathlessness/smoking/heart disease/hypertension/chest pain/cough/hoarseness/fevers
Limitation in mobility/care of feet/limitation of exertion/simple tests of motor function
Sores, growths, discharges/strokes/hospitalization and bed-rest
Hearing/auditory hallucinations
Vision/visual hallucinations
Hypochondriasis
Disfigurement/antisocial behavior
Loss of interest/activities list
History of depression
Organizations and religion/educational and occupational history
Work and related problems/retirement history
Income/health insurance/medical and other expenses/handling of finances/shortages
Housing facilities and related problems
Ability to dress/do chores/help needed or received
Neighborhood and crime
Overall self-rating of satisfaction/happiness/insight
Mute/stuporose/abnormalities of speech
Additional observations of subject and environment/communication difficulties

SOURCE: B. Gurland, J. Kuriansky, L. Sharpe, et al., "The Comprehensive Assessment and Referral Evaluation (CARE)—Rationale, Development and Reliability," *International Journal of Aging and Human Development* 8(11):9-42, 1977-78.

disorders, somatic symptoms, and overall disability (57). Rating scales developed for SHORTCARE have been used to differentiate between depression-induced and primary degenerative dementia.

Reliability and Validity of General Multidimensional Instruments

The comprehensive nature of multidimensional assessment instruments may create the impression that they are more reliable and valid than instruments that measure only one area of functioning. In fact, the segments that measure cognitive status often incorporate instruments such as the MMSE and SPMSQ or use similar instruments. As a result, they are subject to the same reliability and validity questions that apply to instruments that assess only cognitive status. Similarly, segments of multidimensional instruments that measure self-care abilities and other patient characteristics are subject to the same errors as instruments that measure only these characteristics.

The reliability and validity of summary ratings derived from multidisciplinary instruments are uncertain for several reasons. First, the potential for subjective bias is high because summary ratings are based on an interviewer's judgment rather than on the respondent's scores on each segment. With trained interviewers, interrater reliability has been acceptable (17,35,52,57). However, the level of reliability that is acceptable for research purposes may be inadequate for public policy decisionmaking where, for example, eligibility for services might depend on the results of the assessment procedure.

A second problem that affects the validity of summary ratings is that they are based on assumptions about the relative importance of individual items or segments of the questionnaire. Such assumptions are seldom stated explicitly and may not be justified in some cases (74).

Establishing the validity of multidimensional instruments is difficult because there is no accepted alternate procedure for measuring many of the patient characteristics that are assessed. Most attempts to establish validity have compared assessment results with clinical judgments about a patient's status. Although such comparisons may work well for mental health items, they are less satisfactory for self-care abilities and social and environmental items, for which clinical assessment

procedures are less well developed. Some studies have tested validity by comparing findings from one instrument with those from another that may include some identical items. Other studies have used statistical techniques to group test items into discrete domains—a procedure that may not be a meaningful test of validity (74).

Dementia Rating Scales

Dementia rating scales are multidimensional instruments that define levels of patient functioning from least to most impaired. Some purport to track the progression of an underlying disease process from onset to severe impairment; these instruments, usually designed to assess degenerative dementias such as Alzheimer's disease, focus on similarities among patients and the regular progression of dementing illnesses. Others focus on the heterogeneity of persons with dementia; these describe categories of patients, with less emphasis on the regular progression of an underlying disease. The two types of scales (examples of each are described in this section) represent two different views about the nature of dementia, its etiology, and manifestations.

Because persons with dementia vary greatly in their functioning, depending on the severity of the dementia, some method of classifying them is needed for research purposes. For example, studies that compare physiological findings about brain structure or function with patient disability need to characterize patients' conditions as more or less severe. Similarly, research on all types of treatment must categorize patient status in order to measure change in response to treatment (140). Finally, efforts to describe the course of diseases that cause dementia require an agreed-upon method for categorizing patients in terms of severity. As research on dementia increases in response to public concern and more government funding, the need for reliable, valid, and generally accepted dementia rating scales also increases (145).

The Clinical Dementia Rating Scale (CDR) is designed primarily to measure progressive dementias. It describes five stages of dementia in terms of six factors: memory, orientation, judgment and problem solving, community affairs, home and hobbies, and personal care (see table 2-3 in ch. 2). An interviewer rates the subject on each factor on the basis of a medical and psychiatric evaluation, testing with several instruments (the Dementia Scale, the Short Portable Mental Status Questionnaire, and the Face-Hand Test), and an interview with a relative or other informant about the history of the illness and the patient's self-care abilities. Once the interviewer has assigned the subject to a CDR stage on each factor, the ratings are combined according to instructions provided by the authors, and the subject is assigned to a CDR stage overall.

Good interrater reliability has been obtained with this instrument using trained interviewers. Validity has been tested by comparing the results of some parts of the initial evaluation with the final rating and by measuring change in patients over time. However, the authors point out that true validity can only be demonstrated by following patients for a period of years to test the usefulness of the stages and by comparing CDR scores with autopsy data after a patient dies (69).

The Global Deterioration Scale (GDS) describes seven stages of primary degenerative dementia, which the authors describe as "a unique clinical syndrome with a characteristic onset and progression" (141). The GDS focuses on cognitive functioning but also assesses the impact of cognitive deficits on self-care abilities, mood, and behavior. Positive correlations between the GDS and the results of other assessment procedures and physiological measurements based on brain imaging techniques have been reported (140). In addition, anecdotal evidence indicates that families of some dementia patients have found this scale helpful because it describes the course of primary degenerative dementia, allowing family members to understand the disease and anticipate and plan for later stages (143). The scale has been criticized for underplaying the heterogeneity of persons with dementia and variations in the progression of primary degenerative dementia. Its authors suggest, however, that a significant deviation from the progression of stages in the GDS indicates that an individual may not have a primary degenerative dementia or may have other coexisting pathology (142).

The Multidimensional Assessment for Dementia Scale (MAD) (29) adopts a very different approach—emphasizing the heterogeneity of persons with dementia. The MAD scale portrays these differences graphically. For each individual, results of a comprehensive clinical evaluation are charted on seven graphs. Figure 8-4 compares two patients—one with early Alzheimer's disease and one with multi-infarct dementia—on three of the seven MAD scales. Graphs that describe different individuals are compared to identify subsets of dementia patients. The authors have noted different patterns among patients with multi-infarct dementia, Jakob-Creutzfeld disease, and Alzheimer's disease. Differences among Alzheimer's disease patients have also been noted (29).

Other dementia rating scales include the Alzheimer's Disease Assessment Scale (145) and the Criteria for the Diagnosis and Severity of Dementias (56), a scale used with the multidimensional CARE instrument described earlier. These instruments are not discussed in this section because of space limitations, and no implication about their relative value is intended.

Dementia rating scales are used as staging instruments. Staging is useful for describing an individual's condition over time and predicting the course of the illness, for monitoring response to treatment, and for determining the patient's need for services (see ch. 2). Negative aspects of staging are the difficulty of clearly separating one stage from another in progressive dementias and differences in the clinical manifestations and the course of the various diseases that cause dementia. Another major concern from the point of view of assessment technology is the reliability and validity of staging procedures. Questions raised in this chapter about the reliability and validity of instruments that measure cognitive, self-care, and behavioral deficits are also relevant to staging instruments. Combining findings in each of these areas with a staging instrument compounds the potential for error.

Clearly some method of staging is essential for research, and a concept of stages in dementia is useful for treatment decisions and for counseling family members about long-term care plans. **However, despite the obvious theoretical rela-**

Figure 8-4.—Multidimensional Assessment for Dementia (MAD) Scale: Clincal Profile, Course/Disability, and ADLs for an Early Alzheimer's Disease Patient and a Multi-infarct Disease Patient

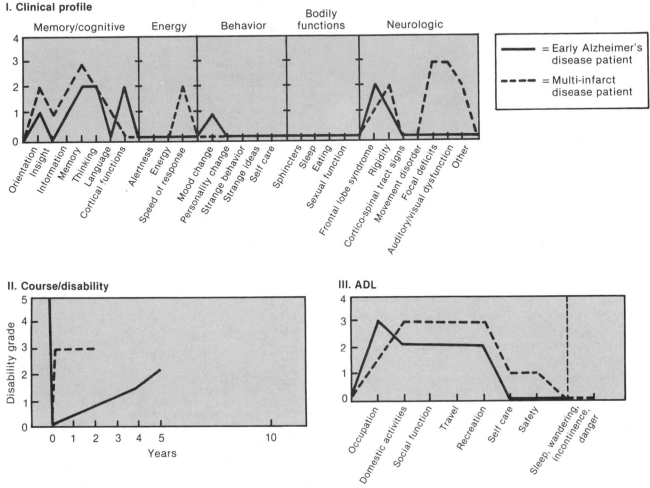

SOURCE: D. A. Drachman, P. Fleing, and G. Glosser, "The Multidimensional Assessment for Dementia Scales," *Alzheimer's Disease: A Report of Progress,* S. Corkin, et al., (eds.) (New York: Raven Press, 1982).

tionship between stages of dementia and each patient's need for health care and social services, the state of the art in assessment is not yet at a point where these scales can be used for public policy purposes.

ASSESSMENT OF CAREGIVER BURDEN

The impact on family members and other informal caregivers of caring for patients with dementia is discussed at length in chapter 4, and findings from studies that define and document caregiver burden are also covered there. This section briefly discusses assessment instruments used to measure caregiver burden and some of the problems that limit their reliability and validity.

Caregiver burden includes the physical, psychological, emotional, social, and financial problems experienced by family members and other informal caregivers (49). A better understanding of these problems is needed because families provide most of the care for dementia patients. Assessment of caregiver burden can provide information about the problems faced by families and can suggest interventions that might provide effective support for them (197).

Instruments To Measure Caregiver Burden

Some instruments to measure caregiver burden focus primarily on the caregivers' subjective or emotional reactions. The Burden Interview (197) is one example (see table 8-15). Others focus on more objective indices, such as changes in the caregiver's physical health, increased use of alcohol and psychotropic drugs, and worsened financial status. Many instruments measure both subjective and objective indices.

Research on caregiver burden is in an early stage, and many studies are primarily descriptive. The assessment instruments are frequently long questionnaires that include questions about the caregiver's physical, mental, emotional, social, and financial status; the relationship between the caregiver and the patient; and the physical, cognitive, self-care, and behavioral deficits of the patient. One example is a 24-page questionnaire used to study families of dementia patients in Michigan (20). A similar instrument was developed to study caregiver burden in families caring for elderly patients with and without cognitive impairment (47).

A different approach to assessing caregiver burden involves in-depth structured interviews with caregivers concerning the problems they face in caring for the patient and their methods of coping with these problems. One group used this method and an Inventory of Hypothetical Problem Situations to study caregiver coping mechanisms (95).

Reliability and Validity of Measures of Caregiver Burden

Many theoretical and practical problems affect the reliability and validity of measures of caregiver burden. Yet most studies do not report on the reliability or validity of the instruments used.

Table 8-15.—The Burden Interview

1. I feel resentful of other relatives who could but who do not do things for my spouse.
2. I feel that my spouse makes requests which I perceive to be over and above what she/he needs.
3. Because of my involvement with my spouse, I don't have enough time for myself.
4. I feel stressed between trying to give to my spouse as well as to other family responsibilities, job, etc.
5. I feel embarrassed over my spouse's behavior.
6. I feel guilty about my interactions with my spouse.
7. I feel that I don't do as much for my spouse as I could or should.
8. I feel angry about my interactions with my spouse.
9. I feel that in the past, I haven't done as much for my spouse as I could have or should have.
10. I feel nervous or depressed about my interactions with my spouse.
11. I feel that my spouse currently affects my relationships with other family members and friends in a negative way.
12. I feel resentful about my interactions with my spouse.
13. I am afraid of what the future holds for my spouse.
14. I feel pleased about my interactions with my spouse.
15. It's painful to watch my spouse age.
16. I feel useful in my interactions with my spouse.
17. I feel my spouse is dependent.
18. I feel strained in my interactions with my spouse.
19. I feel that my health has suffered because of my involvement with my spouse.
20. I feel that I am contributing to the well-being of my spouse.
21. I feel that the present situation with my spouse doesn't allow me as much privacy as I'd like.
22. I feel that my social life has suffered because of my involvement with my spouse.
23. I wish that my spouse and I had a better relationship.
24. I feel that my spouse doesn't appreciate what I do for him/her as much as I would like.
25. I feel uncomfortable when I have friends over.
26. I feel that my spouse tries to manipulate me.
27. I feel that my spouse seems to expect me to take care of him/her as if I were the only one she/he could depend on.
28. I feel that I don't have enough money to support my spouse in addition to the rest of our expenses.
29. I feel that I would like to be able to provide more money to support my spouse than I am able to now.

SOURCE: S.H. Zarit, K.E. Reever, and J.M. Bach-Peterson, "Relatives of the Impaired Elderly: Correlates of Feelings of Burden," *The Gerontologist* 20:649-655, 1980.

One problem that affects validity in some cases is the difficulty of identifying the caregiver. For example, if an adult child assists one parent in caring for the other, it is unclear who the primary caregiver is (49). Although both caregivers can be interviewed for a descriptive research study, public policy applications would require a method for identifying the primary caregiver.

A second problem is the difficulty of identifying a control group, without which it is impossible to determine which caregiver problems are related to the caregiving situation and which pre-date it. Yet deciding who is an appropriate member of a control group raises difficult theoretical and practical problems. For example, instruments developed to measure caregiver burden include many questions about caregiving functions, and therefore the control group cannot include non-caregivers (49). A solution is to use instruments that measure caregiver characteristics, such as physical health, emotional well-being, and financial status, without specific references to the caregiving situation. Many such instruments have been used previously with various population groups so that the problems of identifying an appropriate control group are reduced (49).

Experts have pointed out that many problems reported by caregivers may be unrelated to the caregiving situation. For example, depression could predate a person's caregiving responsibilities (131), and family problems unrelated to caregiving may be blamed on the caregiving situation (115). Moreover, assessments generally rely on self-reports of the caregiver, and accuracy is thus limited by the person's self-awareness, objectivity, and willingness to report problems, feelings, and events accurately.

Public Policy Applications

The many practical and theoretical problems that surround assessment of caregiver burden suggest that these measures should not be used for public policy purposes with legal or quasi-legal impact—for example, allowing publicly funded respite care to some families and denying it to others on the basis of findings from one of the available assessment procedures. Nevertheless, research on caregiver burden is important for government policymaking because it can help to identify programs that support caregivers and that minimize incentives for premature or inappropriate institutionalization of persons with dementia. Development and validation of improved procedures for measuring caregiver burden is an integral part of this research effort.

THE ASSESSMENT PROCESS

This chapter has focused on assessment procedures and instruments, their reliability and validity, and their potential use in establishing eligibility for services, determining level of reimbursement, measuring quality of care, and identifying persons with dementia in health services research. Questions that have not yet been addressed are: Who should do the assessment? Where should it be done? And who pays for it?

Who Should Do the Assessment?

Considerable data, some of which have been discussed earlier, indicate that different observers vary in their judgments about the cognitive, self-care, and behavioral deficits of individuals with dementia. These variations reflect the training and orientation of the observer, his or her relationship to the individual with dementia, and other factors. While assessment instruments provide a common frame of reference for evaluating a pa-tient, interrater reliability is not perfect even using the simplest instruments and is further reduced when the assessment instrument requires a judgment or rating by an observer instead of a simple notation that an individual did or did not answer a question correctly.

The appropriate person or persons to do the assessment depends on its purpose and the instrument that is used. In the simplest case—a research or screening project using an instrument on which an individual's response to specific questions is recorded verbatim and only one answer is correct—an observer who has no clinical training and only a brief orientation to the instrument may be adequate. In the most complex case, in which a multidimensional instrument requiring judgments by an observer is used to plan treatment approaches and identify appropriate long-term care services, a multidisciplinary team, including one or more physicians, a nurse, a social worker, and others, may be needed.

One important question is the amount and type of clinical expertise required for reliable and valid assessment of persons with dementia. While the concept of a brief assessment procedure that can be completed by an individual with no clinical training is attractive in terms of cost and efficiency, the state of the art in assessment of dementia is not sufficiently advanced to support this approach in most situations. Questions about how cognitive test performance is affected by patient characteristics, such as visual, hearing, and speech impairments and educational, ethnic, and cultural background, and about how fluctuations in self-care and behavioral characteristics over time and in different settings affect reliability and validity suggest that considerable clinical expertise is needed for accurate assessment of persons with probable dementia. Such expertise includes knowledge about the physical, cognitive, and behavioral manifestations of dementia, functional mental disorders, and normal aging, in addition to interviewing skills and familiarity with the assessment instruments being used. Untrained observers lack this expertise. In fact, few health care or social service professionals have formal training and experience in all these fields. As a result, many experts advocate the multidisciplinary team approach for both assessment and treatment of persons with dementia (see ch. 9).

With regard to multidimensional assessment instruments, it is unclear whether different results are obtained when one observer evaluates the person in all domains as opposed to a multidisciplinary team in which each professional completes the section of the assessment in his or her area of expertise. OTA is not aware of any research that compares these two approaches to multidimensional assessment.

For purposes of establishing eligibility for services, determining level of reimbursement, measuring quality of care, and identifying persons with dementia in health services research, the question of who does the assessment is extremely important. The clinical knowledge, interviewing skills, and familiarity with assessment instruments of people who perform these functions for Federal, State, and local government agencies vary widely between agencies and in different localities. How that variability affects assessment outcomes and thus access to care, quality of care, and the validity of research findings is an important consideration that has received insufficient attention. Clearly, painstaking procedures for selecting and refining an assessment instrument cannot overcome problems of reliability and validity that arise from the way the assessment is conducted.

Where Should the Assessment Be Done?

Assessment of dementia patients is currently done (formally or informally and with or without the use of assessment instruments) in the offices of individual physicians and other health care and social service professionals; in hospitals, nursing homes, and other residential settings; and in all public and private agencies that provide services of any kind for elderly people. The type and quality of assessment, whether assessment instruments are used, who does the assessment, and how it is paid for are all related to the setting in which it is done.

Research findings indicate that primary care physicians often fail to recognize mental and behavioral disorders in people of all ages, and particularly in elderly people (51,71,104). Studies cited earlier in this chapter show that dementia is frequently not recognized in a variety of in- and outpatient medical care settings. Although data are not available, it is likely that dementia is also frequently not recognized in social service and other community agencies.

Many solutions for these problems have been proposed. First, training in the assessment of persons with dementia could be provided for primary care physicians and other health care and social service professionals and nonprofessionals who interact regularly with people at risk of dementia (see ch. 9). That approach would make assessment available in the places where patients are most likely to be seen. However, training for such a large number of individuals would be costly and difficult to implement. In addition, their other responsibilities and time constraints could limit the quality of assessment some of them would be able to provide.

A second approach is to train primary care physicians and other health care and social service providers to screen for dementia and then refer probable cases to a specialist for comprehensive assessment. Although that might improve the quality of assessment, it would also involve increased cost and at least one additional appointment for the patient and family. Since the specialist is unlikely to know the patient, he or she may be less able than the primary care physician or other care provider to determine whether there has been a change in the patient's cognitive or other abilities. Furthermore, there is disagreement about whether the appropriate specialist is a physician—a neurologist or psychiatrist, for example—or a clinical psychologist, psychiatric social worker, psychiatric nurse, or other mental health professional.

As discussed in chapter 6, fewer elderly than younger people are seen by mental health professionals. Many reasons for this have been cited, including the preference of many such professionals to work with younger patients, negative attitudes about the efficacy of treatment for elderly patients, lack of training programs in geriatric mental health, and the preference of many elderly people to seek treatment from a physical rather than mental health care provider. The extent to which these obstacles can be overcome is unclear, and it is therefore unclear whether government initiatives to increase access to assessment for persons with dementia should focus on increasing referrals from primary care providers to mental health specialists.

Geriatric assessment centers (GACs) are another setting for assessment of persons with dementia. GACs are common in Britain but have been introduced in the United States only in the last 8 to 10 years. They are generally hospital-based and are designed to provide multidisciplinary assessment focused on functional status and medical, psychological, and social needs, in addition to short-term treatment and assistance with long-term care planning for elderly patients (150). Most GACs serve inpatients, but some also provide services on an outpatient basis (105,112,153,188). Both in- and outpatient GACs evaluate persons with dementia. In fact, data from two outpatient centers show that 46 and 32 percent of their patients re-

spectively were diagnosed as having dementia (105,188).

Advantages of GACs for assessment of persons with dementia are the availability of a multidisciplinary team; the focus on physical, mental, emotional, and social aspects of patient functioning and their interrelationship; the emphasis on identification and treatment of physical conditions that frequently cause excess disability; and the availability in the hospital setting of a variety of health professionals, including physical therapists, occupational therapists, dietitians, neurologists, psychiatrists, urologists, and other physician specialists who can assist with diagnosis and treatment for these patients. Possible disadvantages are cost and their relative scarcity.

Until recently, there have been few GACs in this country, so that patients and their families had to travel considerable distances to the nearest center. The number of centers is increasing, and anecdotal evidence and reports in the literature suggest that some hospitals that do not have a GAC instead have a multidisciplinary geriatric consultation team that provides assessment for patients throughout the hospital (19,98,160). In many hospitals, however, such services are not available.

Evaluation and treatment in inpatient GACs is expensive. As a result, some experts have suggested that use of GACs should be limited to certain types of elderly patients for whom its benefits have been clearly demonstrated in terms of longer survival, improved functional status, and decreased use of institutional services (149,152). Patients with severe dementia (defined as those with well-diagnosed dementia who can perform no more than three ADLs) are excluded from one well-known VA geriatric assessment center because research indicates that the GAC intervention has less effect on outcome for them than for other patient groups (150,151). Other VA geriatric assessment centers continue to admit patients with severe dementia, however (117). Geriatric assessment in outpatient centers is less expensive. In addition, the patients are still living in the community—thus allowing a truer impression of their functional status and family supports (105).

The specialized dementia research centers funded by the National Institute on Aging and the

National Institute of Mental Health are another setting for comprehensive assessment of persons with dementia. Expanding the number of these centers will increase access to assessment. In addition, legislation enacted in 1986 authorizes the creation of 5 to 10 Alzheimer's disease diagnosis and treatment centers to provide multidisciplinary assessment in addition to a variety of other services for persons with dementia and their families. The advantages of such centers are the concentration of expertise in one setting and the unitary focus on dementia. One disadvantage is that patients and their families have to travel considerable distances to reach a center. Furthermore, the relatively small number of centers cannot cope with the large number of patients needing assessment.

In some communities, assessment for dementia patients is provided by community mental health centers and public health and social service agencies. However, the extent of such services varies greatly in different localities. Studies cited in chapter 6 suggest that many community mental health centers currently provide no special services for persons with dementia, and no information is available about services provided for these persons by other community agencies. One advantage of providing assessment services in the local community is ease of access by the patient and family. In addition, local agencies may have greater awareness of long-term care services in the community than a regional dementia research, treatment, and education center would.

In addition to the settings already discussed, comprehensive assessment for persons with dementia can be provided in nursing homes and in the individual's home. Some community mental health centers provide outreach services in nursing homes, including patient assessment and consultation with the nursing home staff about medications and management techniques for residents with emotional and behavioral problems (2,99). Some outpatient geriatric assessment centers may provide similar services.

Comprehensive assessment in the patient's home is standard in Great Britain but rarely available in this country. Home health care agencies here routinely provide a general nursing assessment in the home and less frequently an evaluation by a social worker. However, these procedures usually do not focus on cognitive status and self-care and behavioral problems associated with dementia. Physician evaluation is seldom provided at home.

Some reports of comprehensive geriatric assessment in the patient's home have appeared in the literature (27,96). Advantages of this approach are the opportunity to observe the home environment and the interaction of family members directly, and to observe the patient at his or her optimal level of functioning, in the environment that he or she is most familiar with. Disadvantages are the time it takes for highly paid health care professionals to travel to the person's home and the consequent cost of home assessment compared to outpatient assessment in a GAC or a community mental health center.

Who Pays for the Assessment?

Medicare and Medicaid pay for physician diagnosis of disorders that cause dementia and lab tests associated with diagnosis. It has been noted, however, that the level of reimbursement is generally inadequate for the time required to complete a history, physical and neurological examination, to do a mental status exam, and to discuss the problem with the family (78,187). In addition, reimbursement is generally not provided for nonphysician professionals, such as nurses and social workers, who are frequently involved in the assessment process. Changes in these reimbursement policies could increase access to assessment for dementia patients.

Inpatient assessment is not covered directly under the Medicare Prospective Payment System (PPS). Some experts believe that the PPS discourages inpatient geriatric assessment because it creates incentives for shorter hospital stay while inpatient assessment often increases length of stay. (This is because patient conditions are identified that might otherwise have been missed and treatment of those conditions may extend the period of hospitalization (148)). While agreeing with that position, others point out that comprehensive geriatric assessment can improve quality of care for elderly patients and may thus benefit hospitals in communities where there is competition for patients (160). In addition, comprehensive assessment can help to identify patients who may be difficult to discharge (and thus costly for the hospital) so that the discharge planning process can begin early in their hospital stay. No information is available about whether the number of inpatient GACs has increased or decreased since the beginning of PPS in 1983.

ISSUES AND OPTIONS

Although many questions have been raised in this chapter about the reliability and validity of assessment procedures and instruments that measure cognitive, self-care, and behavioral deficits and caregiver burden, it is clear that they address the aspects of patient functioning that are important for determining long-term care needs and identifying appropriate services. In general, they are better indicators of patient functioning and long-term care needs than diagnosis alone or the patient's medical or skilled nursing care needs—thus suggesting that they should be more widely used for research, clinical, and public policy purposes.

Congressional policy options related to the use of assessment instruments to establish eligibility for publicly funded long-term care services and to identify persons with dementia in health services research are discussed here, along with options for increasing access to assessment for persons with probable dementias. Issues and options related to determining level of reimbursement for long-term care services and measuring quality of care are discussed in chapters 10 and 12.

ISSUE 1: Should the eligibility criteria for publicly funded long-term care services be changed to increase access for dementia patients?

Option 1: Retain existing eligibility criteria for publicly funded long-term services.

Option 2: Include a measure of cognitive abilities in the eligibility criteria for some or all publicly funded long-term care services.

Option 3: Include self-care and behavioral measures in the eligibility criteria for some or all publicly funded long-term care services.

Option 4: Develop and test a multidimensional assessment instrument to establish eligibility for publicly funded long-term care services.

The existing eligibility criteria for publicly funded long-term care services focus on medical and health care needs and tend to restrict access to services by persons with dementia who require primarily nonmedical long-term care services, such as personal care and supervision. Option 1 would maintain that situation. The inclusion of a measure of cognitive abilities in the eligibility criteria for Medicare, Medicaid, and VA services (option 2) would increase access to services for these persons. It would also make services available to persons with cognitive deficits resulting from other conditions, including depression, mental retardation, and chronic mental illness, unless these groups were specifically excluded.

Some advocates of increased publicly funded long-term care services for persons with dementia believe that services should also be available to persons with cognitive impairments caused by other conditions. Others maintain that only individuals with dementia or dementia caused by specific diseases should be covered. The requirements for a cognitive assessment instrument to be used for eligibility determination differ depending on which of these positions is chosen. At present, however, the state of the art in cognitive assessment is not sufficiently advanced to serve as a basis for allowing publicly funded services to people with cognitive impairment caused by dementing illnesses but not by other conditions. Such distinctions would be particularly unreliable for elderly patients and ethnic minority groups because of questions about the validity of cognitive assessment procedures and instruments for them.

Nor are currently available procedures and instruments able to differentiate between different diseases and conditions that cause dementia with sufficient accuracy to support Federal programs directed specifically toward those with Alzheimer's disease, multi-infarct dementia, or other designations that have been suggested. At the same time, inclusion of a cognitive measure in the eligibility criteria for publicly funded long-term care services would insure identification of cognitive deficits and generate valuable information about persons with cognitive impairment who apply for these services and about assessment of cognitive status in this population.

Inclusion of self-care and behavioral measures in eligibility requirements (option 3) would increase access to publicly funded long-term care services for persons with dementia. If used alone, these measures would also make services available to individuals with a wide variety of cognitive, emotional, and physical conditions that limit self-care abilities. As with cognitive impairment, some people oppose extension of services to this large group of individuals, while others do not.

Self-care and behavioral deficits are generally easier to measure than cognitive impairments. Some experts argue that they are also more highly correlated with patient care needs than cognitive impairments and that cognitive measures are not needed to establish eligibility for services or determine the appropriate level or locus of care. Others argue that the long-term care needs of persons with cognitive impairments are significantly different from those with physical impairments and that cognitive deficits should be measured in addition to self-care and behavioral deficits. Research is needed to evaluate these opposing views and to define more clearly the relationship between cognitive, self-care, and behavioral deficits, and long-term care needs.

Option 4, the development of a multidimensional instrument for eligibility determination, would also require research on the relationship between patient characteristics and long-term care needs. Development and validation of such an instrument would pose difficult problems of reliability and validity, but its eventual use to establish eligibility for services would reflect current knowledge about the factors that cause a need for long-term care much more closely than existing eligibility criteria do. Such an instrument might also reflect the experience of families and other caregivers about which patient characteristics are most difficult to manage and might therefore be perceived by families and others as fairer than the existing criteria.

ISSUE 2: Should measures of cognitive, self-care, and behavioral deficits or of caregiver burden be required in federally funded surveys of the elderly and long-term care populations?

Option 1: Retain current procedures for selecting survey items to be included in federally funded surveys.

Option 2: Include measures of cognitive status in some or all federally funded surveys of the elderly and long-term care populations.

Option 3: Include measures of cognitive, self-care, and behavioral deficits and of caregiver burden in some or all federally funded surveys.

Congressional involvement in the selection of patient and caregiver characteristics to be measured in survey research would be unusual. Yet many recent federally funded surveys of elderly and long-term care populations have not included measures of cognitive status that permit the identification of people with cognitive deficits. Thus information about the number and proportion of survey respondents with dementia and the severity of their cognitive deficits cannot be derived from survey data. Lack of such information hinders the development of appropriate government policies for the care of these persons.

Many recent federally funded surveys have included measures of self-care and behavioral deficits, and some have included measures of caregiver burden. However, lack of information about the cognitive status of survey respondents means that correlations between cognitive status and self-care and behavioral deficits and caregiver burden cannot be derived from the survey findings. Furthermore, the data cannot be used to determine the relationship between patient characteristics, caregiver burden, long-term care needs, and service utilization.

The Department of Health and Human Services (DHHS) maintains that for Federal policy purposes the long-term care needs of cognitively impaired people are not significantly different from those of physically impaired people. That position may be reflected in the relatively small emphasis on cognitive status v. self-care abilities and other patient characteristics in DHHS-funded research. Although that view may ultimately prove to be correct, available data are insufficient to justify it at present. Thus a congressional mandate may be needed to include cognitive status in addition to other patient and caregiver characteristics in federally funded survey research.

In February 1985, the directors of the five Alzheimer Disease Research Centers funded by the National Institute on Aging agreed to use two cognitive assessment instruments, the Information-Memory-Concentration Test (9) and the Mini-Mental State Examination (39) as part of a common assessment protocol. In October 1985, the directors of the six Alzheimer Disease Diagnostic and Treatment Centers funded by the State of California also agreed to use an instrument that combines the Blessed and MMSE tests as part of their common assessment protocol (78). The combined instrument, which addresses cognitive, ADL, and IADL deficits, is given in appendix C. Although designed for clinical evaluation, it might also be adapted for survey research.

ISSUE 3: What steps, if any, should Congress take to increase access to comprehensive assessment for persons with dementia?

Option 1: Do not take any steps to increase access to comprehensive assessment for persons with dementia.

Option 2: Increase reimbursement through Medicare and Medicaid for assessment by individual physicians and other health care and social service professionals.

Option 3: Increase reimbursement through Medicare and Medicaid for comprehensive

multidisciplinary assessment in geriatric assessment centers or by multidisciplinary geriatric consultation teams on an inpatient or outpatient basis.

Option 4: Set up a program of regional centers to provide comprehensive assessment in addition to other services for persons with dementia and their families.

Option 5: Designate comprehensive assessment of persons with dementia as a mandatory service of existing community-based agencies, such as community mental health centers, and provide supplemental funding for this service.

The VA provides comprehensive multidisciplinary assessment for eligible veterans, and some Alzheimer's disease research centers have negotiated agreements with Medicare and Medicaid for full coverage of comprehensive assessment for their patients. In general, however, Medicare and Medicaid reimburse physicians for diagnosis of dementia, but the level of reimbursement is often not commensurate with the amount of time needed for comprehensive assessment. In addition, reimbursement is frequently not provided for nonphysician professionals who may be involved in the assessment process. Increasing Medicare and Medicaid coverage and reimbursement for assessment by individual physicians and other health care and social service professionals (option 2) would be costly but would also increase access to this important service. Since many health care and social service professionals have not been trained in comprehensive assessment of persons with dementia, federally funded training programs might also be needed to develop the requisite skill base (see ch. 9).

Increasing access to multidisciplinary inpatient assessment would require changes in Medicare coverage or reimbursement policies that might involve:

- exempting inpatient GACs from the Medicare Prospective Payment System,
- creating a special reimbursement category for multidisciplinary assessment,
- designating dementia as a co-morbidity that

would increase reimbursement for hospital stays for persons with dementia in some or all reimbursement categories, or

- allowing inpatient assessment in a GAC or by a multidisciplinary geriatric consultation team as a covered exception for patients who met certain criteria.

Similar changes would be required of Medicaid and private insurance to increase access to inpatient assessment for persons under 65.

Analysis of the feasibility and cost of these alternatives is beyond the scope of this report. However, Congress could direct the Health Care Financing Administration to evaluate these and other alternatives and to report back with recommendations for implementation within a designated period. Instead or in addition, Congress could direct the Health Care Financing Administration to fund demonstration projects to test the efficacy of these and other approaches.

Increasing access to outpatient multidisciplinary assessment would require changes in Medicare, Medicaid, and private insurance that might involve:

- a special funding category for outpatient assessment by a multidisciplinary team;
- a significant increase in the current level of reimbursement for physician diagnosis to cover the cost of multidisciplinary assessment; or
- direct reimbursement for nurses, social workers, and others who are involved in patient assessment but are not usually eligible for direct reimbursement.

Again, analysis of the feasibility and cost of these alternatives is beyond the scope of this report. The analysis could be provided to Congress by the Health Care Financing Administration with options for implementing these or other such changes.

A program of regional Alzheimer's disease or dementia centers (option 4) would provide a locus for professional expertise in assessment and other services for persons with dementia and their families. While many experts endorse this model of service delivery, the number of such centers to be developed is limited by available funding. Requiring patients and their families to travel long distances to a regional center might impose hardship. Ideally, dementia patients should be periodically reevaluated during the course of their illnesses, and travel may become increasingly difficult as the patient's condition worsens. In addition, regional centers may have only limited awareness of the long-term care services available in the patients' own communities.

The provision of comprehensive assessment in existing community agencies, such as community mental health centers (option 5) could solve the problems of travel distances and awareness of local long-term care services that limit option 4. However, most such settings do not have medical staff to diagnose or treat physical problems that cause excess disability. In addition, the Federal role in defining services provided by community mental health centers has decreased greatly in recent years, and Federal funding for community mental health centers has also decreased. Implementation of option 5 would require further analysis of the impact of federally mandated services for dementia patients on the capacity of community mental health centers to provide services for other patient groups. Similar analysis would be needed before mandating the provision of comprehensive assessment for persons with dementia in other community-based agencies.

CHAPTER 8 REFERENCES

1. Abt Associates, Inc., "Analysis of the Maryland Patient Assessment System With Emphasis on the Needs of Behavior Problem Residents," Washington, DC, 1985.
2. Action Committee to Implement the Mental Health Recommendations of the 1981 White House Conference on Aging, American Psychological Association, *Mental Health Services for the Elderly: Report on a Survey of Community Mental Health Centers*, vol. II (Washington, DC, Retirement Research Foundation, 1984).
3. Anthony, K., LeResche, L., Niaz, U., et al., "Limits

of the 'Mini-Mental State' as a Screening Test for Dementia and Delirium Among Hospital Patients," *Psychological Medicine* 12:397-408, 1982.

4. Arenberg, D., and Robertson-Tchado, F., "Learning and Aging," *Handbook of the Psychology of Aging*, J.E. Birren and K.W. Schaie (eds.) (New York, NY: Van Nostrand Reinhold, 1977).

5. Berg, L., Danziger, W.L., Storandt, M., et al., "Predictive Features in Mild Senile Dementia of the Alzheimer Type," *Neurology* 34:563-569, 1984.

6. Blass, J.P., "Mental Status Tests in Geriatrics," *Journal of the American Geriatrics Society* 33:461-462, 1985.

7. Blass, J.P., "NIH Diagnostic Criteria for Alzheimer's Disease," *Journal of the American Geriatrics Society* 33:1, 1985.

8. Blass, J.P., director, Dementia Research Service, Burke Rehabilitation Center, White Plains, NY, statement to the advisory panel for the OTA assessment, Disorders Causing Dementia, Feb. 26, 1986.

9. Blessed, G., Tomlinson, B.E., and Roth, M., "The Associations Between Quantitative Measures of Dementia and of Senile Change in the Cerelral Grey Matter of Elderly Subjects," *British Journal of Psychiatry* 114:797-811, 1968.

10. Botwinick, J., *Aging and Behavior* (New York: Springer-Verlag Publishing, 1973).

11. Botwinick, J., and Birren, J.E., "The Measurement of Intellectual Decline in the Senile Psychoses," *Journal of Consulting Psychology* 15:145-150, 1951.

12. Breen, A.R., Larson, E.B., Reifler, B.V., et al., "Cognitive Performance and Functional Competence in Coexisting Dementia and Depression," *Journal of the American Geriatrics Society* 32:132-137, 1984.

13. Brody, E.M., and Kleban, M.H., "Day-to-Day Mental and Physical Health Symptoms of Older People: A Report on Health Logs," *The Gerontologist* 23:75-85, 1983.

14. Brown, R.G., and Marsden, C.D., "How Common Is Dementia in Parkinson's Disease?" *Lancet*, Dec. 1, 1984, pp. 1262-1265.

15. Buchanan, A., Brock, D., and Gilfix, M., "Surrogate Decisionmaking for Elderly Individuals Who Are Incompetent or of Questionable Competence," contract report prepared for the Office of Technology Assessment, U.S. Congress, 1986, forthcoming in *Milbank Memorial Fund Quarterly*.

16. Bucht, G., Adolfsson, R., and Winblad, B., "Dementia of the Alzheimer Type and Multi-Infarct Dementia: A Clinical Description and Diagnostic Problems," *Journal of the American Geriatrics Society* 32:491-498, 1984.

17. Cairl, R.E., Pfeiffer, E., Keller, D.M., et al., "An Evaluation of the Reliability and Validity of the Functional Assessment Inventory," *Journal of the American Geriatrics Society* 31:607-612, 1983.

18. Calkins, E., "OARS Methodology and the 'Medical Model'," *Journal of the American Geriatrics Society* 33:648-49, 1985.

19. Campion, E.W., Jette, A., and Berkmen, B., "An Interdisciplinary Geriatric Consultation Service: A Controlled Trial," *Journal of the American Geriatrics Society* 31:792-796, 1983.

20. Chenoweth, B., and Spencer, B., "Dementia: The Experience of Family Caregivers, *The Gerontologist* 26:267-270, 1986.

21. Cohen, D., and Eisdorfer, C., "Cognitive Theory and the Assessment of Change in the Elderly," *Psychiatric Symptoms and Cognitive Loss in the Elderly: Evaluation and Assessment Techniques*, A. Raskin and L.F. Jarvik (eds.) (Washington, DC: Hemisphere Publishing Co., 1979).

22. Cohen, D., Kennedy, G., and Eisdorfer, C., "Phases of Change in the Patient With Alzheimer's Dementia: A Conceptual Dimension for Defining Health Care Management," *Journal of the American Geriatrics Society* 32:11-15, 1984.

23. Cole, L.H., "Consideration of Ethnic Variables in the Assessment of Frail Elderly," paper presented at the annual scientific meeting of the Gerontological Society of America, San Antonio, TX, Nov. 16-20, 1984.

24. Corkin, S., "Some Relationships Between Global Amnesias and the Memory Impairments in Alzheimer's Disease," *Aging, Volume 19: Alzheimer's Disease: A Report of Progress*, S. Corkin, et al. (eds.) (New York: Raven Press, 1982).

25. Crook, T.H., "Psychometric Assessment in the Elderly," *Psychiatric Symptoms and Cognitive Loss in the Elderly, Evaluation and Assessment Techniques*, A. Raskin and L.F. Jarvik (eds.) (Washington, DC: Hemisphere Publishing Co., 1979).

26. Cummings, J.L., and Benson, D.F., "Dementia of the Alzheimer's Type: An Inventory of Diagnostic Clinical Features," *Journal of the American Geriatrics Society* 34:12-19, 1986.

27. Currie, C.T., Moore, J.T., Friedman, S.W., et al., "Assessment of Elderly Patient's at Home: A Report of Fifty Cases," *Journal of the American Geriatrics Society* 29:398-401, 1981.

28. DePaulo, J.R., and Folstein, M.F., "Psychiatric Disturbances in Neurological Patients: Detection, Recognition, and Hospital Course," *Annals of Neurology* 4:225-228, 1978.

29. Drachman, D.A., Fleming, P., and Glosser, G., "The Multidimensional Assessment for Dementia Scales," *Aging, Volume 19: Alzheimer's Disease: A Report*

of Progress, S. Corkin, et al. (eds.) (New York: Raven Press, 1982).

30. Duke University Center for the Study of Aging and Human Development, *Multidimensional Functional Assessment: The OARS Methodology* (Durham, NC: Duke University, 1978).

31. Eastwood, M.R., Lautenschlaeger, E., and Corbin, S., "A Comparison of Clinical Methods for Assessing Dementia," *Journal of the American Geriatrics Society* 31:342-347, 1983.

32. El-Ani, D., Schneider, D., and Desmond, M., "The New York State Patient Review Instrument," (Albany, NY: New York State Department of Health, 1985).

33. Escobar, J.I., Burnam, A., Karno, M., et al., "Assessment of Cognitive Impairment in General Population Samples: Educational and Cultural Artifacts," unpublished paper, May 13, 1985.

34. Eslinger, P.J., Damasio, A.R., Benton, A.L., et al., "Neuropsychologic Detection of Abnormal Mental Decline in Older Persons," *Journal of the American Medical Association* 253:670-674, 1985.

35. Fillenbaum, G.G., and Smyer, M.A., "The Development, Validity, and Reliability of the OARS Multidimensional Functional Assessment Questionnaire," *Journal of Gerontology* 36:428, 1981.

36. Fink, M., Green, M., and Bender, M., "The Face-Hand Test as a Diagnostic Sign of Organic Mental Syndrome," *Neurology* 2:46, 1952.

37. Foley, W.J., "Dementia Among Nursing Home Patients: Defining the Condition, Characteristics of the Demented, and Dementia on the RUG-II Classification System," contract report prepared for the Office of Technology Assessment, U.S. Congress, 1986.

38. Folstein, M., Anthony, J.C., Parhad, I., et al., "The Meaning of Cognitive Impairment in the Elderly," *Journal of the American Geriatrics Society* 33:228-235, 1985.

39. Folstein, M.F., Folstein, S.E., and McHugh, P.R., " 'Mini-Mental State': A Practical Method for Grading the Cognitive State of Patients for the Clinician," *Journal of Psychiatric Research* 12:189-198, 1975.

40. Folstein, M., Romanoski, A., and Nestadt, G., "NINCDS Final Report: Differential Diagnosis of Dementia in Eastern Baltimore," prepared for the National Institute of Neurological and Communicative Disorders and Stroke, Baltimore, MD, 1985.

41. Fozard, J.L., "Psychology of Aging—Normal and Pathological Age Differences in Memory," *Textbook of Geriatric Medicine and Gerontology*, 3rd ed., J.C. Brocklehurst (ed.) (New York, Churchill Livingstone, 1985).

42. Fries, B.E., and Cooney, L.M., *A Patient Classification System for Long-Term Care*, report to the Health Care Financing Administration, U.S. Department of Health and Human Services, April 1983.

43. Fuld, P.A., "Behavioral Signs of Cholinergic Deficiency in Alzheimer Dementia," *Alzheimer's Disease: A Report of Progress*, S. Corkin, et al. (eds.) (New York: Raven Press, 1982).

44. Fuld, P.A., "Measuring Components of Memory and Learning," *Assessment in Geriatric Psychopharmacology*, T. Crook, S. Ferris, and R. Bartus (eds.) (New Canaan, CT: Mark Powley Associates, Inc., 1983).

45. Garcia, C.A., Reding, M.J., and Blass, J.P., "Overdiagnosis of Dementia," *Journal of the American Geriatrics Society* 29:407-410, 1981.

46. Garcia, C.A., Tweedy, J.R., and Blass, J.P., "Underdiagnosis of Cognitive Impairment in a Rehabilitation Setting," *Journal of the American Geriatrics Society* 32:339-342, 1984.

47. George, L.K., "The Dynamics of Caregiver Burden, Final Report," submitted to the American Association of Retired Persons, Andrus Foundation, Washington, DC, 1984.

48. George, L.K., and Fillenbaum, G.G., "OARS Methodology: A Decade of Experience in Geriatric Assessment," *Journal of the American Geriatrics Society* 33:607-615, 1985.

49. George, L.K., and Gwyther, L.P., "Caregiver Well-Being: A Multidimensional Examination of Family Caregivers or Demented Adults," *The Gerontologist* 26(3):253, 1986.

50. Gershon, S., and Herman, S.P., "The Differential Diagnosis of Dementia," *Journal of the American Geriatrics Society* 30:S58-S66, 1982.

51. Goldberg, D., Steele, J.J., Johnson, A., et al., "Ability of Primary Care Physicians To Make Accurate Ratings of Psychiatric Symptoms," *Archives of General Psychiatry* 39:829-833, 1982.

52. Golden, R.P., Teresi, J.A., and Gurland, B.J., "Development of Indicator Scales for the Comprehensive Assessment and Referral Evaluation (CARE) Interview Schedule," *Journal of Gerontology* 39:138-146, 1984.

53. Granick, S., Kleban, M.H., and Weiss, A.D., "Relationships Between Hearing Loss and Cognition in Normally Hearing Aged Persons," *Journal of Gerontology* 31:434-440, 1976.

54. Greene, J.G., Smith, R., Gardiner, M., et al., "Measuring Behavioural Disturbance of Elderly Demented Patients in the Community and Its Effects on Relatives: A Factor Analytic Study," *Age and Aging* 11:121-126, 1982.

55. Gurel, L., Linn, M.W., and Linn, B.S., "Physical and Mental Impairment of Function Evaluation in the Aged: The PAMIE Scale," *Journal of Gerontology* 1:83-90, 1972.

56. Gurland, B.J., Dean, L.L., Copeland, J., et al., "Criteria for the Diagnosis of Dementia in the Community Elderly," *The Gerontologist* 22:180-186, 1982.

57. Gurland, B., Golden, R.R., Teresi, J.A., et al., "The SHORT-CARE: An Efficient Instrument for the Assessment of Depression, Dementia, and Disability," *Journal of Gerontology* 39:166-169, 1984.

58. Gurland, B., Kuriansky, J., Sharpe, L., et al., "The Comprehensive Assessment and Referral Evaluation (CARE)—Rationale, Development and Reliability," *International Journal of Aging and Human Development* 8:9-42, 1977-78.

59. Gurland, B.J., and Wilder, D.E., "The CARE Interview Revisited: Development of an Efficient Systematic Clinical Assessment," *Journal of Gerontology* 39:129-137, 1984.

60. Gustafson, L., "Differential Diagnosis With Special Reference to Treatable Dementias and Pseudodementia Conditions," *Danish Medical Bulletin* 32:Supplement 1:55-60, 1985.

61. Haugen, P.K., "Behavior of Patients With Dementia," *Danish Medical Bulletin* 32:Supplement 1:62-65, 1985.

62. Haycox, H.J., "A Simple, Reliable Clinical Behavioral Scale for Assessing Demented Patients," *Journal of Clinical Psychiatry* 45:23, 1984.

63. Heaton, R.K., and Pendleton, M.G., "Use of Neuropsychological Tests To Predict Adult Patients' Everyday Functioning," *Journal of Consulting and Clinical Psychiatry* 49:807-821, 1981.

64. Helms, P.M., "Efficacy of Antipsychotics in the Treatment of Behavioural Complications of Dementia: A Review of the Literature," *Journal of the American Geriatrics Society* 33:206-209, 1985.

65. Hinton, J., and Withers, E., "The Usefulness of the Clinical Tests of the Sensorium," *British Journal of Psychiatry* 119:9-18, 1971.

66. Hoffman, R.S., "Diagnostic Errors in the Evaluation of Behavioral Disorders," *Journal of the American Medical Association* 248:964-967, 1982.

67. Holzer, C.E., Tischler, G.L., Leaf, P.J., et al., "An Epidemiologic Assessment of Cognitive Impairment in a Community Population," *Research in Community and Mental Health* 4:3-32, 1984.

68. Honigfeld, G., and Klett, C.J., "Nurses' Observation Scale for Inpatient Evaluation (NOSIE): A New Scale for Measuring Improvement in Chronic Schizophrenia," *Journal of Clinical Psychology* 21:65-71, 1965.

69. Hughes, C.P., Berg, L., Danziger, W., et al., "A New Clinical Scale for the Staging of Dementia," *British Journal of Psychiatry* 140:566-572, 1982.

70. Jacobs, J.W., Bernhard, M.R., and Delgado, A., "Screening for Organic Mental Syndromes in the Medically Ill," *Annals of Internal Medicine* 86:40-46, 1977.

71. Jencks, S.F., "Recognition of Mental Distress and Diagnosis of Mental Disorder in Primary Care," *Journal of the American Geriatrics Society* 253:1903-1907, 1985.

72. Johansen, A.M., Gustafson, L., Risberg, J., et al., "Psychological Evaluation in Dementia and Depression," *Danish Medical Bulletin* 32:Supplement 1:60-62, 1985.

73. Kahn, R.L., Goldfarb, A.I., Pollack, M., et al., "Brief Objective Measures for the Determination of Mental Status in the Aged," *American Journal of Psychiatry* 117:326-328, 1963.

74. Kane, R.A., "Instruments To Assess Functional Status," *Geriatric Medicine* vol. II, C.K. Cassel and J.R. Walsh (eds.) (New York: Springer-Verlag, 1984).

75. Kane, R.A., and Kane, R.L., *Assessing the Elderly* (Lexington, MA: D.C. Heath and Co., 1981).

76. Katz, S., "Assessing Self-Maintenance: Activities of Daily Living, Mobility, and Instrumental Activities of Daily Living," *Journal of the American Geriatrics Society* 31:721-727, 1983.

77. Katz, S., Ford, A.B., Moskowitz, R.W., et al., "Studies of Illness in the Aged. The Index of ADL: A Standardized Measure of Biological and Psychosocial Function," *Journal of the American Geriatrics Society* 185:914-919, 1963.

78. Katzman, R., Lasker, B., and Bernstein, N., "Accuracy of Diagnosis and Consequences of Misdiagnosis of Disorders Causing Dementia," contract report prepared for the Office of Technology Assessment, U.S. Congress, 1986.

79. Kaufert, J.M., Green, S., Dunt, D.R., et al., "Assessing Functional Status Among Elderly Patients: A Comparison of Questionnaire and Service Provider Ratings," *Medical Care* 17:807-817, 1979.

80. Kay, D.W.K., "The Epidemiology and Identification of Brain Deficit in the Elderly," *Cognitive Disturbance in the Elderly*, C. Eisdorfer and R.O. Friedel (eds.) (New York: Year Book Medical Publishers, Inc., 1977).

81. Kiloh, L.G., "Pseudo-dementia," *Acta Psychiatrica Scandinavica* 37:336-351, 1961.

82. Kittner, S.J., White, L.R., Farmer, M.E., et al., "Methodological Issues in Screening for Dementia: The Problem of Education Adjustment," *Journal of Chronic Diseases* 39:163-170, 1986.

83. Klein, L.E., Roca, R.P., McArthur, J., et al., "Diagnosing Dementia: Univariate and Multivariate Analyses of the Mental Status Examination," *Journal of the American Geriatrics Society* 33:483-488, 1985.

84. Knights, E.B., and Folstein, M.F., "Unsuspected Emotional and Cognitive Disturbance in Medical Patients," *Annals of Internal Medicine* 87:723-724, 1977.

85. Kochansky, G.E., "Psychiatric Rating Scales for Assessing Psychopathology in the Elderly: A Critical Review," *Psychiatric Symptoms and Cognitive Loss in the Elderly*, A. Raskin and L.F. Jarvik (eds.) (New York: Hemisphere Publishing Co., 1979).

86. Kral, V.A., "Benign Senescent Forgetfulness," *Aging, Volume 7: Alzheimer's Disease: Senile Dementia and Related Disorders*, R. Katzman, R.D. Terry, and K.L. Bick (eds.) (New York: Raven Press, 1978).

87. Kral, V.A., "The Relationship Between Senile Dementia (Alzheimer Type) and Depression," *Canadian Journal of Psychiatry* 28:304-306, 1983.

88. Kral, V.A., and Muller, H., "Memory Dysfunction: A Prognostic Indicator in Geriatric Patients," *Canadian Psychiatric Association Journal* 11:343-349, 1966.

89. Kramer, N.A. and Jarvik, L.F., "Assessment of Intellectual Changes in the Elderly," *Psychiatric Symptoms and Cognitive Loss in the Elderly, Evaluation and Assessment Techniques*, A. Raskin and L.F. Jarvik (eds.) (New York: Hemisphere Publishing Corp., 1979).

90. Kuriansky, J.B., and Gurland, B., "Performance Test of Activities of Daily Living," *International Journal of Aging and Human Development* 7:343-352, 1976.

91. LaRue, A., D'Elia, L.F., Clark, E.O., et al., "Clinical Tests of Memory in Dementia, Depression, and Healthy Aging," *Journal of Psychology and Aging* 1:69-77, 1986.

92. Lawton, M.P., Assessing the Competence of Older People," *Research, Planning, and Action for the Elderly*, D. Kent, R. Kastenbaum, and S. Sherwood (eds.) (New York: Behavioral Publications, 1972).

93. Leber, P., "Establishing the Efficacy of Drugs With Psychogeriatric Indications," *Assessment in Geriatric Psychopharmacology*, T. Crook, S. Ferris, and R. Bartus (eds.) (New Canaan, CT: Mark Powley Associates, 1983).

94. Lees, A.J., "Parkinson's Disease and Dementia," *Lancet*, Jan. 5, 1985, pp. 43-44.

95. Levine, N.B., Dastoor, D.P., and Gendron, C.D., "Coping With Dementia: A Pilot Study," *Journal of the American Geriatrics Society* 31:12-18, 1983.

96. Levy, M.T., "Psychiatric Assessment of Elderly Patients in the Home: A Survey of 176 Cases," *Journal of the American Geriatrics Society* 33:9-12, 1985.

97. Lichtenstein, H., and Winograd, C.H., "Geriatric Consultation: A Functional Approach," *Journal of the American Geriatrics Society* 32:356-361, 1984.

98. Light, E., Lebowitz, B., and Baily, F., "CMLTC's and Elderly Services: An Analysis of Direct and Indirect Services and Services Delivery Sites," *Community Mental Health Journal*, in press.

99. Liu, K., "Analysis of Data Bases for Health Services Research on Dementia," contract report prepared for the Office of Technology Assessment, U.S. Congress, 1986.

100. Lockery, S., "Impact of Dementia Within Minority Groups," contract report prepared for the Office of Technology Assessment, U.S. Congress, 1986.

101. Mace, N.L., OTA consultant, personal communication, Aug. 22, 1986.

102. Mahendra, B., "Depression and Dementia: The Multi-Faceted Relationship" (editorial), *Psychological Medicine* 15:227-236, 1985.

103. Manton, K.G., Liu, K., and Cornelius, E.S., "An Analysis of the Heterogeneity of U.S. Nursing Home Patients," *Journal of Gerontology* 40:34-46, 1985.

104. Marks, J.N., Goldberg, D.P., and Hillier, V.F., "Determinants of the Ability of General Practitioners To Detect Psychiatric Illness," *Psychological Medicine* 9:337-353, 1979.

105. Martin, D.C., Morycz, R.K., McDowell, B.J., et al., "Community-Based Geriatric Assessment," *Journal of the American Geriatrics Society* 33:602-606, 1985.

106. Mattis, S., "Mental Status Examination for Organic Mental Syndrome in the Elderly Patient," *Geriatric Psychiatry*, R. Bellack and B. Karasu (eds.) (New York: Grune and Stratton, 1976).

107. McAllister, T.W., and Price, T.R.P., "Severe Depressive Pseudodementia With and Without Dementia," *American Journal of Psychiatry* 139:626, 1982.

108. McCahan, J.F., "Increased Attention to Dementia," *Journal of the American Geriatrics Society* 33:459-460, 1985.

109. McCartney, J.R., and Palmateer, L.M., "Assessment of Cognitive Deficit in Geriatric Patients: A Study of Physician Behavior," *Journal of the American Geriatrics Society* 33:467-471, 1985.

110. Mesulam, M.M., "Dementia: Its Definition, Differential Diagnosis, and Subtypes," *Journal of the American Medical Association* 253:2559-2561, 1985.

111. Mohs, R.C., "Psychological Tests for Patients With

Moderate to Severe Dementia," *Assessment in Geriatric Psychopharmacology*, T. Crook, S. Ferris, and R. Bartus (eds.) (New Canaan, CT: Mark Powley Associates, 1983).

112. Moore, J.T., Warshaw, G.A., Walden, L.D., et al., "Evolution of a Geriatric Evaluation Clinic," *Journal of the American Geriatrics Society* 32:900-905, 1984.

113. Natelson, B.H., Haupt, E.J., Fleisher, E.J., et al., "Temporal Orientation and Education: A Direct Relationship in Normal People," *Archives of Neurology* 36:444-446, 1979.

114. New York State Department of Health and Rensselear Polytechnic Institute, "New York State Long Term Care Case Mix Reimbursement Project: Executive Summary, Derivation of RUG II," 1984.

115. Niederehe, G., Fruge, E., Woods, A.M., et al., "Caregiver Stress in Dementia: Clinical Outcomes and Family Considerations," paper presented in Symposium on "Caring for Dementia Patients: Caregiver Burden and Prospects for Effective Intervention," 36th Annual Meeting of the Gerontological Society of America, San Francisco, CA, 1983.

116. Nolan, B.S., "Functional Evaluation of the Elderly in Guardianship Proceedings," *Law, Medicine, and Health Care* 12:210-218, 1984.

117. Olsen, E.J., director, Development and Management Service, Veterans' Administration Office of Geriatrics and Extended Care, Washington, DC, statement to the OTA Workshop on Health Services Research on Long-Term Care of Patients With Dementia, Washington, DC, Feb. 24, 1986.

118. Omer, H., Foldes, J., Toby, M., et al., "Screening for Cognitive Deficits in a Sample of Hospitalized Geriatric Patients: A Re-evaluation of a Brief Mental Status Questionnaire," *Journal of the American Geriatrics Society* 31:266-268, 1983.

119. Osborne, D.P., Brown, E.R., and Ranadt, C.T., "Qualitative Change in Memory Function: Aging and Dementia," *Aging, Volume 19: Alzheimer's Disease: A Report of Progress*, S. Corkin, et al. (eds.) (New York: Raven Press, 1982).

120. Oswald, W.D., and Fleischmann, V.M., "Psychometrics in Aging and Dementia: Advances in Geropsychological Assessments" *Archives of Gerontology and Geriatrics* 4:299-309, 1985.

121. Overall, J.E., and Gorham, D.R., "Organicity Versus Old Age in Objective and Projective Test Performance," *Journal of Consulting and Clinical Psychology* 39:98-105, 1972.

122. Pattee, J.J., and Gustafson, J.M., "Global Brain Failure in a Nursing Home Resident Population," *Journal of the American Geriatrics Society* 32:308-315, 1984.

123. Perez, F.I., Gay, J.R.A., and Taylor, R.L., "WAIS Performance of Neurologically Impaired Aged, *Psychological Reports* 37:1043-1047, 1975.

124. Perlmutter, M., "What Is Memory Aging the Aging Of?" *Developmental Psychology* 14:330-345, 1978.

125. Pfeffer, R.I., Kurosaki, T.T., Harrah, C., et al., "A Survey Diagnostic Tool for Senile Dementia," *American Journal of Epidemiology* 114:515-527, 1981.

126. Pfeffer, R.I., Kurosaki, T.T., Harrah, C.H., et al., "Measurement of Functional Activities in Older Adults in the Community," *Journal of Gerontology* 37:323-329, 1982.

127. Pfeiffer, E., "A Short Portable Mental Status Questionnaire for the Assessment of Organic Brain Deficits in Elderly Patients, *Journal of the American Geriatrics Society* 23:433-441, 1975.

128. Pfeiffer, E., Johnson, T., and Chiofoio, R., "Functional Assessment of Elderly Subjects in Four Service Settings," *Journal of the American Geriatrics Society* 29:433-437, 1981.

129. Portnoi, V.A., "The Concept of Pseudodementia" (letter to the editor), *Journal of the American Geriatrics Society* 31:321, 1983.

130. Post, F., "Dementia, Depression, and Pseudodementia," *Psychiatric Aspects of Neurological Disease* D. F. Benson and D. Blumer (eds.) (New York: Grune and Stratton, 1975).

131. Poulshock, S.W., and Deimling, G.T., "Families Caring for Elders in Residence: Issues in the Measurement of Burden," *Journal of Gerontology* 39:230-239, 1984.

132. Prigatano, G.P., "Wechsler Memory Scale: A Selective Review of the Literature," *Journal of Clinical Psychology* 34:816, 1978.

133. Rabbitt, P., "Development of Methods To Measure Changes in Activities of Daily Living in the Elderly," *Aging, Volume 19: Alzheimer's Disease: A Report of Progress*, S. Corkin, et al. (eds.) (New York: Raven Press, 1982).

134. Rabins, P.V., Mace, N.L., and Lucas, M.J., "The Impact of Dementia on the Family," *Journal of the American Medical Association* 248:333-335, 1982.

135. Rabins, P.V., Merchant, A., and Nestadt, G., "Criteria for Diagnosing Reversible Dementia Caused by Depression," *British Journal of Psychiatry* 144:488-492, 1984.

136. Radebaugh, T.S., Hooper, F.J., and Greenberg, E.M., "The Social Breakdown Syndrome in a Community Residing Elderly Population," *British Journal of Psychiatry*, in press.

137. Reding, M.J., Haycox, J., and Blass, J.P., "Depression in Patients Referred to a Dementia Clinic: A Three-Year Prospective Study," *Archives of Neurology* 42:894-896, 1985.

138. Reding, M.J., Haycox, J., Wigforss, K., et al., "Follow Up of Patients Referred to a Dementia Service," *Journal of the American Geriatrics Society* 32:265-268, 1984.

139. Reifler, B.V., Larson, E., and Hanley, R., "Coexistence of Cognitive Impairment and Depression in Geriatric Outpatients," *American Journal of Psychiatry* 139:623, 1982.

140. Reisberg, B., "The Brief Cognitive Rating Scale and Global Deterioration Scale," *Assessment in Geriatric Psychopharmacology*, T. Crook, S. Ferris, and R. Bartus (eds.) (New Canaan, CT: Mark Powley Association, 1983).

141. Reisberg, B., Ferris, S.H., DeLeon, M., et al., "The Global Deterioration Scale for Assessment of Primary Degenerative Dementia," *American Journal of Psychiatry* 139:1136, 1982.

142. Reisberg, B., Ferris, S.H., and Franssen, E., "An Ordinal Functional Assessment Tool for Alzheimer's Type Dementia," *Hospital and Community Psychiatry* 36:593-595, 1985.

143. Roach, M., New York, NY, participant, OTA Workshop on Surrogate Decisionmaking on Behalf of Mentally Incompetent Elderly Patients, Washington, DC, Sept. 23, 1985.

144. Roca, R.P., Klein, L.E., Vogelsang, G., et al., "Inaccuracy in Diagnosing Dementia Among Medical Inpatients," *Clinical Research* 30:305A, 1982.

145. Rosen, W.G., Mohs, R.C., and Davis, K.L., "A New Rating Scale for Alzheimer's Disease," *American Journal of Psychiatry* 141:1356-1364, 1984.

146. Roth, L.H., Meisel, A., and Lidz, C.W., "Tests of Competency to Consent to Treatment," *American Journal of Psychiatry* 134:279-284, 1977.

147. Roth, M., and Myers, D.G., "The Diagnosis of Dementia," *British Journal of Psychiatry: Special Publication* 9:87-99, 1975.

148. Rubenstein, L.Z., director, VA Geriatric Research, Education, and Clinical Center, Sepulveda, CA, personal communication, Aug. 20, 1986.

149. Rubenstein, L.Z., and Kane, R.L., "Geriatric Assessment Programs: Their Time Has Come," *Journal of the American Geriatrics Society* 33:646-647, 1985.

150. Rubenstein, L.Z., Abrass, I.B., and Kane, R.L., "Improved Care for Patients on a New Geriatric Evaluation Unit," *Journal of the American Geriatrics Society* 29:531-536, 1981.

151. Rubenstein, L.Z., Josephson, K.R., Wieland, G.D., et al., "Effectiveness of a Geriatric Evaluation: A Randomized Clinical Trial," *New England Journal of Medicine* 311:1664-1670, 1984.

152. Rubenstein, L.Z., Josephson, K.R., Wieland, G.D., et al., "Differential Prognosis and Utilization Patterns Among Clinical Subgroups of Hospitalized Geriatric Patients," *Health Services Research* 20: 881-895, 1986.

153. Rubenstein, L.Z., Rhee, L., and Kane, R.L., "The Role of Geriatric Assessment Units in Caring for the Elderly: An Analytic Review," *Journal of Gerontology* 37:513-521, 1982.

154. Rubenstein, L.Z., Schairer, C., Wieland, G.D., et al., "Systematic Biases in Functional Status Assessment of Elderly Adults: Effects of Different Data Sources," *Journal of Gerontology* 39:686-91, 1984.

155. Rubenstein, L.Z., Wieland, D., English, P., et al., "The Sepulveda VA Geriatric Evaluation Unit: Data on Four-Year Outcomes and Predictors of Improved Patient Outcomes," *Journal of the American Geriatrics Society* 32:503-512, 1984.

156. Salzman, C., and Shader, R.I., "Clinical Evaluation of Depression in the Elderly," *Psychiatric Symptoms and Cognitive Loss in the Elderly: Evaluation and Assessment Techniques*, A. Raskin and L.F. Jarvik (eds.) (New York: Hemisphere Publishing Corp., 1979).

157. Sarno, J.E., Sarno, M. T., and Levita, E., "The Functional Life Scale," *Archives of Physical Medicine Rehabilitation* 54:214-220, 1973.

158. Schneider, D., director, Management Health Systems, Rensselear Polytechnic Institute, letter to OTA, Jan. 28, 1986.

159. Scheuermann, L.W., coordinator, Geriatric Team, Greater Southeast Community Hospital, Washington, DC, personal communication, Aug. 20, 1986.

160. Schneider, D.P, Fries, B.E., Foley, W.J., et al., "Development of the RUG-II Case Mix Measurement System for Long Term Care," Proceedings of the Annual Conference of the Health Services Division, IIE, American Hospital Association, Chicago, IL, February 1986.

161. Shader, R.I., Harnatz, J.S., and Salzman, C., "A New Scale for Clinical Assessment in Geriatric Populations: Sandoz Clinical Assessment Geriatrics (SÇAG), *Journal of the American Geriatrics Society* 22: 107, 1974.

162. Shuttleworth, E.C., "Atypical Presentation of Dementia of the Alzheimer Type," *Journal of the American Geriatrics Society* 32:485-490, 1984.

163. Shuttleworth, E.C., "Memory Function and the Clinical Differentiation of Dementing Disorders," *Journal of the American Geriatrics Society* 30:363-366, 1982.

164. Smith, J.M., "Nurse and Psychiatric Aide Rating Scales for Assessing Psychopathology in the Elderly: A Critical Review," *Psychiatric Symptoms and Cognitive Loss in the Elderly*, A. Raskin and L.F. Jarvik (eds.) (Washington, DC: Hemisphere Publishing Corp., 1979).

165. Smits, H.L., "Incentives in Case-Mix Measures for

Long-Term Care," *Health Care Financing Review* 6:53-59, 1984.

166. Smyer, M.A., Hofland, B.F., and Jonas, E.A., "Validity Study of the Short Portable Mental Status Questionnaire for the Elderly," *Journal of the American Geriatrics Society* 27:263-269, 1979.

167. Staff of the Benjamin Rose Hospital, "Multidisciplinary Studies of Illness in Aged Persons, II: A New Classification of Functional Status in Activities of Daily Living," *Journal of Chronic Disease* 9:55-62, 1959.

168. Storandt, M., Botwinick, R.J., Danziger, W.L., et al., "Psychometric Differentiation of Mild Senile Dementia of the Alzheimer Type," *Archives of Neurology* 41:497-499, 1984.

169. Thal, L.J., Grundman, M., and Golden, R., "Alzheimer's Disease: A Correlational Analysis of the Blessed Information-Memory-Concentration Test and the Mini-Mental State Exam," *Neurology* 36: 262-264, 1986.

170. U.S. Congress, Office of Technology Assessment, *Technology and Aging in America*, OTA-BA-264 (Washington, DC: U.S. Government Printing Office, June 1985).

171. U.S. Congress, Office of Technology Assessment, *Hearing Impairment and Elderly People*, OTA-BP-BA-30 (Washington, DC: U.S. Government Printing Office, May 1986).

172. U.S. Department of Health and Human Services, *Alzheimer's Disease: Report of the Secretary's Task Force on Alzheimer's Disease*, DHHS Pub. No. ADM 84-1323 (Washington, DC: U.S. Government Printing Office, 1984).

173. U.S. Department of Health and Human Services, National Center for Health Statistics, unpublished data from the National Health Interview Survey, 1981.

174. U.S. Department of Health and Human Services, National Institutes of Health, National Institute on Aging, Task Force Report, "Senility Reconsidered, Treatment Possibilities for Mental Impairment in the Elderly," *Journal of the American Medical Association* 244:259-263, 1980.

175. Valle, R., professor, School of Social Work, San Diego State University, personal communication, June 13, 1985.

176. Villardita, C., Cultrera, S., Capone, V., et al., "Neuropsychological Test Performance and Normal Aging," *Archives of Gerontology and Geriatrics* 4:311-319, 1985.

177. Vitaliano, P.P., Breen, A.R., Albert, M.S., et al., "Memory, Attention, and Functional Status in Community-Residing Alzheimer Type Dementia Patients and Optimally Healthy Aged Individuals," *Journal of Gerontology* 39:58-64, 1984.

178. Vitaliano, P.P., Breen, A.R., Russo, J., et al., "The Clinical Utility of the Dementia Rating Scale for Assessing Alzheimer Patients," *Journal of Chronic Disease* 37:743-753, 1984.

179. Weiman, H.M., "Rowing Together: OARS and Teamwork" (letter to the editor), *Journal of the American Geriatrics Society* 34:485, 1986.

180. Weingartner, H., Kaye, W., Smallberg, S., et al., "Determinants of Memory Failures in Dementia," *Aging, Volume 19: Alzheimer's Disease: A Report of Progress*, S. Corkin, et al. (eds.) (New York: Raven Press, 1982).

181. Weintraub, S., Baratz, R., and Mesulam, M.M., "Daily Living Activities in the Assessment of Dementia," *Aging, Vol. 19: Alzheimer's Disease: A Report of Progress*, S. Corkin, K.L. Davis, J. H. Growden, et al. (eds.) (New York: Raven Press, 1982).

182. Weiss, I.K., Nagel, C.L., and Aronson, M.K., "Applicability of Depression Scales to the Old Person," *Journal of the American Geriatrics Society* 34:215-218, 1986.

183. Weissert, W.G., "Innovative Approaches to Long-Term Care and Their Evaluation," paper presented to the Conference on the Impact of Technology on Long-Term Care, Millwood, VA, Feb. 16-18, 1983.

184. Wells, C.E., "Refinements in the Diagnosis of Dementia," *American Journal of Psychiatry* 139:621-622, 1982.

185. Whitehouse, P., assistant professor, Department of Neurology and Neuroscience, The Johns Hopkins University School of Medicine, statement to the OTA Advisory Panel on Disorders Causing Dementia, Washington, DC, Dec. 11, 1985.

186. Wilkinson, I.A., and Graham-White, J., "Psychogeriatric Dependency Rating Scales (PGDS): A Method of Assessment for Use by Nurses," *British Journal of Psychiatry* 137:558-565, 1980.

187. Williams, M.E., Department of Medicine, University of North Carolina School of Medicine, personal communication, Sept. 4, 1986.

188. Williams, M.E., and Williams T.F., "Evaluation of Older Persons in the Ambulatory Setting," *Journal of the American Geriatrics Society* 34:37-43, 1986.

189. Williams, T.F., "Assessment of the Elderly in Relation to Needs for Long-Term Care: An Emerging Technology," *The Impact of Technology on Long-Term Care*, J.M. Grana and D.B. McCallum (eds.) (Millwood, VA: Project HOPE Center for Health Studies, 1986).

190. Williamson, J., Stoke, I.H., Gray, S., et al., "Old People at Home: Their Unreported Needs," *Lancet*, 1964, p. 1117.

191. Winograd, C.H., "Mental Status Tests and the Capacity for Self-Care," *Journal of the American Geriatrics Society* 32:49-55, 1984.

192. Winogrond, I.R., and Fisk, A.A., "Alzheimer's Disease: Assessment of Functional Status," *Journal of the American Geriatrics Society* 31:78-85, 1983.

193. Wolff, M.L., "Determination of Mental Status in an Ambulatory Geriatric Population," *Journal of the American Geriatrics Society* 32:245, 1984.

194. Wolinsky, F.D., Coe, R.M., Miller, D.K., et al., "Measurement of the Global and Functional Dimensions of Health Status in the Elderly," *Journal of Gerontology* 39:88-92, 1984.

195. Yesavage, J.A., "Relaxation and Memory Training in 39 Elderly Patients," *American Journal of Psychiatry* 141:778-781, 1984.

196. Young, R.C., Manley, M.W., and Alexopoulos, G.S., " 'I Don't Know' Responses in Elderly Depressives and in Dementia," *Journal of the American Geriatrics Society* 33:253-257, 1985.

197. Zarit, S.H., Reever, K.E., and Bach-Peterson, J.M., "Relatives of the Impaired Elderly: Correlates of Feelings of Burden," *The Gerontologist* 20:649-655, 1980.

198. Zarit, S.H., Zarit, J.M., and Reever, K.E., "Memory Training for Severe Memory Loss: Effects on Senile Dementia Patients and Their Families," *The Gerontologist* 22:373-377, 1982.

199. Zimmer, J.G., Watson, N., and Treat, A., "Behavioral Problems Among Patients in Skilled Nursing Facilities," *American Journal of Public Health* 74:1118-1121, 1984.

Chapter 9
Personnel and Training

CONTENTS

Personnel and Training

Long-term care is the fastest growing segment of the health services industry in the United States (73). To keep pace with a growing population of elderly Americans the United States will require a 50-percent increase in the number of health care providers by the year 2010, according to the 1981 White House Conference on Aging. Some 2.6 million older persons—almost double the current number—will be in nursing homes by 2030 (87). Noninstitutional long-term care needs have not been estimated.

Attracting and retaining skilled, knowledgeable personnel will continue to be critical to the delivery of quality long-term care. Facilities face several fundamental problems in that regard:

- An inadequate number of health professionals opts for employment in long-term care facilities and programs.
- Professional, paraprofessional, and nonprofessional staff frequently lack prior training and experience in caring for the elderly, chronically ill, and mentally ill served by these facilities and programs.
- The staff turnover rate in long-term care facilities and programs is extremely high (63).

These problems are integrally related. Health professionals' lack of interest for work in long-term care is attributed, in part, to an educational process that stresses acute rather than chronic care and that provides little experience with and information about caring for mentally ill or elderly patients (21,30,40,59). Lack of preemployment training and experience contribute to the high staff turnover experienced by most long-term care programs. Professional, paraprofessional, and nonprofessional employees, whose education has not equipped them with the knowledge and skills to care for long-term care patients, become dissatisfied with work in these settings (63). In addition, the salaries and benefits offered by long-term care facilities and programs are rarely competitive with those available in hospitals and other acute care settings (45,77).

Efforts to project the number of personnel needed to care for demented patients in the United States must consider:

- the Nation's changing demographics,
- the types of services needed, and
- the individuals best qualified to deliver these services.

A brief description of several models of care sets the stage for this chapter's discussion of the various professionals, paraprofessionals, and nonprofessionals who provide services to individuals with dementia, and the overriding issues concerning the education of these personnel. An understanding of the role played by each enables projections of the numbers needed and the training they will require to provide quality care. Educational, institutional, and governmental efforts to prepare individuals for this work and to address the fundamental personnel problems experienced by programs serving individuals with dementia are presented throughout the chapter.

MODELS OF CARE

Selecting an appropriate "model of care" is an important starting point in evaluating the groups and numbers of personnel needed to serve a population. The needs of long-term care patients differ from those of acute care patients. Considerations of personnel needs must account for these differences and determine which individuals are best suited to deliver care. Projections must also take into account the full range of care settings available, and the staffing arrangement appropriate to each.

Three models of care useful in characterizing the delivery of health services are the medical, nursing, and multidisciplinary team approaches to care.

1. The **medical model** of care is the customary basis for estimating personnel needs in

health care. The model emphasizes acute rather than chronic care, diagnostic and treatment services rather than social and rehabilitative services, and the role of the physician over that of other health and social service professionals (48).

2. The **nursing model** focuses on the chronically ill, emphasizing their need for rehabilitative and personal care (e.g., feeding and bathing) services rather than intensive medical care. Nurses function as the primary service providers, working to promote, maintain, and, where possible, restore maximum function and independence in a patient's activities of daily living. In addition, nurses help with events and decisions that confront the patient and family over time (64).

3. The **multidisciplinary team** approach stresses the range of health and social services personnel appropriate to certain care situations. The model suggests that providing quality care to some groups of patients requires the skills and knowledge of a wide variety of professionals and paraprofessionals.

Dementia and the Multidisciplinary Team

The complexity of dementing illnesses makes the team approach to care an appropriate one for individuals with these illnesses. Their unique care needs stem from their combination of medical problems, self-care deficits, cognitive impairments, and social difficulties. Their care requires the skills and knowledge of individuals trained in long-term care, mental illness, and, in most cases, geriatrics. A variety of medical specialists, nurses and nurse's aides, social workers, and rehabilitative and recreational therapists may each contribute components necessary for quality care of persons with dementia.

Although most acute and long-term care facilities rely on a variety of professional, paraprofessional, and nonprofessional personnel, the multidisciplinary team approach, as an actual care strategy, requires both philosophical and formal acknowledgment of the importance of each member's role in the delivery of quality care. Actual training in the theory and practice of the team approach is important for its effective application.

While such training may be a component of on-the-job training or orientation, its incorporation into the formal education of health care and social service providers could enhance their ability to apply this approach.

The Team Approach as a Component of Education

Programs that train health and social service professionals frequently fail to acknowledge that no single group is equipped to meet the diverse needs of most patients. Programs fail to emphasize the valuable knowledge and resources available through professionals in other disciplines. An emphasis, during the educational process, on the role of each professional in conjunction with those in other fields—providing students with experience in working with individuals in a variety of disciplines—might enhance their ability and willingness to do so. Although a few programs have begun to teach this team approach, the majority still focus almost exclusively on a single professional discipline.

One program that attempts to prepare health professionals to apply the team approach is the Veterans Administration's Interdisciplinary Team Training in Geriatrics (described later in this chapter). The program provides clinical experience in geriatrics to students in 40 health-related disciplines from academic institutions throughout the United States (26). In addition to gaining skills and knowledge related to geriatric care, students learn to function as part of a team of caregivers.

Another effort to encourage interdisciplinary cooperation is made through 20 Geriatric Educations Centers (GECs) sponsored by the Bureau of Health Professionals (BHPr) within the Health Resources and Services Administration of the Department of Health and Human Services (also described later). The first four GECs opened in fiscal year 1983; BHPr established 16 more with fiscal year 1985 appropriations (83). The centers aim to disseminate interdisciplinary and discipline-specific information in geriatrics to students of the health and allied health professions. GECs offer training modules for faculty in nursing, medicine, dentistry, social work, psychology, rehabilitation, pharmacy, and long-term care administration in order to aid faculty efforts to establish or augment geriatric education programs at their own institutions.

Multidisciplinary Care in Programs and Facilities

Although most facilities and programs providing long-term care services rely on a variety of health, allied health, and social service personnel, few make a formal commitment to training staff in the theory and practice of multidisciplinary care. Orientation sessions, inservice training programs, and regular team meetings are among the means through which individual facilities and programs instruct staff in the value of and approaches to interdisciplinary cooperation.

Orientation and Inservice Training of Team Members

Facilities and programs that acknowledge a formal commitment to multidisciplinary team care stress the importance of training sessions that incorporate its principles and methods. Orientation and inservice sessions that include all levels of personnel—from physicians to nurse's aides to maintenance and dietary staff—offer opportunities to present information about the patients and the philosophy of the program and to foster mutual respect among staff.

Through these sessions, individuals whose role includes a supervisory function may be apprised of the facility's commitment to treating each employee as an integral member of the care team. In addition, the sessions allow programs to convey to all staff information fundamental to serving their patients. Even housekeeping and maintenance staff, for instance, must know of the tendency for wandering behavior among persons with dementia so as to avoid an inappropriate and potentially harmful response on their part. Technical information regarding skills and treatment procedures may be reviewed separately with the groups of staff responsible for implementing them.

An overriding problem for programs and facilities seeking to train health and social service professionals about caring for patients with dementia is the absence of teaching resources. Several facilities and universities have recognized and

attempted to respond to that need; the Alzheimer's Disease and Related Disorders Association (ADRDA) and the American Health Care Association have published a manual to train nursing home staff about dementia (32).

Another such effort was made by the Hillhaven Corp., a leader in the development of special care units for dementia patients. Hillhaven emphasizes the importance of orientation and monthly inservice training for all staff members. Orientation includes a minimum of 8 hours classroom and 16 hours experiential learning (e.g., role playing and observation). The training manual developed for Hillhaven (60) presents information on the biological, physiological, and social aspects of dementia. Each chapter suggests a lesson plan, including classroom and experiential sessions (15 to 30 minutes each), and possible continuing education activities. Topics include causes of memory loss in the elderly, issues involving the family, and day-to-day nursing care. Tests before and after the training monitor how well the staff integrates the material.

Team Meetings

Facilities that purposefully implement the team approach say that staff meetings are an important way to foster involvement of all levels of personnel in institutional and patient management. Weekly meetings to assess patient status and needs, for instance, include all personnel involved in patient care. Including nurse's aides and other paraprofessionals in these sessions shows an important recognition of their critical role in the delivery of quality care. Of all facility personnel, nurse's aides spend the greatest number of patient contact hours and provide the highest percentage of direct care. Soliciting their input can provide valuable information and may alleviate the intense job dissatisfaction and rapid turnover prevalent among aides in more hierarchical facilities (a problem discussed later in this chapter).

Members of the Multidisciplinary Team

Staff size and composition vary with the number of persons served, the nature of the program, financial resources and management strategy of the program, and State and Federal requirements. The following categories of personnel, however, indicate the range of individuals who may act as team members in a multidisciplinary approach to care (19):

- **management:**
  —board of directors, and
  —administrator;
- **medical staff:**
  —medical director,
  —attending physician,
  —psychiatrist (consultant),
  —neurologist (consultant), and
  —dentist (consultant);
- **nursing staff:**
  —director of nursing,
  —registered nurse,
  —licensed nurse practitioner,
  —nurse's aide, and
  —nurse specialist (e.g., gerontological nurse practitioner);
- **extended care providers:**
  —social worker,
  —physical therapist,
  —occupational therapist,
  —speech therapist,
  —psychologist (consultant),
  —nutritionist (consultant), and
  —pharmacist (consultant);
- **life enrichment personnel:**
  —activities director, and
  —training coordinator.

Budgetary constraints prohibit most facilities and programs from employing such an extensive range of personnel. The majority rely heavily on professionals employed on a contractual or fee-for-service basis (19).

The various groups of professionals and para-professionals frequently employed by long-term care facilities and programs are briefly described here, although greater detail about the roles and educational preparation of each is provided later in this chapter.

- **Physicians:** Aside from the medical director, required for Federal reimbursement of programs, few long-term care facilities employ a full- or part-time physician. Patients needing medical attention must be visited by their personal physician or temporarily transferred to an acute care facility.

- **Nurses and nurse's aides:** The vast majority of full-time employees in most long-term care facilities are registered or licensed practical nurses (RNs and LPNs) and nurse's aides. RNs and LPNs accounted for 22 percent of the full-time staff in U.S. nursing homes in a 1977 survey; nurse's aides, for 68 percent. The shortage of nurses in long-term care, however, is severe (39,73,87).

- **Medical and nursing specialists:** The expertise of medical and nursing specialists (e.g., geropsychiatrists, neurologists, and geriatric nurse practitioners) makes their role in the diagnosis and management of individuals with dementia valuable. Few facilities, however, retain these professionals as part of the permanent staff due to such factors as scarcity and expense.

- **Social workers:** Facilities and programs that serve persons with dementia may employ a social worker on a full-time, part-time, or consultant basis. Their skills in individual and group counseling and their knowledge of local and national resources make them valuable participants in planning and administration of patient care.

- **Recreational and rehabilitative therapists:** A variety of therapists (e.g., physical, occupational, exercise, art, and speech) may work with patients to enhance mobility and fine motor and communication skills. Although few facilities employ therapists from each of these disciplines, many employ one or more specialists on a part-time basis.

- **Pharmacists and nutritionists:** Inpatient facilities may employ experts in pharmacology and nutrition on a contractual basis. These specialists assess individual patient needs and facility programs related to diet and the use of drugs.

- **Psychologists:** Psychologists may provide many direct and indirect services to patients in long-term care settings. Few programs retain a full-time psychologist, although many employ these professionals on a consultant basis. A trained psychologist may assist in developing and evaluating strategies to address behavioral problems manifested by persons with dementia. Psychologists may also provide inservice training for staff and may work with families on how to communicate with and care for persons with dementia.

- **Administrators:** Administrators of facilities and programs caring for persons with dementia play a major role in planning and delivery of care. Their decisions regarding allocation of resources, organizational structure, and program priorities are critical to the quality of service delivered.

ISSUES IN EDUCATION FOR HEALTH AND SOCIAL SERVICE PROFESSIONS

Three factors are important in stimulating interest in caring for specific groups of patients and for work in particular care settings: 1) factual information, 2) clinical experience, and 3) positive faculty role models. The limited interest of many health and social service personnel in geriatrics and long-term care is frequently attributed to the failure of educational programs to address these topics—the emphasis on the role of the professional in acute rather than long-term care situations and the absence of efforts to address negative attitudes toward the elderly (66).

The 1970s marked the beginning of an infusion of material related to care of the elderly and chronically ill into programs for health and social service professionals. The extent to which information about that or any subject or population is included in academic and training programs, however, remains a matter of institutional choice. Variability of institutional priorities and resources results in wide differences in the quality and quantity of educational exposure students receive to any subject area.

Credentialing

Mechanisms to ensure that particular subjects are addressed in the education and training of health and social service professionals include:

1. the establishment of Federal or State requirements in designated subjects and skills for personnel employed by facilities that provide particular services;
2. the inclusion of specific curricular requirements in the accreditation criteria for academic programs; and
3. the incorporation of material related to particular topics on licensure examinations.

No concerted effort has been made to date, however, to ensure knowledge about and experience with dementia patients among personnel employed by facilities and programs serving them.

- **Regulatory requirements:** States and the Federal Government impose few requirements for the training of professionals and paraprofessionals employed by programs and facilities that provide long-term care. They rely on the educational process to provide adequate training in subjects and skills related to patient care. This system fails to account for qualitative and quantitative differences in educational programs that can translate into vastly different levels of preparation among individuals with the same professional title.
- **Accreditation criteria:** Accreditation is one mechanism through which academic training in specific subjects can be standardized for students of particular health or social service professions. At present, however, accreditation committees make few specific curricular requirements. They focus instead on general requirements regarding the overall structure and management of the academic facility. Decisions regarding program requirements, curricular content and format, and allocation of resources are left to individual academic institutions.
- **Professional licensure:** The licensing process is a means of ensuring that professionals seeking employment in particular sectors have a certain degree of related expertise. Licensing examinations and requirements are established and administered primarily by States or professional organizations. State Boards of Nursing, for instance, give examinations developed by the National League of

Nursing; and the American Medical Association's National Board of Medical Examiners develops exams for physician certification. The degree to which certification examinations test for knowledge and skills in areas related to dementia (e.g., geriatrics, long-term care, and mental health) varies among the professions and areas of specialization. Testing specifically about dementia, however, ranges from little to none. Through inclusion of questions testing for knowledge about aging and dementing illnesses, boards that oversee licensure and certification of health and social service professionals may help emphasize the importance of teaching about these subjects.

Resources for Teaching About Dementia

Efforts to educate students and practicing professional and paraprofessional staff about dementing disorders are hindered by a lack of teaching resources, as mentioned earlier. Academic institutions, patient care facilities, and community programs note their need for faculty, textual material, and quality clinical opportunities to provide training in the diagnosis and care of dementia patients.

Recent attention to questions about diagnosis and treatment of persons with dementia has dramatically increased the amount of related written material. While textbooks for health and social service professionals have begun to address the subject, many programs rely on journal articles to provide the latest information about diagnostic and treatment strategies for dementia patients. Journals offer the benefit of exposing students to a variety of perspectives, to current theories about the diseases, and to innovative ideas regarding methods of treatment and care. The transience of the information in periodicals, however, complicates the task of curriculum planning and teaching about dementing illnesses. The absence of a discrete body of information regarding techniques for diagnosis, treatment, and care compounds the difficulties of teaching about the diseases, and may inhibit schools' ability and willingness to formally incorporate teaching about dementia into their curricula.

Opportunities for practical experience with persons with dementia are important in training health and social service professionals and paraprofessionals to work with them. Recognition of the nursing home as an excellent setting for students to gain clinical experience in working with the elderly led to the development of the "teaching nursing home" concept. Universities, particularly those with strong academic programs in geriatrics, have increasingly incorporated clinical rotations and practicum in these facilities as a core part of the curricula for students of health and allied health professions. However, the quality of the facility is critical to determining the quality of students' experience with, understanding of, and interest in working with dementia patients. Geographic factors and absolute numbers of students may make access to facilities with quality programs difficult for academic institutions.

A supply of faculty knowledgeable about and interested in working with dementia patients is critical to teaching students about dementing disorders. The shortage of faculty with expertise in such areas as geriatrics, geropsychiatry, and long-term care is critical. A recent report by the Department of Health and Human Services' Ad Hoc Committee on Enhancement of Training in Geriatrics and Gerontology estimated that only 5 to 25 percent of the numbers of required trained faculty are available to teach geriatrics in health and allied health schools (see table 9-1) (71). In addition, about 450 faculty members with combined expertise in mental health and aging are needed

Table 9-1.—Number of Faculty Members Needed To Teach Geriatrics by 2000[a]

Profession	Number needed
Medical schools—physicians[b]	1,300
Nursing schools	1,300
Social work schools	1,000
Pharmacy schools	300
Clinical psychology programs	450

[a]Figures represent the minimum number of faculty members with a primary commitment to teaching about geriatrics that would be required by the various health and allied health professions. In most cases, the estimates assume a need for three faculty members with expertise in geriatrics for graduate-level programs and two for undergraduate programs.

[b]A 1980 Rand Corp. study of physicians' role in geriatrics estimated a need for 1,350 physician faculty members to teach medical school about aging. Of these, 900 would be geriatricians and 450 would be geropsychiatrists. The numbers were based on a minimum of three faculty members in each school, with additional faculty members to guide medical residency programs (41).

SOURCE: Adapted from U.S. Department of Health and Human Services, National Institute on Aging, Report on Education and Training in Geriatrics and Gerontology, Administrative Document, 1984.

for schools of medicine, nursing, and social work (76).

Fellowships and training grants are effective ways to augment the population of teachers and researchers in a specialized area. The opportunity for physicians to pursue postresidency fellowships in geriatrics, for instance, has increased the number interested in and qualified to pursue research and teach in field of geriatric medicine.

Continuing education is another important way to enhance the knowledge and skills of practicing professionals and paraprofessionals. Its impact on the quality of practice may be more immediate than that of curricular modification at the undergraduate and graduate level (17). It is particularly important in the health professions, where knowledge and understanding of diseases, diagnostic and treatment techniques, and approaches to care are rarely static.

Federal Funding of Education

Much of the impetus for developing programs for preparing health and social service professionals in geriatrics and long-term care has come through Federal funding of education. Title VII of the Public Health Service Act provides institutional and student support for schools of medicine, osteopathy, dentistry, veterinary medicine, optometry, podiatry, pharmacy, public health, and health care administration. Title VIII provides similar support for nursing schools and students. The initial intent of the legislation in 1963 was to respond to reported shortages of health personnel at that time. The program sought to increase enrollment and to ensure the financial viability of health profession schools.

By 1974, the aggregate supply of health personnel had improved significantly. The remaining problem in the supply of health professionals was reportedly one of geographic and specialty maldistribution (78). Congress had revised the program to address these personnel shortages. One effort included the establishment of 11 Area Health Education Centers (AHECs) in 1972. Identifying geriatrics as a field in which trained professionals was in critically short supply, one AHEC was designated to address that gap in 1977. The remaining AHECs are established on a geographical basis rather than topical need.

The Administration has recently sought termination of support for health professional education. Budget proposals in fiscal years 1986 and 1987 recommended no funding for Title VII and Title VIII programs. The Administration contends that Federal subsidy of health professions education is no longer warranted because of the steadily increasing supply and the projected surpluses of professionals (37,56). Geographic and specialty maldistribution are not considered a priority for Federal policy, but would be left to market forces and State and local programs. The Administration's proposal does not address the question of distribution problems in the health professions.

Congressional and academic opponents of the Administration's position point out that the programs no longer seek a universal increase in the number of health professionals. At present, both Title VII and Title VIII are highly specific in their intent to address the shortage of health professionals in particular geographic areas and sectors of health care (e.g., family and internal medicine, or nursing administration) (56). They contend that the loss of funds will impede efforts to address problems of distribution of health professionals.

Support for Medicine and Related Professions

In October 1985, Congress enacted legislation extending primary care training authorities under Title VII of the Public Health Service Act and requiring the Secretary of Health and Human Services to give priority to applicants who demonstrate a commitment to family medicine, general internal medicine, and general pediatrics in their medical education training programs. Public Law 99-129 also extended the Area Health Education Centers program designed to provide training for health professionals in geographically underserved areas and professionally underrepresented sectors of health care. In addition, the law set aside funds for geriatric training programs for health professionals.

Support for Nursing

The 99th Congress also acted to defend nursing education programs from the Administration's proposed cuts. The Administration's fiscal year 1987 budget sought to terminate funding for Title VIII nurse training, reasoning that the present supply of nurses is adequate to meet the Nation's health care needs.

An Institute of Medicine study done in 1982 found, however, that although the number of generalist registered nurses may have increased sufficiently, nursing shortages persist in certain geographic areas and in particular health care settings and nursing specialties (39). (The undersupply of professional nurses in long-term care is described later in this chapter.) In addition, observers note that the demand for nurses with advanced degrees continues to exceed schools' ability to prepare advanced level nurses to work as educators,

administrators, and supervisors (61,67). The Administration's fiscal year 1987 budget would eliminate funding for advanced nurse training programs and nurse practitioner programs.

The Nurse Education Act of 1985 (Public Law 99-92), signed in July 1985, reauthorized the program for nursing special education projects. The legislation emphasized the need for programs that prepare nurses in a variety of settings—acute care, long-term care, ambulatory, and noninstitutional —and for programs that seek to improve the specialty and geographic distribution of nurses in the United States.

PROFESSIONALS AND PARAPROFESSIONALS IN LONG-TERM CARE

This section describes the groups of professionals and paraprofessionals who play a primary role in diagnosis, treatment, and care of persons with dementia in long-term care facilities and noninstitutional programs. It identifies factors that contribute to the difficulties programs and facilities experience in attracting and retaining qualified personnel, and describes various educational, institutional, and governmental efforts to address the problem. The major role played by family members in caring for dementia patients is described in chapter 4.

Nurses

Although the number of nurses working in long-term care has risen significantly since 1972, it has not kept pace with the increase in the number of patients. Between 1972 and 1980, the percentage of nurses working in long-term care facilities rose by 42 percent, and the number employed by home health agencies by 200 percent (11). At present, however, the 18,000 nursing homes in the United States employ a total of 60,000 registered nurses, an average of just over three per facility (22). Because of their central role in providing long-term care, the shortage of nurses and their short job tenure impede the delivery of quality care to the many persons served by these facilities and programs. The average nursing home

resident receives 12 minutes of registered nursing care per day in a skilled nursing facility (SNF) and 7 minutes per day in an intermediate care facility (ICF) (28).

The Health Care Financing Administration predicts that by 1990 there will be a shortfall of 75,000 nurses in nursing homes alone (73). Moreover, the shortage of long-term care nurses may severely limit the potential of home health, adult day, and respite services to offer alternatives to nursing home care for the chronically ill.

Nurses employed by facilities and programs providing long-term care services frequently lack educational training and experience in caring for the chronically ill. That lack is attributed, in part, to an educational process that stresses acute rather than chronic care and that provides little experience with and information about caring for mentally ill or elderly patients.

Several additional factors exacerbate the shortage of nurses in gerontologic and long-term care:

- the growth of the over-75 population, whose high incidence of chronic illness and severe functional impairments creates an increased demand for long-term care services;
- noncompetitive salaries, limited opportunities for career advancement, and unfavorable work conditions for nurses in nursing homes and other long-term care facilities;

- the expansion of nursing roles and functions in long-term care of elderly and chronically ill patients;
- the growth of agencies and programs (e.g., home health and adult day care) providing noninstitutional long-term care;
- decreased enrollment in nurse training programs;
- limited material related to geriatrics and chronic care in basic nursing curricula;
- the limited number of programs providing training in gerontological nursing and long-term care, and low enrollment in these programs; and
- reduced funding to support institutional development and student education in gerontological nursing and related areas (59).

The shortage of professional nurses desiring employment in long-term care may have similar consequences for both inpatient facilities (e.g., nursing homes) and alternative care programs (e.g., adult day care, home health care, and respite care) that serve these individuals. Each may be forced to rely on nurse's aides and other paraprofessionals to function as the primary care providers. Although many day-to-day patient care tasks may be fulfilled by these paraprofessionals, given adequate training and preparation, evidence indicates that they are frequently granted responsibility for procedures that should be performed by professional health care staff (e.g., preparation and administration of intravenous medication, blood transfusion, or insertion of nasogastric tube) (16).

Nurses' Roles in Long-Term Care

The limited number of professional nurses on staff results in increased responsibility for those working in facilities and programs offering long-term care services. For example, in addition to delivering direct patient care, an RN at a nursing home may act as staff supervisor and patient discharge planner, conduct therapeutic socialization groups, coordinate the volunteer program, and conduct staff inservice education programs. Although that approach attempts to gain maximum utilization of a scant resource, the difficulty of fulfilling too broad a range of responsibilities may diminish a nurse's effectiveness, detract from the quality of care, and contribute to the job dissatis-

faction and short job tenure prevalent among registered nurses in this field (19,59,63).

An increasingly important role of nurses, in both institutional and noninstitutional settings, is supervising and training paraprofessional staff and keeping administrative records. Many nurses, particularly in long-term care facilities, spend the majority of their time performing administrative duties rather than in direct patient care. Most basic nursing programs, however, fail to provide training in these duties. The 1985 Invitational Conference on Issues and Strategies in Geriatric Education noted the importance of case management skills and of supervisory and teaching skills for nursing students, given their burgeoning role in long-term care, and encouraged the integration of these skills into basic nurse training programs (14).

Documenting compliance with regulatory requirements for long-term care facilities and programs consumes a vast amount of nursing time. Registered nurses assume primary responsibility for administrative detail and paperwork, leaving direct patient care to nurse's aides, orderlies, and volunteers. Studies indicate that nurse administrators give cost containment a higher priority than quality assurance in their efforts to comply with regulations (42). (The effectiveness of regulatory requirements as a means of assuring the delivery of quality care is described further in ch. 10.)

Recent studies of long-term care facilities and programs in the United States cite the lack of consistent, professional leadership as a major cause of problems related to employee motivation and turnover. Directors of nursing, one study revealed, tend to regard their positions as temporary—few had held their position for longer than 1 year. Instability in facility leadership exacerbates problems of staff turnover and proves damaging to staff morale. Nursing staff show little respect for or responsiveness to a continually changing leadership (42).

Salaries and Benefits

Noncompetitive salaries, limited opportunities for career advancement, and unfavorable work conditions are seen as significant factors in the undesirablity of nursing positions in long-term care facilities and programs. One survey found that staff nurses in nursing homes earned an average of 20 percent less than hospital nurses (45). A comparison of benefits received by nurses employed in different settings revealed that only 9 percent of nursing home nurses received paid vacations and sick leave and that only 11 percent had retirement programs or were provided with health or life insurance plans. The situation is similar for nurses employed by respite, adult day care, and home health programs. By contrast, of hospital nurses surveyed, all received paid vacations and holidays, and almost all had employer-provided health insurance and retirement plans (77).

Nursing Education

Several categories of nurses are licensed to practice. The licensure requirements and scope of responsibility of each category vary with the extent and nature of their educational training.

Registered nurses are professional nurses licensed by individual State boards of nursing. By virtue of their training, RNs are certified to assume nursing roles and duties that other nursing personnel (e.g., LPNs and nurse's aides) are not. Students can prepare for RN licensure in three ways:

1. Baccalaureate programs, offered in 4-year colleges and universities, require 2 years of pre-professional and 2 years of professional study. Graduates receive a baccalaureate degree in nursing, and are eligible to take the State nursing board examination for registered nurses.
2. Diploma programs, offered in hospital schools of nursing, confer a diploma in nursing after successful completion of 2 to 3 years of post-high school study. Graduates of these programs do not receive an academic degree, but are qualified to take the State nursing board examination for registered nurses.
3. Associate degree programs, usually offered in 2-year community technical or vocational colleges, lead to an associate degree in nursing and qualify graduates to take the State nursing board examination for registered nurses.

Recent surveys confirm the low interest among RNs for work in long-term care facilities: Ninety percent of graduates from each of the three types of RN training programs take positions in hospitals; only a small portion opt for nursing home employment (52). The survey did not report on the selection of noninstitutional long-term care nursing positions. Baccalaureate program graduates showed nursing home jobs to be their least preferred employment choice (3.9 percent); diploma and associate degree graduates marked them as the next to least preferred.

A recent Institute of Medicine study found that employment profiles of RNs generally followed that pattern (see table 9-2) (39). The survey was based on responses of nurses aged 35 to 37, an age at which the National League for Nursing believes the career preferences for these professionals are best measured.

Licensed practical nurses are technical nurses licensed by individual State boards of nursing. Most LPNs train in vocational, technical, or community colleges (39). The programs range from 11 to 24 months in length, with the first 2 to 3 months spent in the classroom and the remainder divided between classroom (40 percent) and clinical (60 percent) learning.

Although no national standards differentiate the patient care tasks of LPNs from those of RNs, a recent study identified 78 nursing tasks performed in long-term care facilities. The study asked nurse educators to evaluate which groups of nursing personnel (LPNs, RNs, nurse's aides) were qual-

Table 9-2.—Registered Nurses Aged 35 to 37 in Selected Types of Employment[a]

Type of employment	Degree program		
	Baccalaureate	Diploma	Associate
Hospital	45.4	47.5	67.4
Nursing home	3.9	7.3	6.7
Public and community (health, student, and occupational health)	15.4	9.0	6.1
Nursing education	4.3	1.2	0.6
All others	6.4	10.0	7.5
Not employed in nursing	24.6	25.0	11.7

[a]According to highest levels of educational preparation, November 1980.

SOURCE: Institute of Medicine, *Nursing and Nursing Education: Public Policies and Private Actions* (Washington, DC: National Academy Press, 1983.)

Table 9-3.—Distribution of Nursing Task Responsibilities (in percent)

Task	Nurse's aide	LPN	RN	Task	Nurse's aide	LPN	RN
Administer cardiopulmonary resuscitation	1.3[a]	35.7	28.7	Irrigate vagina (douche)	35.0[a]	28.9	5.6
Administer cough and deep breathing exercises	27.8	28.9	10.6	Make patient's bed: occupied	76.6	6.1	1.0
Administer gavage feedings	2.8[a]	44.8	23.8	Make patient's bed: unoccupied	87.2	3.0	1.5
Administer oxygen therapy	11.9[a]	40.0	15.0	Measure intake and output	63.0	15.5	2.0
Administer oxygen treatment	11.6[a]	38.8	19.0	Place patient in correct alignment	51.9	14.8	3.7
Apply cold treatments	23.8	39.9	5.7	Practice range of motion exercises with patient	44.4	15.0	2.2
Apply elastic bandages	29.7	37.9	5.1	Prepare and give injections	0.0[a]	49.7	6.7
Apply elastic stockings	44.7	27.9	3.6	Prepare and give intravenous medications	1.4[a]	20.7[a]	64.1
Apply heat treatments	18.3	46.1	6.3	Prepare and give oral medications	4.2[a]	46.9	5.2
Apply restraints	58.9	15.3	3.7	Prepare and give rectal medication	7.3[a]	41.7	5.2
Apply sterile dressings/bandages	9.5[a]	50.5	9.5	Prepare and give topical medication	9.3[a]	41.5	5.7
Assist patient dressing/undressing	81.0	4.5	3.0	Provide oral hygiene	80.3	4.4	1.5
Assist patient in/out of bed	80.0	4.5	2.5	Provide perineal care	72.0	9.5	2.0
Assist patient using bedpan	82.4	4.8	2.1	Provide skin care to comatose or paralyzed patients	61.5	13.2	3.3
Assist patient using bedside commode	83.7	3.7	2.1	Record intake of food/fluids	51.0	14.6	2.5
Assist patient using urinal	88.3	3.3	2.7	Record output (feces, urine, vomitus, etc.)	51.3	15.2	55.1
Assist patient walking	73.4	6.5	2.5	Record patients's height/weight	58.2	11.4	2.5
Bathing patient: bed	80.9	8.0	0.5	Remove/clean inner cannula of tracheostomy	1.5[a]	35.3	33.1
Bathing patient: shower	86.5	3.6	1.0	Record temperature, pulse, respiration, and blood pressure	39.7	19.1	5.0
Bathing patient: tub	86.2	3.1	1.0	Regulate blood transfusion	0.0[a]	22.8[a]	49.0
Care for decubitus ulcers (bedsores)	15.1	43.8	5.2	Regulate intravenous flow	2.2[a]	33.3	36.2
Care for patient in isolation	34.7	28.7	7.8	Remove fecal impaction	33.2[a]	29.5	4.7
Check for fecal impaction	39.2	25.8	5.2	Rub patient's back	73.2	4.6	1.5
Collect stool specimen	53.6	16.5	4.1	Serve food trays	75.6	3.5	2.0
Collect urine specimen	56.2	16.3	3.0	Start blood transfusion	4.2[a]	3.4[a]	83.2
Comb patient's hair	83.8	3.5	1.5	Start intravenous fluids	0.0[a]	4.7[a]	85.8
Count apical pulse	30.3[a]	23.4	5.5	Suction patient's nose	25.0[a]	30.6	13.7
Count radial pulse	39.9	17.2	5.6	Suction patient's throat	11.3[a]	44.4	13.1
Count respirations	44.4	16.7	4.0	Suction patient's tracheostomy	2.1[a]	39.2	29.4
Cut patient's finger/toe nails	60.4	17.2	3.6	Take blood pressure	41.2	17.1	3.0
Discontinue blood transfusion	3.7[a]	38.8	34.3	Take temperatures axillary	54.4	15.0	4.1
Discontinue intravenous fluids	10.6[a]	38.3	22.7	Take temperatures orally	55.4	12.4	3.0
Empty/record drainage from tubes	51.2	17.7	9.1	Take temperatures rectally	54.5	15.8	2.5
Engage in OT with patients	55.8	12.8	7.7	Transport patient in wheelchair	70.7	4.5	2.0
Feed patients	68.1	5.9	2.0	Transport patient on stretcher	62.6	12.3	1.8
Give enemas	47.7	26.1	2.0	Test urine for sugar/acetone	56.2	17.0	3.6
Insert naso-gastric tubes	0.0[a]	26.2[a]	49.0	Turn patient	71.1	4.6	2.5
Insert urinary catheter	0.5[a]	51.1	11.3	Weigh/measure patient	67.0	9.9	3.4
Irrigate colostomy	5.4[a]	46.4	16.3				
Irrigate urinary bladder	4.6[a]	48.6	13.9				

[a]Signifies a task for which employee has not received preemployment training.

SOURCE: K.W. Beaver, "Task Analysis of Nursing Personnel: Long-Term Care Facilities in Utah," Ph.D. dissertation, Brigham Young University, 1978.

ified to perform each task, and surveyed nursing personnel in 79 reputable long-term care facilities as to their performance of these tasks (see table 9-3). While nurse educators deemed LPNs qualified to perform 74 of the 78 tasks, LPNs surveyed revealed that they routinely perform all 78 tasks (16). (The four tasks nurse educators deemed inappropriate for LPNs to perform were insertion of nasogastric tubes, preparation and administration of intravenous medication, regulation of blood transfusions, and starting blood transfusions or intravenous fluids.)

Nurse specialists are those who have completed graduate education or fulfilled certification requirements in a particular area of nursing. Such opportunities are generally available only to certified RNs (more specifically, to RNs who have obtained their licenses through a baccalaureate degree program).

The American Nurses Association (ANA) and 12 nurse specialty associations offer specialty certification to RNs who meet their eligibility requirements. Requirements may be practical and/or academic. The American Board of Urologic Allied Health Professionals is the only organization that permits LPNs to apply for specialty certification (39).

Although no specialty association exists for nurses in gerontological practice, the ANA offers a certificate in gerontological nursing to those with 2 years practical experience, and certifies as "gerontological nurse practitioner" those who complete a formal practitioner program outlined in ANA's "Guidelines for Nurse Practitioner Programs" (see description that follows). As of 1985, 49 of 131 institutions with accredited nursing master's programs offered master's training in geriatric nursing. Three offered graduate training in geropsychiatric nursing (53).

Other fields in which the ANA offers specialty certification (e.g., adult clinical specialist, psychiatric and mental health nurse, and adult and family nurse practitioner) address the care of mentally ill, aged, and long-term care patients, and may therefore include information about and experience with individuals with dementia.

Nurse practitioners (NPs) are a subgroup of nurse specialists. They are registered nurses who complete an academic program (approximately 1 year) to obtain skills and knowledge that permit them to collaborate with physicians.

This category of health professional is a new one, but it is developing rapidly. As of 1985, eight accredited programs provided training for geriatric nurse practitioners (GNPs) (53). Several other practitioner programs (e.g., family and adult nurse practitioner, and psychiatric nurse practitioner) include content relevant to serving geriatric and long-term care patients. As of March 1985, the ANA had certified 466 GNPs. By comparison, it certified 4,363 family nurse practitioners and 3,770 adult nurse practitioners (12).

Evaluations of the role NPs might play and the effectiveness of the physician/NP team have been favorable (39). The Congressional Budget Office reports that these professionals are about one-third to one-half as costly as physicians per hour of work, and that they spend more time with each patient (70).

One assessment of present and future personnel needs in caring for the elderly evaluated the role of the geriatric nurse practitioner. The study projected that with moderate delegation of responsibility by physicians to GNPs and physician assistants, the number of primary care physicians needed to care for the elderly in 2010 could be reduced by 25 percent. With maximum delegation to GNPs, the number could drop by 44 percent (see table 9-4) (41). These figures are based on current levels of utilization and assume a role for geriatric specialists and medical subspecialists (e.g., surgeon, cardiologist, or gastroenterologist) in addition to primary care physicians. The study projected a need for 12,000 to 20,000 GNPs by the year 2010. Only 466 GNPs were registered by the ANA as of March 1985 (12).

State law and reimbursement regulations are two influences on the role NPs may play in the delivery of primary care, the tasks they may per-

Table 9-4.—Physician and Nonphysician Personnel (in FTEs) Needed in 2010 to Care for Elderly Population, By System of Delegation[a]

Mode of practice	Moderate delegation[b]					Maximum delegation[c]				
	GS	MS	PCP	GNP/PA	SW	GS	MS	PCP	GNP/PA	SW
Status quo	520	1,109	26,914	11,622	3,766	391	1,109	19,852	19,479	7,532
Consultative	11,702	8,330	21,156	12,169	3,941	8,618	8,330	15,692	20,398	7,882
Primary care	18,205	8,330	17,026	12,169	3,941	13,329	8,330	12,739	20,398	7,882

KEY: FTE full-time equivalent; PCP primary care physician;
GS geriatric specialist; GNP/PA general nurse practioner/physician assistant;
MS medical subspecialist; SW social worker.

[a]based on current utilization levels.
[b]Moderate delegation: Nonhospital care Hospital care
65% MD 90% MD
25% GNP/PA 10% GNP/PA
10% SW 0% SW

[c]Maximum delegation: Nonhospital care Hospital care
40% MD 80% MD
40% GNP/PA 20% GNP/PA
20% SW 0% SW

SOURCE: Adapted from R.L. Kane, D.H. Solomon, J.C Beck, et al., *Geriatrics in the United States: Manpower Projections and Training Considerations* (Santa Monica, CA: Rand Corp., 1980).

form, and the degree to which they must be supervised by a physician. With the evolution of NP training programs, some States amended physician and nurse practice acts to allow NPs to perform some medical procedures previously reserved for physicians. Other activities (e.g., drug prescription, and certain diagnostic procedures) may be done by NPs only under physician supervision, as defined by the State. Under Medicaid and Medicare regulations, certain services are unreimbursable unless supervised or performed by a physician. In this way, the regulations define the role NPs play in patient care and influence the willingness of health care institutions to employ these professionals (62,85).

A Nursing Home Demonstration Project at the University of Utah tested the use of NPs as primary caregivers to long-term care patients. Their responsibilities included:

• definition of observational boundaries or "progress benchmarks" to be used by staff in recognizing and reporting significant change in a patient's condition;
• instruction of nursing staff to foster understanding, skills, knowledge, and values fundamental to quality long-term care;
• evaluation of patient progress;
• assessment of need for, administration of, and interpretation of diagnostic procedures (e.g., hematocrit and urine tests, blood sampling and blood chemistry work-ups, and radiographic studies);
• determination of need for therapy, further assessment, or referral;
• education of patient and family about diagnosis and care plans; and
• 24-hour emergency availability (55).

Nursing Curricula

The importance of cognitive knowledge and clinical experience in determining career preferences is well documented. A greater emphasis on geriatrics and long-term care in nursing education, therefore, is seen as critical to addressing the nursing shortage in these fields (18).

Since the mid-1970s, efforts to include geriatric content into basic (RN and LPN) nursing programs have grown. The Nurse Training Act of 1975 (Public Law 94-63) and its amendments emphasize the problems of providing health care for the elderly and the need for staff development through education. Through the Bureau of Health Professionals' Division of Nursing, the legislation supports efforts to integrate geriatrics into the curricula of both basic and advanced-degree nursing programs (75).

The majority of entry-level programs, however, still include little theoretical or clinical content in geriatrics and long-term care (43). Moreover, because much of the impetus to incorporate geriatrics into basic nursing curricula and to establish programs for advanced training in geriatric nursing has come through federally funded grants and contracts, reduced funding for nursing programs in fiscal years 1986 and 1987 may curtail future progress.

Nursing programs are under no obligation to teach these subjects. Curricular content in nursing programs remains a matter of institutional choice. The National League of Nursing, the accrediting body for academic nursing programs, does not issue written quantitative or minimum curricular requirements (39). Funding constraints and access to resources, faculty, and clinical training sites contribute to the broad disparity in the quality and quantity of material related to geriatrics, mental health, and long-term care in both undergraduate and graduate nursing programs.

Several modifications in standard nursing curricula could facilitate students' preparation for and interest in gerontological and long-term care nursing:

• **Differentiation of acute and chronic illness:** Current nursing education focuses heavily on the acute care patient. Fundamental differences in treatment and prognosis make it necessary to distinguish between acutely and chronically ill persons. An approach that incorporates assessment and management of functional and rehabilitative restrictions of the chronically ill would broaden nursing students' understanding of these patients' care needs.
• **Assessment skills:** Expanding the range of assessment skills taught to nursing students may enhance their ability to contribute to the

diagnosis and care of chronically ill patients. In addition to standard assessment of physical status, nurses who work with the chronically ill may be asked to assess the patient's self-care abilities, cognitive skills, living environment, and social interactions. Particularly in long-term care settings, nurses may be the most appropriate professional to perform a comprehensive assessment of patient status.

- **Case-management:** Because of the wide range of professionals and agencies that can play a role in caring for the chronically ill, it may be useful for nursing programs to prepare nurses to work with patients and families in locating appropriate services and identifying the optimal setting for care.

- **Patient/family education:** Nurses working with the chronically ill may teach patients and families how to perform daily activities and how to modify the physical environment to enhance the patient's comfort, safety, or ability to cope. These skills are often omitted from programs that emphasize disease processes and medical regimens.

- **Training and supervising paraprofessionals:** Because much of the daily care for chronically ill persons in nursing homes is provided by paraprofessional staff, nurses are increasingly expected to train and supervise these employees. To ensure the maintenance of quality care, nurse training programs should include skills necessary for training and supervising paraprofessional and nonprofessional staff.

- **Working within a multidisciplinary team:** As described earlier, the model of care that emphasizes a multidisciplinary team approach to care is different from the physician-based model used in most acute care settings. Clinical exposure to settings where nurses participate in the team approach is important in preparing nursing students for that role.

- **Administrative and supervisory skills:** Finally, because nurses are increasingly expected to supervise and train paraprofessional staff and to assume primarily responsibility for administrative detail and paperwork, these skills should be integrated into basic nurse training programs.

Incorporation of material related to geriatrics and long-term care is fundamental to preparing nurses for work in this increasingly prominent field. The knowledge and skills nursing students acquire in studying and working with elderly and chronically ill persons are an important basis for their ability to work with patients with a dementing disorder. Information about and experience with mentally ill patients may further enhance nurses' capacity to work with individuals who have dementia.

There is no single point in the course of nurse training at which it is "correct" to teach about dementing disorders. The subject may be addressed in a course about aging and disorders prevalent among the aged; it may be incorporated into a unit on psychiatric disturbances or neurologic impairments; it may be described along with other chronic degenerative diseases. However, several topics related to the diagnosis, treatment, and care of dementia patients could be incorporated productively into one or more segments of the required nursing curriculum. These include:

- a list and definitions of dementing disorders;
- assessment techniques (physical, emotional, functional, psychosocial, intellectual);
- common behaviors of persons with dementia (disorientation, wandering, incontinence, drug reactions, aggressiveness);
- interview techniques;
- sensory stimulation and assistance with activities of daily living;
- role of therapeutic techniques (physical, psychological, medical, speech, recreational, occupational);
- clinical progression;
- role of the family;
- environment modification;
- management with minimal restraints (chemical and physical); and
- need for consistent, continual orientation cues (20).

Nurse's Aides

Nurse's aides spend more time with patients and provide more direct patient care than any other group of personnel in long-term care facilities. Recent estimates suggest that 80 to 90 percent of care in nursing homes is given by aides (3,29). This important group of employees, however, also has the lowest level of educational and preemployment training (see table 9-5) and the highest rate of turnover (34,35). Annual turnover rate among nurse's aides averages 75 percent (3).

Lack of preemployment preparation and inservice training, low wages, and the absence of employee benefits, recognition, and opportunities for advancement all contribute to the intense job dissatisfaction and rapid turnover among nurse's aides. A survey of aides at 40 nursing homes in the Detroit area (34) found that:

- only 49 percent were high school graduates;
- only 11 percent had been taught anything concerning geriatrics, gerontology, or problems of the aged;
- 51 percent had received no formal orientation or inservice training (most had been trained by another aide);
- most facilities provided no pay differential in accordance with level of academic achievement or relevant job experience;
- few facilities offered opportunities for career advancement based on experience gained or training pursued during employment;
- monetary rewards and employment benefits (e.g., sick days, paid vacation time, or health insurance) were negligible or nonexistent;
- only 35 percent received pay increases based on seniority; and
- of the aides whose tenure exceeded 5 years, half had received no salary increase and had

been at minimum wage since their initial employment.

In the task anaylsis study of 78 nursing duties described earlier, nurse's aides were found to routinely perform nursing tasks for which nurse educators deem them unqualified (see table 9-4) (16). Although a panel of nurse educators identified 27 tasks for which they deemed aides insufficiently trained, nursing staff of long-term care facilities reported that aides routinely perform 74 of the 78 tasks. For example, facilities indicated that it is not uncommon for nurse's aides to administer oxygen, discontinue intravenous fluids, or give medication, each of which the nurse educators deemed aides insufficiently trained to perform.

Most States have legislative requirements for a specific number of hours of orientation and inservice education for nurse's aides, but the quality and quantity of the training are often limited (1). State requirements regarding preservice education and experience are far less specific for these employees than for administrators and professional staff in long-term care facilities. Because nurse's aides provide the vast majority of direct care in these facilities, the absence of specific training requirements is of particular concern.

Owing in part to the high turnover rate, nursing home administrators are often reluctant to provide the resources, particularly release time and funds, for quality continuing education programs for aides.

Federal Efforts To Improve Training

The Nurse Training Act of 1975, mentioned earlier in conjunction with efforts to incorporate geriatrics into nursing curricula, supports efforts to provide training to paraprofessionals and nurse's aides.

Seeking to upgrade the skills of the paraprofessionals who care for the elderly in nursing homes, the Bureau of Health Professionals' Division of Nursing funded seven basic training programs for nursing home aides and orderlies. Among these, Westbrook College instituted a geriatric nurse assistant program to train students in the basic skills necessary for geriatric nursing care in long-term care facilities, to create a deeper understanding

Table 9-5.—Preemployment Requirements for Nurse's Aides[a]

Requirement	Yes		No		No response	
	Number	%	Number	%	Number	%
High school graduate	2	12.50	12	75.00	2	12.50
Prior training program..........	8	50.00	7	43.75	1	6.25
Nurse's aide experience........	6	37.50	9	56.25	1	6.25
Written application ...	14	87.50	0		2	12.5
Personal interview ...	16	100.00	0		0	
Letters of reference ..	5	31.25	10	62.50	1	6.25

[a]Based on survey of 16 nursing home directors.

SOURCE: M.O. Hogstel, ''Auxiliary Nursing Personnel,'' *Management of Personnel in Long-Term Care*, M.O. Hogstel (ed.) (Bowie, MD: Robert J. Brady Co., 1983).

and awareness of the physical, emotional, social, and religious needs of the elderly. And the Miami Jewish Home and Hospital for the Aged established a regional geriatric training program to upgrade the skills of licensed professional (or vocational) nurses, nurse's aides, and other paraprofessional nursing personnel.

State Efforts To Improve Training

Efforts to improve the training of nursing home personnel are also increasing at the State level. Seventeen States now require training of geriatric nurse's aides (9). To date, however, no State requires that preparatory classes for these individuals include information about dementia and caring for persons with dementia.

The Maryland State Office on Aging designed and administered a project to prepare administrators and nurses in long-term care facilities to train paraprofessional and nonprofessional staff. The project aimed to help these professionals assess the learning needs of their staff and to construct, execute, and evaluate teaching and learning experiences. The group concluded that:

- The morale of paraprofessional and nonprofessional staff members improves when their practice is based on knowledge rather than on tradition or belief.
- Increased knowledge of gerontology is important for facilitating the evolution of new roles in care for the elderly.
- Certification and recognition are important incentives for and expressions of commitment to the importance of formal learning about gerontology for long-term care positions.
- Readily accessible films, books, and other resource materials are important stimuli and supplementary learning tools (8).

The State of Virginia requires that geriatric nurse's aides receive vocational education prior to employment. For a program to be approved, it must meet State requirements. These include a list of minimum competencies to be incorporated into the training program curriculum. Although teaching about dementing diseases is not specifically required, the topic may be addressed under several subjects that are required (e.g., disorientation; physical, psychological, and sociological

changes of aging; and major disorders of the nervous system). Programs are also required to train students to perform a wide range of nursing tasks and to assist patients in activities of daily living, although there is no requirement for training to perform these tasks with an individual with dementia (81).

Physicians

Although it is difficult to assess the actual number of physicians who provide care for chronically ill patients in and out of health care institutions, it has historically been a field of medicine with low appeal. The number of physicians who provide care for nursing home patients is one reflection of this situation.

Few nursing homes in the United States maintain a full-time resident physician, and the number of physicians who report visiting nursing homes over the course of a year is small. In 1981 only 14 percent of physicians reported visiting patients in a nursing home. That percentage is much lower than the 48 percent of physicians who are family practitioners and internists—those most responsible for nursing home visits by physicians—indicating that few physicians continue to provide care once their patients are admitted to nursing homes (58). Even among physicians declaring geriatrics to be their primary specialty, few report doing any work in nursing homes (49).

Work With the Chronically Ill

Several factors have been cited as contributing to physicians' apparent reluctance to work with the chronically ill, particularly with elderly chronically ill patients:

- **Education:** An educational process that stresses acute rather than chronic care and provides little experience with and information about caring for mentally ill or elderly patients contributes to the lack of interest physicians show for working with these patients.
- **Inadequate financial reimbursement:** Medicaid and Medicare reimbursement rates may be too low to offset the costs and inconvenience of travel to facilities in which long-

term care patients reside (not only nursing homes, but also alternative care settings and individual residences). Administrative difficulties in obtaining reimbursement may create further disincentive.

- **Regulatory disincentives:** Certain regulatory requirements may influence physicians' willingness to serve patients residing in long-term care facilities. (Medicare requires one visit per month for patients in SNFs, although State requirements vary. Medicaid requirements call for one visit every 30 days for the first 90 days in an SNF, and every 60 days in ICFs.)
- **Geographical inconvenience:** The geographic isolation of many long-term care facilities adds to the time and inconvenience of physician visits.
- **Ageism:** Societal bias against the elderly and lack of interest in their needs is often cited as a factor contributing to physicians' attitudes toward working with older patients.
- **Lack of professional recognition:** Working with the chronically ill, for whom there may be no treatment or cure, provides little opportunity for the physician to gain recognition as a competent "healer."
- **Therapeutic nihilism:** Physicians express the frustration and lack of professional fulfillment associated with working with patients for whom there is no cure and no treatment that can significantly alleviate symptoms or impede progression of the illness.

Although the relative importance of each factor has not been established, a recent survey of 4,000 physicians in 15 specialties sought to identify factors that influence willingness to provide care for nursing home patients (see table 9-6) (51). The study did not consider the impact of educational and sociological factors on physicians' decisions, but did evaluate the importance of logistical and practical considerations of providing nursing home care.

Because regulatory requirements and reimbursement rates, particularly for Medicaid, vary by State, it is difficult to generalize about their influence on physicians' willingness to serve patients in long-term care facilities. Nevertheless, nationally applied regulations may have an effect.

Table 9-6.—Characteristics of Physicians Who Visit Nursing Homes[a] (% distribution)

Characteristics	Visits per week		
	None	1-4	5+
Board-certified	51.8	28.1	20.1
Noncertified	53.7	19.6	26.7
U.S. medical school graduate	53.5	28.8	23.7
Foreign medical graduate	51.3	14.8	33.9
60 years +	47.1	17.1	35.8
Less than 60	56.7	24.4	19.0
Accepts Medicaid	52.5	22.3	25.6
Does not accept Medicaid	55.2	20.7	24.6
Practice location:			
Large metropolitan	57.5	19.1	23.4
Small metropolitan	5.1	23.1	17.8
Nonmetropolitan	42.8	23.7	33.5
Region:			
Northeast	61.7	20.6	17.7
North Central	45.9	27.1	27.0
South	53.3	20.7	26.0
West	50.3	18.6	31.1

[a]Based on a survey of 4,000 physicians with *office-based* practices. The findings therefore may not be representative of all U.S. physicians. Fifteen medical specialties were respresented.

SOURCE: J.B. Mitchell, ''Physician Visits to Nursing Homes,'' *The Gerontologist* 22:45-48, 1982.

Federal reimbursement programs are structured to avoid excessive payment for what are termed "gang visits" by physicians to nursing facilities—visits during which a physician sees many patients over a brief period and claims reimbursement for each, as if each were a separate call. Medicare reimbursement standards recommend comparing a nursing home visit during which several patients are seen to a routine office visit, whereas a visit during which only one patient is seen be considered a house call. Carriers are advised to assume that multiple patients are visited (i.e., reimburse at the lower rate) unless there is distinct evidence to the contrary. Reimbursement at the level of a routine office visit fails to account for costs in travel and time that such visits entail. Thus, reimbursement standards may create a disincentive for physicians to visit patients in nursing homes.

The impact of such regulations on physicians' reluctance to care for these patients is hard to assess. Surveys indicate, however, that physicians who do visit nursing home patients have high case loads there (an average of 11 patient visits per week), constituting over 7 percent of their weekly patient sessions (51). (Other types of visits include those to office, hospital, emergency room, clinic, and private residence.) It is unclear whether that finding reflects instances in which Medicare restrictions do not apply (e.g., non-Medicare patients in nursing home) or indicates an acceptance of these conditions by physicians working with nursing home residents.

Time spent on nursing home visits does appear to be relevant. Physicians who visit nursing homes report that, including travel time, the average visit takes twice as long (36 rather than 18 minutes) as an office visit (51). The additional time and inconvenience may contribute to physicians' reluctance to care for patients in these facilities.

Educational and sociological factors may influence physicians' professional preferences to an even greater degree than the logistical and practical considerations just described. It is through the educational process that students come to regard particular aspects of medical practice as rewarding, and to recognize those areas of medicine that are professionally and societally esteemed.

As noted, physicians' lack of interest in long-term care is attributed in part to an educational process that emphasizes acute rather than chronic care (23,30). The incurability and slow progression of chronic diseases are a source of frustration to physicians whose training stresses dramatic intervention, treatment, and cure. Working with the chronically ill, for whom there are few split-second decisions or heroic cures, is less gratifying for professionals trained in this manner (23).

Several modifications in medical education may enable schools to address that imbalance and thereby prepare professionals who find satisfaction in serving both chronically and acutely ill patients.

- Greater information about and experience with the chronically ill might enhance students' understanding of the different perspective and skills that are required in caring for these patients.
- Physicians who are knowledgeable about and competent in chronic care may serve as important role models and stimulate students' interest in and respect for the physician's role in long-term care.
- An orientation that does not equate "successful treatment" with "cure" could enable health

care professionals in training to recognize the different expectations that must accompany care for chronically ill patients.
- The value of enhancing the functional capacity and quality of life of patients for whom no cure is possible is an important aspect of chronic care to be conveyed to medical students.

Because dementing diseases are chronic and degenerative in nature, modifications of this sort may be critical to stimulating physicians' interest in working with these patients. In that regard, knowledge about and experience with chronically ill patients—particularly elderly and mentally ill patients—may be of equal importance to lectures and classroom discussion about dementing illnesses.

Didactic Content Related to Dementia.—During the first two years of medical school—the preclinical years—students spend the majority of their academic time in lectures, seminars, and laboratories. The basic medical sciences (e.g., anatomy, physiology, pathology, neurology, immunology, and biochemistry) are conveyed to first- and second-year students using standard didactic teaching methods.

The absence of content related to aging and to geriatric medicine is widely cited as a critical gap in medical education, contributing to physicians' low level of interest in and knowledge about working with older patients. The 1970s marked the beginning of a dramatic increase in the number of schools that incorporated such material into their curricula. A 1983 survey indicated that 91 percent of U.S. medical schools have incorporated some geriatric material into their curriculum (see table 9-7). Seventy-two percent had some required time for geriatric education; 19 percent offered only elective time for geriatrics. (Of 127 accredited medical schools, 114 schools were surveyed and 100 responded (15).)

Continued efforts to include information about aging and medical care of older persons are important for many reasons. Whether geriatrics should be introduced as a separate, required subject or integrated into other core courses remains subject to debate, but teaching medical students

Table 9-7.—Inclusion of Geriatrics in Medical School Curriculum (percentage)[a]

Geriatrics in curriculum	1978	1983
Required curriculum	64	72
Elective curriculum only	36	19
No geriatrics	NR	9

NR: Not reported.
[a]Based on survey of 81 medical schools in 1978 and 100 medical schools in 1983.

SOURCE: P.P. Barry and R.J. Ham, "Geriatric Education: What the Medical Schools Are Doing Now," *Journal of the American Geriatric Society* 33:133-135, 1985.

Table 9-8.—Schools With Geriatric Curriculum: Percentage of Time Each Year of Medical School[a]

Year in school	Required course	Elective course
First	49	21
Second	55	17
Third	9	19
Fourth	3	84

Many schools have curriculum time in more than 1 year.
[a]Based on 1983 survey of 100 medical schools.

SOURCE: P.P. Barry and R.J. Ham, "Geriatric Education: What the Medical Schools Are Doing Now," *Journal of the American Geriatric Society* 33:133-135, 1985.

about dementing disorders does not necessarily require a discrete course about geriatrics.

As with nurse training, there is no "correct" time for teaching medical students about dementing disorders (see table 9-8). Although a course about aging and diseases prevalent among the elderly is an appropriate place for describing the various dementing disorders associated with chronic organic brain degeneration, various aspects of the diseases may be described in any number of courses throughout the curriculum. Physiological aspects, for instance, may be described in a neurology course. Assessment techniques may be discussed in a class about psychiatry. Topics such as community resources and the role of the family may be broached during the study of patient management considerations.

Clinical Experience With Dementia Patients. —The clinical (third and fourth) years of medical education are characterized by practical experience (rotations) in diagnosis, treatment, and care of patients. The elderly and mentally ill are two groups whose specific care needs are frequently overlooked in designing this component.

Because many of the illnesses suffered by older persons are chronic rather than acute, the oppor-

tunity to care for older patients provides students with a different set of experiences. Students gain an understanding of the different role, knowledge, and skills required in caring for the chronically ill. Management of the long-term care patient, for example, may require the physician to head an interdisciplinary team comprising a wide range of health and social service workers. As coordinator, the physician must be able to prescribe drugs as well as services, assess physical as well as emotional needs, and determine the availability and propriety of resources. (Table 9-9 identifies some of the skills relevant to geriatric care that students might be expected to master.)

Table 9-9.—Skills Relevant to Geriatric Care To Be Mastered by Medical Students

Interview and take an accurate medical history of an elderly patient including functional (e.g., the patient's ability to perform daily activities) and psychosocial (e.g., motivation, morale, family and social interaction, household composition, or productivity) factors.

Conduct and record a complete physical examination of an elderly patient, including assessment of normal physical signs of aging and of functional ability (e.g., ability to perform daily activities, or mental status testing).

Distinguish "normal" from pathologic aging (e.g., with respect to cognitive function, psychomotor performance, human sexuality, personality adjustment, and illness behavior).

Demonstrate clinical decisionmaking skills, accounting for altered clinical presentation of disease in the elderly, multiple illness complexes, patient lifestyle, cost-benefit factors, and prognosis.

Apply knowledge of clinical pharmacology in elderly patients (interactions and side effects of specific drugs; patient drug use patterns).

Apply knowledge of rehabilitative medicine in managing the problems of elderly patients (underlying principles, facilities and programs, plan development, and outcome prediction).

Identify available social resources and programs in planning the care of an elderly patient (financial, health, and social supports, including natural support systems).

Coordinate and provide for a continuum of care (delivery of integrated care to elderly persons at differing levels of health and social services, such as hospitals, nursing homes, day care centers, and patient's home).

Participate as part of an interdisciplinary health care team in coordinating assessment and management of elderly patients.

Provide personalized and empathetic care to patients and their families.

SOURCE: J.C. Beck and S. Vivell, "Development of Geriatrics in the United States," *Geriatric Medicine*, vol. 2, C.K. Cassell and J.R. Walsh (eds.) (New York: Springer-Verlag Publishing, 1985).

In addition to the benefits of enhanced knowledge and training gained through caring for the chronically ill, many argue that exposure to these patients heightens students' interest in caring for them. Until recently, medical schools made little effort to provide students with experience with these patients; any experience gained was likely to be incidental. Facilities in which large numbers of elderly or mentally ill persons reside (e.g., nursing homes) came to be considered undesirable working environments.

The most recent data show that of the 127 American medical schools, 99 have required courses that cover geriatrics, including eight that exclusively focus on geriatrics (70). The clinical settings in which students work with the elderly (hospital, nursing home, outpatient clinic, or patient's home) vary according to the affiliations of the particular school. (Table 9-10 indicates the number of schools offering clinical rotations in each of several types of settings.)

The "teaching nursing home," mentioned earlier, is one innovative approach that allows students to gain experience in caring for chronically ill elderly people. Similar in principle to the teaching hospital, it affords medical students and graduates the opportunity to work with patients in a long-term care facility. The National Institute on Aging and the Robert Wood Johnson Foundation both sponsor projects to develop teaching nursing homes in the United States (74,83).

Graduate Medical Education.—For most students, the 4 years of medical school are followed

Table 9-10.—Medical Schools Using Various Training Sites (percentage)

Training sites[a]	Schools
Nursing home	74
Hospital (university or community)	64
Outpatient clinic	63
Veterans Administration hospital	46
Patient's home	43
Other community sites	33
Family practice center	31
Congregate housing	26
Private practice	23
Day care	19

[a]Most schools use more than one site.

SOURCE: P.P. Barry and R.J. Ham, "Geriatric Education: What the Medical Schools Are Doing Now," *Journal of the American Geriatric Society* 33:133-135, 1985.

by a period of internship and residency, during which they gain the additional training necessary to become certified in some branch of medicine. Even those who choose to practice primary care medicine (e.g., internists and family physicians) generally complete a residency program.

The accreditation of residency programs and the certification of physicians completing residency programs provide two avenues for ensuring that physicians in particular medical specialties gain knowledge and experience in the diagnosis and treatment of dementia patients.

Accreditation of a residency program is the process by which the Accreditation Council for Graduate Medical Education (ACGME) grants public recognition to a program providing advanced preparation for physicians in a particular medical specialty. Programs are evaluated by a Residency Review Committee (RRC). Each RRC comprises representatives from the American Medical Association's Council on Medical Education and from professional associations representing that medical specialty (e.g., American Board of Psychiatry and Neurology, or American Board of Internal Medicine) (2).

Certification is the process by which a specialty board grants recognition to an individual physician who has completed a residency program in a particular medical specialty and who has passed an examination of competence in that specialty. Examinations are developed by medical specialty boards within the professional association representing that specialty (2).

Inclusion of material related to dementia is particularly relevent for residents in such specialties as psychiatry, neurology, family medicine, internal medicine, and geriatrics. RRCs for these fields could insist that curricula for residency programs in these specialties include content related to care of persons with dementia. Medical specialty boards in the professional associations representing these medical specialties could design certification examinations that test for knowledge related to diagnosis and treatment of persons with dementia.

At present, no formal board of geriatric medicine exists. Geriatrics is subsumed by other medical specialties, particularly family and internal medicine. Both the American Board of Family Practice and the American Board of Internal Medicine are working to develop examinations that will enable physicians certified in these areas of practice to pursue added qualifications in geriatric medicine (6).

Under a grant from Pfizer Pharmaceuticals, the American Geriatrics Society (AGS) is developing curriculum guidelines for postresidency training in geriatric medicine. The AGS Geriatric Curriculum Development Committee will forward its recommendations to the ACGME's Internal Medicine Residency Review Committee. If the RRC approves the guidelines, it will recommend their inclusion in the ACGME's next *Directory of Residency Training Programs* (7).

Although a limited number of residency programs in geriatrics has become available in the United States since 1972, few physicians pursue graduate training in geriatrics. Because no formal board of geriatric medicine exists, physicians completing a geriatric residency program cannot obtain formal certification similar to that available in other medical specialties. The absence of opportunities for professional recognition may significantly influence individuals' willingness to pursue training in geriatrics after medical school. The debate about designating geriatrics as a separate area of medical expertise or whether competence in geriatric care should be required of all physicians is widely discussed in the literature.

Postgraduate Medical Education.—Opportunities for geriatric fellowships are increasing. One of the first fellowship programs in geriatric medicine was instituted by the Veterans Administration in July 1978 (26,86). Candidates must be certified in internal medicine, family medicine, or psychiatry.

The Federal Council for Internal Medicine has suggested that such advanced training may generate teachers and researchers in geriatric medicine and care, and may also develop expertise in physicians who wish to become medical directors for long-term care facilities or consultants to those caring for elderly patients with complex medical or psychosocial problems (27).

Social Workers

Social workers' skills in individual and group counseling and their knowledge of local and national resources make them valuable partners in planning and administering care for persons with dementia. They may participate in:

- client intake interviews,
- preadmission counseling of client and family,
- postadmission counseling and followup services for patient and family,
- financial needs assessment,
- utilization of and referral to community resources,
- coordination of volunteer programs,
- case management, and
- discharge planning (19).

Social workers may provide consultative services to other members of the health care team, and in some facilities may act as team leader. In identifying and meeting the psychosocial needs of patients and families, social workers may become involved in client advocacy inside and outside of long-term care facilities (19).

A social worker may also serve as case manager for individuals with dementia and their families. Community referral programs, as well as programs and facilities providing services, may employ a social worker for that purpose. As case manager, a social worker may help patient and family locate appropriate services, identify sources of funding, and monitor services delivered. In consultation with the appropriate health care staff, a social worker may also help identify the optimal setting for care and evaluate the effectiveness of services delivered.

Although social service staff may hold any variety of undergraduate or graduate degrees, this assessment focuses on the educational preparation of those with a master's degree in social work. A master's degree generally requires a minimum of 2 years postgraduate work. During the first year, students complete core courses in social work practice. The foundation material aims to provide students with fundamental knowledge, skills, and guidelines for practice that can be applied across practice settings, population groups, and problems. Course content includes material related to human behavior and the social environment, social welfare policy and services, special population groups, values and ethics, social work practice, and research methods.

On completion of the fundamental course work, students select a field of concentration (see table 9-11). Common concentrations are in:

- children and youth services,
- family services,
- gerontology,
- health,
- mental health, and
- social and economic development.

Within these fields, many programs allow students to select a mode of practice (e.g., clinical, administration, programming and supervision, or research) in which to specialize. Through a combination of classroom and experiential learning, students gain knowledge and skills specific to their area of concentration and mode of practice.

In September 1983, the Council on Social Work Education (CSWE) was awarded a 14-month grant by the Administration on Aging to promote the development, adoption, and infusion of geronto-

logical curricula and teaching materials into social work programs. The project was intended to expand the number of social workers equipped to plan and deliver services to the elderly (46). CSWE surveyed all 89 graduate social work education programs regarding their course offerings in gerontology; the information was reviewed and updated in late 1983 and early 1984 (25).

Gerontological social work programs generally require a course in social policy related to aging (e.g., housing, transportation, or medical assistance) and in direct service to the elderly (e.g., skills, knowledge, and resources needed in serving the elderly). Students select additional courses that combine their concentration in gerontology and the mode of practice that they have chosen. Clinicians, for example, might take a course in clinical social work with the aged and their families, while administrators might take a course in senior center administration or administrative issues in financing health care for the elderly.

A large portion of the social work student's academic time—about 3 days per week—is devoted to work experience. Many gerontological programs stress the importance of experience with diverse segments of the elderly population in a variety of settings—those who are relatively healthy and independent, those who are homebound, those in acute care settings and long-term care facilities, and those who are terminally ill. These programs may require students to rotate through a variety of practice settings, including a senior center, nursing home, a hospital outpatient department, and a State, county, or city office on aging. Students learn to evaluate, assess, and manage service, to establish treatment plans, and to counsel older adults and their families.

The curriculum of the gerontological social work program at Syracuse University illustrates the degree to which the core courses and field opportunities may provide information about and exposure to dementia patients:

Processes of Aging: covers organic brain syndromes including comparison with acute dementias, strategies for management, and theories of causation.

Direct Service to the Elderly: 1 class session of 14 devoted to dementia. Texts and journals are the written source materials used.

Table 9-11.—Concentrations Chosen By Master of Social Work Students[a]

Concentration	Percent
Gerontology	2.5
Alcohol, drug, or substance abuse	1.2
Child welfare	4.4
Community planning	1.4
Corrections, criminal justice	1.2
Family services	6.5
Group services	0.6
Health	7.2
Industrial social work	0.8
Mental health/community mental health	11.6
Mental retardation	0.7
Public assistance/public welfare	1.0
Rehabilitation	0.5
School social work	1.5
Other fields of practice of social problems	5.0
Combinations	2.0
Not yet determined	21.4
None	30.7

[a]Based on 1983-84 survey of 21,569 students enrolled in U.S. master of social work programs.

SOURCE: Council on Social Work Education, "Statistics on Social Work Education," Washington, DC, 1984.

Field Practice: 16 hours per week. Settings include long-term care facilities, psychiatric and general hospitals, senior centers, and State and local agencies on aging. Each may involve students in services for elderly individuals with dementia (68).

Other social work concentrations may also include course material and field experience related to the care of individuals with dementia. Students concentrating in mental health, for instance, take courses in chronic mental illness, psychopathology, social policy related to the mentally ill, and group methods in clinical social work or family therapy. Field work in such settings as psychiatric hospitals, community mental health centers, and psychiatric departments of general hospitals may involve them in caring for persons with chronic dementias.

Rehabilitative and Recreational Therapists

Facilities and programs that provide care for persons with dementia may employ one or more rehabilitative or recreational therapists on a part-time or consultant basis. Individuals with training in any number of specialties—occupational, physical, exercise, art, music, or speech therapy—may enrich the quality of care provided. Programs note the positive impact that physical and creative outlets have for persons with dementia—diminishing problematic behavioral tendencies such as wandering, agitation, and agression:

Exercise Therapy: The opportunity for physical exertion proves particularly important to persons with dementia, many of whom are still quite physically able. Programs note that simple, daily exercise periods significantly diminish patients' restlessness, agitation, and wandering behaviors. In addition, exercises offer a time for group recreation, and help maintain patients' mobility and fitness. Exercise programs may be led by an individual with training in movement therapy. Alternatively, a movement therapist may teach staff how to facilitate an exercise program.

Art Therapy: Art therapy may enhance a program for persons with dementia, offering the opportunity for creative expression, and enabling individuals to gain satisfaction through tangible accomplishment. While a facility may institute an arts and crafts program without the services of a designated art therapist, a specialist's ability to gain insights into patients' personalities and needs from their creative endeavors may assist staff to serve these individuals better.

Physical Therapy: Larger facilities, particularly nursing homes, may employ a physical therapist to assist individuals with specific mobility problems. For instance, physical rehabilitation may be necessary for a person with dementia who has suffered a hip fracture.

Occupational Therapy: A certified occupational therapist (OT) or certified occupational therapy assistant (COTA), like an art therapist, may contribute to program quality by providing creative and productive projects for persons with dementia. In addition, an individual trained in occupational therapy may design reality orientation programs and sensory stimulation activities for persons with dementia. These programs may be conducted by an OT, a COTA, or another member of the staff trained by one of these specialists.

Speech Therapy: Swallowing difficulties are a common and potentially fatal problem among persons with dementia. The skills of a speech therapist may be particularly important for these individuals.

It is critical that those who provide rehabilitative or recreational therapy for persons with dementia understand the nature of dementing illnesses—the extent to which persons with dementia may profit from therapeutic techniques and from physical, creative, and emotional outlets despite their cognitive and physical deficits. Educational programs in different therapeutic specialties may address these issues to varying degrees, and students may gain clinical experience related to care of persons with dementia. It remains important, however, for facilities and programs employing a rehabilitative or recreational therapist to provide basic training to ensure the adequacy of a professional's knowledge about dementing disorders and skills in communicating with and managing those with dementia.

Psychologists

Psychologists can play an important role in multidisciplinary team care for persons with dementia. They can assist in developing and evaluating strategies that address behavioral difficulties frequently encountered with persons with dementia. Psychologists can provide inservice training for staff and can help family members learn ways to communicate with and care for individuals with dementia more effectively.

Psychologists offer many direct and indirect services to those in long-term care settings. These can include:

Direct Services: As a staff member or consultant to a facility or program that provides care or refers individuals to appropriate care settings, a psychologist may assist in evaluating and planning individual care needs. Psychologists may perform the initial assessment of a patient's cognitive, intellectual, and behavioral functioning, in order to evaluate the extent of services required and the type of setting that would be appropriate (13). Those skilled in neuropsychological assessment can provide valuable information regarding diagnosis, nursing care, and rehabilitation approaches for older individuals (31,47).

Staff Training: A professional psychologist may provide quality inservice training to staff in long-term care facilities or in programs that provide care for persons with dementia. The need for such training has been emphasized and is evidenced by one national sample of nursing homes that indicated that only 4 percent of long-term care staff ever attended a course on mental or social problems (44). The psychologist can provide substantive information about aging, age-related psychosocial changes, psychopathology in older persons, and intervention techniques for improving patient care and functioning. In addition, this professional may provide insights on the role and function of the mental health specialist in long-term care settings. As a team care coordinator or consultant, the psychologist may further train long-term care staff in carrying out certain treatment processes and objectives (13).

Program Development: A psychologist in the long-term care setting may also assist in facility- or program-wide planning (e.g., milieu therapy or reality orientation), evaluation of existing programs, and policy formulation. The psychologist's knowledge and insights may help identify undefined or unmet needs of older individuals.

A survey done in 1979 of all accredited doctoral and internship programs in clinical and counseling psychology revealed a substantial increase in content related to aging (24). A previous study of 101 doctoral programs in clinical psychology found only one that offered formal training in the psychology of aging (see table 9-12) (65). A greater number of programs offered training opportunities in the field of aging, though none had classes and practicum as part of the required curriculum. The 1979 survey found that:

- 4 of 104 responding doctoral programs in clinical psychology offer formal programs in the psychology of aging;
- 46 programs carried courses with some content directly applicable to clinical psychology of aging (e.g., neuropsychology, psychological assessment, or developmental psychology);
- 60 programs cited one or more geriatric practicum facilities with which they were associated; five programs required students to work in one of these settings; and
- 64 programs reported faculty interest in or knowledge about the clinical psychology of aging.

Issues related to persons with dementing disorders—assessment and care; the role of the family and role of health care staff caring for those with dementia—are likely to be addressed by advanced degree programs for psychologists specializing in aging, although no formal documentation exists.

Program and Facility Administrators

Administrators of facilities and programs caring for persons with dementia play a major role in planning and delivering care. Their decisions regarding the allocation of resources (e.g., the number and type of staff hired), organizational structure, and program priorities are critical determinants of the quality of services delivered. Therefore, their understanding of the nature of dementing illnesses and patients' needs is a key to the quality of care provided.

It is quite likely, however, that the administrator of a long-term care facility or program has no prior experience with or training related to the care of persons with dementia. Even those who have formal education in health care administration may have received no training on the nature of dementing disorders and patients' specific care needs. Programs that train health care administrators emphasize management skills and responsibilities. They often provide little or no in-

Table 9-12.—APA-Accredited Doctoral Clinical Programs and Internship Programs, 1975 and 1979

Program	1975		1979	
	Number	Percent[a]	Number	Percent[b]
Doctoral clinical:				
Accredited programs	101	—	120	—
Replies	76	75	104	87
Formal programs in clinical psychology and aging	1	1	4	4
Informal programs in clinical psychology and aging	N/A	N/A	15	14
Programs with at least 1 course in aging	25	33	46	44
Programs with 1+ practicum facility in aging	34	45	60	58
Programs with 1+ faculty interested/knowledgeable in aging	38	50	64	62
Internship training:				
Accredited programs	118	—	169	—
Replies	97	82[b]	138	82[b]
Programs providing formal experience in aging	22	23	56	41
Programs with some contact in aging	42	43	33	24
Programs with staff interested/knowledgeable in aging	31	32	58	42

[a]Percentages based on total number of replies received, except where otherwise rated (see note b).
[b]Percentage of programs surveyed.
NOTE: N/A means not available.

SOURCE: L.D. Cohen and S.G. Cooley, "Psychology Training Programs for Direct Services to the Aging (Status Report: 1980)," *Professional Psychology: Research and Practice* 14:720-728, 1983.

formation about specific diseases and individual patient needs.

Formal preparation of nursing home administrators is just beginning to conform to traditional accreditation procedures (84). The Council on Post Secondary Accreditation's Commission on Health is responsible for accreditation of programs that train these administrators. The Association of University Programs in Health Administration is currently developing a proposal to examine the educational needs of nursing home administrators. The result may be a model curriculum that would eventually be reflected in educational programs and licensing examinations (84).

A 1984 survey of State licensure requirements found that 11 jurisdictions require only a high school diploma, 19 require a baccalaureate degree, 15 require an associate degree, and 6 have no educational requirements for nursing home administrators (84). Requirements for directors of noninstitutional programs (e.g., respite or adult day care) are even less stringent than those for nursing home administrators. In Virginia, for instance, an individual need only be of sound physical and mental condition to operate a day care facility for persons with dementia (82).

The American College of Health Care Administrators (ACHCA), however, reports recent that States are now making educational requirements for nursing home administrators more rigorous.

ACHCA's 1985 survey found that 42 States require between 15 and 30 hours of continuing education per year for the periodic renewal of licenses (5).

A national licensure examination for nursing home administrators also exists. States establish their own pass/fail standards for the examination. Categories on the test include patient care, personnel management, financial management, marketing and public relations, laws and regulations, and resource management. Approximately one-quarter of the questions are in the category of patient care, addressing such topics as nursing, social, physician, and pharmaceutical services and recreational activities for long-term care patients. The National Association of Boards of Examiners for Nursing Home Administrators reports that the most recent examination contained at least one question about dementia (50).

Volunteers and Survey Staff

Many long-term care facilities and programs rely on volunteers to help provide services to their patients. Volunteers may assist staff in managing patients during mealtime or recreation periods, may help to transport patients within a facility, or may simply visit with patients in the facility or in their home. No Federal or State requirements govern the training of these volunteers. Nonetheless, it is critical for youngsters and adults whose volunteer work brings them in direct contact with persons with dementia to have a basic understanding of the nature of dementing disorders and training in appropriate communication with and response to behavioral problems exhibited by these persons. The facility or program using their services or a designated community resource may provide such basic training for volunteers.

Agencies that inspect long-term care facilities and programs are subject to few Federal or State regulations or requirements regarding staffing levels and qualifications. Among the States there are wide variations in the experience and educational background of surveyors and in the composition of survey teams. Nationally, about half the surveyors are nurses, one-fifth sanitarians, and most others engineers, administrators, and generalists (38).

Surveyor training is particularly important where measures of quality involve assessing actual care provided rather than simply reviewing facility records and structural features. Resident-focused evaluations, like those in the newly developed Patient Care and Services system, are described in chapter 10. Health Care Financing Administration data on surveyors indicate that many States are not adequately trained to conduct surveys that focus on resident care. In 1983, for example, eight States had only one or two licensed nurses on staff. In addition, Federal training programs have been cut back substantially in recent years due to budget constraints. A recent survey revealed that one-quarter of State surveyors had fewer than 10 hours of training, and that one-third of those had none (38).

FEDERAL AND STATE STAFFING REQUIREMENTS

States assume primary responsibility for enacting laws and promulgating standards for nursing homes, respite facilities, adult day care centers, and home health care programs. Medicaid and Medicare impose additional requirements on participating long-term care facilities.

Regulatory mechanisms that seek to ensure the delivery of quality care may be classified as structural, procedural, or outcome-oriented (see ch. 10). Federal and State requirements for long-term care facilities and programs have been primarily structural—establishing standards regarding the physical plant, recordkeeping, and staffing of nursing facilities (1,38).

Classification of Staffing Requirements

Staffing requirements may be categorized broadly as either quantitative or qualitative. Quantitative requirements specify the number of personnel that must be on duty for a given number of residents or beds in a facility. Qualitative requirements specify the number of personnel that must be on duty for a given number of residents or beds in a facility. Qualitative requirements specify the types of personnel who must be em-

ployed, the patient care tasks that must be performed, and the professional qualifications of those who perform them. The degree to which either type of regulation can ensure the delivery of quality care, however, may be limited by the absence of training requirements for nursing home personnel.

Substantive and qualitative differences in the education and training of individuals with the same title result in vast differences in the degree to which they are prepared to work with particular groups of patients. Without standards to define specific skills and subjects in which they must be trained—prior to or during employment—there may be little assurance that individuals are equipped to provide quality care.

Federal and State regulations do not address this issue. No Federal requirements for staff training apply to all nursing facilities, and only 22 States have defined training provisions. The required amount of time, format, and content of training vary substantially among States and most address training related primarily to health and safety precautions (e.g., fire prevention, evacuation procedures, sanitation). Requirements for training in specific subjects and skills related to patient care are left to the discretion of each facility (1). Federal standards on staff training are defined for facilities seeking participation in the Medicare program. Where these exist, they are similar to State regulations: they address training related to health and safety precautions, not subjects and skills related to patient care.

Quantitative Staffing Requirements

The degree to which quantitative requirements can ensure the delivery of quality care is controversial. Many contend that other characteristics of the labor force (e.g., staff training, staff mix, job satisfaction) may be at least as important as staff size in determining the quality of care delivered (1).

In a contract commissioned by the Health Care Financing Administration, Abt Associates, Inc., reviewed State laws on nursing home staffing, compared State and Federal requirements, and analyzed the effect of these requirements on actual staffing patterns. The study confirmed several points about quantitative requirements:

- There are no federally defined quantitative staffing requirements for nursing homes.
- Thirty-eight States have quantitative staffing requirements for SNFs; 24 for ICFs. The majority of these are stated as a staff-to-patient rather than a staff-to-bed ratio. The rules may or may not be supplemented by qualitative staffing requirements such as those specifying a particular mix of employees.
- In most cases quantitative staffing requirements appear to be the result of legislative or administrative compromise between consumer groups, the nursing home industry, and the State budget office, rather than a decision founded on firm evidence that a particular ratio assures quality care. To date, no evidence for such figures exists.
- In the majority of States, the State-defined minimum staffing requirement has been adopted by the State Medicaid program as the maximum staff level reimbursable by the program. The regulations in California, Massachusetts, New York, and Wisconsin are examples of that situation.

Qualitative Staffing Requirements

Although qualitative staffing requirements attempt to establish structural and procedural standards conducive to the delivery of quality care, they do not account for inadequacies in education and training of nursing home personnel, or for individual differences in competence and motivation. Mandatory staff training in specific subjects and skills may be of some value, but even these measures cannot compensate for differences among people. Thus quality assurance, as it relates to facility staffing, is particularly difficult to address through regulatory mechanisms.

The types of qualitative staffing requirements used by the States include:

- **Shift-specific requirements:** States may require personnel with particular professional qualifications to be on duty at certain times. Several, for instance, specify that an RN be on duty during each day shift, and that either an RN or an LPN be present during evening and night tours of duty (1). These provisions assume that the presence of staff with particular professional qualifications ensures the delivery of quality care.
- **Staff mix requirements:** States may outline "staff mix" requirements that specify the types of personnel a facility must employ. These may take into account such factors as facility classification (SNF or ICF), shift time (day or night), and number of persons served by the facility. Such provisions, again, may be of limited value where personnel are insufficiently knowledgeable about, or poorly motivated to provide, quality care.
- **Role-specific requirements:** States may require a particular level of academic achievement for personnel in specific roles within a facility. Thirty-seven States, for example, require that the Director of Nursing Services (DNS) of a skilled nursing facility be an RN. Ten States require the DNS to have specialty training (e.g., in geriatrics) in addition to RN licensure (1).
- **Task-specific requirements—patient care:** States that require the performance of particular tasks may or may not specify the level

of training required for personnel who will perform them. The Abt study indicates that where tasks related to patient care are required (e.g., bathing, or turning bed-ridden patients), States do not specify the qualifications or training necessary for staff performing them. Task-specific requirements may be of diminished value as a quality assurance mechanism without provisions that ensure training commensurate with responsibilities delegated.

- **Task-specific requirements—administrative:** Tasks for which States delegate responsibility to specific staff persons appear to be primarily administrative. Twenty-four States, for instance, specify tasks for which the DNS is responsible (e.g., hiring staff, coordinating staff activities, developing patient care plans, and providing inservice training and orientation for new staff). That can mean that a DNS is granted responsibilities for which he or she may lack prior training. The DNS of a nursing facility is a licensed nurse—either RN or LPN—but most nurse training programs include little or no training in managerial and administrative skills. Without an accompanying requirement that nurses supplement their basic education to acquire these skills before assuming a managerial role, States delegate responsibilities that the DNS may be ill-prepared to fulfill.

- **Substantive training requirements:** Nurse's aides are the only group for which any State requires training in subjects and skills related to patient care. (The only subjects in which nursing homes are required to train employees, however, are those related to safety and sanitation within the facility.) For other groups of employees, States rely on the accreditation and education process to provide adequate preparation for work with nursing home residents. Recognizing the vast role that nurse's aides play in direct patient care, and the absence of formal educational training—including high school—among a large percentage of these employees, 17 States have instituted mandatory job-training requirements for nurse's aides. The number of classroom and clinical teaching hours, the content, and the timing vary, but most require that training be completed within the first 6 months of employment (9).

Actual v. Required Staffing Patterns

The Abt survey of actual staffing patterns in nursing facilities reveals that median staffing levels in virtually every State meet or exceed the State-defined minimum. Even States without quantitative staff requirements have median staffing levels that compare favorably with those elsewhere (1).

These findings do not appear to be the result of any discrepancy between requirements for facility licensure and those for participation in reimbursement programs, for, as noted earlier, most State Medicaid programs have adopted the State-defined minimum as the maximum staffing level reimbursable by the program (1).

Two factors may contribute to the disparity between the required and actual level of staffing in many facilities. First, Medicare and private pay financing mechanisms may have enabled facilities, at the time of the Abt study, to employ greater numbers and more highly trained staff than regulations required. Unlike Medicaid, the Medicare program does not define a maximum reimbursable staffing level. The cost reimbursement system, along with the elasticity of rates with private pay patients, may have allowed facilities to exceed State and Federal staffing requirements.

Second, technical considerations may dictate the need for a larger or more professional staff than requirements stipulate. State staffing requirements may be more the product of legislative compromise and administrative guesswork than a reflection of evidence that a particular staffing pattern can ensure quality care (1). Staffing patterns that exceed minimum requirements may therefore reflect institutional decisions about the actual number and mix of staff necessary to operate a facility.

Neither qualitative nor quantitative requirements are statistically significant in explaining actual median staffing levels in nursing facilities. Nursing homes apparently make their staffing decisions on the basis of technical and economic considerations rather than in response to regulations (1).

FEDERAL PROGRAMS FOR EDUCATION AND CURRICULUM DEVELOPMENT

An understanding of the principles and practices related to interdisciplinary health care, long-term care, geriatrics, and mental illness is an important component in the preparation of health and social service personnel who work with persons with dementia. Much of the impetus for including these topics in training programs for health and social service professionals has come through federally funded grants and contracts in education.

Recent efforts by the Administration to terminate funding for programs that train health care personnel have been mentioned throughout this chapter. These actions have been based on reports of the current supply and projected surpluses of health professionals. However, while Federal funding efforts have succeeded in increasing the aggregate supply of health care personnel, problems related to geographic and specialty distribution remain (39,57,78).

Since the mid-1970s, Congress has sought to redirect funding of education for health-related professions in order to address reported shortages of personnel in particular sectors of health care and particular regions of the country. Geriatrics and long-term care are among the fields where knowledgeable professionals are reported to be in critically short supply. Federal efforts to address this issue are described in this section. Because the Federal Government has been instrumental in initiating and supporting education in these fields, elimination of Federal funds could seriously impede continued efforts in that regard (59).

Administration on Aging

The Older Americans Act (OAA) of 1965 (42 U.S.C. 3001 et seq.) established the Administration on Aging (AOA) within the Department of Health, Education, and Welfare (now Department of Health and Human Services) as the coordinator of grants and contracts to the States for the development of new or improved programs for older persons. Title IV of the OAA addresses "Training, Research, and Discretionary Projects

and Programs" for the elderly. Administration of title IV is delegated to the Administration on Aging with assistance and cooperation, as necessary, from the Department of Education, the National Institutes of Health, and other appropriate agencies and departments of the Federal Government.

Part A of title IV—Education and Training—deals with the need to attract a greater number of qualified personnel to the field of aging and to upgrade the training of personnel working on this issue. It directs the AOA Commissioner to make grants and enter into contracts to achieve these purposes. Activities may include support and development of education, training, and curricula for practitioners in health and social service professions; inservice training for personnel in offices and agencies that administer programs related to aging; and dissemination of information about aging to the public (79).

Training Related to Care of Dementia Patients

A 1984 amendment to the OAA recognizes the increasing need for personnel knowledgeable about the treatment and care of persons with Alzheimer's disease and related disorders. It requires that:

> In making grants and contracts under this part, the Commissioner shall give special consideration to the recruitment and training of personnel, volunteers, and those individuals preparing for employment in that part of the field of aging which relates to providing custodial and skilled care for older individuals who suffer from Alzheimer's Disease and other neurological and organic brain disorders of the Alzheimer's type and providing family respite services with respect to such individuals.

A 1984 amendment to Part B requires the AOA Commissioner to make grants and contracts that address the needs of these persons.

> In making grants and contracts under this section, the Commissioner shall give special consideration to projects designed to meet the supportive service needs of elderly victims of Alzheimer's

disease and other neurological and organic brain disorders of the Alzheimer's type and their families, including home health care for such victims, adult day health care for such victims, and homemaker aides, transportation, and in-home respite care for the families, particularly spouses, of such victims.

Training in Interdisciplinary Health Care Delivery

The Older Americans Act also directs the AOA Commissioner to make grants for the establishment and support of multidisciplinary centers of gerontology and gerontology centers of special emphasis. Language added to the law in 1984 requires, among other things, that the multidisciplinary centers shall:

- recruit and train personnel;
- conduct basic and applied research related to aging;
- stimulate the incorporation of information on aging into the teaching of biological, behavioral, and social sciences at colleges and universities;
- help to develop training programs in the field of aging at colleges and universities; and
- provide information and consultation to the public and voluntary organizations that serve the needs of older individuals in planning and developing services under other provisions of the OAA.

In accordance with these requirements, AOA supports nine Long-Term Care Gerontology Centers (80). A primary objective of these centers is the development of professional and paraprofessional staff for delivery of health care, personal care, and other services through career and continued education and training. Through research, education, and service activities involving university faculty members, agency planners, administrators, and practitioners, the centers assist local communities, States, and regions in developing and implementing more cost-effective and efficient long-term care policies, programs, and systems.

Several centers provide opportunities for professional training in geriatrics and long-term care. The Pacific Northwest Regional Center in Seattle, Washington, for example, has developed several interdisciplinary training sites where students of medicine, nursing, social work, public health, pharmacy, dentistry, dietetics, and physical therapy work in teams to plan and deliver care to functionally impaired elderly individuals (4).

Alzheimer's disease has been of major interest to the Long-Term Care Gerontology Centers. Related activities at various centers include development, testing, and evaluation of approaches to delivery of service and care to Alzheimer patients; development of model support groups for families; and development of training models to assist service providers in working with caregivers (80).

Health Resources and Services Administration

The Health Professions Educational Assistance Act of 1976 (Public Law 94-484) and the Nurse Training Act of 1975 (Public Law 94-63) exemplify the genesis of legislative attention to the need for geriatric training among health professionals and paraprofessionals. The former authorized the Secretary of Health, Education, and Welfare to award grants and contracts for interdisciplinary training and for curriculum development for the "diagnosis, treatment, and prevention of diseases and related medical and behavioral problems of the aged" (54).

The Health Resources and Services Administration's Bureau of Health Manpower (now Bureau of Health Professionals, or BHPr) was designated to administer the legislation. BHPr provides national leadership in coordinating, evaluating, and supporting the development and employment of U.S. health personnel. It assesses the supply and requirements of the Nation's health professions and develops and administers programs to meet those requirements; collects, analyzes, and disseminates information on the characteristics and capacities of health professions' education systems; and develops, tests, and demonstrates new approaches to the education and employment of health personnel within various patterns of health care delivery and financing systems. BHPr provides financial support to institutions and individuals for health education programs; it also administers Federal programs for development and deployment of targeted health personnel and for the institutional development, training, employment, and evaluation of such staff (80).

Geriatric Education Centers

Beginning in 1983, BHPr supported the development of regional geriatric education centers (80). In that year and in fiscal year 1984, four GECs were funded. A total of 20 GECs were funded for fiscal year 1985. GECs are intended to serve as prototypical resources in multidisciplinary training for health professionals in geriatric care. Each center offers training to a range of health professionals, including doctors, dentists, nurses, pharmacists, and social workers. The main functions of the GECs are to:

- conduct faculty training programs to prepare key resource persons in schools of the various health profession;
- serve as a clearinghouse for information on multidisciplinary geriatric education programs and instructional resources;
- provide educational services in support of geriatric training to academic centers, professional associations, and State and local health agencies;
- assist schools of the various health professions to select, install, implement, and evaluate appropriate geriatric course materials and curriculum improvements; and
- establish organized multidisciplinary units to provide a critical mass of resources for geriatric leadership and coordination (83).

Other BHPr Projects Supporting Study of Geriatrics

The Bureau of Health Professionals also funds:

- training grants to support geriatric activities for residents in family and internal medicine;
- projects to integrate geriatrics into programs for physician assistants;
- area health education centers programs seeking to develop didactic information and clinical experiences in geriatrics for students of dentistry, nursing, pharmacy, social work, and related areas;

- gerontological nursing concentrations in master's and doctoral nursing programs;
- training of geriatric nurse practitioners; and
- the development of continuing education gerontology training programs for nurse educators and practicing nurses (80).

Veterans Administration

In 1973 the Veterans Administration (VA) initiated an effort to encourage health care professionals to specialize in geriatric medicine.

Geriatric Research, Education, and Clinical Care Centers

Through an integrated approach, the VA's geriatric research, education, and clinical care centers (GRECCs) train practitioners, teachers, and researchers in the field of geriatrics. Fifteen centers have been authorized by Congress; 10 are operating. Each center focuses on the clinical treatment of a particular aspect of geriatrics that has implications for improved care and for the education of health professionals. Several focus primarily on neurological disorders and organic brain disease (80).

Physican Fellowships

VA supports 20 physician fellowships in geriatrics. Participants gain expertise in geriatrics and gerontology through clinical training at VA medical centers that have medical school affiliations. Each of the 10 GRECCs offers fellowship positions to postresidency physicians interested in geriatrics and long-term care. The VA geriatric fellowship program began in 1978 (33).

Interdisciplinary Team Training in Geriatrics

The VA Interdisciplinary Team Training in Geriatrics program provides clinical experience in geriatrics to students in health disciplines from academic institutions throughout the country. Approximately 50,000 students participated in 1985. VA provides funding support for about 2,400 to 2,500 of these students. Participants include master's students in psychology, social work, audiology and speech therapy; residents in optometry and podiatry; clinical nurse specialists in geriatrics; and students of pharmacology and occupational therapy. Students gain knowledge and skills related to geriatric care and learn to function as part of a team of caregivers (80).

Training and Support for Nursing Students

The VA Health Professional Scholarship Program supports students enrolled in accredited baccalaureate nursing programs and accredited master's degree programs offering specialties needed by the agency. In fiscal year 1982, more than 25 percent of the awards to master's degree students were for geriatric/gerontological nursing. In return for the financial assistance, recipients provide a minimum of 2 years' service in a VA medical center (80).

VA also provides training for clinical nurse specialists in geriatrics. The program, established in 1981, enables master's-level nursing specialists to complete their clinical practicum at the VA medical center affiliated with their academic institution. In fiscal year 1983, VA supported 106 master's clinical nurse specialist students—40 in geriatrics, 53 in psychiatric mental health, and 13 in rehabilitation (80).

Continuing Education

VA provides funds to each of its medical centers to provide continuing education programs for its employees. The agency also funds programs for continuing education at the local, regional, and national level. A recently conducted regional program focused on Alzheimer's disease and other dementias (80).

National Institute of Mental Health

Through the Center for Studies of Mental Health of the Aging, the National Institute of Mental Health addresses training and personnel needs among the aging. Its related activities include:

- faculty development awards to prepare expert faculty in the field of geriatric mental health;

- postgraduate (fellowship) specialty training in geriatric mental health; and
- design of geriatric training models to provide training experience to the nonspecialist in geriatrics and to stimulate the development of model materials and curricula for the incorporation of geriatric mental health skills and knowledge in the general training of professionals in the four core mental health disciplines (psychiatry, psychology, social work, and nursing) (80).

Approximately 50 awards were made through these three programs in fiscal year 1983. Other activities identified for program support include continuing education in mental health and aging for clinicians already in practice, inservice, or setting-specific training in mental health and aging, and curriculum development addressing these and other needs (80).

Health Care Financing Administration

Some funding of geriatric education comes through the Medicare program, managed by the Health Care Financing Administration. The money is allotted to teaching hospitals—facilities in which graduate medical students gain clinical experience in patient care while working under the supervision of qualified physician-faculty—to compensate them for the costs incurred in patient care. The provisions do not specify reimbursement practices for facilities and programs other than hospitals (e.g., teaching nursing homes) that serve as clinical training sites for students of health professions. For the most part, services provided in long-term care facilities and programs are not reimbursable under Medicare. Thus, there would be no compensation for health professionals training in these settings.

Before the October 1983 Medicare revisions, hospitals were reimbursed retrospectively for patient care on a cost or charge basis. Under that system, direct and indirect costs of graduate medical education programs (residencies) were included in the reimbursement calculations. Under the new prospective payment system, reimbursement is allocated at fixed rates for each diagnostic category (diagnostic-related group). Educational costs are considered separately. Both direct and indirect costs are identified.

When the prospective payment system was designed, Congress and the Administration identified several factors that generate increased financial burden for teaching hospitals, but that should be compensated. These include:

- direct educational costs (e.g., stipends for residents or salaries for physician supervisors);
- indirect educational costs (e.g., additional test ordered by, and additional services provided by residents as part of their learning experience);
- the greater load of severely ill patients attracted to teaching hospitals; and
- the greater level of charity care provided by teaching hospitals (368 teaching hospitals—6.4 percent of all hospitals in the country—provided 49 percent of the hospital charity care in 1984 (10).

The Administration's budget proposals for 1986 and 1987 sought dramatic reductions in education payments through Medicare. The proposals were meant to freeze payments for direct medical education expenses and to halve the indirect medical education subsidy. Such financing mechanisms, the Administration hoped, would begin to discourage the trend toward specialized medicine.

In its action on the 1986 and 1987 budgets, however, Congress retained Medicare provisions for reimbursement of direct and indirect medical education costs incurred by teaching hospitals (72).

Although leaders in medical education agree that a greater supply of primary care physicians is important and that some policy incentive may be necessary to slow the trend toward specialization, they suggest less drastic measures than those proposed by the Administration. By defining a limited period during which graduate medical students could receive Federal funds, the program might encourage students to enter primary care rather than specialized medicine. Primary care residencies generally take 12 to 36 months, while more highly specialized fields (e.g., surgery and neurology) may require up to 7 years of residency training. Those who seek to discourage medical specialization contend that, because specialized medicine inflates the cost of medical care, the additional training costs of these programs should be borne by the trainees, institutions, and programs themselves (36).

ISSUES AND OPTIONS

The dementing disorders described in this assessment demarcate the differences between services needed by individuals with dementia and those needed by patients with acute conditions. Consideration of present and future personnel needs must account for these differences and determine which individuals are best suited to deliver care. Projections must consider the full range of care settings available, and the type of staffing arrangements appropriate to each.

Programs and facilities serving individuals with dementia and their families confront several fundamental problems in attracting and retaining knowledgeable and experienced personnel. Many of these problems—the limited number of health and social service professionals interested in long-term care; the lack of prior training and experience related to care of elderly, chronically ill, and mentally ill patients; and the high staff turnover rates—may be related to issues in the education and training process.

Educational programs that prepare health and social service professionals and paraprofessionals continue to emphasize the role of working with individuals with acute rather than long-term care patients. In doing so, they establish a set of expectations that may diminish the appeal and satisfaction of working with chronic care patients. Positive faculty role models are an important way to convey interest in and raise the esteem of professionals in long-term care. In addition, students require substantive information about the clinical experience with chronically ill patients.

The absence of teaching resources is an overriding problem for programs and facilities seeking to train personnel in working with chronic care patients. Although there is an abundance of information related to the diagnosis and treatment of persons with dementia in recent journals for health and social professionals, the absence of a discrete, consensual body of information complicates the task of curriculum planning and teaching about dementia.

ISSUE 1: Should the Federal Government play a role in the coordination of institutions and programs that train health and social services professionals?

Option 1: Do not get involved in the accreditation of academic institutions and programs that train health and social service professionals.

Option 2: Establish curricular requirements to be included as criteria for accreditation of academic programs and institutions preparing individuals for health and social service professions

Under option 2, legislation could designate the number of hours, the format, and subjects to be incorporated into programs training personnel in these fields. In that way, Congress could ensure the inclusion of content related to the care of persons with dementia (e.g., long-term care, geriatrics, and mental health) in programs that train health and social service professionals.

ISSUE 2: Should the Federal Government establish standard definitions and licensure requirements for health and social service professionals?

Option 1: Continue to allow individual States to establish definitions and licensure requirements for health and social service occupations.

Option 2: Direct the Department of Health and Human Services or another appropriate Federal agency to formalize definitions and licensure requirements for health and social service professions.

Option 2 would allow the Federal Government to ensure uniform standards for experience and training of individuals with a particular professional title. Licensure requirements could specify subjects and skills to be addressed and the number of hours of clinical and classroom training to be designated to each. In addition, requirements could specify particular topics to be addressed on standardized licensing examinations.

ISSUE 3: Should government establish qualitative personnel requirements for programs and facilities caring for persons with dementia?

Option 1: Define the number and type of personnel to be employed by facilities and programs serving individuals who need long-term care.

Option 2: Allow personnel requirements to be defined by Federal and State reimbursement programs.

Under option 1, requirements could be based on such criteria as the number of patients, type of facility (e.g., inpatient, home-care, adult day care), and illness classification of patients served. Under option 2, any requirements would be applicable only to facilities and programs seeking eligibility for Federal or State reimbursement for services provided.

ISSUE 4: Should the Federal Government define training requirements for the various types of personnel employed by facilities and programs caring for persons with dementia?

Option 1: Continue to allow States to define training requirements for staff of programs and facilities caring for persons with dementia.

Option 2: Establish specific preemployment, inservice, and continuing education requirements for personnel employed by facilities and programs caring for persons with dementia.

Under option 1, standards on orientation, in-service training, and continuing education would continue to apply primarily to programs seeking reimbursement through State or Federal programs (Medicare or Medicaid). Option 2 would allow Congress to specify standards on the number of hours, the format, and particular subjects required for each personnel group employed by facilities and programs caring for persons with dementia.

ISSUE 5: Should the Federal Government provide financial support to academic institutions and programs, and to students training for health and social service careers?

Option 1: Eliminate support for educational programs that prepare health and social service professionals in fields related to care of persons with dementia.

Option 2: Sustain general support for programs preparing health and social service professionals through existing legislation.

Option 3: Specify that funds be used for health and social service education to enhance opportunities for training related to care of persons with dementia.

Option 4: Retain support for programs sponsored by Federal agencies that train health and social service personnel in fields related to care of persons with dementia.

Option 2 would continue to rely on legislation such as Title VII and Title VIII of the Public Health Services Act to support programs preparing health and social service professionals. Under option 3, funds could be used to enhance institutional resources (e.g., curriculum, clinical training, faculty) for teaching about topics related to care of individuals with dementia, such as long-term care, geriatrics, neurology, and mental health. Option 4 would involve supporting programs such as Interdisciplinary Team Training in Geriatrics, Geriatrics Education Centers, and Long-Term Care Gerontology Centers.

Options 2 through 4 could be exercised by devoting attention to dementia in existing geriatric training programs. Increased funding for geriatric training was authorized for physicians and dentists in the Omnibus Health Act of 1986 (P.L. 99-660). Such training could be encouraged, either directly through legislation or indirectly through hearings and congressional inquiries, to include a focus on dementia. Additional initiatives for nurses and nurse's aides would more directly improve the daily care of the majority of those suffering from dementia.

CHAPTER 9 REFERENCES

1. Abt Associates, Inc., "Study of Appropriate Staffing Ratios of Daily Nursing Hours for the Purpose of Establishing Federal Requirements in Nursing Homes: A Review of State Requirements for Nursing Home Staffing," Contract No. HCFA 500-80-0072, 1981.
2. Accreditation Council for Graduate Medical Education, "Directory of Residency Training Programs," Chicago, IL, May 1984.
3. Almquist, E., and Bates, D., "Training Program for Nursing Assistants and LVN's in Nursing Homes," *Journal of Gerontological Nursing* 6:622-627, 1980.
4. American Association of Medical Colleges, "The Long-Term Care Gerontology Center Program: First Annual Yearbook," under Cooperative Agreement with the Administration on Aging, 1982.
5. American College of Health Care Administrators, Licensure Information by State, compiled from 1985 statistics of National Association of Boards of Examiners for Nursing Home Administrators, 1985.
6. "American Geriatrics Society Education Committee Update: Review Boards," *American Geriatrics Society Newsletter* 14:5, April 1986.
7. "American Geriatrics Society Receives Curriculum Guidelines Grant," *American Geriatrics Society Newsletter* 14:5, April 1986.
8. American Health Care Association, "Trends and Strategies in Long-Term Care," Washington, DC, 1985.
9. American Health Care Association, "1985 Mandatory Nurse's Aide Training," unpublished list, Washington, DC, 1985.

10. American Hospital Association Annual Survey of Hospitals, 1984.
11. American Nurses Association, *Fact Sheet on Registered Nurses* (Washington, DC: Government Relations Division, ANA, 1980).
12. American Nurses Association, *Facts About Nursing: 1984-85* (Kansas City, MO: June 1985).
13. American Psychological Association, "Geropsychology in Long-Term Care Settings," *Professional Psychology*, August 1979, pp. 475-484.
14. Archbold, P., "Evolving Curricular Developments in the Health Professions" (panel discussion), *The Report of the National Invitational Conference on Issues and Strategies in Geriatric Education: 1985*, U.S. Department of Health and Human Services, Health Resources and Services Administration, Bureau of Health Professions, Mar. 4-6, 1985, The Circle Inc., McLean, VA, pp. 78-80.
15. Barry, P.P., and Ham, R.J., "Geriatric Education: What the Medical Schools Are Doing Now," *Journal of the American Geriatric Society* 33:133-135, 1985.
16. Beaver, K.W., "Task Analysis of Nursing Personnel: Long-Term Care Facilities in Utah," dissertation presented to the Department of Educational Administration, Brigham Young University, April 1978.
17. Besdine, R.W., "Evolving Curricular Developments in the Health Professions" (panel discussion), *The Report of the National Invitational Conference on Issues and Strategies in Geriatric Education: 1985*, U.S. Department of Health and Human Services, Health Resources and Services Administration, Bureau of Health Professions, Mar. 4-6, 1985, The Circle Inc., McLean, VA, pp. 73-77.
18. Brower, H.T., "The Nursing Curriculum for Long-Term Institutional Care," *Creating a Career Choice for Nurses: Long-Term Care* (New York: National League for Nursing, 1983).
19. Browning, M.A., "An Interdisciplinary Approach to Long-Term Care," *Management of Personnel in Long-Term Care*, M.O. Hogstel (ed.) (Bowie, MD: Robert J. Brady Co., 1983).
20. Burnside, I.M., "Organic Mental Disorders," *Handbook of Gerontological Nursing*, B.M. Steffl (ed.) (New York: Van Nostrand Reinhold Co., 1984).
21. Butler, R.N., "Geriatrics and Internal Medicine," *Annals of Internal Medicine* 91:903-908, 1979.
22. Butler, R.N., and Seymour, S.K., "The Changing Demography and Its Challenges for the Academic Medical Center," *Journal of the American Geriatric Society* 31:525-528, 1983.
23. Cassel, C.K., and Jameton, A.L., "Dementia in the Elderly: An Analysis of Medical Responsibilty," *Annals of Internal Medicine* 94:802-807, 1981.
24. Cohen, L.D., and Cooley, S.G., "Psychology Training Programs for Direct Services to the Aging (Status Report: 1980)," *Professional Psychology: Research and Practice* 14:720-728, 1983.
25. Council on Social Work Education, "Statistics on Social Work Education," Washington, DC, 1984.
26. Feazell, J., Veterans Administration, Office of Academic Affairs, Washington, DC, personal communication, 1986.
27. Federal Council for Internal Medicine, "Geriatric Medicine: A Statement for the Federated Council for Internal Medicine," *Annals of Internal Medicine* 95:372-376, 1981.
28. Flagle, C.D., "Issues of Staffing Long-Term Care Activities," *Nursing Personnel and the Changing Health Care System*, M.L. Millman (ed.) (Cambridge, MA: Ballinger Publishing Co., 1978).
29. Geriatric Nursing Assistant Training Task Force, "Geriatric Nursing Assistant Training in Virginia," Final Report, Department of Education of Commonwealth of Virginia, January 1982.
30. Gillick, M.R., "Is the Care of the Chronically Ill A Medical Prerogative?" *New England Journal of Medicine* 310:190-193, 1984.
31. Golden, C.J., *Diagnosis and Rehabilitation in Clinical Neuropsychology* (Springfield, IL: Charles C. Thomas Publisher, 1978).
32. Gwyther, L.P., *Care of Alzheimer's Patients: A Manual for Nursing Home Staff*, Alzheimer's Disease and Related Disorders Association and American Health Care Association, 1985.
33. Haber, P., Veterans Administration, personal communication, 1985.
34. Handshu, S.S., "Profile of the Nursing Aide," *The Gerontologist*, Part I, Autumn 1973, pp. 315-317.
35. Hogstel, M.O., "Auxiliary Nursing Personnel," *Management of Personnel in Long-Term Care*, M.O. Hogstel (ed.) (Bowie, MD: Robert J. Brady Co., 1983).
36. Iglehart, J.K., "Federal Support of Graduate Medical Education," *New England Journal of Medicine* 312:1000-1004, 1985.
37. Iglehart, J.K., "Federal Support of Health Manpower Education," *New England Journal of Medicine* 314:324-328, 1986.
38. Institute of Medicine, *Improving the Quality of Care in Nursing Homes* (Washington, DC: National Academy Press, 1986).
39. Institute of Medicine, *Nursing and Nursing Education: Public Policies and Private Actions* (Washington, DC: National Academy Press, 1983).
40. Institute of Medicine, *Report of a Study: Aging and Medical Education* (Washington, DC: National Academy Press, 1978).
41. Kane, R.L., Solomon, D.H., Beck, J.C., et al., *Geriatrics in the United States: Manpower Projections and*

Training Considerations (Santa Monica, CA: Rand Corp., 1980).

42. Kayser-Jones, J.S., "A Comparison of Care in a Scottish and a United States Facility," *Geriatric Nursing* 2:44-50, 1981.

43. Kayser-Jones, J.S., "Gerontological Nursing Research Revisited," *Journal of Gerontological Nursing* 7:217-223, 1981.

44. Kramer, M., Taube, C.A., and Redick, R.W., "Patterns of Use of Psychiatric Facilities by the Aged: Past, Present, and Future," *The Psychology of Adult Development and Aging*, C. Eisenforfer and M.P. Lawton (eds.) (Washington, DC: American Psychological Association, 1973).

45. Levine, E., and Moses, E.B., "Registered Nurses Today: A Statistical Profile," *Nursing in the 1980s: Crises, Opportunities, Challenges*, L.H. Aiden (ed.) (Philadelphia: J.B. Lippincott Co., 1982).

46. Levine, P., "A Directory of Gerontology Study Opportunities at Graduate Schools of Social Work," Council on Social Work Education, Washington, DC, 1984.

47. Lezak, M., *Neuropsychological Assessment* (New York: Oxford University Press, 1976).

48. Lindeman, C., "Manpower in Nursing Homes: Implications for Research," *Mental Illness in Nursing Homes: Agenda for Research* (Rockville, MD: U.S. Department of Health and Human Services, 1984).

49. Maklan, C.W., "Geriatric Specialization in the U.S.: Profile and Prospects," dissertation submitted in partial fulfillment of the requirements for the degree of Doctor of Philosophy, University of Michigan, Ann Arbor, 1984.

50. Miller, J., Executive Director, National Association of Boards of Examiners for Nursing Home Administrators, personal communication, 1986.

51. Mitchell, J.B., "Physician Visits to Nursing Homes," *Gerontologist* 22:45-48, 1982.

52. National League for Nursing, *Nursing Data Book 1981*, 1982.

53. National League for Nursing, *Masters Education in Nursing: Route to Opportunities in Contemporary Nursing*, 1986.

54. Panneton, P.E., Moritsugu, K.P., and Miller, A.M., "Training Health Professionals in the Care of the Elderly," *Journal of the American Geriatrics Society* 30:144-149, 1982.

55. Pepper, G.A., Kane, R., and Teteberg, B., "Geriatric Nurse Practitioner in Nursing Homes," *American Journal of Nursing* 76:62-64, January 1976.

56. Price, R.J., "Health Services and Resources Programs: FY86 Budget," *Issue Brief*, Congressional Research Service, Library of Congress, Washington, DC, Feb. 1, 1986.

57. Price, R.J., "Health Professions Education Programs, Title VII of the Public Health Service Act," *Issue Brief*, Congressional Research Service, Library of Congress, Washington, DC, Feb. 1, 1986.

58. Rabins, D.L., "Physician Care in Nursing Homes," *Annals of Internal Medicine* 94:126-8, 1981.

59. Reif, L., "The Critical Need for Nurses in Long-Term Care: Implications for Geriatrics Education," *Gerontology and Geriatrics Education* 3:145-153, winter 1982.

60. Reifler, B.V., and Orr, N. (eds.), *Alzheimer's Disease and the Nursing Home: A Staff Manual* (Tacoma, WA: Hillhaven Corp., 1985).

61. Robb, S.S., and Malinzak, M., "Knowledge Levels of Personnel in Gerontological Nursing," *Journal of Gerontological Nursing* 7:153-158, 1981.

62. Romeis, J.C., Schey, J.M., Marion, G.S., et al., "Extending the Extenders: Compromise for the Geriatric Specialization-Manpower Debate," *Journal of the American Geriatrics Society* 33:559-565, 1985.

63. Sbordone, R.J., and Sterman, L.T., "The Psychologist as a Consultant in a Nursing Home: Effect on Staff Morale and Turnover," *Professional Psychology: Research and Practice* 14:240-250, 1983.

64. Shields, E.M., and Kick, E., "Nursing Homes: A National Problem," *Nursing in the 1980's, Crises, Opportunity, Challenges*, L.H. Aiken (ed.) (Philadelphia: J.B. Lippincott Co., 1982).

65. Siegler, I.C., Gentry, W.D., and Edwards, C.D., "Training in Geropsychology: A Survey of Graduate and Internship Training Programs," *Professional Psychology* 10:390-395, 1979.

66. Spence, D.L., Feigenbaum, E.M., Fitzgerald, F., et al., "Medical Student Attitudes Toward the Geriatric Patient," *Journal of the American Geriatrics Society* 16:976-983, 1968.

67. Stanley, K.R., "Staff Development and Training," *Management of Personnel in Long-Term Care*, M.O. Hogstel (ed.) (Bowie, MD: Robert J. Brady Co., 1983).

68. Syracuse University, Undergraduate Catalog 1984-85 (Syracuse, NY, 1984).

69. Toy, S., Research Associate, Association of American Medical Colleges, personal communication, Sept. 10, 1986.

70. U.S. Congress, Congressional Budget Office (CBO), *Physician Extenders: Their Current and Future Role in Medical Care Delivery* (Washington, DC: U.S. Government Printing Office, 1979).

71. U.S. Congress, *Executive Summary: The Report of the National Invitational Conference on Issues and Strategies in Geriatric Education: 1985*, U.S. Department of Health and Human Services, Health Resources and Services Administration, Bureau of Health Professions, Mar. 4-6, 1985, The Circle Inc., McLean, VA.

72. U.S. Congress, House of Representatives, The Com-

mittee of Conference, "Conference Report to Accompany H.R. 3128, *Consolidated Omnibus Budget Reconciliation Act of 1985*," Report 99-453 (Washington, DC: U.S. Government Printing Office, 1985).

73. U.S. Department of Health and Human Services, Health Care Financing Administration, *Long-Term Care: Background and Future Directions* (Washington, DC: U.S. Department of Health and Human Services, 1981).

74. U.S. Department of Health and Human Services, National Institutes of Health, National Institute on Aging, "Recent Developments in Clinical and Research Geriatric Medicine: The NIA Role," NIH Pub. No. 79-1990, Washington, DC, 1979.

75. U.S. Department of Health and Human Services, Public Health Service, "Gerontological Nursing Programs Offered in the U.S.," October 1984.

76. U.S. Department of Health and Human Services, Public Health Service, *Report on Education and Training in Geriatrics and Gerontology*, February 1984.

77. U.S. Department of Health, Education, and Welfare, Health Resources Administration, *The Supply of Health Manpower: 1970 Profiles and Projections to 1990* (Washington, DC: Bureau of Health, Education, and Welfare, Bureau of Health Resources Department, 1974).

78. U.S. Senate, Special Committee on Aging, "Developments in Aging: 1983," Vol. 2-Appendices, Report 98-360 (Washington, DC: U.S. Government Printing Office, 1984).

79. U.S. Special Committee on Aging, "Compilation of the Older Americans Act of 1965 and Related Provisions of Laws, As Amended Through October 9, 1984," S. Prt. 99-53 (Washington, DC: U.S. Government Printing Office, June 1985).

80. U.S. Senate Committee on Labor and Public Welfare, *Health Manpower 1974: Part V*, hearings before the Subcommittee on Health, June 25, 1974 (Washington, DC: U.S. Government Printing Office, 1974).

81. Virginia Department of Education, "The Nursing Assistant Task/Competency List," Health Occupations Education Service, Virginia Department of Education, Richmond, VA, July 1983.

82. Virginia Department of Social Services, Division of Licensing Programs, "Standards and Regulations for Licensed Adult Day Care Centers," *The Code of Virginia*, Title VI, Ch. 9, Sec. 63.1-174, Richmond, VA, 1984.

83. Walkington, R.A., "Sources of Funding," *The Report of the National Invitational Conference on Issues and Strategies in Geriatric Education: 1985*, U.S. Department of Health and Human Services, Health Resources and Services Administration, Bureau of Health Professions, Mar. 4-6, 1985, The Circle Inc., McLean, VA.

84. Weisfeld, N., "Acccreditation, Certification, and Licensure of Nursing Home Personnel: A Discussion of Issues and Trends," prepared for the Institute of Medicine, National Academy of Sciences, Washington, DC, Dec. 31, 1984.

85. Weston, J.L., "Ambiguities Limit the Role of Nurse Practitioners and Physician Assistants," *American Journal of Public Health*, 74:6-7, 1984.

86. Whitcomb, M.E., "The Federal Government and Graduate Medical Education," *New England Journal of Medicine* 310:1322-1324, 1984.

87. White House Conference on Aging, *Final Report the 1981 White House Conference on Aging*, Nov. 30-Dec. 3, 1981, vol. 1, Washington, DC, 1981.

Quality Assurance in Long-Term Care: Special Issues for Patients With Dementia

CONTENTS

Table

Quality Assurance in Long-Term Care: Special Issues for Patients With Dementia*

With a burgeoning population of elderly individuals at risk of needing long-term care, the most rapidly increasing inflation ever in the health care sector, and continuing scandals about substandard care, the Nation's long-term care program faces serious challenges. It faces the demand for more and better nursing home care and an expanded, effective range of alternatives to institutional care. It also faces significant fiscal constraints, as growth in expenditures threatens to undermine the fiscal viability of Medicare and to bankrupt State budgets that provide a share of Medicaid funds. It faces the challenge of eliminating discrimination against individuals most in need of competent and caring long-term services—the "heavy care" patients who require substantial supervision and "hands-on" care (particularly individuals with dementing illnesses), and those individuals, impoverished by age and illness, who must rely on Medicaid for assistance in paying for nursing home care.

Despite considerable improvement, inadequate quality of long-term care nationwide remains a serious problem. These failings are the product of many factors and exist despite government regulation. In general, the regulatory system for institutional care is criticized for having inadequate and inappropriate standards, an ineffective monitoring or inspection system, and insufficient compliance mechanisms for enforcing even minimal standards. For noninstitutional long-term care, quality assurance is in its infancy, with less well-developed standards, more significant monitoring problems, and a general absence of compliance mechanisms and remedies for inadequate care or services.

These problems reflect difficulties in regulating services like home health care, home chore assistance, and respite care in standard ways. Many programs are so small or localized that regulatory controls could appear cost-ineffective or impractical. Complex regulatory requirements could act as a disincentive to individuals offering these services, thereby undermining efforts to encourage further development of noninstitutional care. Nonetheless, formal delivery of long-term care services in noninstitutional settings creates a need for some mechanism to assure the delivery of quality care.

Policymakers seeking to assure high-quality long-term care must consider three major questions: What are the appropriate goals for long-term care? How can quality be measured and assessed? And how can its provision be assured? This chapter examines the problems and issues involved in assuring quality long-term care, with a special focus on the care needs of individuals with a dementing disorder.

The first section of the chapter describes major conceptual issues in defining and measuring quality in long-term care. The second section discusses problems in long-term care quality, describes the current regulatory system, and presents major criticisms of the standards, inspections, and enforcement mechanisms for assuring acceptable quality. The final section suggests mechanisms for improving quality in long-term care during an era of fiscal constraints.

Much of the chapter focuses on quality assurance in nursing homes, as public policy currently has a more extensive role in paying for and establishing standards in these settings. Some discussion of quality assurance for other long-term care services (e.g., adult day care, respite care, home health services) is included.

---

*This chapter is based largely on a contract report by Catherine Hawes, and research assistant Linda L. Powers, Center for Social Research and Policy Analysis, Research Triangle Institute, Research Triangle Park, North Carolina.

DEFINING QUALITY IN LONG-TERM CARE

The first step in assuring delivery of quality care is to define the term "quality." The customary emphasis on the effect of care on a person's physical health is difficult to apply in the case of those needing long-term care. Long-term care is aimed at persons with diseases and disabilities that are chronic and often degenerative. It typically encompasses both health care and social support services that enable an individual and his or her family to cope with multiple impairments over time, but cure is rarely a feasible objective.

The Relevant Domains of Long-Term Care Quality

From a quality assurance perspective, quality in long-term care revolves around two principal factors: the characteristics of individuals, and their care needs. A salient characteristic of most people needing long-term care is the multiplicity of their impairments. The average nursing home resident, for example, is an 83-year-old widow suffering from three or more chronic diseases and disabilities (174). Individuals residing in domiciliary care facilities (DCFs) (e.g., board and care homes) also have multiple physical and mental impairments. And older persons who use other long-term care services commonly also have multiple chronic diseases and disabilities that interfere with their ability to function independently. These individuals differ in many ways, such as in their informal supports, the type and severity of primary medical conditions, and the length of time they require care. However, they have a number of important similarities that are central to a definition of long-term care quality:

- They require services that may involve care of acute or subacute illness but in which chronic care needs predominate.
- They have multiple diseases and disabilities for which care and services are needed. Medical diagnosis is but one component of assessing their care needs.
- Their physical, mental, and social well-being are closely related—mental and emotional status both affect and are affected by physical health. Substantial research indicates that

environments that foster autonomy, integration, and personalized care are related not only to satisfaction but to improved health outcomes (16,35,83,131). Social isolation is associated with declining physical health status and premature mortality (9,60,61,125).

- They can benefit from efforts to improve, maintain, or prevent decline in physical functioning. The ability to function more or less independently in activities of daily living, despite disease and disability, is central to individuals' well-being.

Quality of long-term care is thus a complex and multidimensional concept. Long-term care should address the physical, functional, mental, and emotional needs of individuals with multiple chronic diseases and disabilities. Moreover, it should be aimed not only at improving individuals' physical health, but also at enhancing the quality of their daily lives (126). Even if the relevant dimensions of appropriate long-term care are known, however, evaluating the quality of care provided can be an elusive goal.

Difficulties in Defining Quality

An inherent difficulty in defining quality involves the **multidimensionality of long-term care**. For many individuals, achieving one aspect of high-quality long-term care may impinge on another aspect. Take the case of an elderly woman whose mobility is slightly impaired but who enjoys walking about a nursing home unattended, valuing control and autonomy in this small area of her life. Because the woman is somewhat unsteady on her feet and has had one fall, the nursing home staff and her physician feel that she should be prevented from walking around without a staff member to assist her. Because she resists this suggestion, she is frequently restrained. The goal of the nursing home and physician is to prevent a negative health outcome—a fall, and possible serious complications. Yet the impact, from the resident's perspective, is to seriously erode personal control, freedom, and quality of life. Complicating the situation is the fact that her enforced immobility may contribute to further loss of functional ability and to other adverse conditions, such as skin breakdown and pneumonia.

This hypothetical case illustrates the potential in long-term care for direct conflict between one aspect of quality and another—an incompatibility seen most clearly in relation to quality of life issues. It points out that quality of care is not necessarily synonymous with quality of life (120).

Another difficulty in establishing a single definition of long-term care quality involves the **variability of individual needs and preferences**. What is high quality for one patient may not be for another. Moreover, those who provide long-term care and those who receive it often differ in their concept of what constitutes high-quality care. The views of health care professionals and providers have dominated in the delivery of services, despite indications that they may differ from the views of patients. In one study, nursing home residents, their families, nursing home administrators, nurses, and other staff were asked to identify factors that best capture their concept of quality (43). The study demonstrated that the relative importance of various components varies from group to group:

- Nursing home administrators responded that "self-worth" was the most salient aspect of quality, with lighting and environmental stress as the two other most important dimensions.
- Families chose resident treatment plans, preventive health care, and recreational activities as the three most significant dimensions of quality.
- Residents rated personal identity as the most important component of overall quality, with food appeal and staff attitudes as the other two most important dimensions.

In short, there is no simple, elegant way to define quality or to determine objectively the extent to which all of its many facets are present. For purposes of quality assurance, therefore, quality must be defined in relation to those things that can be reliably measured and that a quality assurance system can reasonably achieve.

Measuring Quality of Care

One model for assessing quality that has received considerable attention identifies three aspects of health care to be evaluated—input, process, and outcome measures of quality (46):

1. **Inputs and structural components of care** describe the quantity and quality of resource inputs (e.g., personnel, services, and equipment), as well as structural variables that characterize the environment in which care is provided. Current Federal standards and licensure laws are based largely on such measures.

2. **Process measures** encompass the activities or procedures involved in actually providing care. Process-based quality is typically defined in terms of commonly accepted professional norms or standards regarding the types of services and procedures individuals require based on an assessment of their needs. The evaluation of process focuses on whether appropriate services are provided and on the manner in which they are performed.

3. **Outcome measures of care** focus on positive and negative personal characteristics that can be attributed to the care provided (47). The argument for using outcomes to define and measure quality of care is based on the premise that the ultimate goal of health care systems and procedures is improving or maintaining individuals' health. Proponents argue that outcome measures form the conceptual basis for defining quality and that outcomes are the ultimate validation of all other possible measures of quality (26,27,46,78,88,90, 148).

There has been considerable debate over which way of conceptualizing and measuring quality— input, process, or outcome—is most appropriate for long-term care (3,103,110,111,188). Most observers argue against relying totally or largely on input measures and are critical of regulations and research that do (88,97,132). Proponents of outcome measures argue that focusing on outcomes avoids arguments about which processes and inputs are most effective by letting the results— individual outcomes—speak for themselves. Further, a focus on outcomes might allow providers and policymakers flexibility in determining the most cost-effective means of achieving the desired outcomes.

Specifying appropriate and achievable outcomes for recipients of long-term care is beset with conceptual and measurement problems, however:

- Outcomes used in most health care evaluations, such as mortality, rehabilitation, and discharge, may be incomplete or inapplicable for long-term care (85,96,103,160).
- Information about appropriate or achievable outcomes is scarce and inconclusive (96).
- Accuracy of prognostic judgments—expected outcomes—is quite low for long-term care. One study reported only 50 percent accuracy in prognostic judgments regarding expected changes in functional status (191).

Thus, a major task is to identify realistic, achievable outcomes for individuals needing long-term care.

Perhaps the most significant limitation of using outcome measures as regulatory standards is the difficulty in relating individual outcomes to the structure and process of care received (96). Even care of outstanding quality (by input/structure or process standards) does not always produce favorable outcomes. For most individuals needing long-term care, the enormous range and complexity of individual health problems, the limitations of medical knowledge about the course and care of chronic degenerative diseases, and the effect of individual characteristics are such that negative outcomes such as death or deterioration in function often cannot be prevented—no matter how skilled and extensive the care provided (160).

Use of outcome measures for regulatory purposes thus requires that regulators have substantial information about the impact of variables beyond a provider's control. Outside variables to be considered include recipients' characteristics (e.g., age, sex, diagnosis, and functional disabilities) and their effect on outcomes of care. Further, the degree to which the course of chronic diseases and

disabilities can be predicted, given prescribed care of acceptable quality, must be considered. Without awareness of these factors, a definition of quality, sets of criteria, and regulatory requirements based solely on desirable individual outcomes would be unworkable and unrealistic (66,96).

These difficulties are particularly pronounced when attempting to define quality and developing outcome-oriented measures of care for persons with dementia. Although evidence indicates that the rate of deterioration *can* be moderated through a strong social and medical support system, statistically significant associations between the process of care and individual outcomes have not been established. Variability in the speed and course of individual cases of dementia makes it difficult to specify outcomes as measures of quality. Again, many of these variables appear to be unrelated to the quality of care received. In addition, the chronic, degenerative nature of dementing disorders makes traditionally used health outcome measures inappropriate indicators of quality.

The fact that there are difficulties in specifying appropriate, achievable outcomes does not mean that quality assurance systems—whether regulatory or voluntary—cannot specify some outcome-oriented, recipient-focused measures of quality. These can be developed, and providers can be more effectively monitored and held accountable for the care individuals receive. Outcome-oriented measures may be most applicable to long-term care in nursing homes, since these providers generally oversee a greater portion of recipients' lives than nonresidential care providers do. However, outcome measures also have potential for use in other settings (e.g., home care).

Measures of individual status and process quality that are related to care received and are relevant for persons with dementia are discussed later in this chapter. Many of the outcome-oriented measures discussed in the next section apply primarily to monitoring nursing homes. Because day care, respite care, and home care are usually limited to one type of intervention and occur for only a limited time each day or week, attributing outcomes solely to the quality of a provider's care or services is difficult. For such long-term care services, outcome measures that are problem-specific and related directly to the care provided are more appropriate. These are discussed later in this chapter.

Developing Outcome Measures of Quality

Monitoring positive outcomes, such as curing infections and decubiti (bedsores), restoring physical functioning, and minimizing deterioration, might be appropriate for evaluating the performance of long-term care providers. Alternatively, a system like that in New York, focusing on preventable *negative* outcomes or "sentinel health events," could be useful. This section identifies examples of process and outcome-oriented indicators of poor quality care that are particularly appropriate for persons with dementia.

- **Dehydration and Malnutrition:** These are outcomes that are not only considered undesirable but also generally preventable. Dehydration, for example, has been suggested as an indicator of poor quality care or sentinel health event—a generally preventable negative outcome (54,69,107,149). The condition usually indicates inadequate attention to fluid intake, and thus may serve as a measure of a facility's provision of care (69). Monitoring the occurrence of dehydration may be particularly relevant for persons with dementia, who may neglect or be unaware of their need for fluids. Dehydration can worsen the mental condition of someone with a dementing illness (92).

  Malnutrition is another generally reliable outcome measure of quality. In most cases, unexplained and excessive weight loss or gain is an indicator of inadequate dietary services. The situation for someone with dementia, however, is more complex. In the second stage of Alzheimer's disease, for instance, people often experience motor hyperactivity. Even when adequate nutrition and meal assistance or supervision are provided, some individuals lose weight and become emaciated (13,44,68), and may be misinterpreted as a result of inadequate nutrition. Thus, if malnutrition is used as an outcome quality measure, surveyors must carefully consider residents'

characteristics in conjunction with dietary services.

- **Drugs and Medications:** Excessive use of psychotropic drugs, medication errors, and adverse drug reactions among nursing home and board and care residents have been cited as common problems and examples of poor quality of care (14,74,84,142,144,145,179, 197). For persons with dementia, such medication errors and overreliance on psychotropic drugs are particularly troublesome. Sedatives, blood pressure drugs, and heart medications are just a few of the medications that can worsen the functional capacity of such individuals (92,140). Further, because reports indicate that some facilities rely on chemical restraints as a substitute for staff and on psychotropics to control wandering and other behavioral problems associated with dementia, excessive use of psychotropics and adverse drug interactions may be useful quality-of-care measures.

  Protocols or process standards for proper use of psychotropic drugs and survey procedures for monitoring facility performance have been developed and could be incorporated in regulations and in a revised Federal certification process (21,94,99,130,156).

- **Decubitus Ulcers:** Another potential indicator of poor quality of care is the development of decubiti (bedsores), particularly as residents become less mobile (117,198). Protocols have been developed for identifying and measuring the severity of such skin breakdowns and pressure sores (100,117,130). For physically dependent residents (e.g., those who are bed- and chair-fast), the outcome measure would be the incidence and severity of decubiti. Surveyors would have to determine whether the decubiti occurred while the individual was in the nursing home, and whether, given the resident's condition, the development or worsening of the decubiti was avoidable.

- **Urinary Incontinence, Urinary Tract Infections, and Overuse of Indwelling Catheters:** Urinary incontinence is common in the later stages of many dementing illnesses. When it develops, however, a medical evaluation is indicated. Potentially treatable causes (e.g., infections or an enlarged prostate gland) may be found. Numerous strategies exist to manage incontinence due to Alzheimer's disease, and standards can be developed for proper treatment of the condition. Fluid restriction is *not* an acceptable treatment for urinary incontinence (92).

Another indicator of quality might be the use of indwelling catheters as opposed to bladder training programs and staff attention for management of incontinence. Many view the excessive use of indwelling catheters as a sign of poor care, and process standards have been developed for their proper use (22,57,118,130, 135,192,198). Among nursing home residents who have indwelling catheters, the development of infections is also a sign of poor care (57,80,135,136,139). One measure of outcome quality, therefore, would be the incidence of urinary tract infections among residents who are catheterized.

- **Restraints:** Use of physical and chemical (psychotropic drugs) restraints to control disruptive behavior (e.g., wandering, screaming, or agitation) among residents with dementia may indicate inadequacies in provision of care. Where restraints are used as a substitute for staff supervision, activities, and treatment, they may be considered a negative outcome or sentinel health event, preventable through appropriate care. Guidelines for the use of restraints, which can be developed as appropriate process standards of care, have been suggested (42).

- **Nursing and Personal Care:** These are very relevant to the quality of life experienced by nursing home residents, and to their sense of well-being, satisfaction, and mental and social functioning (15,62). The Iowa Department of Health, for example, evaluates 17 nursing and personal care services as part of each facility's licensure survey (21,99). Two other instruments also assess personal care and grooming, New York's Sentinel Health Events (11), and one used by the Kane Group (89). These could be used to develop standards for appropriate personal care and grooming outcomes.

For residents with dementia, interviews may not be feasible, but direct observation may be an effective way to determine the quality of their personal care. Observations could focus on such things as cleanliness of resident's clothing and oral and physical hygiene (e.g., hair and nails). Surveyors might also observe such features as the promptness with which call lights and other resident requests for assistance are acknowledged, cleanliness of assistive devices (e.g., indwelling catheter tubes), and the manner in which personal care is delivered.

- **Mental Status:** The need for greater attention to mental health aspects of care, including appropriate assessment and management techniques for mental and behavioral problems and specialized activities programs, is well documented (25,152,175,199). The two most frequent diagnoses among nursing home residents are depression and intellectual impairment (e.g., organic brain syndrome, confusional states, or dementia) (25,178,199). Appropriate treatment is essential since depression, demoralization, and social isolation have been measured and associated with social functioning (18,62), physical health status, premature mortality (9,61), and activity levels (98). Moreover, particularly for depression, elderly individuals are at least as responsive to psychiatric treatment as other groups (36). Although it is not known how measurement of cognitive or behavioral factors can be incorporated into assessments of quality, it is clear that these factors are important.

- **Quality of the Living Environment:** This is a prime component of residents' definition of quality (126). Quality of the living environment includes residents' physical safety, facility cleanliness, and comfort (e.g., the ability of residents to have personal possessions and furnishings in their rooms). Standards could define expectations for the condition of residents' rooms, bathrooms, and common areas. Inspections could focus on such "outcomes" as safety, sanitation, and comfort. The Iowa instrument, mentioned above, provides a scoring procedure for evaluating several aspects of the living environment in nursing homes. A similar instrument could be developed for board and care facilities.

In summary, outcomes representing changes in patient status over time and those representing "benchmark" indicators of quality can serve as measures of quality of care. More often, however, given the current paucity of knowledge about expected outcomes for persons with dementia and the complex relationship between individual's characteristics, treatment interventions, and health outcomes, outcome measures might more appropriately be used as potential indicators of poor quality of care. Negative outcomes that appear to have been preventable could prompt examination of facility process and structure. The development of appropriate process and structural standards to define acceptable quality of care is discussed later in this chapter.

THE FAILURE TO ASSURE ACCEPTABLE QUALITY IN LONG-TERM CARE

Long-term care has been provided, with more or less skill and resources, in various forms for decades—first in mental institutions, poorhouses, and poorfarms, and later in converted houses, farms, and motels. Home health care, by visiting nurses or by "practical nurses" hired by families, also has a relatively long history. But significant expansion of formal long-term care services really began only within the last quarter-century, particularly since the passage of Medicaid in 1965. Institutional long-term care, primarily in nursing homes, was the first to flourish under these new payment systems. Home health care, home chore services, adult day care, and respite care have emerged much more recently, and their services and quality assurance systems are both in their infancy, as noted earlier. A common factor for all these long-term care services is the difficulty of ensuring or measuring the delivery of quality care.

Concern About Quality

Concern about quality of long-term care arises from a variety of factors:

- **Demographics:** An increasing number of elderly persons will require some form of long-term care, and those at risk of needing long-term care are rapidly growing in number, as described in chapter 1.
- **Debilitation of Patients:** Evidence suggests that individuals seeking nursing home and home health services are increasingly frail and disabled. The growth in the number of individuals with dementia is particularly relevant, since they are exceptionally vulnerable to poor care and least able to assert and protect their own rights.

- **Information About Quality:** Available evidence about the quality of care is troubling. Little systematic information is available about the quality of programs outside nursing homes (e.g., home health care, respite care, adult day care). Long-term care in nursing homes, while improved, still has substantial quality problems.
- **Cost Containment:** The overwhelming preoccupation with cost containment may detract from efforts to improve quality or to assure even a uniformly acceptable minimum level of quality in long-term care services.

Demographics and Patient Debilitation

An important reason for concern about quality is the increasingly debilitated condition of individuals needing long-term care. Within the last decade, people admitted to nursing homes have been older and suffer from more chronic diseases and functional disabilities (174). That trend may escalate because of recent changes in Medicare's hospital payment policies that tend to encourage earlier discharge of patients (104). In addition, testimony at recent hearings before the U.S. Senate Special Committee on Aging and a survey of agencies by the Aging Health Policy Center suggest that Medicaid's Prospective Payment System for hospitals has also increased the demand on home health agencies (184,195). Agencies report the greatest increase in demand is among those 75 to 84 years old (195). Limitations on nursing home bed supply may increase the debility of individuals seeking home health and other informal long-term care services. Thus, throughout the system, providers are encountering a demand for more skilled services in addition to the widespread need for nontechnical care and assistance with activities of daily living.

Troubling Evidence About the Quality of Long-Term Care

Despite the considerable progress that has been made, and the outstanding performance of many providers, quality of care continues to be a concern. Media attention and awareness of nursing home negligence has been more intense than that for other long-term care providers. Likewise, State and Federal studies of the quality of care delivered have focused on nursing homes.

Noninstitutional Long-Term Care.—Little systematic evidence is available about the quality of long-term care for such services as home health, home chore, respite, and adult day care. In part, this lack of knowledge is because of the relative paucity of government funding, weak standards of care, and the difficulties of monitoring the performance of these providers. In addition, because of the policy emphasis on the cost containment potential of noninstitutional care, most studies of programs such as home health and adult day care have focused on cost and utilization issues and on the potential of these programs for delaying or preventing nursing home placement (76). Little attention has been directed to the quality of services such agencies provide in general.

Information on the quality of these services for individuals with dementia is even more scarce. The one consistent finding across the few studies done confirms the general impression that home health, home chore, and adult day care agencies typically do not serve individuals with the kinds of cognitive impairment, behavioral problems, and incontinence that are typical of persons with dementia (93,106).

In addition, little is known about the quality of noninstitutional services because of the scarcity of the services themselves (92; see also 73,165). The range and scope of most programs are a function of federally sponsored efforts, but relatively little Federal funding is directed to establishing or expanding noninstitutional long-term care services (101,161).

Several studies have found that home health, home chore, and adult day care services increase contentment and satisfaction among those who receive them compared with those who do not (57,194). In addition, there is evidence that home health care can produce measurable improvements in functional status (e.g., 91,123) and some clinical outcomes (28,59). These findings, however, tell more about the potential for desirable outcomes from noninstitutional services than about the actual level and range of quality among the broad spectrum of providers.

Observers generally indicate that the quality of services, as well as the scope of what is provided, varies from agency to agency. Studies have found striking inconsistencies among agencies in the types of client needs that are identified and the types of service provided (150,191). One researcher, for example, found substantial disagreement about the type and frequency of home care services needed by a group of 50 individuals assessed by five multidisciplinary teams (physicians, social workers, and nurses) (151). Similar studies found little consistency among providers with respect to services actually used by people receiving home care (8,34).

The scarcity of studies focusing on the quality of noninstitutional long-term care and the lack of clear criteria for assessing these services make judgments about their quality difficult. Some evidence, largely anecdotal, suggests widespread disparity of in-home services provided (e.g., 179,183). No comprehensive effort has been made to determine how pervasive the poor quality of care is.

The General Accounting Office (GAO) studied Medicare's home health services (173). The primary focus of that study, like others, was on utilization and substitution of aide services for care previously provided by family and friends. The study also identified factors that adversely affected proper use, and that have implications for the quality of services. GAO found that physicians who authorize home health services do not take an active oversight role in the program. GAO also found that medical documentation in the agencies' client records is often incomplete. These findings indicate the difficulties of effectively monitoring the quality of home care.

The initial lack of systematic, comprehensive information on the quality of noninstitutional long-term care services is also troubling because of the changing "dogma of home care" (190). During the early 1970s, it was widely asserted that in-home services were less costly than nursing home care for frail and disabled elderly people. Indeed, while advocates for older Americans asserted that community-based long-term care was preferable to nursing home care, it was the cost containment argument that most attracted policymakers. As time passed and the number of empirical studies focusing on costs grew, the discussion moved toward the position that, while costs could go either way, noninstitutional care was always preferable.

As noted, recent evidence indicates there is reason to believe that expansion of home health, adult day care, and other alternatives is not likely to reduce aggregate nursing home use (193). Moreover, the assertion that in-home services are most cost-effective or preferable is open to question. There is, some observe, a concern that policies to discourage use of nursing homes are creating a "class of isolates" (190). For individuals with dementia and their families, this concern is particularly worrisome, since the isolates may include not only the ill person but also the primary caregiver. Given the lack of information and the difficulty of monitoring the quality of services, there is concern that "a substantially unregulated home care industry will outdo the nursing home scandals of the 1970s" (190).

Nursing Homes and Domiciliary Facilities.—Information about the quality of nursing homes and board and care facilities is considerably more extensive and better documented. Preliminary findings of studies at Duke University's Center for the Study of Aging and Human Development suggest that most families seek and receive in-home or community-based services only immediately before nursing home placement of someone with dementia. Thus, nursing home and domiciliary care are the primary types of formal long-term care most persons with dementia experience (63).

The development of health and safety regulations incorporated in State licensure laws and Federal certification standards for Medicare and Medicaid, combined with increased professionalism

and expertise in the nursing home industry, have contributed to significant improvements in the quality of several aspects of long-term care. Perhaps most dramatic is the improved safety of nursing homes, as regulators concentrated their inspection and enforcement activities on securing facility compliance with building and fire safety codes. Despite such advances, most observers acknowledge that even today the quality of care nursing homes provide varies significantly. The quality of life is superior in a relatively small percentage of homes—perhaps 15 percent nationwide—and seriously substandard in an estimated 20 to 30 percent (79,87,113,133,184).

In 1975, the U.S. Senate Subcommittee on Long-Term Care estimated that at least 50 percent of the Nation's nursing homes were substandard, with one or more life-threatening conditions (184). Based on a national inspection of nursing homes in 47 States and interviews with 3,458 residents in the mid 1970s, the Department of Health, Education, and Welfare (DHEW) found widespread deficiencies—overdrugging of residents, inadequate medical attention, insufficient diets, and a widespread failure by homes to provide needed therapies. DHEW found, for example, that only 31 percent of the residents needing physical therapy received it, and that 80 percent of medications were improperly administered (180).

Although conditions have improved in many nursing homes, more recent studies by State commissions and independent researchers confirm many of these earlier findings. One of the most common criticisms concerns overmedication with antipsychotic drugs and tranquilizers (86,133,142, 188). Other significant problems in care are noted. In fact, during the last decade State studies have found significant and troubling signs of poor-quality care:

- Virginia, which prides itself on having the best nursing homes in the country, found an average of 23 deficiencies in minimum health and safety standards per home (188).
- Missouri found that 25 percent of its nursing homes failed to meet minimum health standards (122).
- A Texas study revealed that 33 percent of the facilities violated minimum dietary standards (169), and a subsequent task force that visited

113 facilities found that 25 percent had "inadequate interior maintenance" (cracked or peeling paint, signs of water leaks, broken windows in resident rooms, etc.) and 33 percent had "offensive odors" in residents' rooms (168).

- Ohio found that 25 percent of its nursing homes spent less per resident per day on food than the amount considered by the U.S. Department of Agriculture and a panel of consultant dietitians to be the minimum necessary to meet the essential nutritional needs of an elderly person (133).

Other problems continually cited as problems in nursing home care include overuse of psychotropic drugs, misadministration of medications, excessive use of physical restraints, inadequate medical care, inattention to residents' rights and mental health needs, inadequate or inappropriate food and food service, failure to provide needed therapies, and inattention to care that restores or minimizes functional decline (10, 30,31,37,38,39,52,57,69,77,79,80,85,113,116,121, 1,127,128,129,133,134,141,168,169,188). The combination of physical, functional, and cognitive disabilities suffered by individuals with dementia makes them particularly vulnerable to these problems.

Quality problems in formal long-term care services are not limited to nursing homes. Studies and reports about domiciliary care facilities also have been the subject of studies and reports that reveal a number of serious quality problems. Identifying problems in such facilities and remedying them through a systematic quality assurance system, however, is much more complex than with nursing homes. As described in chapter 6, domiciliary care facilities include everything from board and care homes and residential facilities to adult foster care homes and halfway houses. Facilities vary substantially in size, population, services provided, and source and level of payment. No direct Federal regulation of domiciliary care exists, and States vary enormously in the number of facilities they regulate and the extent of the regulatory structure. Given that diversity, the role and purposes of any particular domiciliary care facility are not always clear and cannot be generalized. Thus, establishing quality standards

for their performance is complex. Despite the large numbers of individuals residing in such facilities, relatively little is known about them.

Domiciliary care facilities (DCFs), as described in this chapter, are categorized as board and care homes. These facilities primarily serve an older population and are intended to provide food, shelter, and some degree of protection, supervision, or personal care that is generally nonmedical in nature (29,95,112,143). The "personal care and oversight" responsibilities of board and care operators are established by State regulations, and vary substantially (143). Usually these include assistance with the activities of daily living (ADLs) (e.g., eating, bathing, grooming), assistance in obtaining needed medical and social services, supervision of residents' medications, and help in transportation and shopping (168). Despite State requirements, board and care homes vary in the quality and extent of services and care they provide.

Board and care facilities have received less sustained attention and study than nursing homes, but a series of fatal fires and stories of abuse and neglect during the 1970s focused national attention on their problems. The studies and investigations found widespread and serious safety and quality problems—at the same time State and Federal policies were encouraging the expansion of this sector. States were "deinstitutionalizing" patients from State mental hospitals. State and Federal policies under Medicare and Medicaid were encouraging the reclassification of nursing home residents from higher to lower levels of care, often out of the nursing home altogether.

Extension of the Federal Life Safety Code for intermediate care nursing homes forced many facilities out of Medicaid, and many converted to board and care or boarding homes. States could reduce their financial burden by moving individuals from licensed nursing homes and State hospitals to boarding homes and board and care facilities. The U.S. Senate Special Committee on Aging reported in 1975 that the result was increasing numbers of elderly people being "relegated to facilities which were unsafe and in which poor care, inadequate nutrition, negligence, physical abuse, and unsanitary conditions were rampant" (186).

Despite a series of Federal initiatives, in 1982 the Inspector General of the Department of Health and Human Services reported a continuing low level of State regulation and oversight of board and care facilities (177). Other studies, cited below, echo this finding, supplementing it with a litany of reported abuses and citations of substandard care.

Residents of board and care facilities suffer from a variety of physical, functional, and mental impairments and require substantial assistance and supervision on a regular basis. As described in chapter 6, memory defects and disorientation are common problems among elderly residents of board and care facilities. Evidence suggests that the living conditions, care, and services experienced by many residents is deficient. One common finding is that a majority of elderly people in DCFs are living in large, old, often dilapidated facilities, in mixed residential and business neighborhoods that are decaying. Further, they are doing nothing but watching television, sitting, staring at the walls while waiting for the next meal, or wandering the streets (45,115).

Rehabilitation programs or those designated to prevent avoidable decline in either mental or functional (ADL) capacity are rare, despite high levels of disability (45,115,137,154). Even where therapeutic and social services are available, comparisons of assessed needs to services received revealed serious deficits in dental, medical, nutritional, and transportation services, as well as in socialization and recreation activities (45,115,137). Finally, mental health services are rare relative to need for all but mentally retarded residents.

The findings of these studies have been supported by Federal reports and congressional studies and testimony. The Department of Health and Human Services (DHHS) conducted a study of board and care homes and found an erratic level of personal care and a lack of supportive services for residents (178). Subsequent studies by the U.S. House Select Committee on Aging and GAO revealed evidence of resident abuse, substandard health care, unsanitary conditions, and unsafe facilities (172,181,182). As the House Select Committee on Aging reported, its investigations and hearing testimony revealed "widespread instances of poor living conditions and negligent care" (182).

Cost Containment and Quality of Care

Efforts by policymakers to reduce public expenditures draw additional attention to questions regarding long-term care; increasing pressure at State and Federal levels to contain costs may be problematic from a quality perspective. One Medicaid director describes long-term care as "the black hole of State budgets," and throughout the Nation, cost containment is the central long-term care issue. As several observers note, there is potential conflict between cost containment and quality (41,71,97).

Empirical research has not directly addressed the relationship between a provider's costs or reimbursement levels and the quality of long-term care provided. Some studies suggest a weak relationship between cost and quality of care (151). Others, however, report that certain cost containment policies correspond to reduced quality of care (19,20,32,33,71,151). The actual relationship between resident's characteristics (case mix), quality of care, and costs remains difficult to assess.

State reimbursement rates for nursing homes (see table 10-1) and reimbursement methodologies vary widely. Lack of conclusive information regarding the relationship between cost and quality of care, however, makes it difficult to estimate the significance of these differences. Many argue that strong quality assurance mechansims are essential to compensate for discrepancies in reimbursement levels provided by different States (79,151).

Similar arguments are made with respect to domiciliary care. The drive for cost containment in State nursing homes and mental health facilities often results in shifting individuals with relatively significant dependencies and care needs out of intermediate care facilities and State mental hospitals into less well-monitored board and care facilities (65,163). Several studies suggest that the current reimbursement method for board and care housing is inadequate to encourage the upgrading of DCFs to meet even the existing minimal safety and quality of care standards (163,164,

Table 10-1.—Nursing Home Per Diem Reimbursement Rates, By State, 1978-83

State	SNF[a] reimbursement rates (rate in dollars)						ICF[b] reimbursement rates (rate in dollars)
	1978	1979	1980	1981	1982	1983	1982
Alabama	—	114.93	114.13	107.35	105.27	119.31	104.26
Alaska	22.85	26.95	29.33	30.79	33.38	37.61	25.81
Arizona	—	—	—	—	—	—	—
Arkansas	—	20.97	23.35	25.53	27.39	—	25.35
California	—	30.81	31.65	36.35	37.36	38.09	28.90[c]
Colorado	—	23.14	26.03	28.24	30.78	—	30.92
Connecticut	26.16	30.17	33.22	36.50	41.60	46.78	26.57[c]
Delaware	30.40	35.68	36.96	41.59	44.49	29.59	44.28[c]
District of Columbia	—	52.38	66.93	65.90	—	—	50.87[c]
Florida	—	18.79	21.13	23.82	26.01	—	33.21
Georgia	—	23.38	25.93	28.63	34.32	25.94	
Hawaii	—	55.05	62.11	71.56	79.45	—	58.18[c]
Idaho	21.93	22.00	21.19	25.35	27.61	28.72	31.33
Illinois	22.14	24.93	27.40	28.61	30.24	30.76	34.04
Indiana	—	—	34.90	38.27	42.32	45.86	32.68
Iowa	28.75	29.75	33.56	44.62	59.51	73.55	25.89
Kansas	20.14	23.83	25.48	27.80	31.75	32.44	22.16[c]
Kentucky	—	37.50	45.00	45.00	51.31	49.35	31.95
Louisiana	23.58	23.58	26.73	31.85	29.65	34.80	26.62[c]
Maine	—	54.98	56.20	61.15	65.93	71.20	40.30
Maryland	26.21	29.30	31.52	36.14	39.53	—	36.14[c]
Massachusetts	—	32.71	39.57	41.06	44.40	—	33.24
Michigan	—	29.20	31.50	35.56	36.72	38.98	36.72
Minnesota	29.50	32.07	38.25	44.81	47.36	51.32	35.88[c]
Mississippi	—	—	28.59	31.43	34.09	36.22	32.53
Missouri	15.55	18.37	26.80	30.00	35.00	40.00	29.12
Montana	—	30.20	33.85	36.75	39.58	—	36.75[c]
Nebraska	—	—	—	41.23	44.64	49.27	26.07
Nevada	—	30.15	37.72	40.25	47.50	47.50	43.61
New Hampshire	—	27.13	29.84	36.26	44.88	59.22	44.54
New Jersey	36.26	38.73	41.83	46.13	51.91	58.05	43.81
New Mexico	—	58.93	—	60.86	73.41	82.10	32.08
New York	49.65	55.35	62.17	67.63	73.98	78.70	49.21
North Carolina	34.19	36.58	41.78	45.56	48.98	52.03	33.49
North Dakota	—	26.44	31.91	37.87	43.40	45.02	30.00
Ohio	—	—	—	35.39	38.22	39.39	36.80
Oklahoma	—	21.00	26.00	29.00	32.00	32.00	26.53
Oregon	24.82	28.61	34.23	39.79	45.15	50.12	32.85
Pennsylvania	25.50	25.50	32.47	33.15	—	—	37.62
Rhode Island	29.75	36.43	40.86	47.33	49.23	53.71	38.95
South Carolina	—	35.29	39.84	44.25	40.77	40.77	32.05
South Dakota	19.10	20.94	23.33	26.36	30.08	33.39	26.88
Tennessee	32.80	32.50	36.20	40.50	42.60	46.36	27.40[c]
Texas	24.74	28.07	30.86	33.66	35.67	38.25	26.79
Utah	—	32.30	36.52	39.32	42.26	44.96	34.06[c]
Vermont	28.86	31.49	34.84	39.25	44.07	—	44.07
Virginia	—	42.54	46.43	51.26	61.90	—	42.66
Washington	—	23.33	28.92	31.68	35.25	35.92	34.37[c]
West Virginia	28.11	30.57	32.89	36.15	41.21	44.38	37.46
Wisconsin	31.85	35.00	38.00	42.00	42.52	44.22	32.00[c]
Wyoming	23.13	26.30	29.90	33.71	38.12	40.85	33.71[c]

[a]SNF—skilled nursing facility.
[b]ICF—intermediate care facility.
[c]Data for 1981.

SOURCES: SNF data for 1978, 1982, and 1983 from telephone interviews with State Medicaid agencies conducted by the Aging and Health Policy Center (AHPC); SNF data for 1979, 1980, and 1981 from AHPC and LaJolla Associates; ICF data for 1982 from LaJolla Associates.

172,180). At the same time, budgetary pressures make it difficult for States to increase payments to DCFs—or to increase funds allocated to monitoring the adequacy of services. Much the same can be argued about payment levels and resources for monitoring quality in other in-home and community-based long-term care services. A study by the Aging and Health Policy Center indicates that home health agencies are experiencing or anticipating a decrease in Medicaid reimbursement (195), and that funds for monitoring performance and assuring quality are scarce.

Inadequacy of the Current Regulatory System

Given the documented problems in long-term care quality, particularly in nursing homes and DCFs, and the concern about the adequacy of in-home and other long-term care services, the obvious question is whether the current regulatory structure is adequate to remedy problems in quality.

Historical Perspective

Despite 20 years of Federal regulation, the problem of quality in long-term care has been addressed incompletely and only episodically, for several reasons. At the outset, policymakers' most immediate concern was securing widespread participation by health care providers in Medicare and, to a lesser extent, Medicaid (50). They feared that imposing strict quality of care standards on health care institutions would severely restrict program beneficiaries' access to health care. Although nearly 6,000 facilities applied to participate in Medicare by December 1966, only 740 were able to achieve compliance by July 1967 (187).

As a result, at both Federal and State levels, policymakers chose not to demand full compliance with the health and safety standards established for hospitals and nursing homes participating in Medicare and Medicaid. Instead, institutions that were in "substantial" compliance were allowed to participate and receive reimbursement only if they had acceptable plans to correct deficiencies. That approach persists today. Few nursing homes, for instance, are in full compliance with Federal

health and safety standards. Many continue to operate with waivers of some standards and with plans to come into compliance for others.

The historical context for government regulation of health care also helps to explain the absence of policy focus on quality. Government-mandated health and safety standards originated in programs providing funds to institutions caring for children (67). These regulations were as much a product of concern that government receive good value for its money as they were of worry about the quality of life and care for the institutions' residents. The evolution of nursing home standards at the Federal level followed much the same pattern, emerging in conjunction with Medicare and Medicaid funding. The result was the promulgation of health and safety standards that sought less to define and assure high quality of care and life for nursing home patients than to ensure that government funds were not expended for obviously substandard care.

The Federal role in assuring long-term care quality thus has three components: 1) the formulation and promulgation of health and safety regulations; 2) the inspection of providers to determine the level of compliance with regulations; and 3) the enforcement of regulatory standards and administration of sanctions for noncompliance. The effectiveness of each of these components—regulatory standards, monitoring, and enforcement—is the subject of continuing debate.

The Regulatory System for Nursing Homes

States promulgate health and safety standards that nursing homes must meet in order to receive an operating license. Any home that wishes to participate in Medicare or Medicaid must meet additional Federal and State standards (i.e., "conditions of participation" for skilled nursing facilities and "standards of care" for intermediate care facilities). Once certified as being "in substantial compliance" with these standards, a nursing home qualifies for reimbursement by Medicare or Medicaid for the care provided to program beneficiaries. More than 80 percent of all nursing homes participate in one or both programs. Medicaid assists in paying for the care of at least 70 percent of all nursing home residents, and over 80 percent of those in homes in some States (82).

The following are some of the more common criticisms of the regulatory system, as it applies to nursing homes:

- **Minimums Become Status Quo:** The standards themselves have been acknowledged to represent "minimums," and many critics argue that these minimums, particularly in staffing and mental health support, are too low to assure acceptable quality of care. That may be particularly problematic for persons with dementia, who require substantial assistance and supervision.
- **Structural Characteristics Emphasized:** Regulations focus almost exclusively on structural characteristics and "inputs" that facilities must provide (e.g., door widths, square feet of room per resident, and staff/resident ratios). The assumption underlying the specification of these inputs is that they are associated with the provision of at least minimally acceptable care. In effect, the Federal regulations and survey forms measure the capacity of a facility to provide certain kinds of inputs and infer that the outcome will be acceptable care (180). State reports have been critical of that focus in Federal standards. While the necessity of structural and input standards is not questioned, most States argue for an enhanced focus on actual facility performance and resident outcomes (37,77, 128,129,133).
- **Ambiguous Terminology:** State reports also criticize Federal regulations for a lack of clarity on certain key elements in the standards. For instance, the lack of clear guidelines about what constitutes "imminent danger" or "adequate" staffing to meet the needs of residents places a substantial burden on surveyor judgment. It also makes enforcement more difficult, since such individual judgments are less likely to be accepted in court (31,37,77,129, 133,188).
- **Medical Model of Care Emphasized:** The regulations are widely criticized for being largely a product of a medical model of long-term care. Although nursing home residents need expert medical care and benefit from

restorative or rehabilitative therapies, current regulatory standards tend to ignore many other important aspects of long-term care. As the New York Moreland Act Commission argued, existing regulations do not capture many of the essential requirements of nursing homes as *homes* (128). Others note that the social and psychological needs of residents are inadequately addressed by regulations. These concerns are particularly important given the extent of mental and cognitive impairment among nursing home residents.

Inspections.—While the responsibility for enacting laws and promulgating standards is clearly divided between the States (for licensure) and the Federal Government (for certification to participate in Medicare and Medicaid), the relationship with respect to inspections is somewhat more complex. Licensure inspections are solely the responsibility of the States, most commonly the State department of health or its equivalent. Inspection of homes participating in Medicare is the responsibility of the Federal Government, which contracts with State agencies for these surveys. Under Medicaid, inspection and certification responsibility rests with the State department handling public assistance programs. Usually that agency subcontracts with the State facility licensing agency to perform the Federal surveys. Alternatively, the public assistance agency may perform the surveys with one of its own divisions, subject to Federal approval.

For both Medicare and Medicaid, the Federal Government has "look behind" authority. That is, Federal surveyors may conduct independent inspections of certified nursing homes to audit or validate the States' certification activities, and the Federal Government can decertify substandard facilities directly. The Federal certification survey process is intended to measure provider performance and identify deficiencies that result in poor quality care. It is also meant to produce sufficient documentation of deficiencies to support the Government's case in contested enforcement actions.

Both State and Federal inspections have been criticized on two major points:

1. **Primary Focus on Records:** Studies find nursing home records are often incomplete

Box 10-A.—Judicial Review of Nursing Home Inspection Process

The original suit, *Smith* v. *O'Halloran* (159), was filed on behalf of a group of nursing home residents in a Denver, CO, facility. The suit alleged poor care and violations of residents' rights, but more importantly it charged the Federal Government with failing to adequately monitor the performance of providers. During the trial, residents proved a variety of violations of Federal regulatory standards, including theft of personal funds, overuse of psychotropic drugs, inadequate care resulting in bedsores, inadequate skin and nail care, inadequate bowel assistance, and unsanitary conditions.

The case against the government agencies was based on the theory that Title XIX of the Social Security Act requires a Federal nursing home survey process that determines whether residents are actually receiving care they need, not merely whether facilities have the potential or capacity to provide needed care. In 1978, the Colorado Health and Medicaid agencies joined the plaintiffs, arguing that the mandatory Federal survey process was inadequate to determine whether residents receive needed care.

A Federal district court found that: 1) serious deficiencies exist in some nursing homes; 2) the current survey system is facility-oriented rather than resident-oriented; and 3) it is feasible for DHHS to develop a survey system focusing on resident needs and care delivery. The court held, however, that DHHS had no legal obligation to develop such a resident-focused survey system.

In *Smith* v. *Heckler*, the Federal Tenth Circuit Court of Appeals reversed the lower court's decision, holding that the Medicaid law does impose a duty upon the Secretary of DHHS "to establish a system to adequately inform herself as to whether the facilities receiving Federal money are satisfying the requirements of the Act, including providing high quality patient care."

The appeals court returned the case to the district court to determine what survey system would satisfy the Secretary's duty. The Health Care Financing Administration indicated to the court that it would implement a resident-oriented survey system in August 1986. The court is holding hearings to determine whether HCFA's proposed changes in the survey system, known as the Patient Care and Services (PaCS) survey, will meet the appeals court standard.

and tend not to reflect actual care and conditions (58,87,102,119). Thus, surveys generally measure only the homes' "paper compliance" with input and structural standards—not the care actually provided or the impact on residents' well-being (77,127,128,134,180). Of several hundred items on current Federal survey forms, for example, fewer than 20 require surveyors to actually observe residents. A New Jersey report on nursing home quality argues that this can contribute to poor care:

> If the surveyors simply rely on written documentation . . . and do not physically check the patients, many problems, such as bedsores, poor circulation, dehydration, etc., may remain uncorrected and undiscovered (127).

2. **Predictable Timing of Surveys:** Survey agencies routinely notify facilities in advance of annual certification inspections. Even without formal notification, the regular scheduling of annual inspections may give facilities sufficient warning of when to expect a visit. That aspect of the survey process is criticized for yielding inaccurate evaluations. Several States note that facilities correct deficiencies only immediately prior to expected surveys (10,31,37,116,121,128,134).

The Health Care Financing Administration (HCFA) has tested a resident-focused quality assurance survey system, Patient Care and Services (PaCS), in three States—Connecticut, Rhode Island, and Tennessee—and in select facilities nationwide. The system was to be fully implemented in each State by August 1986. PaCS aims to redirect the survey process from emphasizing facility structure and theoretical caregiving capacity toward evaluating actual delivery of care and its outcomes. PaCS requires surveyors to directly observe and document specific aspects of the physical environment, specific care procedures, and a representative sample of residents. Several features of the system require further development (e.g., a formal protocol for sampling of residents and for evaluating the proportion of undesirable outcomes attributable to care provided). However, the focus on outcomes of care rather than facility structure and written records of care has been commended as a potentially promising way to improve quality assurance (79).

Additional weaknesses of the survey process include inadequate staffing, training of survey staff, and inconsistencies between surveyors. During the last decade, some 15 State studies of nursing homes and the regulatory process have been conducted. Six reported inadequate resources for survey staff to be a significant problem (Arkansas, California, Colorado, Illinois, New Jersey, and Ohio); seven State commissions argued that survey staff training was inadequate (Arkansas, California, Colorado, Illinois, Michigan, New Jersey, and New York). Several studies argued that inadequate resources directed to the critical task of monitoring facility performance result in disparities in the performance of surveyors and inconsistencies in the numbers and types of deficiencies cited from State to State.

One analysis of data on Federal certification deficiencies found that the proportion of a State's skilled nursing facilities having more than 25 deficiencies in 1981 varied form none in Delaware to 100 percent in the District of Columbia (176). Another study found substantial variation from State to State in the most frequent types of deficiencies cited (166). Although such variations may in part reflect genuine differences in facility performance between States, they are also, to some degree, the result of unacceptable differences between States in the focus and accuracy of surveys (79).

Weaknesses in the survey process have been the focus of a protracted legal battle (see box 10-A), settled by the 1984 decision of the 10th Circuit Court of Appeals (158). The court's decision requires the Federal Government to modify the Federal certification survey process so as to assure quality of care in nursing homes more effectively.

Enforcement.—Even if the Federal standards were improved and the revised survey process complies with the decision in *Smith* v. *Heckler*, inadequate enforcement of standards could remain an impediment to improving quality of care.

Federal procedures for dealing with nursing homes found to be out of compliance are oriented toward helping them improve rather than toward enforcing certification standards. Current policies permit States to certify facilities in "substantial compliance" or those with "plans of correction." Policies encourage States to consult with and "persuade" facilities to come into compliance, rather than to punish them. In fact, under Federal regulations, State agencies cannot punish a violation immediately. Survey agencies must issue a notice to the operator of a substandard nursing home, giving the facility time (usually 30 to 60 days) in which to correct deficiencies. The HCFA Provider Certification State Operations Manual specifically instructs the survey agency to try to resolve cases before they are referred to the formal administrative enforcement agency for sanctions for noncompliance.

That posture may appear both reasonable and beneficial in some cases, but its overall effect is to allow States to continue certifying facilities that provide poor or marginal care. Studies find large numbers of "in-and-out" facilities: marginal or substandard long-term care facilities that are chronically out of compliance when surveyed temporarily eliminate deficiencies under a plan of correction, then quickly lapse into noncompliance until the next inspection, often a year later (31,77, 79,128,134). In other cases, nursing homes may be decertified (see next section) but quickly correct deficiencies to be promptly recertified for Medicare or Medicaid participation (4).

Even when State licensure and certification agencies and HCFA regional offices proceed with decertification, facilities still re-enter the program relatively easily. Federal Medicare regulations call for "reasonable assurance" that deficiencies that led to termination will not recur (42 CFR 489.57). In practice, however, State agencies feel they have no authority to deny certification to a facility that is in substantial compliance with Federal standards—whatever its prior record (4,124).

Decertification.—Termination of a provider's contract to participate in Medicaid or Medicare is the primary Federal method for securing compliance or punishing noncompliance. Representatives of consumers, providers, and regulators consistently criticize decertification as an enforcement tool; the absence of intermediate enforcement mechanisms is seen as a problem. Consumers and regulators advocate the introduction and implementation of a broader range of sanctions. During the last decade, nine State reports have argued that although decertification is the only authorized sanction, it is ineffective and rarely used (Arkansas, Colorado, Illinois, Minnesota, New Jersey, New York, Ohio, Texas, and Virginia) (also see refs. 6,29).

Concentrating enforcement on a mechanism that, if imposed, generally means closing a facility, is regarded by many as excessively severe and counterproductive. Decertification, particularly for minor deficiencies, may appear inappropriately harsh, and therefore not be used. As a result, providers may have little incentive to correct deficiencies.

Decertification is also criticized for the burden it imposes on residents and on State agencies to find placement for residents removed from substandard facilities. In addition to problems of bed scarcity, transferring individuals needing long-term care to a new facility may be traumatic, particularly for those with dementia, and can be harmful to their health (138). Thus, even in States where beds are available (e.g., Texas), decertification may appear an undesirable, if not unworkable, sanction (79,124).

Other problems with decertification as an enforcement mechanism are the cost and time involved in the legal proceedings associated with closing facilities or terminating provider contracts. Courts have held that a license to operate a nursing home and, in some cases, the contract to participate in Medicaid, are property rights. Thus, homes can challenge these sanctions, first in administrative hearings and then through a series of court appeals. That process is costly for State regulatory agencies. The facilities, however, can report the proceedings as an expense of doing business and be reimbursed through Medicaid or Medicare (134). The process often results in years of delay before sanctions are imposed (10,37,52, 127,129,133). Agencies typically drop all action if a facility comes into compliance at any time during the appeals process (134). The result is that nursing homes often receive no penalty for even the most severe violations of Federal health and safety standards.

Two intermediate Federal sanctions could be used in place of decertification. The issuance of time-limited provider contracts, pending correction of deficiencies, is available for certification violations. Second, the Omnibus Budget Reconciliation Act of 1981 (Public Law 97-35) authorized an intermediate Federal sanction: suspension of Medicare payments for patients admitted to facilities not in compliance with Federal conditions of participation but in which the deficiencies do not pose imminent threat to patients' health. Similar authority was granted to the States for Medicaid-only facilities. DHHS published the proposed regulations for this sanction in the Federal Register, July 3, 1986. The regulation became effective August 4, 1986 (51 FR 24484).

The inappropriateness of decertification and the failure of the Secretary to implement the intermediate sanction authorized by Congress 6 years ago have contributed to continued reliance by State regulatory agencies on attempts to *persuade* providers to come into compliance with Federal standards. Faced with an unworkable sanction, the dominant model of enforcement activity resorted to by States is "consultation" with facilities that fail to meet Federal certification standards. For instance, surveyors may choose not to record deficiencies, attempting to use this discretion to persuade facilities to correct the failure in a "reasonable" period of time. Even in cases where deficiencies are reported on a Federal survey report, State agencies still attempt to use education and consultation to achieve facility compliance with minimum Federal health and safety standards.

Most State studies are critical of the "consultation" model, arguing that it often results in inaccurate survey reports and fails to assure uniform and continual compliance with Federal regulations. In particular, it fails to address the problem of facilities that are habitually substandard, coming into compliance only to prevent decertification but reverting to noncompliance as soon as the threat is removed for another year.

Thus, although States are given the responsibility of enforcing Federal standards, they lack meaningful and workable Federal sanctions. That failing is a constant source of discontent and of criticism from the States (6,29,30,77,128,134,169).

Regulation of Board and Care Facilities

The regulatory structure for board and care facilities has been characterized as more fragmented and weaker than that for nursing homes. In general, Congress has maintained that it has little financial leverage over such facilities and, thus, little authority to demand Federal health and safety standards. Congressional actions aimed at improving board and care facility quality have been largely indirect.

The 1976 Keys amendment to the Social Security Act was the first attempt to exert some Federal pressure. The amendment gives States complete regulatory authority over DCFs, requiring them "to establish, maintain and insure the enforcement of standards" concerning admission policies, life safety, sanitation, and civil rights protection in facilities where three or more recipients of Supplemental Security Income (SSI) reside.

Three weaknesses have been identified in this Federal initiative:

1. Although the legislation encourages many States to clarify the language in their standards and regulations, State regulations largely exclude specifications about residents' personal care and social needs (45,114,142,162, 163).
2. The amendment is worded so that it applies only to board and care facilities that provide some form of medical or remedial care. That language has been interpreted as covering board and care homes that provide protective oversight or supervision, but not those that provide only food and shelter. That distinction dramatically narrows the universe of facilities covered by the Keys amendment, excluding an estimated 300,000 boarding homes in which large numbers of SSI recipients may reside (137,162,177).

3. The "penalty provision" of the Keys amendment has been widely criticized as inappropriate and unworkable (177). Under Keys, the Federal Government is authorized to reduce a recipient's Federal SSI payment by the amount of any State supplement "for medical or remedial care" if the recipient resides in a facility not approved by the State as meeting State domiciliary care standards. The intent is to provide an incentive for SSI recipients to move out of substandard or unlicensed facilities into ones that meet State standards. In theory that should force owners of substandard facilities to upgrade their facilities to meet State standards, but in practice it ignores the fact that many SSI recipients lack the physical or mental capacity to find alternative housing—even if it were available. Further, the penalty is taken directly against recipients rather than against substandard facilities or noncomplying States. The DHHS Inspector General has noted that this is "a position which has few—if any— defenders" (177). For these reasons, the "penalty provision" has never been invoked.

Subsequent Federal initiatives have been similarly unsuccessful in assuring improved quality in domiciliary care facilities. The 1978 Amendments to the Older Americans Act (OAA) encouraged nursing home ombudsman programs to include advocacy for board and care residents. Under that voluntary provision, few States expanded the scope of their ombudsman programs (170). The 1981 Rinaldo amendment to OAA, therefore, required State nursing home ombudsmen programs to investigate complaints about board and care homes. However, as several directors of ombudsman programs observe, without a substantial increase in State or Federal funding, they have insufficient staff to implement this provision effectively (53,72,146).

As a result of findings about inadequate quality and the weakness of existing regulatory structures, DHHS developed recommendations and a strategy to remedy what it felt were significant problems in board and care homes (180). The strategy includes an attempt to develop model State statutes, a grant to the National Bureau of Standards to develop fire safety standards, establishment of a central unit within DHHS to monitor board and care issues, and partial withholding of OAA funds from States that fail to certify that they maintain and enforce safety and quality of care standards as part of their OAA plan. No additional Federal funds have been made available to the States, however, to improve standards, monitoring, or enforcement of existing regulations; nor have any penalties been imposed on States for failure to uphold quality of care standards. Thus, the burden of improving quality of care and life in board and care homes continues to rest entirely on the States, whose efforts in that regard have been limited, despite their relatively long history of regulating board and care facilities.

States have made little progress in developing uniform and comprehensive standards of care or in developing an effective monitoring and enforcement system. Although each State has some regulations for licensing or certifying board and care facilities, significant variations exist in these regulations and in the level of effort States invest in inspecting facilities and enforcing standards of care and safety (5,64,164).

Variation in State regulatory policies reflect variations in the types of facilities defined as domiciliary care facilities. Programs and facilities specifically for mentally retarded adults tend to be the most formally and strictly regulated. Board and care facilities housing an elderly or mixed adult population have traditionally been subject to only minimal standards and surveillance. A survey of 31 States' board and care regulations noted that regulations focusing on board and care for elderly residents emphasize maintenance (food and shelter) and "bricks and mortar," rather than rehabilitation or other therapeutic services (45,154).

Given the characteristics and care needs of board and care residents, State regulatory standards may be insufficient to guarantee quality care. A comprehensive review of board and care standards identified the types of regulations that are the most common nationwide (143):

- **Structural Requirements:** The majority of regulations address structural (e.g., physical plant) rather than procedural (e.g., care) requirements. Given the level of functional and

mental impairment among DCF residents, these standards may be insufficient.

- **Staffing Requirements:** Staffing patterns and staff training requirements are another source of concern. Seventy percent of States that regulate board and care require that a responsible person be present in the facility at all times; but specific staffing standards, including staff/resident ratios, are stipulated in only 28 percent of State regulations. One-quarter of the regulations require some form of training for all staff, and another 27 percent mandate training for only some positions. Half the regulations do not require any staff training.

- **Procedural Requirements:** Regulations regarding actual provision of care were also sparse. Only half the States require board and care facilities to develop individual treatment plans and needs assessment for residents. Fewer than half oblige the operator to ensure that residents have periodic visits or examinations by physicians or nurses. And fewer than half mandate that facilities maintain relations with social service, welfare, or mental health agencies on behalf of residents. One-fourth of the States have regulations requiring that facility operators assist residents in obtaining dental care; one-tenth, eye care; and one-third, mental health services.

- **Residents' Rights:** The issue of resident's rights has been recognized as a pervasive problem in board and care facilities and, by its absence, in regulatory standards. Only a little more than half the States specify that residents have the right to privacy or visitation rights. Only half require facility operators to be accountable for residents' funds. (GAO found that operators frequently abuse residents rights by taking complete control of SSI checks and refusing to give residents private spending money (172).) Complaint and grievance procedures for residents are specified in only 37 percent of the regulations, and nearly all regulations have only minimal standards referring to the removal, relocation, or discharge of residents.

Monitoring Compliance.—Under the Keys amendment, States have sole responsibility for setting standards and inspecting DCFs. Within States, that responsibility is variously assigned, often to State health departments or mental health agencies. Thus, inspection is even more decentralized, and problems of fragmentation and poor coordination between agencies within States are frequently cited as major problems (163). Further, as previously described, State agencies say inadequate numbers and training of surveyors are major impediments to effective inspection. In addition, inspections of board and care facilities appear to focus almost exclusively on physical characteristics, fire safety, and other structural features rather than on the quality of care provided.

A 1982 survey by the Aging and Health Policy Center (AHPC) describes factors cited by State agencies as barriers to effective quality assurance in board and care facilities (164). Seventy-five percent of the regulatory agencies surveyed reported inadequate funds or personnel to license, inspect, and enforce board and care regulations. Some commentators suggest that understaffing of regulatory programs has been prevalent for some time (147). An investigation of board and care regulations in New York and New Jersey noted that staff shortages hamper surveillance and enforcement of licensed facilities and identification of unlicensed ones (137,162,167). Studies suggest, however, that even if agencies were adequately staffed, inspectors are generally poorly trained and ill prepared to evaluate the quality of care in DCFs or nursing homes (147,164). Further, fewer than one-fourth of State regulations provided for inspection of board and care facilities without prior notice to the operator.

Enforcement.—Enforcement of board and care standards is also lax. Although 87 percent of State regulations require facility operators to correct violations of the standards (143), imposition of sanctions for such violations is rare (147). While States often have the authority to issue a fine, revoke the operator's license, or remove residents, few agencies have used these powers. In the AHPC survey, State agencies argued that the absence of intermediate sanctions, such as civil penalties and fines that are not subject to lengthy administrative or judicial review, impedes their enforcement capabilities and explains the lack of enforcement activity (5,164).

Perhaps the greatest impediment to improved quality assurance activities by the States, however, is the fear that imposing and enforcing more stringent regulations would drive many board and care facilities out of business (137,163). When Michigan began licensing board and care facilities and imposing higher standards of care and safety, for instance, an estimated one-fourth of the facilities dropped out of the program. Ombudsmen in that State suggest that many facilities continued to house the same residents (with the same personal care and oversight needs), but simply converted to "boarding homes," unlicensed and unregulated (16).

Although the burden for assuring acceptable safety and care in board and care homes rests with States, they have few incentives to undertake this task, particularly given the lack of Federal initiatives and funds to match Federal mandates to improve the quality of care in and regulation of domiciliary care facilities. Facing pressure to curtail their Medicaid expenditures on nursing homes and anxious to reduce State-only expenditures on patients in State hospitals, for example, States may have a strong incentive not to impose higher standards on board and care facilities that house people who might otherwise be in costlier facilities.

Regulation of Noninstitutional Long-Term Care Services

As discussed earlier, Medicaid and Medicare were intended to contain the costs of hospital and nursing home services. That concern is apparent in the content of regulations, particularly for Medicare. Reflecting that intention, the Federal definition of services was narrowly circumscribed and medically oriented. Under Medicare, home health services are reimbursable only if they are skilled care services; health-related social support services for chronically ill individuals were excluded from coverage unless the person required some form of skilled care at the same time. Eligibility requires that a Medicare beneficiary be confined to his or her residence, be under a physician's care, and need skilled nursing care or physical or speech therapy. These restrictions, aimed primarily at containing costs, are reflected in the Medicare certification standards.

Home Health Agencies.—In order for a home health agency to provide services that are reimbursable by Medicare, the agency must be certified as being in compliance with Federal standards. Of the more than 12,000 home health agencies, some 6,000 are Medicare-certified (56,75). Federal "conditions of participation" mandate that each agency provide both skilled nursing care and at least one other service from among physical therapy, speech therapy, occupational therapy, medical social services, and home health aide services. The agency may contract with other providers for services it does not directly provide. Other Federal certification conditions relate primarily to operating policies, administrative structure and budgeting, clinical recordkeeping, staffing, and, where applicable, State licensure requirements (183).

The Medicaid program also pays for certain home health services. States have wide latitude in establishing eligibility criteria for individuals and reimbursable services, for establishing reimbursement rates, and for defining standards Medicaid-certified agencies must meet.

The conditions a provider must meet to participate in the Medicaid program are generally less extensive than those for Medicare-certified agencies (7). Under Title XIX, the State Medicaid agency determines whether a home health agency can be a contractor or vendor under the Medicaid program. In general, Medicaid agencies contract only with providers certified to participate in Medicare, in effect piggybacking on the Federal standards and survey process. States that do not have sufficient numbers of Medicare-certified agencies to meet the demand for Medicaid home health services may contract with agencies that meet only State licensing law. Nineteen States, however, have no home health agency licensure requirements (7,56). In these cases, the State Medicaid agency may simply let the contract to the lowest bidder who provides the desired services (7).

In addition to Medicare and Medicaid, the Federal Government has provided funds through the Social Services Block Grant and title III of the Older Americans Act. Like Medicaid, these programs generally contract with Medicare-certified home health agencies for the provision of home health services or, where insufficient numbers of Medicare-certified providers are available, rely on State licensing for quality assurance.

Thirty-three States and the District of Columbia have licensure laws pertaining to home health agencies. Licensure is a tool that allows States to specify quality standards, and is viewed as particularly important for regulating those agencies that provide services only to self-paying clients. For approximately 6,000 non-Medicare certified agencies (and industry experts estimate the number is actually larger), the only requirements they must meet are those imposed by the States. In the States without licensure laws, such agencies are virtually unregulated (7).

Among States that regulate licensure of home health agencies, substantial variation can be found in the content and specificity of the laws.

- Some States have essentially "pro forma" licensing laws that merely define what constitutes a home health agency and the administrative structure required for the agency to qualify as a home health provider.
- Other States have laws that incorporate service standards, often modeled on Medicare's, but in some cases more detailed and explicit about staffing, training, services to be provided, assessment of recipient of care, care planning, recordkeeping, and coordination with other agencies.
- In most States, the standards focus largely on the agency's presumed capacity to provide appropriate services.

Perhaps the most significant deficit in the current regulatory system for home health providers is the absence in nearly half the States of any regulatory quality assurance system for non-Medicare certified home health agencies. Non-Medicare agencies in those States are subject to no required standards and to no monitoring of their performance—even of their capacity to provide acceptable services. Members of industry trade associations note that these agencies have few incentives to engage in a costly quality assurance system on their own, and they are concerned that such agencies may provide unacceptable quality of care. The associations further observe that such agencies tend to have lower charges, since they are not required to be certified, licensed, or to have internal quality assurance reviews. Because Medicare generally does not cover the kinds of home health services persons with dementing disorders may routinely require, these individuals are at particular risk; if seeking lower cost services, they may turn to unregulated home health agencies.

Like nursing homes, home health agencies receiving Federal reimbursement are inspected at least yearly to determine their compliance with the program's conditions of participation. In States that require licensure for home health agencies, inspections are generally done by the State licensing agency. Alternatively, the State health department, under contract to DHHS, may conduct the inspections. HCFA has the authority to conduct validation surveys to measure the accuracy of the State agency surveys. The impression of home health trade association officials is that these surveys have recently become more detailed, including occasional visits to the agencies (56).

As with regulations for nursing homes, home health regulations represent a structural and resource input approach to standard setting, in which the primary focus is limited to the agency's capacity to provide appropriate services based on its administrative organization and staffing patterns, rather than its actual provision of care. Inspections, too, focus on agency documents and client records, including reports of the agency's internal evaluation of its performance. Thus, the survey process, like that for long-term care in nursing homes, is able to measure only the agency's paper compliance with structural and resource input standards.

Other Services.—Regulatory standards to assure high-quality care are even sparser for other types of long-term care (e.g., adult day care and respite care). Thirty-nine States have established licensing laws for adult day care programs, but the regulations range from specifying only standards for receiving public funding to specifying staffing and services requirements. Home chore services and respite care programs, whether at a facility or in homes, are largely unregulated by local, State, or Federal agencies. In general, only those programs that provide services under Medicaid waivers are subject to any regulation or per-

formance monitoring (141). Thus, relatively little is known about the quality of these programs, and existing licensing bodies do little to assure quality of care. As with home health care, perhaps the greatest potential for identifying appropriate standards and monitoring systems rests with the Medicaid waiver programs and peer review systems.

Among peer review and trade associations, substantial work is being done to develop quality-of-care and service standards. Further, particularly for individuals with dementia and their families, the experience of some States with Medicaid waivers for community-based services provides the greatest potential for developing both voluntary and regulatory quality assurance programs. (These are discussed at greater length later in this chapter.)

Lack of Coordination.—One significant quality problem is that home health and other related home- and community-based services for elderly Americans are not being effectively coordinated, and regulation tends to exacerbate the problem rather than resolve it. For each program, State, Federal, and usually local administration is different; eligibility is different; reimbursement is different; and the programs are targeted at different subgroups. Such targeting often occurs with little regard for the reality of the multiple and complex disabilities and care needs of the chronically ill older population. Medicare is aimed at the "highly skilled care patient," Medicaid at the indigent patient, and social service programs at the relatively well older person. There are at least three problems with this kind of targeting:

1. It ignores the fundamental reality that, for the chronically ill older person, health care and social support needs not only overlap but often compound one another.
2. Classification tends to become arbitrary. The needs of an elderly person may be perceived as social or medical based largely on the program for which the client is eligible or for which the person applies.
3. There is a tendency for the older person to receive only those services that a particular agency directly provides.

Although government regulations and voluntary standards set by agencies both often emphasize requirements for multidimensional needs assessment, care planning, and service coordination, the reality seldom matches the requirement. Services are rarely provided or even accessible through a single entry point, and, except for special demonstration projects, the formal requirements of interagency arrangements have not proved uniformly effective in coordinating services to older persons. While requirements may exist and be fulfilled on paper, they are not enforced in practice (171,179). Effective case management and agency coordination are still not widespread, and frail elderly individuals and their families are left to wander through a bureaucratic maze in search of needed and ostensibly available services.

POSSIBILITIES FOR REFORM

Defining, measuring, and assuring quality continue to be vexing problems throughout the field of human services. Formal licensing, certification, and accreditation procedures, although useful in assuring minimum capability among service providers, do not address actual performance or ensure that client well-being is effectively protected. Most standards used to evaluate provider performance represent minimal compliance thresholds. They generally focus on provider capacity and are relatively static, changing little with regard to the state of the art in service delivery.

Further, as the number of providers has grown in relation to the number of regulatory staff, the process of monitoring providers has deteriorated. Extensive reliance by regulatory agencies on written documentation of provider compliance has become standard practice. The emphasis on paper compliance grew out of management systems theory, recognition of practical constraints on regulatory agencies, and difficulties involved in monitoring services in a decentralized system. With a multitude of providers and relatively few inspectors, the system allows regulators to rely on documentation rather than observation of the quality of services or measurement of outcomes. The practice has been widely criticized as unreliable (10,129,134).

Also, traditional quality assurance systems tend to use techniques that are more reactive than proactive, particularly regarding compliance mechanisms. Reactive mechanisms investigate service problems and rely on enforcement remedies or sanctions ensure compliance. Proactive mechanisms emphasize monitoring and assisting providers in improving practice and preventing problems.

Observations and criticisms of quality assurance mechanisms in the human services field are particularly relevant to long-term care. Demographic trends and increased need for long-term care, an increasingly debilitated population of older persons, fiscal constraints, and continuing concern about quality of care present serious challenges to policymakers, regulators, and providers alike. Although the existing regulatory system and increasing knowledge and skill among providers have led to improvements, much remains to be done to assure acceptable long-term care quality.

Several themes are central to a discussion of the possibilities for reform of the Nation's quality assurance system:

- **Structural and Process Standards:** Structural and process standards of care have contributed to improved long-term care quality and remain important components of a quality assurance system.
- **Outcome-Based Standards:** Quality assurance can be improved, both in terms of defining standards and monitoring compliance, by using quality measures that are resident-focused and more process- and outcome-oriented. In addition to specifying provider behavior in terms of expected structures and processes of care, standards and inspections could focus on the quality of care actually provided. One way of achieving that goal is to monitor and assess resident outcomes and, ultimately, specify desired outcomes.
- **Quality of Life:** Standards could address outcomes and processes related to the quality of life, in addition to the quality of health and habilitative care. These may be particularly applicable to nursing homes and domiciliary care facilities.

- **Information:** A central element of a more effective quality assurance system is improved information. Both providers and regulators need substantial information about residents' characteristics:
  - —Data about residents' conditions and needs are essential for determining necessary levels of resource inputs and appropriate processes of care, and for specifying and evaluating resident outcomes.
  - —Such data are needed for effectively monitoring provider performance, for identifying factors leading to potential problems and unacceptable performance, and for correcting identified deficiencies.
  - —For many outcome and process measures, the necessary data are identifiable, measurable, and accessible. Additional information is needed, however, to establish criteria for evaluating provider performance.
  - —Information must be more systematically applied in developing standards of care and evaluation criteria.
  - —A system for generating feedback of information on provider performance and state-of-the-art care is essential to a dynamic and evolutionary set of standards and criteria.
  - —More information is also important for efforts to improve existing regulations. As noted, relatively little is known about the performance of home health agencies, adult day care programs, and respite care. Further, there is little systematic, empirical information about what interventions are effective, particularly in terms of the care and management of individuals with dementia. Thus it is difficult to determine whether existing standards, inspections, and enforcement mechanisms are effective—or what kinds of quality assurance mechanisms would be more effective.
- **Enforcement:** Currently neither the regulatory system nor market mechanisms is effective for ensuring high-quality care. Regulatory compliance mechanisms have proved ineffective in enforcing standards. And consumers are hindered both by third-party payment systems and general inaccessibility to the legal process.

Several methods are available for assuring quality in long-term care, as discussed in the remainder of this chapter. Market forces, including competition and consumer empowerment, are one possible means. Provider quality assurance activities and professional peer review are other options. Improved regulatory systems are also possible, even in an era of fiscal constraints and deregulation.

Market Forces To Assure Quality

In a competitive "free" market, the issue of defining and regulating long-term care quality would be largely academic, interesting but not critical for assuring that people received high-quality care. In such a competitive market, consumers would be informed, able to switch easily from one provider to another, and would allocate resources in such a way as to maximize their well-being. For long-term care, however, this model seems largely inapplicable.

Although reducing regulation and relying on competitive market forces are increasingly popular ideas, these mechanisms are seriously limited for ensuring quality care. Individuals who need nursing home or domiciliary care generally suffer from a bewildering array of physical, functional, and mental disabilities. Their ability to choose rationally among providers and, if dissatisfied with the quality of care, to switch from one provider to another, is hampered by several factors, including:

1. poor access to information;
2. limited ability to understand information;
3. restricted mobility;
4. a financing system biased toward institutional care; and
5. a vendor payment system that removes much of the decisionmaking from the consumer.

Once admitted to a nursing home or board and care facility, a resident is, in a very real sense, part of a "captive" population (193). That is, residents have little access to information and are generally unaware of other options. Further, with multiple disabilities and limited mobility, they can seldom exercise the option of leaving. This problem is exacerbated by the tight nursing home bed supply in most States (51,65). Occupancy rates that average better than 95 percent make it difficult to find another facility, even when residents are capable of moving. Because of their restricted ability to leave, residents have little leverage even when they choose to complain to providers (70). For individuals with dementing illnesses, the problem of being an effective consumer is especially severe.

Families provide most long-term care themselves. When formal long-term care services are required, however, families are also hampered in their efforts to act as effective consumers. One significant difficulty they encounter is the absence of useful comparative information on the cost and quality of various long-term care settings. Such judgments are difficult even for professionals; for a family unschooled in measuring the quality of health care and under pressure to find help, meaningful evaluations are exceedingly difficult. Although trial and error is a theoretical solution to finding the best provider, it is inappropriate for someone needing long-term care.

Families are hindered by a variety of other factors, including financial constraints, the unwillingness of many long-term care providers to accept and properly care for individuals with dementing illnesses, and the general unavailability of appropriate long-term care services aside from nursing homes (134,185). In addition, families are often pressured to make quick decisions about a long-term care provider, particularly when a hospital is seeking to discharge an elderly patient as quickly as possible.

These factors create serious difficulties for consumers of long-term care and their families who hope to use traditional market forces to assure the quality or accessibility of long-term care. Problems may be compounded for those who have no close relatives to assist them in pressuring providers to improve quality.

Given these problems, particularly the vulnerability of consumers, some argue that government has a fundamental role in assuring improved quality in long-term care. Further, they note, as the primary payer for most long-term care, especially for nursing homes and indirectly for board and care, the government has an obligation to ensure that public monies are well-spent, that public funds are not spent on substandard care, and that public beneficiaries have access to long-term care of acceptable quality.

The practical difficulties of regulating and monitoring providers, however, give consumers an indispensable role in quality assurance. Regulatory standards, inspections, and enforcement mechanisms remain important, but the practical difficulties encountered by regulatory agencies, particularly in a decentralized system, mean that consumers and their advocates must take a strong role in quality assurance. Informed, empowered, and assertive consumers and advocates may hold the greatest potential for assuring quality in long-term care. Several mechanisms could strengthen the role of consumers and enhance their ability to use more traditional market mechanisms to assure acceptable long-term care quality.

Inspection/Survey Process

Consumers could be included in the inspection/survey process. Their views on the quality of care they receive from licensed and certified long-term care providers could be actively solicited by inspectors. That approach is most feasible in institutional settings; however, it is also possible for surveyors to telephone or visit a sample of home health and adult day care clients. For consumers with a dementing disorder, the surveyor could interview the person's family or, in an institution, members of the residents' council.

Consumer Advocates and the Legal Process

The role and powers of consumer advocates could be enhanced. That would be particularly appropriate for nursing home ombudsmen, whose legal authority covers both nursing homes and DCFs. Adequate funding for such ombudsmen, however, has not matched the expansion in their formal roles or the numbers of individuals who need their assistance in resolving disputes between long-term care providers and consumers. A recent Institute of Medicine report specified several recommendations for increased involvement of consumers and consumer advocates in quality assurance (79).

Consumer advocates might also be given the broader role of assisting consumers with all long-term care providers, including home health agencies, home chore service, adult day care, and in-home respite care.

The ability of long-term care consumers to use the legal process to enforce their rights to appropriate care and treatment could be enhanced through additional funding of legal services for elderly individuals.

Information Dissemination

The ability of consumers and their families to be informed and effective could be enhanced by more systematic and widespread dissemination of information about case management, about evaluating the quality of care and services provided by long-term care institutions and agencies, and about mechanisms to remedy problems they encounter.

Revision of Residents' Rights

Federal nursing home regulations could be revised so that residents' rights are elevated to a condition of participation. The Institute of Medicine recommended such revisions and specified standards in some detail (79). Of course, the case of persons with dementia is especially difficult, since cognitive impairment inhibits their ability to assert and protect their rights. However, protection from transfers or discharges, and assertion of the rights of residents, their legal guardians, and their families, could enhance the effectiveness of long-term care consumers and their advocates.

Congress could amend the Social Security Act's requirement that States establish and maintain standards for facilities in which three or more SSI recipients reside. In addition to standards specified in the Keys amendment, Congress could require that States establish residents' rights for individuals in DCFs.

Provider Self-Review, Peer Review, and Professional Review

Another mechanism for improving and assuring the quality of long-term care involves the activities of providers and other health care professionals. Improved management among providers, more extensive training of direct care staff, and increased involvement of health professionals in nursing homes, for example, have had beneficial effects over the last two decades. Many long-term care providers are independently establishing internal quality assurance systems to monitor and improve their performance (see ch. 9). Further, professional groups, peer review organizations, and industry trade associations have made significant strides in encouraging long-term care providers to improve the quality of their services and the effectiveness of their monitoring systems.

Provider Self-Review

Several multistate nursing home organizations, including the National Health Corp., Hillhaven, Beverly Enterprises, and Ohio Presbyterian Homes for the Aged, have developed internal quality assurance programs (79). These systems typically monitor some quality indices (e.g., staffing patterns, patient case mix, changes in patient status) that might suggest quality problems in their facilities. Some, such as Ohio Presbyterian Homes, have developed detailed quality reviews that they routinely conduct in each of their facilities. These reviews include both resource input and process measures of quality. Hillhaven has been particularly active in attempting to develop standards for appropriate care and management of individuals with Alzheimer's disease.

Trade Association Review

Trade associations have begun encouraging members to establish standards for acceptable quality of care and to review their performances in a more systematic manner. The American Health Care Association's "Quest for Quality," for example, specifies matters that ought to be evaluated by nursing homes, suggests goals for quality performance, and provides quality review instruments.

The National Association for Home Care is also developing model standards to assist members in assuring that the care they provide meets acceptable professional standards of quality (56). At the State level, at least one State industry association has refused membership to two providers whose nursing homes did not pass the association's peer review.

Professional Organization Review

Professional organizations have also been active in long-term care quality assurance activities. The Joint Commission on Accreditation of Hospitals (JCAH) has had a voluntary accreditation program for nursing homes since 1966. Home health agencies that are hospital-based may also seek JCAH accreditation (56). The JCAH process emphasizes voluntary participation by providers, independent peer review, and professional responsibility, and includes continuing educational and consultation for providers seeking such accreditation (200).

The National League for Nursing (NLN) and the American Nurses Association's Division of Gerontological Nursing have been active in promulgating standards for long-term care nursing. Home health agencies seeking NLN accreditation must comply with standards defined by that organization. NLN also retains input and process measures for use in its ongoing evaluation of each agency's performance (56).

Associations like the National Council on Aging (NCOA) have become active in developing model standards for some long-term care providers. NCOA has developed a variety of suggested standards for adult day care programs. These are designed to augment adult day care licensure standards established in 39 States, which vary in content (from funding criteria to quality standards) and specificity. The NCOA standards address appropriate staffing patterns, structural and facility guidelines, and issues such as activities and administration. They specifically address issues related to appropriate care of individuals with dementia (141).

In some instances, private foundations have initiated efforts to improve quality of long-term care. The Robert Wood Johnson Foundation, for example, sponsors a teaching nursing home program to establish ties between nursing homes and schools of nursing and medicine. The foundation hopes the program will stimulate nursing facilities to improve their delivery of quality care and to develop internal quality assurance standards (2).

Data Collection Efforts

While self-regulatory activities by pr peer review agencies, and health care profes sionals represent potentially beneficial developments in voluntary quality assurance, little is known about the efficacy of these programs (96). Of all the activities described, only the teaching nursing home program is being systematically evaluated in terms of its impact on quality of care (153). Although such efforts should be encouraged, reliance on them for quality assurance is probably misplaced until their impact has been empirically evaluated.

Regulation and Quality Assurance

Like the concept of "quality" itself, quality assurance in long-term care is complex and multidimensional. Quality of care is the product of many factors, including provider willingness and capacity to provide care, consumer characteristics and behavior, the role of consumer advocates, involvement of other health care professionals, third-party reimbursement policies, and the state of knowledge about effective treatment and care. It is also, in no small measure, the result of government policies aimed at assuring uniformly acceptable quality of care to elderly and chronically ill individuals.

Conceptual Model of a Regulatory Quality Assurance System

The primary components of a regulatory system for quality assurance are: 1) establishing standards of care; 2) monitoring compliance; and 3) enforcing compliance. The three are inextricably related. Without an adequate inspection system and mechanisms for enforcing compliance, standards of care can become meaningless. In addition, standards themselves must allow consistent, objective assessment and must be clear and fair enough to be enforceable in legal proceedings when necessary.

Several mechanisms have been suggested for strengthening the regulatory system for purposes of quality assurance. First, a richer definition of quality—one that is multidimensional, resident-focused, and outcome-and-process-oriented— would be valuable. Second, criteria for evaluating the performance of long-term care providers might be defined. Third, an inspection system capable of assessing and rating quality of care could be established. Fourth, regulators could implement a system of incentives and disincentives for inducing compliance with at least minimal standards of care. Fifth, a process of collecting information for monitoring providers and modifying normative criteria could be implemented.

Developing Process and Structural Standards of Care

Professional and public perceptions of illnesses shape management and treatment (48,196). Because there is no cure for Alzheimer's disease and most other chronic dementing disorders, and because no single treatment has proved effective, many health care professionals and providers assume that relatively little can be done for persons with dementia other than providing food and shelter. That assumption leads to "warehousing" of these individuals, and contributes to the overuse of physical and chemical restraints.

Dementing disorders, like other chronic illnesses for which there is no cure, require careful management and planning. Although systematic research on the effectiveness of various management strategies is notably absent (81), the experience of many health care professionals and providers supports the argument that good management improves the functional, behavioral, and health status of individuals with dementia (see ch. 7).

Chapters 2 and 7 discuss management and treatment processes believed to be effective for persons with dementia (see box 10-B). These are important because, as discussed earlier in this chapter (in the section on defining quality), patient outcomes cannot be the only measure of quality in long-term care. These procedures could form the basis of recommendations for structural and process quality standards of care for a variety of long-term care settings, from nursing homes to adult day care programs.

Yet there is a dearth of research on the effectiveness of these techniques. They are largely the product of experience, often by trial and error,

---

Box 10-B.—Management and Treatment Procedures Effective With Individuals With Dementia

Medical Care.—All patients need an interested and informed physician, although frequent physician visits to patients with dementia may be unnecessary. Some researchers suggest that for persons with Alzheimer's disease, 4 to 6 months is an appropriate interval between examinations in the absence of a change in status or behavior (23,92). Current Federal standards specify that a nursing home is responsible for ensuring that appropriate physician visits are made to Medicare and Medicaid patients.

Diagnosis.—An adequate diagnosis is essential in order to rule out other factors that may cause memory loss and to ensure that, where Alzheimer's disease is present, other treatable disorders are identified and treated.

Hearing and Vision Care.—Decreased sensory input, resulting from poor vision or deafness, may aggravate existing confusion among persons with dementia. Medicare and Medicaid often do not cover hearing and vision examinations, or reimburse the purchase of sensory aids (e.g., eyeglasses and hear-

ing devices). Hearing and vision evaluations could be made standard components of medical care to be provided for those receiving long-term care.

Drugs.—Many different drugs (e.g., antidepressants, antipsychotics, and sleeping pills) are used to treat dementia and accompanying symptoms. Extreme caution and vigilance are imperative in administering drugs to someone with dementia, as many can have negative side effects (e.g., insomnia, confusion, hallucinations, agitation, or motor difficulties). It may be prudent to require that a physician or nurse authorize and monitor any drug administered to persons with dementia, eliminating prescription of drugs on an "as needed" basis.

Assessment and Individualized Care Plans.—Individualized assessment and care plans are important elements of adequate care. Ideally, these should be done by a multidisciplinary team and include an evaluation of the person's cognitive, functional, physical, mental, and emotional status. Periodic updates are important to monitor status and identify effective features of care.

Communication.—Individuals with dementia can suffer from several types of communication deficits. Caregivers must learn how to communicate with the individuals and how to interpret what could otherwise be considered inappropriate or deliberately assaultive behavior. Specific techniques have been suggested for improving communication with persons with Alzheimer's disease (13,55).

Activity and Exercise.—Many physicians prescribe active therapy rather than pharmacological approaches to the behavioral problems prevalent among persons with dementia, and recommend exercise and increased physical activity during the day to reduce restlessness and tension (23,92). Studies suggest that activity and exercise are vital not only to reduce wandering and restlessness, but also for physical health (44).

Maintaining Functional Capacity.—Minimizing functional decline delays and helps prevent the physical problems associated with inactivity, in addition to contributing to psychological well-being (44,68). A goal of long-term care, therefore, is to improve, maintain, or prevent avoidable decline in an individual's functional abilities, particularly in activities of daily living (e.g., eating, walking, and toileting).

Mental and Social Stimulation.—Memory training and reality therapy are used in a number of settings in an attempt to offset cognitive deterioration experienced by persons with dementia. Techniques include review of names, date, and time; reminiscence exercises; and music therapy. These activities are thought to contribute to recipient's self-confidence and to enhance alertness (13,44,55,105).

Environment.—Environmental factors appear to be crucial to behavior management for persons with

dementia. Judicious management of the environment is thus an important consideration in optimizing a person's functioning and reducing behavioral problems (13,17,49).

Safety Measures.—Both institutional and family caregivers are often overwhelmed by the need to keep someone with dementia under constant surveillance. Numerous precautions could be implemented to prevent falls, injuries, and other mishaps. Safety measures include having residents wear identification bracelets; placing locks at the bottom of room doors; affixing bells to exit doors; storing medications out of residents' reach; keeping cleaning fluids and other toxic substances locked up; supervising residents who smoke, to prevent fires; keeping furnishings in the same places; and removing extension cords, footstools, and other objects that may be hazardous to someone with limited mobility (55).

Staff Training.—Many observers argue that current standards for staff training in nursing homes, board and care facilities, and community-based settings are seriously inadequate (79), and that improved training, particularly in relation to care and management of individuals with dementia, is essential to improve the quality of care of these residents (106).

Staffing Levels.—Federal regulations regarding staffing levels are not specific, requiring only that staffing be "adequate" to meet the needs of nursing home residents. Most nursing homes, however, are not staffed at a level that many experts believe is appropriate for individuals with Alzheimer's disease and other cognitive disorders. A recent analysis suggests that a staff aide/resident ratio of 1 to 5 is appropriate for the care of individuals with Alzheimer's disease in nursing homes (63). The Institute of Medicine reports current ratios in U.S. nursing homes to be between 1 to 10 and 1 to 15 (79).

among nurses, social workers, physicians, other health professionals, and family caregivers who have been providing care and services to persons with dementia over a period of years. Therefore, it is premature to suggest that these and similar techniques be incorporated into Federal regulations as mandatory procedural standards. But experience to date does suggest several options for congressional action:

• Federal regulations or State licensure laws could require every long-term care provider to conduct a multidimensional needs assessment and develop an individual care plan for each resident. The assessment could focus on physical health, mental status, and physical functioning. It could also include evaluation of sensory status; the care plan could include appropriate referrals.

- Every long-term care provider could be required to ensure that each person who exhibits signs of cognitive impairment be referred to an appropriate health care provider for further assessment and to a physician for a comprehensive physical examination (unless the person has already been seen by a physician).

- Every long-term care provider could be required to refer to a physician any person with dementia who exhibits sudden changes in physical, functional, or cognitive status. Further, the resident's chart/care plan should report such behavioral changes and the provider's course of action.

- Federal policy on payment for hearing, vision, and dental care (through Medicare and Medicaid) could be revised to mandate payment for needed appliances.

- Federal certification standards for nursing homes and State licensure laws for DCFs could be revised to include specific process of care standards on the appropriate use of physical and chemical restraints.

- Although exhorting States to improve licensure standards for DCFs is one possibility, Congress could also amend the Social Security Act, adding more specific guidelines to the requirement that States establish and maintain standards for facilities in which three or more SSI recipients reside. In addition to the items specified by the Keys amendment (admission policies, life safety, sanitation, and civil rights), the States could be required to ensure that each DCF resident receives appropriate personal and health care. Such an amendment could mandate that States require all licensed DCFs to: 1) conduct a routine needs assessment and develop a simple care plan for all residents; 2) establish relationships with social service and mental health agencies on behalf of residents; 3) assist residents in obtaining care for dental, vision, and hearing problems. States could also be required to develop process standards for the appropriate use of physical restraints and psychotropic drugs in DCFs.

- Federal certification standards could be revised to mandate preemployment staff training for nurse's aides. Further, the standards could more explicitly define the content of that training. The training could include specific information about dementias and effective management and treatment of individuals with dementing disorders.

- The Social Security Act could be amended to require that States establish training requirements for all supervisory and resident care staff in DCFs. (Only 25 percent of State regulations for DCFs require some form of staff training, and 27 percent require training for only some positions.) The training could include information on care and management of individuals with dementia (e.g., appropriate use and risks associated with psychotropic drugs and physical restraints, and effective treatment of communication and sleep disorders, wandering, agitation, and combative behavior).

- The Federal Government could encourage States and professional organizations to promulgate standards on appropriate staffing levels and training for noninstitutional long-term care programs (e.g., adult day care, respite care). Staffing standards that are case-mix sensitive may be particularly useful, since not all such programs serve clients with cognitive impairment and associated behavioral problems.

- Federal standards for staffing of nursing homes could be revised to require at least one registered nurse on duty in every nursing home for at least one shift every day. That requirement has been recommended by the Institute of Medicine (79).

- Federal nursing home standards could also be revised to eliminate the distinction between skilled nursing facilities (SNFs) and intermediate care facilities (ICFs). That is one of the most significant Institute of Medicine recommendations. The original perception was that ICFs and SNFs would serve distinct populations with significantly different care needs. In practice, that has not occurred; most facilities serve a mix of patients with varying disabilities and care needs. Moreover, individuals with dementia are typically cared for in ICFs. Yet, as discussed, while they do not typically require daily skilled nursing care, they do require the services of skilled nurses, particularly in assessment, care planning, and supervision of care. The current guidelines for staffing in ICFs do not seem adequate to meet the complex care and supervision needs of residents with dementia.

- Federal standards for minimum nursing aide-to-resident ratios in nursing homes could be made more explicit. Current standards require staffing to be "adequate" to meet the needs of residents; but studies reveal that staffing levels seldom approach the 1 to 5 ratio suggested as appropriate for the care of someone with Alzheimer's disease (63). Alternatively, guidelines for State survey agencies could specifically address the care needs of particular groups and methods of determining whether staffing is adequate, given a facility's mix of residents.

- Congress could amend the Social Security Act to require that States establish staffing standards for DCFs. For example, Congress could require that DCFs hire a geriatric nurse practitioner or psychiatric nurse for a specified number of hours per week or month to review residents' needs, to develop care plans, to review the use of any drugs or physical restraints, and to develop and coordinate arrangements with other social service or mental health agencies that provide services needed by the DCF residents.

- Congress could require that States report the results of their DCF admission policies and the findings of inspections. That would help determine whether individuals who require more supervision or nursing and personal care than DCFs can provide are nevertheless being housed in board and care facilities.

- Congress could establish a "look behind" authority for the Department of Health and Human Services to inspect DCFs in the States. In particular, DHHS could focus on whether some individuals who require nursing home care are being inappropriately housed in DCFs. Since most States have adopted measures to reduce the number of Medicaid recipients in nursing homes, they may have little incentive to prevent such inappropriate placement. Therefore, Congress might also consider monetary penalties against the States for any failure to adequately monitor DCF resident admission and retention.

Improving the Monitoring of Long-Term Care Providers

Monitoring providers' performance in relation to standards is the second critical component of a regulatory quality assurance system. The relationship between standards and inspection is reciprocal. Standards—the first component—must be amenable to objective measurement by inspectors, and must be administratively feasible for State and Federal agencies to implement. Similarly, many characteristics of the inspection system are influenced by the nature of the standards selected. Process or outcome quality standards, for instance, would demand considerably more of inspectors than structural or input-based standards, as the latter are relatively easy to quantify and measure objectively.

One suggestion for reform is the professionalization of agencies that perform facility inspections (12). That would be particularly critical if standards were based on process or outcome quality measures for which some subjective determinations would be unavoidable. Some aspects of the inspection system, however, are important regardless of the type of standards used. These include: timing, frequency, and type of inspection (e.g., announced/unannounced); size and composition of inspection teams (e.g., multidisciplinary teams, generalists); frequency and nature of surveys that validate inspections; and administrative structure and norms that support inspectors.

Reforming the survey process for nursing homes is the prerogative of the Federal Government, while States are responsible for DCF inspection standards. Several reforms could improve the inspection system for both types of institutions. Most of these reforms have been uniformly recommended in a decade's worth of State reports.

As noted, as a result of *Smith* v. *Heckler*, the Federal Government is under court order to develop a survey process that is more resident-focused, and was to have introduced the Patient Care and Services (PaCS) System in August 1986. Several States have attempted to modify their licensure inspections, and Iowa has developed a resident-focused, outcome-oriented survey that is currently being evaluated (21,99,100). In general, however, such surveys do not include items directly related to the special care and service ls of individuals with dementia. They could, however, be appropriately modified, particularly given the large and growing size of the nursing home population with some type of cognitive impairment (1080.

Surveys or inspections could be unannounced and scheduled to reduce the likelihood that providers could anticipate them. Some inspections, for example, could be conducted during the evening or on weekends, when they are unexpected and when deficiencies, such as short staffing, are thought to be most common (77,128,134,169).

Surveys, like regulations and performance standards, could be resident-focused and outcome- and process-oriented, rather than concentrating on structural features, facility records, and the capacity to provide appropriate care. Inspections could thus focus more on the care and services needed by and provided to residents And, to the degree possible, they could focus more on residents' outcomes as initial indicators of quality of care and life in the facility. Surveys could include direct observation of residents (e.g., their personal grooming, use of physical restraints) and the care and services they actually receive (79).

Surveys may be made both shorter and more effective if they focus on key indicators of quality of care and quality of life. The outcome-oriented measures described earlier in this chapter could be used as some key indicators. Several States have experimented with a shortened, more focused survey process, and evaluations suggest that, to a large extent, such surveys are at least as effective in identifying deficiencies as the current process (40,99,109,130). A more effective survey process would allow agencies to concentrate inspection and enforcement resources on facilities with a history of poor care. Although all facilities ought to be inspected at least annually, poor facilities could be inspected more frequently (79).

One concern is that the key indicators of quality identified by those surveys may not be sufficiently comprehensive, particularly in describing mental health needs and care, quality of life, and process quality that are especially relevant to the care and management of individuals with dementia. Each of the existing systems could be evaluated to determine whether it includes significant indicators of the care needed and received by someone with dementia. For such persons, the key indicators of quality that are outcome-oriented could include the items discussed in this chapter (e.g., overuse of physical restraints, overuse of psychotropic medications, personal care and grooming, dehydration). In addition, the survey could include some process measures of quality, since proper procedures of care and management for this population seem to be better developed than outcome-quality measures.

Under the current survey process, each facility receives the same inspection as all other facilities in the Medicaid or Medicare program with the same certification level (SNF or ICF). Given the diversity of facilities and of resident populations, such a system prohibits an effective orientation to individuals. For a more efficient and effective survey process, the survey instrument could be adjusted from facility to facility, based on the characteristics of the residents. Thus, for example, a facility with a high mix of individuals needing rehabilitative care would receive a slightly different survey from one with a high mix of persons with dementia. The outcome-oriented measures of quality for a stroke patient might focus on functional improvement, while for someone with dementia it might focus on drugs, restraints, and so on. A revised survey process and instruments could allow and encourage surveyors to focus on outcome and process measures specific to the nature and extent of individuals' disabilities and the resident mix of a given facility.

Although shorter, more focused surveys may be appropriate, a more extensive survey might be useful when inspections reveal quality problems. Identification of particular characteristics or outcomes may indicate where underlying problems exist in a facility. Negative outcomes—those not predicted given the residents' status or the mix of disabilities—could trigger a more extensive examination of a facility's resource inputs and processes of care. For instance, regulations may specify appropriate protocols for administering medications. If overmedication is discovered, further inspection might identify staff inadequacies or inappropriate processes of care as an underlying cause.

In most States, surveys are done by nurses or generalists. Only a few States have standard survey teams that include dietitians, physical and occupational therapists, pharmacists, physicians, social workers, psychiatrists or psychiatric social workers, and other professionals. Where surveys reveal problems in particular areas of care, specialists could be available to conduct more in-depth inspections. (For example, where an inspection team identifies problems in nutritional services, the agency could have a dietitian conduct a complete survey of resident's nutritional status and the facility's dietary services.) Such specialists need not be included in every survey but could be on staff or under contract to the inspecting agency. The availability of psychiatrists, psychiatric social workers, and geriatric nurse practitioners experienced in assessing the care needs of persons with dementia would be particularly useful.

While such a process would entail increased inspection costs in some States, the increases could be minimal. Surveys that are more resident-focused and outcome-oriented are likely to be shorter than the current Federal survey process. Thus, some resources could be redirected to a more efficient and comprehensive survey of those facilities with quality problems.

Staff training could be improved, teaching surveyors/inspectors how to expand their focus beyond review of facility records to the direct observation of residents' conditions, care needed, and care received. In addition, training could include specific information on the state of the art in the care and management of individuals with dementia, including information assessment, care planning, and relevant outcome and process measures of quality.

The Federal Government could take more responsibility for the adequacy of survey staff, in terms of numbers, training, and experience. Alternatively, the government could provide funding to the States to monitor care in programs and facilities participating in Medicaid and Medicare.

Mere exhortation by the Federal Government has apparently been insufficient to elicit significant improvement in the inspection activities at State agencies. Increased Federal funding for these purposes could raise State capabilities and give the Federal Government more authority and ability to demand improved performance. Although that would increase Federal costs, the increase would be a relatively small proportion of the funds now spent through Medicare, Medicaid, and SSI for care, and it would reduce the likelihood that those funds are being used to pay for substandard care.

Improving Enforcement Mechanisms

Even with improved regulatory standards and a more effective survey and inspection process, effective enforcement—the third element of a quality assurance system—may be critical to improvements in marginal or substandard facilities. Inadequate enforcement appears to be national in scope. State survey agencies may apply formal sanctions only if a facility remains in violation beyond the deadline for compliance in the plan of correction (79). Formal sanctions thus become the last step in a long series of followup visits and plans of correction designed to induce compliance. Facilities are not punished for violating health and safety standards, but rather for failing to carry out an administrative order to correct violations. The result is that substandard homes may operate without penalty for more than a year even with serious violations of minimum standards.

Federal and State enforcement procedures could be modified to enhance the Federal role in ensuring the quality of nursing home care. Some options for more effective enforcement are authorized under Federal law and regulations. Others do not exist under Federal oversight authority but have been used in a variety of States and could be incorporated into Federal regulations. These options include creating a range of sanctions or remedies that could be used in place of or in addition to consultation and decertification.

The Federal Government could encourage States to adopt a stronger enforcement posture and could make this feasible by: 1) separating the consultant and surveyor roles; 2) making survey followup procedures more specific; 3) creating a workable range of Federal sanctions and applying them more rigorously; and 4) increasing both Federal oversight and Federal support of State enforcement activities.

Consultation.—Federal regulations currently require survey agencies to advise facilities on how to improve their performance. In many States, surveyors are responsible for both consulting with and disciplining providers, despite the potential conflict in these roles. Several States, notably Washington, New York, and Connecticut, use separate agencies for consultation and enforcement; they consider the procedure successful. Survey agencies could examine their policy role and reorient the program toward enforcement rather than consultation.

Suspension of Payment for New Admissions.—The Omnibus Budget Reconciliation Act of 1980 gave authority to the Secretary of Health and Human Services to deny Medicare payments for new admissions to providers that are out of compliance with conditions of participation, so long as the deficiencies do not pose an immediate threat to the health and safety of the residents in the facility. The act assigns similar authority for Medicaid-only facilities to State agencies.

HCFA issued regulations to implement the law, which became effective in August 1986. These so-called intermediate sanctions regulations suggest that a State agency may recommend suspension of payments for *new* Medicare and Medicaid admissions for up to 11 months in a facility that has deficiencies that do not pose immediate threats to the residents' health and safety but do "require more emphasis than just a plan of correction." HCFA's New York regional office reports ·this mechanism to be effective in securing compliance with certification regulations. However, the regulation on suspension requires a full set of administrative hearings before the sanction takes effect (79). That makes the intermediate sanction nearly as difficult and slow to implement as decertification.

Before the regulations for bans on admission became final, a surveyor who found that a facility was consistently or repeatedly violating certification standards could choose only one sanction under the Federal programs: decertify the facility and recommend termination of a provider's contract. For the reasons previously cited, surveyors and State agencies hesitate to do that. Even with the intermediate sanctions in place, however, reform of enforcement process is badly needed.

Several options are possible. One of these is to examine and consider a facility's past record

Consideration of Past Record.—Federal regulations could be modified to allow States to sanction a facility by taking into account both the survey findings from prior years and those from the most recent survey. That modification would address the problem of the chronically substandard facility. States also need a method of weighting the seriousness of offenses that define repeat violations, matching sanctions to violations, and determining liability for offenses in order to effectively sanction repeat offenders. Statutory authority would be necessary to enable HCFA to prescribe procedures for States to follow in dealing with chronic or repeat violators. In addition, HCFA would have to develop criteria for determining who is responsible for repeat offenses. In determining such liability, HCFA and the States could use the definition of ownership applied under current Medicaid fraud statutes: any party having 5 percent or more interest in the facility, land, or deed. The current Minnesota State statute is a good example.

Many States have authority to use a variety of intermediate sanctions under State licensing laws. Some of these could be considered for adoption at the Federal level for violations of Medicare and Medicaid health and safety regulations. These include:

- **Suspension of Admissions:** Thirty-two States have the authority to deny payment or to prohibit new admissions to a facility. These sanctions can apply to all admissions, or only to Medicaid admissions, depending on the State.
- **Civil Fines:** Twenty-six States have the authority to assess a civil fine against a facility that fails to meet licensing standards. The amount of the fine varies according to the severity of the deficiency. Fines range from a few hundred to several thousand dollars. Of these States, 13 said they assessed fines in 1983; Florida, Wisconsin, and California were the most active. In general States view such penalties favorably, arguing that they are effective. Some State studies, however, report concerns that the amount of the fine would simply be made up by reduced expend-

itures on patient care (e.g., ref 134). Further, the exceptional length of the appeals process has limited the effectiveness of fines in some States.

- **Receivership:** In 21 States, when conditions pose an imminent threat to the health or safety of residents, a facility can be sanctioned by appointing a receiver to operate the facility. That is, the authority to operate a facility can be temporarily or permanently removed from the current owner or operator and granted by the courts to another person or group.

- **Conditional, Provisional, and Probationary Licenses:** In several States a conditional or provisional license can be given for a limited time, during which time the facility is to correct licensing violations. The license is terminated if required corrections are not made.

- **Monitorships:** Seven States have authority to appoint a facility monitor. A monitor is assigned by the State licensure agency for a specified period to ensure that the facility's plan of correction is being implemented and that care of acceptable quality is being delivered to residents during the correction period.

- **Suspension/Withholding of Payment, Reduced Rates:** Suspension or withholding of payment, or reducing a facility's Medicaid rates, are ways of imposing financial sanctions. The period of suspension or reduction depends on when the facility comes into compliance. Texas uses "vendor hold" to stop all Medicaid payments to a facility that has serious, uncorrected deficiencies.

- **Criminal Penalties:** Thirty States have criminal penalties for violations of licensing laws. Generally, these penalties apply to violations of residents' rights and abuse of residents. Thirty-eight States also have laws making reporting of resident abuse mandatory. In a survey by the Institute of Medicine, only five States reported having used criminal penalties in 1983, when 376 actions were taken. Most of the actions took place in New York (79). In its 1984 survey of State licensure and certification agencies, the institute found that a total of 2,000 actions were taken against

some 15,000 facilities in 1983. Most of these (85 percent) were taken in 13 States. This statistic probably indicates that some States are more enforcement-oriented than others, not that facilities in these 13 States are consistently poorer providers than facilities in other States.

The Institute of Medicine findings regarding variations in the enforcement mechanisms used by States are significant for quality assurance. The institute found that the use of sanctions by a State is associated with several factors, including: 1) higher State appropriations for the State survey agency; 2) special training for surveyors in how to inspect nursing homes and gather evidence for enforcement proceedings; 3) a wider range and number of available sanctions; and 4) survey procedures that require greater numbers of facility visits or inspections each year. In essence, the situation appears to be a self-fulfilling prophecy: States committed to strong enforcement—in terms of personnel, resources, and procedures—were the most likely to develop and use sanctions. Thus, while Federal regulations could authorize a wider range of enforcement remedies and facilitate their use, the States must have some incentive to make effective use of these tools. Options:

- Congress could consider providing additional funds to the States for enforcement activities. That procedure was quite successful with the 1976 Fraud and Abuse Amendments in encouraging States to set up special Medicaid vendor fraud units.

- Congress could consider developing a more meaningful way to sanction States that do not effectively monitor the performance of nursing homes and enforce compliance with Federal standards. The current provision, which involves cutting off all Medicaid funding, has the same limitations as nursing home "decertification"; it is too harsh for some violations and, because of its enormous consequences, it is not used even for serious failings. A more appropriate penalty might be a percentage reduction in the Federal share of Medicaid payments.

As noted, the weakest part of the Keys amendment to the Social Security Act board and care provisions is that the penalty is taken against the SSI recipients—not against the facility that is violating minimum standards. Given the lack of direct Federal oversight, establishing effective enforcement mechanisms is difficult.

- Congress could consider modifying the Social Security Act to require that States develop an effective range of enforcement sanctions. Some of the sanctions previously discussed as options for nursing homes might also be effective for DCFs.
- Congress could also consider how it might encourage States to inspect DCFs effectively and enforce standards. Since monetary penalties seem to provide powerful incentives, some sort of fiscal incentive for States could be considered.
- Congress could consider providing special funds for States to upgrade their quality assurance system for DCFs. Specifically, funds could be targeted to training of inspectors, expansion of the inspection staff, and the development or expansion of existing enforcement staff (including both administrative hearing and prosecutorial staff).

Research and Quality Assurance

Research knowledge on issues of treatment and management of dementia is incomplete. Although individuals with dementia are widely believed to constitute the majority of long-term nursing home residents, and although most such individuals eventually need nursing home care, little is known about which management techniques are most effective. Health services research is needed if appropriate standards are to be developed for long-term care providers. Research on the following kinds of questions would be helpful in identifying problems, developing standards, and improving the quality assurance system in long-term care:

- **How many nursing home residents suffer from Alzheimer's disease and other dementias?** Currently this question cannot be answered with any precision, since families are reluctant to inform facilities of such a diagnosis, fearing the facility will discriminate in admission. Further, many residents are not accurately diagnosed.

- **What kinds of behavioral problems (e.g., wandering, agitation, and combative behavior) are associated with dementia?** More specifically, do they occur in combination? Do they occur only at certain times or in response to certain external stimuli (e.g., does wandering increase immediately after admission to a nursing home)? Answers to these questions would be helpful in informing nursing homes and adult day care programs, for example, about what kinds of behavior to expect and when is it most likely to occur.
- **What kinds of interventions are most effective in dealing with behavioral problems?** Interventions would include drugs, appliances, and management techniques. How might interventions vary by type of long-term care provider (e.g., nursing home v. community-based)?
- **What kinds of interventions are most effective in dealing with other aspects of dementia (e.g., communication disorders, incontinence, and loss of functional abilities)?** Although some information is available, there has been no systematic examination of the techniques used or comparison of the effectiveness of various approaches in long-term care settings.
- **What staffing patterns are most effective for treating and managing individuals with a dementing disorder?** More specifically, are different types of staff and staff/patient ratios needed at different stages in the course of diseases?

Little information is available on the number of individuals with dementia in facilities other than nursing homes. Perhaps of greatest concern are board and care facilities and unlicensed board and care homes, since regulatory standards and oversight of these institutions are sparse. Substantial research on both incidence and appropriate management would be appropriate:

- What proportion of individuals in DCFs have cognitive impairment, and how significant is that impairment?
- What other impairments (e.g., physical health and functioning) do cognitively impaired persons in DCFs have? How severe are those impairments?

- Do cognitively impaired persons in DCFs also have behavioral problems (e.g., wandering) that might place them at physical risk?
- Given the nature and severity of these impairments, what defines appropriate care (e.g., staffing, activities, drug review and administration, physical therapy)?
- Can DCFs currently provide appropriate care for the cognitively impaired persons residing there?
- How widespread is the use of physical and chemical restraints in DCFs? Are they used appropriately? Are residents at risk because DCFs are not equipped to deal with conditions or behaviors associated with dementia—except through physical restraints and psychotropic drugs?
- Are cognitively impaired persons transferred to nursing homes (or some other more appropriate setting) if and when the DCF cannot provide appropriate care?

In addition, the problem of individuals with fairly serious physical and cognitive impairments residing in unlicensed and unregulated homes, board and care homes could be addressed.

- Congress could mandate an investigation of the nature and seriousness of the problem, using the addresses of SSI recipients to identify unlicensed facilities.

It would also be useful to have more precise information about the effectiveness of various inspection processes and enforcement remedies. There is significant variation among the States in the numbers and types of individuals included in survey teams for nursing homes, DCFs, home health agencies, and adult day care programs; in how frequently inspections are conducted; in whether inspections are announced or unannounced; and in the focus of the surveys. Yet no study has compared the effectiveness of these approaches in accurately and completely identifying the nature and extent of violations or deficiencies. Similarly, though States vary in the availability and utilization of sanctions, no systematic comparison has been done of the effectiveness of various sanctions and enforcement attitudes on provider performance.

- Congress could consider requiring HCFA to provide funds to study the effectiveness of various inspection and enforcement processes.

CHAPTER 10 REFERENCES

1. AFL-CIO Executive Council, "Nursing Homes and the Nation's Elderly: America's Nursing Homes Profit in Human Misery," Statement and Report Adopted by the AFL-CIO, Bal Harbour, FL, Feb. 25, 1977.
2. Aiken, L.H., Mezey, M., Lynaugh, J., et al., "Teaching Nursing Homes: Prospects for Improving Long-Term Care," *Journal of the American Geriatrics Society* 33(3):196-201, March 1985.
3. Alaszewski, A., "Problems in Measuring and Evaluating the Quality of Care in Mental Handicap Hospitals," *Health and Social Service Journal* 89:A9-A15, 1978.
4. Allen, G., Chief, Division of Facility Certification, Texas Department of Human Resources, Austin, TX, personal communication, 1985.
5. American Bar Association, *A Model Act Regulating Board and Care Homes: Guidelines for the States*, Chicago, IL, 1983.
6. American Bar Association, Commission on Legal Problems of the Elderly, *Analyses of 1982 Draft Conditions of Participation and Decertification Procedures*, Washington, DC, Mar. 19, 1982.
7. American Bar Association, Commission on the Legal Status of the Elderly, "The Black Box of Home Care Quality." Testimony before U.S. House of Representatives, Select Committee on Aging, July 19, 1986.
8. Anderson, N.N., Patten, S., and Greenberg, J., *A Comparison of Home Care and Nursing Home Care for Older Persons in Minnesota*, vols. I and II, (Minneapolis, MN: Institute of Public Affairs and Center for Health Services Research, University of Minnesota, 1980).
9. Anderson, N., and Stone, L., "Nursing Home Research and Public Policy," *The Gerontologist* 9:214-218, 1969.
10. Arkansas General Assembly, *Nursing Home Study, 1978: Evaluation of State Regulation*, vols. 2 and 3, The Legislative Joint Performance Review Committee, Little Rock, AR, 1978.
11. Axelrod, D., and Sweeney, R.D., *Report to the*

Governor and the Legislature on the New Surveillance Process for New York Residential Health Care Facilities, New York State Department of Health, Albany, NY, May 1, 1984.

12. Bardach, E., "Enforcement and Policing," paper presented at the Association of Public Policy and Management, Philadelphia, PA, October 1983.

13. Bartol, M.A., "Nonverbal Communication With Patients with Alzheimer's Disease," *The Journal of Gerontological Nursing* 5(4):21-31, July-August 1979.

14. Basen, M.M., "The Elderly and Drugs—Problem Overview and Program Strategy," *Public Health Reports* 92:43-48, January/February 1977.

15. Bennett, C., *Nursing Home Life: What It Is and What It Could Be* (New York: Tiresias Press, 1980).

16. Bennett, R., "The Meaning of Institutional Life," *The Gerontologist* 3:117-125, 1963.

17. Bennett, R., and Eisdorfer, C., "The Institutional Environment and Behavior Change," *Long-Term Care: A Handbook for Researchers, Planners and Providers*, S. Sherwood (ed.) (New York: Spectrum Books, 1975).

18. Bennett, R. (ed.), *Aging, Isolation and Resocialization* (New York: Van Nostrand Reinhold Press, 1980).

19. Birnbaum, H., Bishop, C., Jensen, G., et al., *Reimbursement Strategies for Nursing Home Care: Developmental Cost Studies* DHEW Contract No. 600-77-0068, (Cambridge, MA: Abt Associates, 1979).

20. Birnbaum, H., Bishop C., Lee, A.J., et al., "Why Do Nursing Home Costs Vary? The Determinants of Nursing Home Costs," *Medical Care* 19:1095-1107, November 1981.

21. Bisenius, M.F., *Quality of Health Care in Iowa Nursing Homes: Results From the ICF Outcome Oriented Survey, December 1, 1982 - November 30, 1983* (Des Moines, IA: Iowa State Department of Health, Division of Health Facilities, April 1984).

22. Bjork, D.T., Pelletier, L.L., and Tight, R.R., "Urinary Tract Infections With Antibiotic Resistant Organisms in Catheterized Nursing Home Residents," *Infection Control* 5:173-176, April 1984.

23. Blazer, D., comments summarized in *The Caregiver: Newsletter of the Duke Family Support Network of the Alzheimer's Disease and Related Disorders Association*, fall 1985.

24. Booz-Allen & Hamilton, "Overview of Domiciliary Care: Programs in Each of the Fifty States," working paper, Baltimore, MD, 1975.

25. Brody, E.M., Lawton, M.P., and Liebowitz, B., "Senile Dementia: Public Policy and Adequate Institutional Care," *American Journal of Public Health* 74:1381-83, December 1984.

26. Brook, R.H., "Studies of Process-Outcome Correlations in Medical Care Evaluation," *Medical Care* 17:868-877, 1979.

27. Brook, R.H., Davies, A.R., and Kamberg, C.J., "Selected Reflections on Quality of Medical Care Evaluation in the 1980s," *Nursing Research* 29(2):127-133, March-April 1980.

28. Bryant, N.H., Candland, L., and Lowenstein, R., "Comparison of Care and Cost Outcomes for Stroke Patients With and Without Home Care," *Stroke* 5:54-59, January-February 1974.

29. Butler, P., "Nursing Home Quality of Care Enforcement: Part II: State Agency Reinforcement Remedies," *Clearinghouse Review* 665-701, October 1980.

30. California Auditor General, Department of Health Services, *Long-Term Care Facilities*, Sacramento, CA, 1982.

31. California Commission on State Government Organization and Economy, *The Bureaucracy of Care: Continuing Policy Issues for Nursing Home Services and Regulation* (Sacramento, CA: State of California, August 1983).

32. Caswell, R.J., and Cleverly, W., *Final Report: Cost Analysis of Ohio Nursing Home*, report to the Ohio Department of Health, Columbus, OH, February 1978.

33. Caswell, R.J., and Cleverly, W.O., "Cost Analysis of the Ohio Nursing Home Industry," *Health Services Research* 18:359-382, Fall 1983.

34. Chow, R.K., "Development of a Patient Appraisal and Care Evaluation System for Long-Term Care," *The Journal of Long-Term Care Administration* 5:21-17, 1977.

35. Coe, R.W., Self-Conception and Institutionalization, *Older People and Their Social World*, A. Rose and W. Peterson (eds.) (Philadelphia, PA: F.A. Davis, 1965).

36. Cohen, G.D., "Approach to the Geriatric Patient," *Medical Clinics of North America* 61(4):855-866, July 1977.

37. Colorado Attorney General's Office, *Report of the Attorney General Concerning the Regulation of the Nursing Home Industry in the State of Colorado*, Denver, CO, 1977.

38. Connecticut, Governor's Blue Ribbon Nursing Home Commission, *Report of the Blue Ribbon Committee to Investigate the Nursing Home Industry in Connecticut*, Hartford, CT, 1976.

39. Connecticut, Governor's Blue Ribbon Nursing Home Commission, *Report of the Blue Ribbon Committee to Investigate the Nursing Home Industry in Connecticut*, Hartford, CT, 1980.

40. Connelly, K., et al., "Targeted Inspections of Nurs-

ing Homes," *Quality Review Bulletin* 9:239-242, August 1983.

41. Cotterill, P.G., "Provider Incentives Under Alternative Reimbursement Systems," *Long-Term Care: Perspectives From Research and Demonstrations*, R.J. Vogel and H.C. Palmer (eds.) (Washington, DC: Health Care Financing Administration, U.S. Department of Health and Human Services, 1983).

42. Covert, A.B., Rodrigues, T., and Soloman, K., "The Use of Mechanical and Chemical Restraints in Nursing Homes," *Journal of the American Geriatrics Society* 25:85-89, 1977.

43. DiBerardinis, J., and Gitlin, D., *Identifying and Assessing Quality Care in Long-Term Care Facilities in Montana*, report submitted to the Department of Social Rehabilitation Services, State of Montana, under Contract No. 80-070-0016, Center of Gerontology, Montana State University, Bozeman, MT, November 1979.

44. Dietsche, L.M., and Pollmann, J.N. "Alzheimer's Disease: Advances in Clinical Nursing," *Journal of Gerontological Nursing* 8(2):97-100, February 1982.

45. Dittmar, N.D., and Smith, G., *Evaluation of the Board and Care Homes: Summary of Survey Procedures and Findings*, report to the Assistant Secretary for Planning and Evaluation, U.S. Department of Health and Human Services, Denver Research Institute, University of Denver, Denver, CO, 1983.

46. Donabedian, A., "Evaluating the Quality of Medicare Care," *Milbank Memorial Fund Quarterly* 44:166-206, July 1966.

47. Donabedian, A., *Explorations in Quality Assessment and Monitoring, Vol. 1: The Definition of Quality and Approaches to Its Assessment* (Ann Arbor, MI: Health Administration Press, 1980).

48. Eisdorfer, C., and Cohen, D., "Management of the Patient and Family Coping With Dementing Illness," *The Journal of Family Practice* 12(5):831-837, May 1981.

49. Eisdorfer, C., Cohen, D., and Preston, C., "Behavioral and Psychological Therapies for the Older Patient With Cognitive Impairment," *The Clinical Aspects of Alzheimer's Disease and Senile Dementia*, G. Cohen and N. Miller (eds.) (New York: Raven Press, 1982).

50. Feder, J.M., *Medicare: The Politics of Federal Hospital Insurance* (Lexington, MA: Lexington Books, 1977).

51. Feder, J., and Scanlon, W., "Regulating the Bed Supply in Nursing Homes," *Milbank Memorial Fund Quarterly* 58(1):54-88, 1980.

52. Florida Department of Health and Rehabilitative Services, Office of the Inspector General, *Nursing Home Evaluative Report*, Tallahassee, FL, September 1981.

53. Freeman, I., Director, Nursing Home Residents Advocates, Minneapolis, MN, Board of Directors, National Citizens Coalition for Nursing Home Reform, personal communication, 1985.

54. Freidler, T.M., Koffler A., and Kurokawa, K., "Hyponatremia and Hypernatremia," *Clinical Nephrology* 7:163, 1977.

55. Friedman, F.B., "It Isn't Senility—The Nurses' Role in Alzheimer's Disease," *The Journal of Practical Nursing* 38:17-19, February 1981.

56. Galton, R., Director of Clinical Services, National Association for Home Care, Washington, DC, personal communication, 1986.

57. Garibaldi, R.A., Brodine, S., and Matsumiya, S., "Infections in Nursing Homes, Policies, Prevalence, and Problems," *New England Journal of Medicine* 305:731-35, September 1981.

58. Geboes, K., Hellemans, J., and Bossaert, H., "Is the Elderly Patient Accurately Diagnosed?" *Geriatrics* 91-96, May 1979.

59. Gerson, L.W., and Collins, J.F., "A Randomized Controlled Trial of Home Care: Clinical Outcomes for Five Surgical Procedures," *Canadian Journal of Surgery* 19:519-23, 1976.

60. Granger, C.V., and MacNamara, M.A., "Functional Assessment in Program Evaluation for Rehabilitation Medicine," *Functional Assessment in Program Rehabilitation Medicine*, C. Granger and G. Gresham (eds.) (Baltimore, MD: Williams & Wilkins, 1984).

61. Greenfield, S., Solomon, N., Brook, R., et al., "Development of Outcome Criteria and Standards To Assess the Quality of Care for Patients With Osteoarthrosis," *Journal of Chronic Diseases* 31:375-388, 1978.

62. Gurland, B., Dean, L., and Cross, P., "The Effects of Depression on Individual Social Functioning in the Elderly, *Depression in the Elderly: Causes, Care, and Consequences*, L. Breslau and M. Haug (eds.) (New York: Springer Publications, 1983).

63. Gwyther, L., *Care of Alzheimer's Patients: A Manual for Nursing Home Staff*, American Health Care Association and Alzheimer's Disease and Related Disorders Association, Washington, DC, 1985.

64. Harmon, C., *Board and Care: An Old Problem, A New Resource for Long-Term Care*, Center for the Study of Social Policy, 1982.

65. Harrington, C., and Grant, L., "Nursing Home Bed Supply, Access, and Quality of Care," unpublished paper, University of California Aging and Health Policy Center, San Francisco, CA, 1985.

66. Hawes, C., *Defining, Measuring and Assuring*

Quality in Long-Term Care, final report to the Robert Wood Johnson Foundation, Princeton, NJ, November 1983.

67. Hawes, C., "Politicians, Patients, and Providers: The Politics of Long-Term Care," dissertation submitted as partial fulfillment of requirements for degree of Doctor of Philosophy, University of Texas, Austin, 1981.

68. Hayter, J., "Patients Who Have Alzheimer's Disease," *American Journal of Nursing* 748:1460-1463, 1974.

69. Himmelstein, D.U., Jones, A.A., and Woolhandler, S., "Hypernatremic Dehydration in Nursing Home Patients: An Indicator of Neglect," *Journal of the American Geriatrics Society* 31:466-472, August 1983.

70. Hirshman, A., *Exit, Voice and Loyalty: Response to Decline in Firms, Organizations and States* (Cambridge, MA: Harvard University Press, 1977).

71. Holahan, J., *How Should Medicaid Programs Pay for Nursing Home Care?* Report 3172-12 (Washington, DC: The Urban Institute, January 1985).

72. Hornbustle, R., nursing home ombudsman, Cleveland, Ohio; Board of Directors, National Citizens Coalition for Nursing Home Reform; personal communication, 1985.

73. Horowitz, A., "Families Who Care: A Study of the Natural Support Systems of the Elderly," paper presented at the 31st Annual Meeting of the Gerontological Society of America, Dallas, TX, 1978.

74. Howard, J., "Medication Procedure in a Nursing Home: Abuse of PRN Orders," *Journal of the American Geriatrics Society* 25:83-4, 1977.

75. Hoyer, R., Director of Research, National Association for Home Care, Washington, DC, personal communication, 1986.

76. Hughes, S., "Apples and Oranges? A Review of Evaluations of Community Based Long-Term Care," *Health Services Research* 20:461-488, October 1985.

77. Illinois Legislative Investigating Commission, *Regulation and Funding of Illinois Nursing Homes*, Springfield, IL, 1984.

78. Institute of Medicine, *Assessing Quality in Health Care: An Evaluation* (Washington, DC: National Academy Press, 1974).

79. Institute of Medicine, *Improving the Quality of Care in Nursing Homes* (Washington, DC: National Academy Press, 1986).

80. Irvine, P.W., Van Buren, N., and Crossley, K., "Causes for Hospitalization of Nursing Home Residents: The Role of Infection," *Journal of the American Geriatrics Society* 32:103-7, February 1984.

81. Jarvik, L.F., and Kumar, V., "Update on Treatment: Most Approaches Still Prove Disappointing," *Generations* 9(2):10-11, Winter 1984.

82. Jazwiecki, T., Director, Office of Reimbursement and Financing, American Health Care Association, personal communication, 1986.

83. Kahana, E., Liang, S., and Felton, B., "Alternative Models of Person-Environment Fit: Prediction of Morale in Three Homes for the Aged," *Journal of Gerontology* 35:584-595, 1980.

84. Kalchtaler, T., Caccaro, E., and Lichtiger, S., "Incidence of Poly-Pharmacy in a Long-Term Care Facility," *Journal of the American Geriatrics Society* 25:308-313, 1977.

85. Kane, R., "Assuring Quality of Care and Quality of Life in Long-Term Care," *Quality Review Bulletin* 7:3-10, October 1981.

86. Kane, R., and Kane, R., "Care of the Aged: Old Problems in Need of New Solutions," *Science* 200:913-919, 1978.

87. Kane, R., Kane, R., Kleffel, D., et al., *The PSRO and the Nursing Home, Volume I: An Assessment of PSRO Long-Term Care Review*, report submitted to the Health Care Financing Administration, U.S. Department of Health, Education, and Welfare, under contract No. 500-78-0040, 1979.

88. Kane, R.L., Bell, R.M., Hosek, S.D., et al., *Outcome-Based Reimbursement for Nursing Home Care*, prepared for the National Center for Health Services Research (Santa Monica, CA: The Rand Corp., December 1983).

89. Kane, R.L., Bell, R., Riegler, S., et al., *Assessing the Outcomes of Nursing-Home Patients* (Santa Monica, CA, The Rand Corp, 1982).

90. Kane, R.L., Bell, R., Reigler, S., et al., "Predicting the Outcomes of Nursing Home Patients," *The Gerontologist* 23(2):200-206, Apr. 23, 1983.

91. Katz, S., Ford, A.B., Down, T.D., et al., *Effects of Continuity Care: A Study of Chronic Illness in the Home*, U.S. Department of Health, Education, and Welfare, Health Services and Mental Health Administration, National Center for Health Services Research and Development, DHEW Publication No. (HSM) 73-3010, 1972.

92. Kennie, D.C., and Moore, J.T., "Management of Senile Dementia," *American Family Physician* 22:105-109, 1980.

93. Kethley, A.J., and Parker, M.K., *A National Inventory of Services To Help Families Care for Older Family Members and Family Support and Long-Term Care* (Excelsior, MN: InterStudy, 1984).

94. Kidder, S., "Survey Methodology for Detecting Medicare Errors," Department of Health and Human Services, *State Operations Manual*, Health Care Financing Administration, 1985.

95. Kochar, S., "SSI Recipients in Domiciliary Care Fa-

cilities: Federally Administered Optional Supplementation," *Social Security Bulletin* 17-28, 1977.

96. Kurowski, B., and Breed, L., *A Synthesis of Research on Client Needs Assessment and Quality Assurance Programs in Long-Term Care* (Denver, CO: Center for Health Services Research, University of Colorado Health Sciences Center, March 1981).

97. Kurowski, B., and Shaughnessey, P.W., The Measurement and Assurance of Quality, *Long-Term Care: Perspectives From Research and Demonstrations*, R.J. Vogel and H.C. Palmer (eds.) (Washington, DC: Health Care Financing Administration, U.S. Department of Health and Human Services, 1983).

98. Larson, R., "Thirty Years of Research on the Subjective Well-Being of Older Americans," *Journal of Gerontology* 33:109-125, 1978.

99. Lee, Y.S., "Nursing Homes and Quality of Health Care: The First Year of Result of an Outcome-Oriented Survey," *Journal of Health and Human Resource Administration* 7(1):32-60, summer 1984.

100. Lee, Y.S., and Braun, S., "Health Care for the Elderly: Designing a Data System for Quality Assurance," *Computers, Environment, and Urban Systems* 6:49-82 (spring 1981).

101. Levit, K.R., Lazenby, R.H., Waldo, D.R., et al., "National Health Expenditures, 1984," *Health Care Financing Review* 7:1-35, fall 1985.

102. Linn, M.W., "Predicting Quality of Patient Care in Nursing Homes," *The Gerontologist* 14:225-227, 1974.

103. Linn, M.W., Gureland, L., and Linn, B.S., "Patient Outcome as a Measure of Quality of Nursing Home Care," *American Journal of Public Health* 67:337-344, April 1977.

104. Lyles, Y.M., "Impact of Medicare Diagnosis-Related Groups (DRGs) on Nursing Homes in the Portcamp, OR, Metropolitan Area," *Journal of the American Geriatrics Society* 34:573-578, 1986.

105. Mace, N., "Day Care for Demented Clients," *Hospital and Community Psychiatry* 35(10):979-984, October 1984.

106. Mace, N.L., and Rabins, P.V., "Day Care and Dementia," *Generations* 9(2):41-44, winter 1984.

107. Mahowald, J.M., Himmelstein, D.U., "Hypernatremia in the Elderly: Relation to Infection and Mortality," *Journal of the American Geriatrics Society* 29:177, 1981.

108. Manton, K., "Changing Health Status and Need for Institutional and Noninstitutional Long-Term Care Services," paper prepared for the Institute of Medicine Committee on Nursing Home Regulation

(Durham, NC: Duke University, Center for Demographic Studies, December 1984).

109. Mathematica Policy Research, Inc., *Evaluation of the State Demonstrations in Nursing Home Quality Assurance Processes*, Final Report to the Health Care Financing Administration, U.S. Department of Health and Human Services, January 1985.

110. McAuliffe, W.E., "Measuring the Quality of Medical Care: Process Versus Outcome," *Milbank Memorial Fund Quarterly* 57:118-152, 1979.

111. McAuliffe, W.E., "Studies of Process-Outcome Correlations in Medical Care Evaluations: A Critique," *Medical Care* 16:907-930, November 1978.

112. McCoy, J.L., "Overview of Available Data Relating to Board and Care Homes and Residents," unpublished memo, U.S. Department of Health and Human Services, Washington, DC, 1983.

113. Mech, A.B., "Evaluating the Process of Nursing Care in Long-Term Care Facilities," *Quality Review Bulletin* 6:24-30, March 1980.

114. Meiners, M.R., et al., "Incentive Reimbursements for Nursing Homes: San Diego Controlled Experiment," paper presented at the Western Economics Association Meetings, Las Vegas, NV, 1984.

115. Mellody, J.F., and White, J.C., *Service Delivery Assessment of Boarding Homes: Technical Report*, (Philadelphia, PA: U.S. Department of Health, Education, and Welfare, 1979).

116. Michigan Department of Public Health, *Division of Health Facilities Certification and Licensure Management and Operations Review*, report to the Bureau of Health Care Administration, Plante and Moran, Consultants, Inc., Lansing, MI, 1981.

117. Michoki, R.J., and Lamy, P.P., "The Problem of Pressure Sores in a Nursing Home Population: Statistical Data," *Journal of the American Geriatrics Society* 24:323-8, July 1976.

118. Miller, M.B., "Iatrogenic and Nursigenic Effects of Prolonged Immobilization of the Ill Aged," *Journal of the American Geriatrics Society* 23:360-69, August 1975.

119. Miller, M.B., and Elliott, D.F., "Errors and Omissions in Diagnostic Records on Admission of Patients to a Nursing Home," *Journal of the American Geriatrics Society* 106-16, March 1976.

120. Miller, M.C., and Knapps, R.C., *Evaluating the Quality of Care: Analytic Procedures and Monitoring Techniques* (Germantown, MD: Aspen Systems Corp., 1979).

121. Minnesota Senate and House Select Committee on Nursing Homes, Final Report, Minnesota State Legislature, St. Paul, MN, January 1976.

122. Missouri State Senate, Health Care Committee,

Nursing and Boarding Home Licensing in Missouri, Jefferson City, MO, 1978.

123. Mitchell, J.B., "Patient Outcomes in Alternative Long-Term Care Settings," *Medical Care* 16:76-77, June 1978.

124. Moden, M., Special Assistant to the Texas Attorney General, personal communication, 1985.

125. Morris, J.N., and Granger, C., "Assessing and Meeting the Needs of the Long-Term Care Person," *Adult Day Care: A Practical Guide*, C. O'Brien (ed.) (Monterey, CA: Wadsworth Health Service Press, 1982).

126. National Citizens Coalition for Nursing Home Reform, *A Consumer Perspective on Quality Care: The Residents' Point of View*, Washington, DC, 1985.

127. New Jersey State Nursing Home Commission, *Report on Long-Term Care* (Trenton, NJ: 1978).

128. New York State Moreland Act Commission, *Regulating Nursing Home Care: The Paper Tigers* (New York, NY: 1975).

129. New York State Moreland Act Commission on Nursing Homes and Residential Facilities, *Long-Term Care Regulation: Past Lapses, Future Prospects: Summary Report* (New York, NY: 1976).

130. New York, *Report to the Governor and the Legislature on the New Surveillance Process for New York State Residential Health Care Facilities*, New York State Department of Health, Office of Health Systems Management, Albany, NY, May 1984.

131. Noelker, L., and Harel, Z., "Predictors of Well-Being and Survival Among Institutionalized Aged," *The Gerontologist* 19:562-567, 1978.

132. O'Brien, J., Saxberg, B.O., and Smith, H.L., "For Profit or Not-For-Profit Nursing Homes: Does it Matter?" *The Gerontologist* 23(4):341-48, 1983.

133. Ohio Nursing Home Commission, *A Program in Crisis: Blueprint for Action, Final Report of the Ohio Nursing Home Commission*, Ohio General Assembly, Columbus, OH, 1979.

134. Ohio Nursing Home Commission, *A Program in Crisis: Interim Report*, Ohio General Assembly, Columbus, OH, 1978.

135. Ouslander, J.G., and Kane, R.L., "The Costs of Urinary Incontinence in Nursing Homes," *Medical Care* 22:69-79, January 1984.

136. Ouslander, J.G., Kane, R.L., and Abrass, I.B., "Urinary Incontinence in Elderly Nursing Home Patients," *Journal of the American Medical Association* 248:1194, 1982.

137. Palmer, H.C., "Home Care," *Long-Term Care: Perspectives From Research and Demonstrations*, R. Vogel and H. Palmer (eds.), Health Care Financing Administration, U.S. Department of Health and Human Services, Washington, DC, 1983.

138. Pastalan, L., *Forced Relocation: A Study of Involuntary Change of Patients From One Sociophysical Environment to Another*, report for the National Institute of Mental Health, U.S. Department of Health, Education, and Welfare, 1974.

139. Platt, R., Polk, B.F., Murdock, B., et al., "Mortality Associated With Nosocomial Urinary-Tract Infection," *New England Journal of Medicine* 307:637, 1980.

140. Rabins, P.V., "Management of Irreversible Dementia," *Psychosomatics* 22(7):591-594, July 1981.

141. Ransom, B., Director, National Institute on Adult Daycare, and National Institute on the Rural Elderly, National Council on Aging, personal communication, 1986.

142. Ray, W.A., Federspiel, C.F., and Schaffner, W., "A Study of Anti-psychotic Drug Use in Nursing Homes: Epidemiological Evidence Suggesting Misuse," *American Journal of Public Health* 70:485-91, May 1980.

143. Rechstein, K.J., and Bergofsky, L., "Domiciliary Care Facilities for the Aged: An Analysis of State Regulations," *Research on Aging* 5(1):25-43. 1983.

144. Requarth, C.H., "Medication Usage and Interaction in the Long-Term Care Elderly," *Journal of Gerontological Nursing* 5:33-7, March-April 1979.

145. Reynolds, M.D., "Institutional Prescribing for the Elderly: Patterns of Prescribing in a Municipal Hospital and a Municipal Nursing Home," *Journal of the American Geriatrics Society* 32:640-645, September 1984.

146. Rourke, S., Director, Citizens for Better Care, Detroit, Michigan; Board of Directors of the National Citizens Coalition for Nursing Home Reform; personal communication, 1985.

147. Ruchlin, H.S., "An Analysis of Regulatory Issues and Options" *Long-Term Care, Reform and Regulation in Long-Term Care*, V. LaPorte and J. Rubin (eds.) (New York: Praeger Publishers, 1979).

148. Ruchlin, H.S., "A New Strategy for Regulating Long-Term Care Facilities," *Journal of Health Politics, Policy and Law* 2:190-211, 1977.

149. Rutstein, D.D., Berenberg, W., Chalmers, T.C., et al., "Measuring the Quality of Medical Care: A Clinical Method," *New England Journal of Medicine* 194:582-88, March 1976 (tables revised 9/1/77).

150. Sager, A., *Learning the Home Care Needs of the Elderly: Patient, Family, and Professional Views of an Alternative to Institutionalization* (Waltham, MA: Levinson Policy Institute, 1979).

151. Schlenker, R.E., *Nursing Home Reimbursement, Quality, and Access—A Synthesis of Research*, prepared for the Institute of Medicine Conference on Reimbursement, Anaheim, CA, Nov. 10, 1984.

152. Schmidt, L.J., et al., "The Mentally Ill in Nursing

Homes: New Back Wards in the Community," *Archives of General Psychiatry* 34:687-691, June 1977.

153. Shaughnessy, P., et al., evaluation at the Robert Wood Johnson Foundation Teaching Nursing Home Demonstrations, at the University of Colorado, Center for Health Services Research, Denver, CO, 1986.

154. Sherwood, C.C., and Seltzer, M.M., *Task III Report—Board and Care Literature Review: Evaluation of Board and Care Homes* (Boston, MA: Boston University School of Social Work, January 1981).

155. Sherwood, S., and Gruenberg, L., "Domiciliary Care Management Information System" (mimeo) (Boston, MA: Boston Massachusetts Department of Social Gerontological Research, 1979).

156. Simpson, W., *Medications and the Elderly: A Guide for Promoting Proper Use* (Rockville, MD: Aspen Systems, 1984).

157. Skelly, F.A., Mobley, G.M., and Coan, R.E., "Cost-Effectiveness of Community-Based Long-Term Care: Current Findings of the Georgia Alternative Health Services Project," *American Journal of Public Health* 72:353-357, April 1982.

158. *Smith v. Heckler*, 747 F.2nd 583 (10th Cir., 1984).

159. *Smith v. O'Halloran*, 557 F.Supp. 289 (D. Colo., 1983), rev'd sub. nom.

160. Smits, H., "Quality Assurance of Long-Term Care," *World Hospitals*, 1982, pp. 37-39.

161. Somers, A.R., "Financing Long-Term Care for the Elderly: Institutions, Incentives, Issues," Institute of Medicine, *America's Aging-Health in An Older Society* (Washington, DC: National Academy Press, 1985).

162. Steinbach, L., Holmes, M., and Holmes, D., *Domiciliary Care in New York and New Jersey*, contract report for the Office of the Principal Regional Official, DHEW, Region II, Contract No. 120-76-0002, New York, NY, 1978.

163. Stone, R., and Newcomer, R.J., "Board and Care Housing: The State Role," *Long-Term Care of the Elderly: Public Policy Issues*, C. Harrington, et al. (Beverly Hills, CA: Sage Publishers, 1985).

164. Stone, R., Newcomer, R.J., and Saunders, M., *Descriptive Analysis of Board and Care Policy Trends in the 50 States*, Aging and Health Policy Center, University of California, San Francisco, CA, September 1982.

165. Sussman, M.B., "Family, Bureaucracy and the Elderly Individual: An Organizational/Linkage Perspective," *Family, Bureaucracy and the Elderly*, E. Shanas and M. Sussman (eds.) (Durham, NC: Duke University Press, 1977

166. Systemetrics, Inc., *The MMACS Long-Term Care Data Base: Construction of a New Research File and Assessment of Its Quality and Usefulness*, report to the Health Care Financing Administration, U.S. Department of Health and Human Services, Washington, DC, December 1983.

167. Temple University, Center for Social Policy and Community Development, *Board Homes in Philadelphia: Summary of Findings and Implications for Policy*, Philadelphia, PA, January 1978.

168. Texas Nursing Home Task Force, *Report on Nursing Homes to the Attorney General of the State of Texas*, Austin, TX, 1979.

169. Texas Senate, Subcommittee on Public Health and Welfare, Office of the Attorney General of the State of Texas, *Report on Texas Nursing Homes to John Hill, Attorney General*, Austin, TX, 1977.

170. U.S. Administration on Aging, Office of Program Development, *The Long-Term Care Ombudsman Program: Development From 1975-1980*, Administration on Aging, Washington, DC, January 1981.

171. U.S. Congress, General Accounting Office, *Home Health: The Need for a National Policy to Better Provide for the Elderly*, Washington, DC, 1977.

172. U.S. Congress, General Accounting Office, *Identifying Boarding Homes Housing the Needy, Aged, Blind, and Disabled: A Major Step Toward Resolving a National Problem*, HRD-80-1, Washington, DC, Nov. 19, 1979.

173. U.S. Congress, General Accounting Office, *Medicare Home Health Services: A Difficult Program To Control*, Washington, DC, 1981.

174. U.S. Congress, General Accounting Office, *Medicaid and Nursing Home Care: Cost Increases and the Need for Services Are Creating Problems for the States and the Elderly*, Washington, DC, 1983.

175. U.S. Congress, General Accounting Office, *The Elderly Remain in Need of Mental Health Services*, HRD-82112, Gaithersburg, MD, 1982.

176. U.S. Department of Health and Human Services, Health Standards Quality Bureau, unpublished analysis of 1981 (Medicare and Medicaid Automated Certification Survey) data, Washington, DC, 1981.

177. U.S. Department of Health and Human Services, Office of the Inspector General, *Board and Care Homes: A Study of Federal and State Actions To Safeguard the Health and Safety of Board and Care Home Residents* (Washington, DC: Department of Health and Human Services, April 1982).

178. U.S. Department of Health and Education and Welfare, *Boarding Homes Assessment* (Washington, DC: U.S. Government Printing Office, 1979).

179. U.S. Department of Health, Education and Wel-

fare, Health Care Financing Administration, "From Simple Idea to Complex Execution: Home Health Services Under Titles XVIII, XIX, and XX," draft report, Washington, DC, 1977.

180. U.S. Department of Health, Education and Welfare, Office of Nursing Home Affairs, *Long-Term Care Facility Improvement Study: Introductory Report*, Washington, DC, July 1975.

181. U.S. House of Representatives, Select Committee on Aging, *Hearing: Fraud and Abuse in Boarding Homes*, No. 97-295 (Washington, DC: U.S. Government Printing Office, June 25, 1981).

182. U.S. House of Representatives, Select Committee on Aging, *Oversight Hearing on Enforcement of the Keys Amendment*, No. 97-296 (Washington, DC: U.S. Government Printing Office, July 1, 1981).

183. U.S. House of Representatives, Select Committee on Aging, Hearing, "The Black Box of Home Care Quality," July 29, 1986.

184. U.S. Senate, Special Committee on Aging, Quality of Care Under Medicare's Prospective Payment System, Hearings Before the 99th Congress, 1st Session, *Medicare DRGs: Challenges for Quality*, Sept. 26 (vol. 1), *Medicare DRGs: Challenges for Post-Hospital Care*, Oct. 24 (vol. II), *Medicare DRGs: Government Role in Ensuring Quality*, Nov. 12 (vol. III), Nov. 12, 1985.

185. U.S. Senate, Special Committee on Aging, Subcommittee on Long-Term, *Nursing Home Care in the United States: Failure in Public Policy* (Washington, DC: U.S. Government Printing Office, 1974).

186. U.S. Senate, Special Committee on Aging, *Nursing Home Care in the United States: Failure in Public Policy, Supporting Paper No. 7. The Role of Nursing Homes in Caring for Discharged Mental Patients (and the Birth of a For-Profit Boarding Homes Industry* (Washington, DC: U.S. Government Printing Office, March 1975).

187. U.S. Senate, Committee on Finance, *Medicare and Medicaid: Problems Issues and Alternatives*, 91st Cong., 2d sess. (Washington, DC: U.S. Government Printing Office, 1970).

188. Virginia Joint Legislative Audit and Review Commission, *Long-Term Care in Virginia* (Richmond, VA: The Virginia General Assembly, Mar. 28, 1978).

189. Vladeck, B., *Unloving Care* (New York: Basic Books, 1980).

190. Vladeck, B., and Freeman, I., "The Nursing Home Conundrum," *Reshaping Health Care for The Elderly: Recommendations for National Policy*, C. Eisdorfer (ed.) (forthcoming).

191. Wan, T., Weissert, W.G., and Livieratos, B.B., "The Accuracy of Prognostic Judgments of Elderly Long-Term Care Patients," paper presented at the American Public Health Association Meeting, New York, NY, November 1979.

192. Warren, J.W., Muncie, H.L., Berquist, E.J., et al., "Sequelae and Management of Urinary Infection in the Patient Requiring Chronic Catheterization," *Urologist* 125:1, 1981.

193. Weisbrod, B.A., and Schlesinger, M., "Public, Private, Non-Profit Ownership and the Response to Asymetric Information: The Case of Nursing Homes," discussion paper No. 209, Center for Health Economics and Law, University of Wisconsin at Madison, 1983.

194. Weissert, W.G., " Estimating the Long-Term Care Population: Prevalence Rates and Selected Characteristics," *Health Care Financing Review* 6(4), 1985.

195. Wood, J., "The Effects of Cost Containment on Home Health Care Agencies," *Home Health Care Services Quarterly* 6(4):59-78, winter 1985.

196. Zarit, S., Orr, N., and Zarit, J., *Working With Families of Dementia Victims: A Treatment Manual*, UCLA Long-Term Care Gerontology Center, Los Angeles, CA, 1984.

197. Zawadski, R.T., Glazer, G.B., and Lurie, E., "Psychotropic Drug Use Among Institutionalized and Noninstitutionalized Medicaid Aged in California," *Journal of Gerontology* 33:825-34, November 1978.

198. Zimmer, J.G., "Medical Care Evaluation Studies in Long-Term Care Facilities," *Journal of the American Geriatrics Society* 27:62-72, 1979.

199. Zimmer, J.G., Watson, N., and Treat, A., "Behavioral Problems Among Patients in Skilled Nursing Facilities," *American Journal of Public Health* 74:1118-21, October 1984.

200. Zwick, D., "The HCFA Proposal to Accord 'Deemed Status' to Nursing Homes Accredited by JCAH," unpublished paper prepared for the Institute of Medicine, Committee on Nursing Home Regulation, 1984.

Chapter 11

Medicaid and Medicare as Sources of Funding for Long-Term Care of Persons With Dementia

CONTENTS

Medicaid and Medicare as Sources of Funding for Long-Term Care of Persons With Dementia*

When the legislation that created the Medicare and Medicaid programs was being considered by Congress in 1965, it was the object of wildly differing predictions. Some legislators predicted that the bill, if enacted, would "destroy private initiative for our aged to protect themselves with insurance against the costs of illness,"[1] and characterized the proposed health insurance coverage as "the 'smack of socialism' implicit in a coverage-for-all program without avail." Others described the bill as the "greatest advance in social legislation ever presented to the Congress of the United States,"[2] and predicted that through the Medicare provisions "public assistance would be relieved of much of its present burden."

The truth has fallen somewhere between. The Medicare and Medicaid programs today represent an important health insurance resource for millions of the aged and disabled, including persons with dementia.

Those who qualify for Medicare have at least some assurance that a significant portion of their hospital and physician bills will be reimbursed. At the same time, however, many services are not covered under Medicare and even covered services are subject to coinsurance, deductibles, and fee limits that increase the financial burden on program beneficiaries.

The Medicaid program has different benefits and disadvantages. Millions of low-income persons eligible under Medicaid, including many with dementia, can qualify for reimbursement for medical bills incurred for covered services. Nursing home care for persons with dementia, for example, is largely dependent on the availability of Medicaid reimbursement. But categorical and financial eligibility requirements exclude millions of other indigent persons, and those who do qualify often discover that needed services are not covered or that health care providers will not accept Medicaid reimbursement.

Thus, while the two programs are critically important for many persons with dementia, numerous constraints limit their impact. Some of these constraints are inherent in the legislative structure of the programs. Others are products of interpretations by the Federal and State agencies charged with their administration. Additional factors, especially regarding Medicaid, represent conscious political choices by legislators and administrative officials between various populations seeking government assistance from limited budgets.

Although Medicaid expenditures constitute a relatively small portion of total State budgets, they are perceived as consuming a significant portion of State discretionary funds (10). That perception was heightened during the 1970s as nearly every State experienced at least one period during which Medicaid expenditures rose far beyond budget allocations. These increases led to cutbacks in eligibility, scope of services, and reimbursement, and they resulted in greater legislative watchfulness of Medicaid administration.

That increased scrutiny has resulted, in many cases, in a "status quo" approach to administration. So long as no significant changes are proposed, State officials run little risk of being called to account before legislative budget and appropriations committees. Short-term fiscal planning becomes the rule, rather than the exception. As a result, only a few States have been willing to in-

---

*This chapter is a contract report by David F. Chavkin, Directing Attorney, Maryland Disability Law Center, Baltimore, Maryland.

[1]Individual views of Senators Harry F. Byrd, John J. Williams, Wallace F. Bennett, Carl T. Curtis, and Thruston B. Morton opposing enactment of the Medicare provisions of H.R. 6675 as amended by the Senate Finance Committee, 1 *U.S. Code Cong. & Admin. News* 2214-2215 (89th Cong., 1st sess., 1965.

[2]Supplemental views of Senators Abe Ribicoff and Vance Hartke to H.R. 6675 as reported by the Senate Finance Committee, 1 *U.S. Code Cong. & Admin. News* 2215-2216 (89th Cong., 1st sess., 1965).

novate in their Medicaid programs over the past few years.

The reluctance to experiment is often reinforced by the competition between various groups for limited funding. The two most significant of these groups are advocates for maternal and child health programs and those for programs for the elderly. Growing concern over infant mortality and morbidity rates has led many States to consider efforts to improve access to prenatal care, labor and delivery services, and neonatal care. At the same time, the increased numbers of elderly persons, especially those over the age of 80, have resulted in pressures for increased funding for long-term care services in the community and in nursing homes. Most States have struggled in attempting to balance these two significant but competing priorities.

Even within the specialized delivery system that serves primarily elderly persons, there is often competition for limited funds. For example, persons with dementia are not the only elderly who need long-term care, although they are perhaps the largest group. The mentally alert frail elderly have equally valid needs for services. Thus, specialized residential care units for persons with de-

mentia must often vie for funds with adult day care programs for mentally alert frail elderly persons.

No attempt is made here to resolve these competing priorities. Rather, this chapter reviews the impact of Federal programs on funding for care and services for persons with dementia. It is based on a review of the existing Federal and State laws, regulations, and policies. In addition, during the fall of 1985 and winter of 1986, interviews were conducted with State administrators, health care providers, program beneficiaries, advocates, and family caregivers in 15 States. These interviews helped highlight the special problems created for persons with dementia due to differences between the theory of Federal and State policies and their actual implementation.

The review also highlighted some of the aspects of these programs that adversely affect persons with dementia. These aspects suggest changes in the programs that could be implemented to improve services for this population. The chapter then concludes by identifying major issues that should be resolved before reform is undertaken. These changes may then be implemented within an overall resolution of program priorities.

EVALUATING THE PROGRAMS

The Medicare and Medicaid programs are largely "disease-neutral" (see figures 11-1 and 11-2). Applicants need not suffer from a particular debilitating illness in order to qualify for assistance. (The major exception to this rule is the special eligibility program under Medicare for persons suffering from end-stage renal disease (42 U.S.C. 1395c(3)). Services provided under the programs are also generic in nature and are not directed at particular diseases or conditions. (The Medicaid regulations go even further by prohibiting limitations on the "amount, duration, or scope of a required service . . . solely because of the diagnosis, type of illness, or condition" (42 CFR 440.230(c)).

Despite that underlying philosophy, apparently neutral provisions may have a special impact on persons suffering from particular illnesses or conditions. For example, a 14-day limit on inpatient

hospital services may be more than adequate for a pregnant woman who will experience a low-risk delivery. It is far less adequate for a multihandicapped elderly recipient suffering from cancer.

Although the Medicare program now reimburses hospitals on the basis of diagnosis-related groups, the basic scope of services is still disease-neutral. Moreover, under Medicaid, States impose limits on the amount, duration, and scope of services that do not vary based on the diagnosis, type of illness, or condition. As a result, even if a State reimburses hospitals on the basis of diagnosis-related groups, a restrictive limit on the scope of inpatient hospital service may discourage access.

In identifying the factors that affect the role Medicare and Medicaid play in financing long-term care for persons with dementia, it is therefore

Figure 11-1.—Medicare in a Nutshell

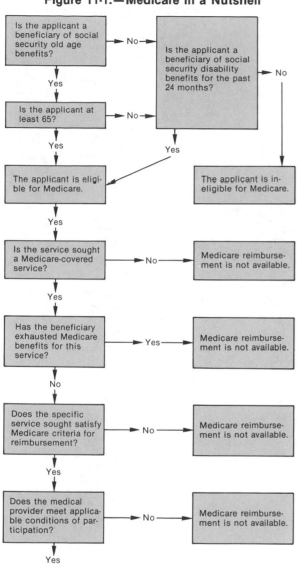

applicable to a single disorder. For example, the current inability to positively diagnose Alzheimer's disease creates special eligibility difficulties that do not arise for persons with brain tumors. In reviewing program impact, four factors that can influence the availability of financing must be considered—eligibility, scope of services, reimbursement practices, and administrative procedures.

For example, a restrictive eligibility policy may prevent an individual from ever qualifying for benefits. Similarly, even if eligible, an individual may be denied needed care because of the restrictive scope of services covered. Moreover, even if someone is eligible for reimbursement for a covered service, restrictive reimbursement practices may discourage providers from rendering the needed service. Finally, restrictive administrative procedures may inhibit the ability of eligible beneficiaries to receive covered services from participating providers.

By contrast, a State with liberal income and resource standards will permit more individuals to qualify for assistance. A broad scope of services that includes both institutional and noninstitutional care will encourage the delivery of needed care and services in the least restrictive environment appropriate to each patient's needs. Similarly, reimbursement practices may be modified to encourage the growth of specific classes of providers and thereby improve access to appropriate, high-quality, cost-effective services. Finally, smooth and timely processing of providers' requests for prior authorization of services can help encourage provider participation and thereby also improve access to services. All these incremental changes will also increase costs of the programs, however.

The factors that affect the current availability of financing for long-term care under Medicare and Medicaid are reviewed in turn in this chapter. Some will have a unique impact on beneficiaries with dementia. Others may adversely affect those with dementia along with other elderly and disabled persons.

important to look beyond the words of a requirement and examine the actual impact on program beneficiaries. Although the term dementia generally refers to Alzheimer's disease and to various related disorders, certain problems are more

Figure 11-2.—Medicaid in a Nutshell

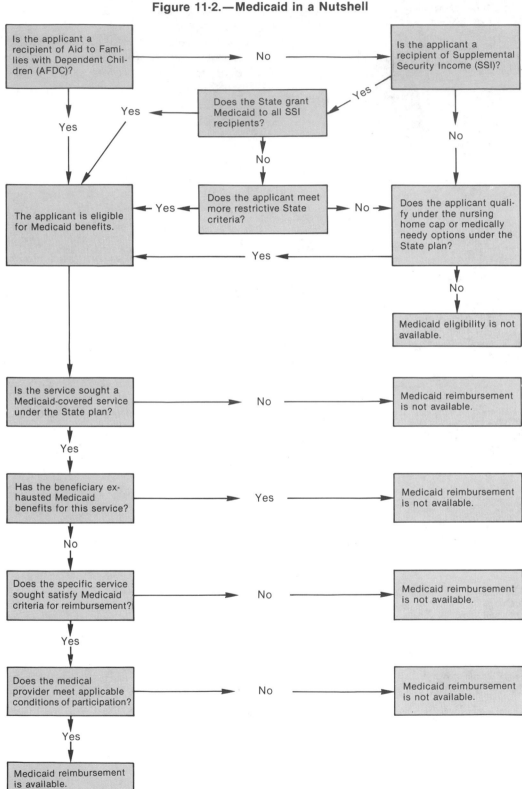

ELIGIBILITY

Medicare

Individuals can establish eligibility for Medicare in several ways. The vast majority of beneficiaries qualify at age 65 based on their eligibility for social security retirement benefits. (Several special eligibility provisions for those age 65 or over extend the definition of "covered employment" to include, for example, those who would be eligible if certain Federal employment were considered to be covered employment (42 U.S.C. 1395c(1)). The process of establishing eligibility for applicants age 65 or over generally presents no major difficulties.

By contrast, the major basis of Medicare eligibility for persons with dementia under the age of 65 is fraught with complexities. Those under 65 can establish eligibility if they have been entitled to social security benefits or to railroad retirement benefits because of disability for at least 24 months (42 U.S.C. 1395c(2)). Special problems arise for persons with dementia in establishing eligibility for these disability benefits.

Definition of Disability

Problems arise with the very definition of disability under the social security and railroad retirement programs: Disability is specified as an "inability to engage in any substantial gainful activity by reason of any medically determinable physical or mental impairment that can be expected to result in death or which has lasted or can be expected to last for a continuous period of not less than 12 months" (42 U.S.C. 416(i)(1)).

The first problem arises from the language "medically determinable." Although Alzheimer's disease is an organic brain disorder, it cannot be positively diagnosed during a person's lifetime using current techniques. Until the individual's death, when an autopsy can verify the existence of Alzheimer's disease, diagnosis depends on the exclusion of all other "diagnosable" causes for the symptoms. These problems of diagnosis exist even though recent studies indicate that approximately 90 percent of all diagnoses of Alzheimer's disease are corroborated through autopsy (see ch. 3).

Apparently the inability to point to a single dispositive medical test is part of the reason for the problem.

The present disability definition therefore makes it quite difficult for someone with Alzheimer's disease to establish eligibility. The burden of proof is on the applicant to demonstrate the existence of a disability by a preponderance of evidence. Since the diagnosis of this disease, especially in its early stages, is a matter of educated conjecture, many applicants will be initially denied assistance since they cannot meet this burden (14).

Listing of Impairments

The simplest way of establishing disability is to demonstrate that an applicant's condition is described in the "Listing of Impairments" (20 CFR 404P App 1). The listing describes impairments that are severe enough to preclude someone from engaging in any substantial gainful activity (the "severity" requirement) and that are expected to result in death or to last for a continuous period of not less than 12 months (the "duration" requirement).

Unfortunately, Alzheimer's disease and other forms of dementia are not explicitly reflected in the listing as either neurological or mental disorders. In 1985, the Department of Health and Human Services (DHHS) issued a revised listing of impairments to address, at least in part, the criticism by Congress and others of the treatment of mentally disabled applicants. But DHHS again explicitly rejected the inclusion of specific criteria for the evaluation of Alzheimer's disease and related disorders (50 FR 35038).

Since dementia is not expressly listed as an impairment, the simplest route for establishing eligibility is therefore barred for an applicant with dementia. The person must then demonstrate that all of the elements of the definition of disability are satisfied. The difficulty of doing that is compounded by the varying levels of functional disability demonstrated by persons with dementia at different times. A single brief interview with a consultative medical examiner may not elicit even the deficits in affect and behavior that are all too apparent to family members and co-workers. That failure contributes to the high likelihood that someone with a dementing disorder will be denied benefits on initial application (14).

Mental Impairment

The problems encountered by mentally disabled beneficiaries during the Social Security Administration's continuing eligibility reviews have received extensive national exposure. Congress responded (Public Law 98-460) by establishing a moratorium on periodic reviews until new standards could be developed that would treat mentally disabled beneficiaries more fairly. Now that the revised Listing of Impairments has been issued, the continuing disability investigation process has started again.

Although the moratorium provided significant relief for many current beneficiaries by maintaining their eligibility during an interim period, it provided no help for new applicants suffering from dementia. They continue to have their eligibility determined on the basis of policies that have been found by the courts to discriminate against mentally impaired persons (5). As a result, denials of eligibility are still a common response to such applications.

The treatment of dementia as a mental disorder in the Listing of Impairments also creates special problems. Although individuals suffering from the various dementing disorders sometimes display behaviors similar to someone with mental illness, dementia remains an organic brain disorder. The effect of including dementia as a mental disorder may be to discourage applications and to unfairly limit eligibility for needed benefits, care, and services.

Waiting Period

When an applicant is found to be eligible, disability benefits generally do not begin immediately. The Social Security Act imposes a "waiting period" of five consecutive calendar months before benefits can be initiated (42 U.S.C. 416(i)(2)(A)).

Although the waiting period is designed to ensure that temporarily disabled applicants will not be certified for social security disability benefits, it works a special hardship on applicants with dementia. As described earlier, it is usually impossible to establish eligibility until many months after the onset of symptoms. The 5-month waiting period is then applied in establishing the beginning date of eligibility for social security disability benefits. Once the waiting period has elapsed, an additional 24 months must pass before Medicare benefits will be initiated (42 U.S.C. 426(b)(2)(A)).

The cumulative effect of these provisions is therefore to delay the onset of Medicare eligibility until long after the benefits are most needed. By the time Medicare eligibility does begin, the applicant's condition may have deteriorated sufficiently so that only custodial long-term care may be needed. As the discussion of services later in this chapter indicates, the value of Medicare eligibility will at that point be greatly diminished.

Medicaid

Whereas eligibility under Medicare is largely determined by the governing legislation, eligibility under Medicaid is largely a matter of political choices by State governments. Although the Medicaid statute requires States to provide coverage for certain categories of persons, most coverage decisions are left to the States, within the categories of persons eligible for Federal matching funds.

As noted earlier, although Medicaid expenditures make up a relatively small portion of total State budgets, they are seen as consuming a significant portion of State discretionary funds (10). As a result, especially in relatively tight fiscal times, State proposals to expand coverage often pit one population of potential recipients against another. The result is frequently a political impasse that prevents any changes in the scope of State programs.

Confusing Eligibility Criteria

As confusing as the Medicare eligibility process sometimes seems, it is relatively straightforward compared with the complexities of establishing eligibility for Medicaid. Eligibility in this case builds on the complexities of the federally assisted welfare programs and then adds some special wrinkles of its own. The result is a complicated system of rules and regulations that leaves applicants, recipients, providers, advocates, State agency officials, and, frequently, Health Care Financing Administration staff uncertain over the appropriate interpretation of Federal statutes, regulations, and interpretive rules.

The confusion created by these regulations was noted in the decision in *Friedman* v. *Berger*. In that decision, while attempting to interpret the legal requirements, the judge noted:

> As program after program has evolved, there has developed a degree of complexity in the Social Security Act and particularly the regulations which makes them almost unintelligible to the uninitiated. There should be no such form of reference as "45 CFR [sec] 248.3(c)(1)(ii)(B)(2)" discussed below; a draftsman who has gotten himself into a position requiring anything like this should make a fresh start. Such unintelligibility is doubly unfortunate in the case of a statute dealing with the rights of poor people (13).

Since that decision, Medicaid regulations have been further complicated by the enactment of the Omnibus Budget Reconciliation Act of 1981, the Tax Equity and Fiscal Responsibility Act of 1982, and the Deficit Reduction Act of 1984 (Public Laws 97-35, 97-248, and 98-369). Each piece of legislation altered aspects of the Medicaid statute, frequently in a quest for simplification. Their cumulative effect in many areas of the law, however, has been to further confuse and complicate interpretation.

Welfare Piggybacking

One overriding issue that must be confronted by applicants with dementia is the fact that the Medicaid program "piggybacks" its eligibility requirements on the criteria for the Supplemental Security Income (SSI) and Aid to Families with Dependent Children (AFDC) programs. Unlike Medicare, which is a social insurance program, Medicaid is a welfare program with strict means tests. The overall effect of that linkage is to require most applicants to be impoverished before eligibility can be established. That approach is one of the major criticisms of the Medicaid program by families caring for a relative with dementia.

The problem is magnified because of the unique effects of dementia on middle-class families. The availability of health insurance for most such families means that the majority of medical problems will be paid for in whole or in part by third-party coverage. Few private insurance plans cover the services required by a person with dementia, however. Thus, many middle-class families turn to a welfare program—Medicaid—for partial assistance in financing the costs of care and treatment for a family member with dementia.

Medicaid/AFDC Linkage.—The AFDC program provides financial support for children under the age of 18 deprived of parental support or care by reason of the death, continued absence from the home, unemployment, or physical or mental incapacity of a parent (42 U.S.C. 606(a)). Financial support to the child includes payments to meet the needs of the caretaker relative(s) with whom the child is living (42 U.S.C. 606(b)).

Although the onset of dementia usually occurs late in life, it may happen to someone who still has children under the age of 18. In such a situation, the family may be able to establish AFDC eligibility based on the mental incapacity of the parent suffering from dementia. Demonstrating that a parent is incapacitated by dementia is not usually difficult, for the AFDC program's standards for incapacity are far more lenient than the social security disability standards. Establishing eligibility, however, may still be quite difficult.

AFDC is intended for use by indigent families. Financial requirements under the program are set by the States and are generally far more restrictive than under the adult welfare programs. For example, the AFDC eligibility income standard for a family of three in many States is lower than the SSI eligibility standard for an individual (see table 11-1). Similarly, the resource standard permits a family of six to own less than half as much liquid assets as a couple under SSI. AFDC eligibility is thus available only to very poor families.

Once eligibility is established, all family members included in the AFDC grant will also be certified for Medicaid eligibility (42 U.S.C. 1396a(10)(A)(i)(I)). That certification will be provided without a separate application for each family member as long as the family remains eligible for AFDC (42 CFR 435.909(a)).

Table 11-1.—Aid to Families with Dependent Children FDC Maximum Benefit and Need Standard for a Family of Three

State	Maximum benefit[a]		Standard of need[b]	
	1984[c]	1985[d]	1985[d]	Percent
Alabama	118	118	384	31
Alaska	696	719	719	100
Arizona	233	233	233	100
Arkansas	164	164	234	70
California	526	555	555	100
Colorado	336	346	421	82
Connecticut	529	546	546	100
Delaware	287	287	287	100
District of Columbia	299	327	654	50
Florida	231	240	400	60
Georgia	202	208	366	57
Hawaii	468	468	468	100
Idaho	305	304	554	55
Illinois	302	302	632	48
Indiana	258	256	307	83
Iowa	360	360	497	72
Kansas	364	373	373	100
Kentucky	188	197	197	100
Louisiana	190	190	538	35
Maine	341	370	510	73
Maryland	295	313	433	72
Massachusetts	379	396	627	63
Michigan (Washington Co.)	445	447	592	76
Michigan (Detroit)	418	417	557	75
Minnesota	500	524	524	100
Mississippi	96	96	286	34
Missouri	261	263	312	84
Montana	332	332	401	83
Nebraska	350	350	350	100
Nevada	228	233	285	82
New Hampshire	341	378	378	100
New Jersey	360	385	385	100
New Mexico	258	258	258	100
New York (Suffolk Co.)	579	579	579	100
New York (N.Y.C.)	474	474	474	100
North Carolina	202	223	446	50
North Dakota	357	371	371	100
Ohio	276	290	627	46
Oklahoma	282	282	282	100
Oregon	368	386	386	100
Pennsylvania	350	364	614	59
Rhode Island	462	479	479	100
South Carolina	142	187	187	100
South Dakota	321	329	329	100
Tennessee	127	138	246	56
Texas	148	167	555	30
Utah	362	363	685	53
Vermont	530	558	852	65
Virginia	310	327	363	90
Washington	462	476	768	62
West Virginia	206	206	275	75
Wisconsin	513	533	628	85
Wyoming	325	265	265	100

[a]Maximum benefit is the amount paid for a family of three with no countable income. Family members include one adult caretaker. In States with area differentials in benefits, figure shown is for area with the highest benefit. Maximum benefits are identical to payment standards in all States except Colorado, Indiana, Mississippi, and Utah, where the payment standards are higher.
[b]Standard of need is the amount of money the State determined a family of three needs per month to achieve a minimum standard of living in that State. The standard of need is used to determine initial eligibility for AFDC. Benefits levels do not have to equal a State's need standard.
[c]As of Jan. 1, 1984.
[d]As of Jan. 1, 1985.

SOURCE: U.S. Congress, House Committee on Ways and Means, ''Background Material and Data on Major Programs Within the Jurisdiction of the Committee on Ways and Means,'' Washington, DC, February 1984 and February 1985.

Medicaid/SSI Linkage.—Until 1974, Federal law authorized grants-in-aid for States wishing to provide assistance to aged, blind, or disabled persons. Within Federal requirements, States were permitted a wide range of discretion in defining financial and nonfinancial eligibility requirements for these programs. All recipients of aid to the aged, blind, or disabled also received Medicaid coverage (42 U.S.C. 1396a(a)(10) prior to the changes enacted through Public Law 93-233).

Effective January 1, 1974, Congress "federalized" these adult grant-in-aid programs through the enactment of the Supplemental Security Income program as Title XVI of the Social Security Act. (A few jurisdictions still utilize a grant-in-aid program of Aid to the Aged, Blind, and Disabled (AABD).) The SSI program established a minimum national benefit level and uniform national eligibility criteria. Administration of the adult welfare programs was also shifted from the State welfare agencies to the Social Security Administration.

Because SSI eligibility criteria were generally more liberal than the State welfare criteria they replaced, it was anticipated that thousands of people would suddenly become eligible for SSI benefits. That was not, in itself, of concern to the various States because the grants and administrative costs of the basic SSI program were to be paid by the Federal Government. Thus, States that used to share in the costs of adult welfare programs would now realize some savings.

However, a related aspect of this federalization did cause concern. Because many States used relatively restrictive adult welfare eligibility criteria prior to 1974, the number of persons who automatically received Medicaid benefits was also relatively small. The expected huge increase in eligible persons in 1974 therefore also portended a considerable rise in the number of Medicaid recipients once the new Federal SSI program was fully implemented.

States share the costs of the Medicaid program with the Federal Government. Federal financial participation varies from 50 percent in the wealthier States to a maximum of 83 percent in the poorer States (42 U.S.C. 1396d(b)), so States must fund between 17 and 50 percent of the costs. Fears of huge increases in Medicaid costs in some States resulted in requests for legislative changes in this linkage requirement between SSI and Medicaid.

Congress responded by altering the linkage through legislation now known as the 209(b) option (as it was added as Section 209(b) of the Social Security Amendments of 1972). That option permits States to no longer grant Medicaid automatically to all SSI recipients. Instead, they can apply more restrictive eligibility criteria than those used by the SSI program (42 U.S.C. 1396a(f)).

One other provision has lessened the traditional linkage between adult welfare eligibility and Medicaid eligibility. That provision is known as the 1634 option after Section 1634 of the Social Security Act (42 U.S.C. 1383c; 20 CFR 416.2101-416.2119). Once the SSI program was enacted, Congress authorized the Social Security Administration to contract with States to have the Social Security Administration make eligibility determinations for Medicaid. States electing that option receive a computer tape from the Social Security Administration of SSI/Medicaid eligibles. These individuals are then automatically certified for Medicaid without having to apply separately.

States using SSI criteria that elect to execute 1634 agreements provide Medicaid automatically to all eligible persons. Other States require Medicaid-eligible SSI recipients to request medical benefits separately. Such a requirement for a separate request must be approved under Federal law. The experience in States without 1634 agreements is that some eligible persons will never seek benefits and that some monies can thereby be saved. These savings are supposed to balance out the additional administrative costs of processing separate requests for medical assistance. However, studies commissioned by the Health Care Financing Administration cast significant doubt on the existence of any savings (29).

Applicants suffering from dementia must therefore deal with one of three possible administrative schemes (see table 11-2). In the majority of States participating in the Medicaid program, Medicaid is granted automatically to anyone receiving SSI benefits. In a second group, applicants must separately request Medicaid benefits even if they are receiving SSI benefits. However, they must be found eligible based on that request. Finally, in the third group of States, SSI recipients must separately apply and will be determined eligible only if they meet a State's potentially more restrictive categorical and financial eligibility criteria.

Table 11-2.—Medicaid Benefits for Aged, Blind, and Disabled Persons

Medicaid jurisdiction	SSI[a] criteria 1634 Agreement[c]	SSI criteria state determination	209[b] Criteria
Alabama	X	....	....
Alaska	....	X	....
Arizona	b	....	....
Arkansas	X	....	....
California	X	....	....
Colorado	....	X	....
Connecticut	....	....	X
Delaware	X	....	....
District of Columbia	X	....	....
Florida	X	....	....
Georgia	X	....	....
Guam	d	....	....
Hawaii	....	....	X
Idaho	....	X	....
Illinois	....	....	X
Indiana	....	....	X
Iowa	X	....	....
Kansas	....	X	....
Kentucky	X	....	....
Louisiana	X	....	....
Maine	X	....	....
Maryland	X	....	....
Massachusetts	X	....	....
Michigan	X	....	....
Minnesota	....	....	X
Mississippi	X	....	....
Missouri	....	....	X
Montana	X	....	....
Nebraska	....	....	X
Nevada	....	X	....
New Hampshire	....	....	X
New Jersey	X	....	....
New Mexico	X	....	....
New York	X	....	....
North Carolina	....	....	X
North Dakota	....	....	X
North Marianas	X	....	....
Ohio	....	....	X
Oklahoma	....	....	X
Oregon	....	X	....
Pennsylvania	X	....	....
Puerto Rico	d	....	....
Rhode Island	X	....	....
South Carolina	X	....	....
South Dakota	X	....	....
Tennessee	X	....	....
Texas	X	....	....
Utah	....	....	X
Vermont	X	....	....
Virgin Islands	d	....	....
Virginia	....	....	X
Washington	X	....	....
West Virginia	X	....	....
Wisconsin	X	....	....
Wyoming	X	....	....
Total—55	35	6	14

[a]SSI = Supplemental Security Income.
[b]Arizona's program is based on a Section 1115 demonstration project waiver.
[c]Based on data from 1982.
[d]In these jurisdictions, Medicaid is provided to recipients of Old Age Assistance (OAA), Aid to the Blind (AB), Aid to the Permanently and Totally Disabled (APTD), and Aid to the Aged, Blind and Disabled (AABD). The SSI program does not operate in these jurisdictions.

SOURCES: Supplemental Security Income 1634 agreements from Urban Systems Research and Engineering, ''Short-Term Evaluation of Medicaid: Selected Issues,'' contract report prepared for Health Care Financing Administration, U.S. Department of Health and Human Services, Baltimore, MD, 1984.

The confusion created by that variability does not disproportionately affect applicants with dementia compared with others applying for services covered by Medicaid. However, the severity and duration of dementing conditions and the limitations of private health insurance coverage mean families coping with such an illness are much more likely than families dealing with other diseases to seek Medicaid coverage.

SSI Eligibility

The SSI program began in January 1974 with a monthly benefit level of $140 for an eligible individual (42 U.S.C. 1382(b)(1)), which had been adjusted for cost-of-living increases even prior to the implementation of the program. Today, the national benefit level for an individual is $336, with allowances for regular cost-of-living increases (42 U.S.C. 1382). In addition, some States, at their option, provide State-funded cash supplements for some recipients (42 U.S.C. 1382(e)). These optional State supplementary payments are generally limited to those States with higher living costs. These are also generally the States that had relatively more liberal adult welfare programs prior to 1974.

Certain grandfathered recipients also receive mandatory supplements under the SSI program. Section 212 of Public Law 93-66, for example, was designed to ensure that no recipient of aid to the aged, blind, or disabled prior to 1974 would receive a smaller grant under the new SSI program. In addition, certain individuals who were eligible under the State welfare plans in effect prior to January 1, 1974, but who are ineligible under current definitions of disability, are considered to meet current standards (42 U.S.C. 1382c(a)(3)(E)).

To establish SSI eligibility, an applicant with dementia must satisfy both "nonfinancial" and "financial" eligibility requirements. The former are those special characteristics that an applicant must possess in order to establish "linkage" to the SSI program (such as being 65 or older, blind, or disabled). Most applicants with dementia will attempt to establish "linkage" on the basis of either disability or old age. "Financial" eligibility requirements include strict income and resource requirements.

Listing of Impairments.—The SSI program relies on the same disability criteria as the social security disability program (42 U.S.C. 1382c(a)(3)(A); 20 CFR 416.925). The criteria under both programs are supposed to be uniform nationally; significant interstate differences in criteria have arisen, however, because of DHHS's policy of "nonacquiescence." Under that policy, DHHS decides which decisions of the U.S. district courts and courts of appeal it will apply in cases other than those involving the specific applicant or class of applicants of the case. That policy has been the subject of numerous congressional hearings. The variations in the criteria to be applied also necessarily affect the evidence that can be submitted by an applicant for benefits in attempting to demonstrate disability.

The same problems facing applicants with dementia under the social security disability program therefore must also be confronted when applying for SSI. However, someone found not to meet social security disability standards as applied by the Social Security Administration may still qualify under those same standards as applied by the State Medicaid agency. The Health Care Financing Administration has traditionally argued that such findings of nondisability are binding on the States. A Federal district court recently found that the Medicaid statute granted States the right to make independent Medicaid disability determinations for medically needy and optionally categorically needy persons (24).

A major difference between the two programs is that SSI applicants do not have to meet the earnings requirements of the social security disability insurance program. To be eligible for social security disability benefits, an applicant must have worked 20 of the 40 calendar quarters before becoming disabled (42 U.S.C. 416(i)(3)(B)). That requirement of recent "connection to the labor force" creates additional problems for persons with dementia. If it takes too long for the applicant to demonstrate disability, the applicant may no longer meet the 20/40 requirements. Once that eligibility period has been exhausted, the applicant cannot again qualify for Social Security disability benefits without reestablishing a connection to the labor force.

Financial Eligibility Criteria.—Applicants for SSI must meet strict income and resources criteria. Individuals with net income or net assets in excess of those standards (after allowable exclusions) are ineligible for SSI.

From 1974 until 1985, the Federal resource standards for SSI permitted an applicant or recipient to own $1,500 in nonexcludable resources (42 U.S.C. 1382(a)(1)(B)(ii)). (That level was increased to $1,600 on Jan. 1, 1985; to $1,700 on Jan. 1, 1986; to $1,800 effective Jan. 1, 1987; to $1,900 effective Jan. 1, 1988; and to $2,000 effective Jan. 1, 1989 (Public Law 98-369).) An applicant or recipient with an eligible spouse could own $2,250 in nonexcludable resources (42 U.S.C. 1382(a)(1)(B)(i); 42 U.S.C. 1382(a)(2)(B)). Although such assets as a home are excluded from consideration, these limited resource standards deny eligibility for individuals and families with savings until those funds have been practically exhausted.

The rules determining which resources are not counted for eligibility may cause some anomalous and potentially inequitable results. For example, although a recipient may own a home worth $500,000, an applicant with a savings account of $1,701 is completely ineligible for benefits in 1986. The same result would occur if the applicant owned life insurance with a face value of more than $1,500 and a cash surrender value of $1,701.

An applicant living in the community must have a net monthly income under $336. Since that income places a recipient below the national poverty level, most applicants will by definition be impoverished both before SSI eligibility can be established and after it is certified.

Although the SSI standards do exempt some income from consideration—for example, up to $30 of earned income in a calendar quarter is disregarded if it is received infrequently or irregularly (20 CFR 416.1112(c)(1))—recipients with pension and similar outside income are not generally eligible because of these low income standards. SSI income standards exempt up to $60 of unearned income in a calendar quarter (42 U.S.C. 1382a(b)(2)(A); 20 CFR 416.1124(c)(12)). Unearned income includes social security benefits, public and private pensions, alimony, dividends, and interest. Computed on a monthly basis, that means

that someone with income of $357 in most States will be ineligible for any SSI benefit and may therefore be ineligible for Medicaid as well.

The SSI income eligibility standard for persons living in nursing homes is even lower. Since 1974, the SSI program has limited such eligibility to those persons who have net income, after applying the income disregards, of less than $25 per month (42 U.S.C. 1382(e)(1)(B)(i)) on the assumption that Medicaid will pay room and board for a recipient in a nursing home. That amount has not been changed since the SSI program began, in January 1974.

The $25 grant is supposed to be adequate to pay for personal needs within the facility, such as toiletries, clothing, reading materials, and other items not included within the Medicaid reimbursement rate. In some States, nursing homes charge residents for additional utility costs attributable to a personal television. As in the community, then, a wide gap exists between the allowance and the actual need.

Medicaid Eligibility for Non-SSI Recipients

People who cannot establish SSI eligibility because they are not at least 65 or do not meet social security disability criteria generally cannot qualify for Medicaid regardless of the extent of their medical bills (42 U.S.C. 1396a(a)(10)). (A few States provide payments to medically indigent adults out of State funds, however. These medically indigent adult programs vary significantly from State to State in both the financial criteria for eligibility and the scope of services available to the recipient.) That inability to qualify occurs because Federal financial participation under the Medicaid statute is generally limited to those persons who are receiving aid or assistance under the AFDC or SSI programs or who would be eligible to do so but for excess income or resources (42 U.S.C. 1396a(a)(10)(C), 42 U.S.C. 1396d(a)).

Two special eligibility provisions are available for use by applicants with dementia as well as other aged or disabled persons—the nursing home cap program and the medically needy option. These assist persons who are recipients of neither AFDC nor SSI.

Nursing Home Cap Program.—Under the nursing home cap program (42 U.S.C. 1396a(a)(10)(A)(ii)(V) and (VI)) a fixed income test is established for residents of nursing homes. The results of that fixed income test cannot exceed 300 percent of the supplemental security income benefit rate (42 U.S.C. 1396b(f)(4)(C)).

Through the nursing home cap program, a nursing home resident with a 1986 income under $1,009 in a State using the maximum allowable level could be eligible for coverage of the costs of nursing home care and other medical services while residing in the home. This option permits a State to provide some reimbursement for nursing home care without opening up its Medicaid program to all disabled or aged persons with high medical bills.

Since the nursing home cap program uses a fixed income test, an applicant with gross monthly unearned income of $1,029 would be ineligible for benefits, regardless of medical expenses, since the net monthly income of $1,009 ($1,029 minus $20 per month income disregard) would exceed the eligibility level of $1,008. Someone with $1,028 in gross monthly unearned income, however, would be eligible for medical assistance toward the costs of care.

The amount of assistance to be provided is determined through a two-step eligibility process. First, the recipient's net income is compared with the eligibility standard of $1,008. If the net income after disregards is $1,008 ($1,028 minus $20 income disregard) and the applicant meets resource standards, the person is eligible for Medicaid.

Second, the recipient's obligation to pay for care is determined. The recipient is permitted to retain income equal to the personal needs allowance recognized in that State (at least $25 per month). In a State allowing the minimum, the recipient keeps $25 of income and pays the remainder ($1,028 minus $25, or $1,003) to the nursing home. The State Medicaid agency reimburses the nursing home for the remainder of its costs up to the maximum Medicaid reimbursement allowed in the State.

Medically Needy.—When the Medicaid program was enacted in 1965, one of its major features was a flexible income test, included because of widespread dissatisfaction with the fixed income test used under the Kerr-Mills program, the predecessor to Medicaid. Under a fixed income test, as in the nursing home cap program, applicants with incomes over a certain level cannot be aided even if they have high medical bills that reduce their available income. Under a flexible income test, those with even relatively high incomes can be helped with such medical expenses.

States choosing to establish medically needy programs may provide Medicaid eligibility to applicants who would qualify for AFDC or SSI but for excess income or resources. By incurring medical expenses, such applicants may "spend down" to an income level established by the State. The medical expenses are then deducted from the applicant's net income. Medical expenses incurred after that point may then be covered by the State.

Thirty-nine jurisdictions have elected to take advantage of the medically needy option (see table 11-3). (Some States, however, do not cover disabled or aged adults under this program.) It therefore represents an important program for persons with dementia and currently is an important funding source for care. Several factors affect the scope of the medically needy program, where available.

(1) Income Levels.—Federal law prohibits States from using medically needy income standards that exceed 133.33 percent of the AFDC payment standard for an equivalent size family (42 U.S.C. 1396b(f)(1)(B)(i)). Thus, if the AFDC payment standard for a family of four is $180, the medically needy income level cannot exceed $240.

AFDC payment standards are generally the lowest welfare payments in a State. In many States, moreover, they equal only a percentage of the standard of need for that size family. As a result, the medically needy income level artificially depresses an applicant's income far below the amount required to live on. Thus, to be eligible under the medically needy program the family of someone with dementia will have to reduce its available income far below the SSI benefit level. Only then will Medicaid pay for the remaining costs of care.

These limitations can lead to some seemingly anomalous results. In a State electing the medically needy option and using an income level of

Table 11-3.—Medicaid Eligibility Coverage in the States

State	Categorically needy	Medically needy
Alabama	X	....
Alaska	X	....
Arizona	X	X
Arkansas	X	X
California	X	X
Colorado	X	....
Connecticut	X	X
Delaware	X	....
District of Columbia	X	X
Florida	X	*
Georgia	X	*
Hawaii	X	X
Idaho	X	....
Illinois	X	X
Indiana	X	*
Iowa	X	*
Kansas	X	X
Kentucky	X	X
Louisiana	X	X
Maine	X	X
Maryland	X	X
Massachusetts	X	X
Michigan	X	X
Minnesota	X	X
Mississippi	X	....
Missouri	X	....
Montana	X	X
Nebraska	X	X
Nevada	X	....
New Hampshire	X	X
New Jersey	X	*
New Mexico	X	....
New York	X	X
North Carolina	X	X
North Dakota	X	X
Ohio	X	....
Oklahoma	X	X
Oregon	X	X
Pennsylvania	X	X
Puerto Rico	X	X
Rhode Island	X	X
South Carolina	X	a
South Dakota	X	....
Tennessee	X	a
Texas	X	a
Utah	X	X
Vermont	X	X
Virginia	X	X
Washington	X	X
West Virginia	X	X
Wisconsin	X	X
Wyoming	X	....

aMedically needy program does not cover all aged and disabled persons.

SOURCE: Office of Technology Assessment, 1986.

$300 for an individual, a disabled applicant with unearned income of $355 per month would be eligible for SSI and Medicaid benefits. That is true because the applicant's net income (after applying the $20 per month income disregard) is $335, or $1 less than the SSI benefit level of $336.

With a gross income of $357 per month, however, the person would be ineligible for SSI since net income would exceed the SSI benefit level by $1. The applicant would also be ineligible for Medicaid, since net income under the medically needy program would exceed the medically needy income level by $37. The $37 figure is calculated by comparing the applicant's net income ($357 gross income minus $20 income disregard equals $337) with the medically needy income level in the State of $300.

In this example, the applicant would have to incur medical expenses of $37 per month before Medicaid coverage would begin to pay for any remaining bills. A "notch" is thus created in the Medicaid eligibility process whereby an applicant who is ineligible by $1 for SSI loses $26 in available income because of the limitations on the medically needy income level.

(2) Deeming.—"Deeming" is a concept that affects applicants for both SSI and medically needy coverage. It is also an eligibility factor often encountered by persons with dementia.

One of the principles underlying the administration of most welfare programs is the notion that only income and resources actually available to an applicant or recipient will be considered. Deeming is used to permit the consideration of income and resources that may not actually be available to the applicant or recipient. Instead that income is defined to be available.

For example, pension income received by one spouse may be considered available to the other spouse applying for Medicaid. In determining the spouse's Medicaid eligibility the "deemed" income will be added to the applicant's own income. This is true even if the nonapplicant spouse fails to actually make any income available to the applicant.

In States using SSI criteria, deeming considers the availability of income and resources of a spouse or of the parents of a child under the age of 21. Thus, with some exceptions, the income and resources of one spouse will be considered available to the other spouse regardless of their actual availability.

Two common effects of deeming have been noted. The first is felt when the income and resources belong to the nonapplicant spouse, in which case they are considered available to the applicant spouse. The "deemed" income or resources may thereby either result in a finding of ineligibility or increase the amount of medical expenses that must be incurred before eligibility is established. At the same time, the nonapplicant spouse will be impoverished since he or she will be forced to live at the SSI benefit level in most States.

The second effect is felt when the income and resources belong to the applicant. In that case, a portion of that spouse's income and resources will be considered available to the nonapplicant spouse. If, for example, the nonapplicant spouse has no income in his or her own name, the "deemed" income will be used to support the nonapplicant.

This "backwards deeming" from a spouse in a nursing home to family members outside it is critical if family members are going to have some income to meet their needs for food, clothing, and shelter. However, Federal limits on the amount of income that can be deemed to the nonapplicant spouse ensure that impoverishment will occur.

For example, in the case of an individual in a nursing home with only a spouse at home, the amount that may be set aside for that person's needs may not exceed the highest of the SSI benefit standard, the optional State supplement (if any), or the medically needy income standard (42 CFR 435.832). In most States, this means that the spouse in the community must live on $336 per month. These limited set-asides have been upheld by the courts (21).

The effect is potentially worse in States using more restrictive eligibility criteria. Under the Federal deeming rules, 209(b) States are required to deem income at least to the extent required in States using SSI criteria. However, these more restrictive States also have the option of deeming to the extent that they did before 1972. The amount of deemed income and resources may therefore be significantly greater in 209(b) States than in those using SSI criteria.

The deeming requirements in 209(b) States are somewhat unsettled. In 1979, the United States Court of Appeals for the District of Columbia invalidated the Federal deeming rules then in effect for 209(b) States (16). The Court of Appeals

decision was then overturned by the United States Supreme Court (25). During the period between the two decisions, the Secretary of Health and Human Services had rescinded the 1977 deeming rules invalidated by the Court of Appeals and approved by the Supreme Court. The Secretary has since proposed reinstating the 1977 rules.

One of the perverse effects of deeming is to encourage the separation of families through placement of a family member in a nursing home or through divorce. In States using SSI criteria, for example, when a spouse moves to a nursing home deeming must end with the beginning of the first day of the first full month of residency (20 CFR 416.1167(a)). (Some States had deemed income indefinitely prior to the promulgation of SSI standards. This limitation lessens some of the harshest effects of deeming in States utilizing SSI criteria, but has also been cited as a reason some States elect to use the 209(b) option.) Similarly, if a husband and wife are divorced, only actual contributions will be considered between husband and wife.

Since these incentives run contrary to traditional governmental policies, two approaches have been developed to discourage the results. The first permits waiver of the deeming rules on a case-by-case basis when costly nursing home care could be avoided by the availability of Medicaid funding for home-based care. This waiver is referred to popularly as the "Katie Beckett" waiver after the name of the child whose case led to the waiver authorization (42 CFR 435.734(b)). The second approach permits States to provide home- and community-based services to individuals who, in the absence of such services, would require institutional care and would be eligible for Medicaid if they moved to nursing homes (42 U.S.C. 1396n).

The waiver language includes deeming both from parent to child and from spouse to spouse, but its limited use has been directed almost entirely to the first situation. Nothing would prevent it from being used more extensively to encourage home-based care for persons with dementia, however, especially during the early stages of the disease, when home management is frequently realistic.

Although the deeming process appears to be sex-neutral, it frequently has a disproportionately adverse effect on women. At least for the near future, most husbands will earn more than their wives and therefore will have a greater entitlement to pension benefits. Although both spouses may intend to have these benefits available to support them in retirement, serious problems occur when the man is placed in a nursing home first.

In SSI States, for example, the income of the person in the nursing home will be deemed to the spouse living in the community. From her husband's deemed income, a woman will be allowed as her living standard a maximum amount equal to the SSI benefit level or $336; she is limited indefinitely by Federal law to an amount far below the poverty standard. By contrast, if the man is the spouse still in the community, his obligation to pay any portion of his income to the wife would end with the beginning of her first full month in the nursing home.

Because of widespread dissatisfaction with these outcomes, some exceptions are being carved out. Some States with community property laws as well as other jurisdictions are attempting to divide income and resources more equitably between spouses in nursing homes and in the community. Those attempts have been met with great resistance from the Health Care Financing Administration. In California, for example, the Health Care Financing Administration disapproved a State plan amendment to use the State's community property rules to determine eligibility (ref. 6, Report Letter 487).

In community property and noncommunity property States, courts have begun carving out additional exceptions. (See, for example, *Purser* v. *Rahm*, 1985; similar cases have been brought in California, New York, and other States.) Under the judicial approach, a less than truly adversarial support lawsuit may be initiated by the spouse in the community against the spouse in the nursing home to define the former's property rights. Such a suit usually results in an allowance for the spouse in the community far in excess of $336 per month. Attempts by the State Medicaid agencies to disregard this judicial determination have generally not been successful (23).

(3) Residency.—Another problem that frequently arises for applicants with dementia is the issue of residency. Under Federal law, States are only obligated to provide medical assistance to eligible persons residing in the State. The problem arises in determining the State of residence under those regulations. For example, assume that an adult had been living in one State for his or her life. Now, after the onset of dementia, adult children decide to move the parent closer to their homes in another State. Under Federal law, the State in which the children live would now have an obligation to provide medical assistance coverage.

Federal regulations indicate that the residence of an adult is ordinarily where the adult is living with the intent to remain indefinitely (42 CFR 435.403(i)(1)(i)). The previous regulations, however, indicated that the residency of an adult no longer capable of stating intent was the State in which the person was living when that capability was lost (49 FR 13526; 47 FR 27078). A disabled parent therefore frequently remained in the State of origin, far from the children, since Medicaid reimbursement was often such a critical factor.

The current regulations constitute a significant change. Instead of linking the disabled parent to the home State, the regulations now provide that an adult incapable of stating intent is a resident of the State in which the person is living (42 CFR 435.403(i)(1)(i)). This change makes a significant difference in encouraging adult children to provide some care and support for disabled parents. In practice, however, interviews with State agency staff and reviews of State policies indicated that many States are still following the previous rules (4).

(4) Accounting Periods.—Another issue that affects Medicaid eligibility for applicants with dementia is the length of the accounting period for determining it. Under Federal law, States electing to establish medically needy programs may use accounting periods of up to 6 months (42 CFR 435.831). Thus, instead of determining eligibility on a month-by-month basis, States can determine an applicant's status for a 6-month period.

For example, if it is determined that an applicant exceeds the medically needy income level by $135 each month in a 6-month accounting period (because the person's net income equals $455 in a State using a $300 eligibility level), the applicant would have a total spend-down liability of $810 in medical expenses (six times $135 per month). Only after the applicant incurred $810 in medical bills would Medicaid eligibility be established and additional covered expenses reimbursed.

The longer the accounting period, the more medical expenses must be incurred and the more difficult it is for an applicant to establish eligibility. Few health care providers are willing to extend credit to permit an applicant to incur sufficient expenses. Thus, the applicant must pay out of pocket to the provider a substantial amount even though the applicant's income is already far below the poverty level.

The other effect of a longer accounting period is to make it more difficult for an applicant to establish eligibility in the community. An applicant who became ill in a single month might generate enough medical bills to satisfy the $135 spend-down obligation and thereby establish Medicaid eligibility for remaining bills in that month. However, it is extremely unlikely that the same applicant would generate $810 in medical expenses (the spend-down liability if a 6-month accounting period is used) without some institutional care.

Attempts to challenge accounting periods exceeding 1 month have been unsuccessful (1,11,18). In *Hogan* v. *Heckler*, the Court of Appeals for the First Circuit described the impact of the 6-month accounting period on one of the applicants, a veteran with quadriplegia, in the following language:

> Receiving Veterans and Social Security benefits that bring his spend-down up to nearly $2,300, the applicant is assertedly forced to operate on credit, depending on the willingness of his attendant to go unpaid for months at a time, while his medical expenses accumulate to reach the required amount. At some point, the applicant was abandoned by his attendant and was forced to seek emergency care at a hospital for a short spell to increase his medical expenses. Other members of the plaintiff class are in a similar situation (18).

Despite recognizing the hardships longer accounting periods work on applicants, the courts have ruled that the Federal regulation authorizing 6-month accounting periods is not illegal. Any change would therefore require congressional action.

(5) Responsibility of Relatives.—Medicaid policy regarding the financial responsibility of relatives is one of the areas of greatest confusion among applicants and recipients. In some cases this confusion leads to unnecessary separation or divorce. In others the result is needless delays in applying for assistance.

The Social Security Act restricts the circumstances in which relative responsibility can be applied to spouse for spouse and to parent for minor child or adult child who is disabled or blind (42 U.S.C. 1396a(a)(17)). Thus, an adult child is not liable under the Medicaid statute for the support of elderly or disabled parents. Even in those circumstances in which relative responsibility is possible, it is seldom pursued. Under Federal law, "deeming" is the only form of relative responsibility mandated on the States (see, for example, 42 CFR 435.723 and 435.724). Few States go beyond that requirement.

A few States do aggressively pursue relative responsibility by enforcing general support laws. In these cases, requests for contributions may be sought from responsible relatives who are not actually supporting recipients at levels established by the State. Court actions may also be filed to compel support payments from noncontributing relatives.

A closely related approach involves the use of liens. The Medicaid statute had traditionally barred most use of liens by States to recover Medicaid payments that had been properly paid (see Section 121(a) of the Social Security Amendments of 1965 (Public Law 89-97), as amended by Section 13(a)(8) of Public Law 93-233 and Section 132(a) of the Tax Equity and Fiscal Responsibility Act of 1982)). That restriction has now been changed to permit the use of liens against the real property of certain elderly recipients and certain recipients under 65 who are in a nursing home and not expected to return home (42 U.S.C. 1396p). However, even in these circumstances, liens are prohibited against a home occupied by the recipient's spouse, by a minor child, or by a blind adult or disabled child (42 U.S.C. 1396p(a)(2)).

These statutory changes in the lien provisions are relatively recent and few States have amended their plans to include this requirement. Many, however, are considering such changes as part of a comprehensive plan to target limited financial resources while permitting more liberal allowances for the needs of spouses and children of applicants.

(6) Transfer of Assets.—In part because of the low resource standards under Medicaid, the specter of wealthy individuals transferring assets for less than fair consideration in order to qualify for Medicaid benefits has haunted the program almost since its inception. Anecdotes, whether true or false, have been widely circulated of people transferring hundreds of thousands of dollars in order to be covered by Medicaid in a nursing home.

Few data are available to support these anecdotes. Moreover, several incentives under Medicaid would discourage such transfers. A person who gave up substantial assets in order to qualify for Medicaid would have to live on a personal needs allowance of $25 per month. At the same time, the recipient would be limited to nursing homes willing to accept Medicaid patients. These two factors would operate to discourage most truly consensual transfers. Nevertheless, the specter still persists.

Initially, the Medicaid program, by incorporating the resource requirements of the SSI program into the adult medically needy program, prohibited States using SSI criteria from penalizing individuals who transferred assets for less than fair consideration. A 209(b) State applying more restrictive criteria could include a transfer of asset prohibition so long as such a requirement was validly part of the State's 1972 Medicaid plan. Most State efforts to impose such requirements prior to 1980 were unsuccessful (see, e.g., 2,12).

That situation was changed in 1980 by the Boren-Long Amendments to the Social Security Act (Public Law 96-611, sections 5(a)-(c)). That legislation amended the SSI program to prohibit transfers of assets for less than fair market value within 24 months of applying for assistance where the purpose of the transfer was to qualify for SSI or to establish continuing eligibility. States were also authorized to impose similar or even more restrictive requirements under their Medicaid programs (see 42 U.S.C. 1396p(c) as added by Section 132(b) of the Tax Equity and Fiscal Responsibility Act of 1982 (Public Law 97-248), and as amended by the Technical Corrections Act of 1982 (Public Law 97-448)).

Although these provisions attempted to deal with what was perceived to be a significant problem, they opened as many loopholes as they closed. Any applicant with substantial assets to protect could simply transfer those assets with impunity more than 2 years in advance of applying for assistance. Federal law could have used a longer period than 2 years for prohibiting transfers. As the period increases, however, it becomes more and more difficult to demonstrate that the transfer was for the purpose of qualifying for assistance. States that have tried to use longer periods have not achieved great success in discouraging transfers. The 2-year provision is especially relevant for persons with dementia, because the illness is protracted and years may pass between the onset of symptoms and the need for nursing home care.

Most recently, a further attempt was taken to deal with this problem through the Consolidated Omnibus Budget Reconciliation Act of 1985 (COBRA) (Public Law 99-272, Section 9506(a)). Most States do not consider assets placed in a discretionary trust in determining the eligibility of an applicant or recipient. A discretionary trust is one in which the assets are to be spent in the sole discretion of the trustee for the benefit of the beneficiary. The trust assets are therefore not actually available to the beneficiary although trust payments to that person would be considered as income. The act of placing assets in a discretionary trust, within 2 years of applying for assistance or while a recipient, might also trigger a State's transfer of asset provision, however.

The COBRA legislation amended Federal law to declare that discretionary trusts, referred to as Medicaid qualifying trusts, are no longer exempt from consideration as an asset. These amendments are therefore designed to discourage the practice regardless of when the trust was created.

In actuality, however, the effect of these amendments will likely be to encourage applicants wishing to qualify for Medicaid to make outright gifts of assets that would otherwise be placed in a discretionary trust. Since many States succeeded in requiring beneficiaries to petition courts to invade such trusts, the short-term effect of these amendments may be counterproductive by reducing the assets that States might otherwise reach.

For persons with dementia, transfer-of-asset provisions may block steps that could be taken to ease the hardship on spouses in the community without outside income. If the spouse in a nursing home has all of the income in his or her name, the amount allocated to the spouse in the community will vary between approximately $72 and $336, depending on the State involved. To ease the hardship created by that limitation, a spouse in a nursing home might attempt to transfer income-generating assets to the sole ownership of the spouse outside the nursing home. Such

an approach would be barred by existing law unless the transfer takes place more than 2 years before the spouse in the nursing home needs Medicaid reimbursement for care.

On the other hand, families with a relative with dementia may actually be less disadvantaged by the transfer-of-asset prohibition than other families. The current provision tends to reward families that seek legal and financial advice early. Because of the time that may pass between onset of symptoms and the need for nursing home care for a patient with dementia, a family that transfers assets early will be able to protect those assets for the use of other family members and still maximize Medicaid eligibility.

SCOPE OF SERVICES

Medicare

The Medicare program covers primarily acute medical care and does not cover protracted long-term care. Moreover, while hospital services, physician services, and skilled nursing care are included, some basic acute medical services, such as prescription drugs, are excluded. The limitations on the scope of services therefore have a direct impact on the importance of the Medicare program for beneficiaries with dementia.

The coverage of a service, however, does not necessarily imply that reimbursement will be available for beneficiaries with dementia. In interviews conducted during the course of this assessment, Medicare beneficiaries uniformly decried what they described as "misleading" Federal brochures —pamphlets, for example, that indicate that Medicare beneficiaries can receive up to 100 days of nursing home care (4). Although that statement is factually correct, few people who receive Medicare ever receive this reimbursement for nursing home care.

Those who were interviewed felt that they had been led into a false sense of security by the brochure explanations of coverage. The two most dramatic examples of this problem occur with regard to two exclusions from coverage under

Medicare—the "not reasonable and necessary" exclusion and the "custodial care" exclusion.

"Not Reasonable and Necessary" Exclusion

The Social Security Act excludes from reimbursement under Medicare "any expenses incurred for items or services which . . . are not reasonable and necessary for the diagnosis or treatment of illness or injury or to improve the functioning of a malformed body member" (42 U.S.C. 1395y(a)(1)(A)). The exclusion thus places the burden on the beneficiary to show that the particular item or service for which reimbursement is sought will "treat" the disease. Since the services required by a patient with dementia, for example, will not cure the disease but only manage its symptoms, reimbursement is uncertain. Yet, most chronic diseases of the elderly are not "cured" by medical care and treatment. For example, a patient with coronary heart disease will frequently require care and treatment designed to manage the symptoms of the disease even though the underlying disease will not be cured. Because there is no similar medical protocol for patients with Alzheimer's disease, however, and because the services required by patients with dementia are not purely medical, the standard excludes coverage for many services for many patients with dementia.

This exclusion problem is similar to the drafting difficulties encountered in legislative attempts to cover hospice care under Medicare (42 U.S.C. 1395d(d)). (Section 122(h)-(k) of the Tax Equity and Fiscal Responsibility Act of 1982 added hospice care as a covered service.) It was not sufficient to simply amend the Social Security Act provisions defining scope of services. Since hospice care is not a cure-oriented service, but rather a supportive maintenance one, the "not reasonable and necessary" exclusion's focus on treatment would have presented coverage problems.

Congress opted to modify the "not reasonable and necessary" exclusion to permit coverage of hospice care that is reasonable and necessary for "the palliation or management of terminal illness" (42 U.S.C. 1395y(a)(1)(C)). This standard differs significantly from the "diagnosis or treatment" standard and thereby authorizes coverage that would not otherwise be available.

"Custodial Care" Exclusion

The Medicare program also excludes items or services that "are for custodial care" (42 U.S.C. 1395y(a)(9)). This exclusion is similar to and often overlaps the "not reasonable and necessary" exclusion. Indeed, the 1982 amendments authorizing reimbursement for hospice care also had to modify the "custodial care" exclusion by denying reimbursement for "custodial care (except, in the case of hospice care, as is otherwise permitted under paragraph [1862(a)] (1)(c)" (42 U.S.C. 1395y (a)(9)).

The "custodial care" exclusion is perhaps most often used with regard to nursing home care. Since only skilled nursing and rehabilitation services are covered under Medicare, "custodial care" is defined to include all services that do not qualify as "skilled nursing and skilled rehabilitation services" (42 CFR 405.310(g)).

"Skilled nursing" services:

1. are ordered by a physician;
2. require the skills of technical or professional personnel such as registered nurses, licensed practical (vocational) nurses, physical ther-

apists, occupational therapists, and speech pathologists or audiologists; and
3. are furnished directly by, or under the supervision of, such personnel (42 CFR 409.31(a)).

That definition has been applied restrictively to deny reimbursement for many otherwise covered services. (Many of these initial denials have been overturned at the administrative law judge hearing stage or in judicial review; see ref. 6, para. 4115). Such denial of coverage has occurred because insufficient weight has been given to such factors as when a technical or professional person's skills are required to observe and assess the patient's changing condition.

Although the regulations expressly recognize the needs of "patients who, in addition to their physical problems, exhibit acute psychological symptoms such as depression, anxiety, or agitation, etc., [and therefore] may also require skilled observation and assessment by technical or professional personnel to assure their safety and/or the safety of others" (42 CFR 409.33), Medicare reimbursement for extended nursing home care is nonetheless unusual. One aggravating factor for persons with dementia is the limited rehabilitation potential. As noted earlier, the Medicare program remains "cure-oriented." With regard to nursing home care, the Federal regulations acknowledge that "even if full recovery or medical improvement is not possible, a patient may need skilled services to prevent further deterioration or preserve current capabilities" (42 CFR 409.32(c)).

However, even the best skilled services will frequently not prevent, but will only slow, further deterioration under current treatment protocols for persons with dementia. And the best skilled services will generally not preserve current capabilities, but will only slow their loss.

Medicaid

Although the Federal Medicaid statute permits substantial State flexibility in identifying which services will be reimbursed for which populations, it also imposes some uniform requirements. Those persons who are described as "categorically needy" must be reimbursed for the following services: inpatient hospital services, outpatient hospital services, rural health clinic services, other laboratory and x-ray services, skilled nursing facility services, early and periodic screening diagnosis and treatment services, family planning services and supplies, physician services, and nurse-midwife services (42 U.S.C. 1396a(a)(10)(A) and 1396d(a)). Home health services must also be provided for any person entitled to skilled nursing facility services (42 U.S.C. 1396a(a)(10)(D)).

The term "categorically needy" is not used in the Social Security Act. It has become a term of art under the Federal Medicaid regulations (42 CFR 435.500). It refers to those persons receiving SSI and AFDC (the mandatory categorically needy) as well as those special groups (the optional categorically needy) who display special characteristics, such as the nursing home cap population, that entitle them to eligibility. Most of the optional categorically needy groups were added to the Medicaid rolls after 1965 without express statutory authorization. Starting in 1981, many of these groups were expressly added to the Social Security Act.

If a State plan covers the "medically needy," separate service requirements are imposed. Furthermore, if a State covers the "medically needy" and reimburses for services in institutions for mental diseases or in intermediate care facilities for the mentally retarded (or both), then it must also cover either the services required for the "categorically needy" or an assortment of the services for which Federal reimbursement is available.

Uncovered Services

The initial problem confronted by a recipient with dementia may be that the services needed are not covered by the State plan, for one of two reasons. First, some services are not eligible for Federal financial participation under the Federal Medicaid statute, which only authorizes reimbursement for "medical care" and "remedial care" (42 U.S.C. 1396d(a)). (These terms have been expanded in recent years to include services authorized pursuant to home- and community-based waivers.) Services such as respite care, which may be important for the maintenance at home of a person with dementia, are not covered. Minor structural changes to a home that would delay

or avoid institutionalization of a person with dementia are also not covered.

Second, the Federal Government has chosen not to make the Medicaid program uniform in the 55 jurisdictions administering the program. States continue to possess the discretion to decide what services are to be covered for which populations.

Amount, Duration, and Scope

Inclusion of a service in the State plan for a particular population does not automatically ensure coverage. States are permitted to impose limitations on the amount, duration, and scope of covered services that may greatly reduce availability. For example, a State may cover physician services, but may permit only one visit per month. Similarly, inpatient hospital services may be covered, but only for 12 days of coverage per fiscal year.

Legal challenges to such limitations have been largely unsuccessful. Federal regulations require that services must be sufficient in amount, duration, and scope to reasonably achieve their purpose (42 CFR 440.230(b)), yet most courts have ruled that no violation is present even if many medical procedures reasonably require services in excess of the limitation (3,8,17).

Similarly, although Federal regulations prohibit States from arbitrarily denying or reducing the amount, duration, or scope of a required service to an otherwise eligible recipient solely because of the diagnosis, type of illness, or condition (42 CFR 440.230(c)), most courts have ruled that limitations due to fiscal reasons are not arbitrary and do not discriminate even if certain diagnoses, illness, or conditions generally require services in excess of the limitation (3,8,17). Moreover, although Federal regulations authorize State Medicaid agencies to place limits on a service based only on such criteria as medical necessity or on utilization control procedures (42 CFR 440.230(d)), most courts have upheld across-the-board limits that are not based on these considerations (3,8,17).

Institutions for Mental Diseases

Another possible influence on the availability of nursing home care for Medicaid recipients with dementia is the Federal exclusion of services in institutions for mental diseases except for persons at least 65 and for inpatient psychiatric hospital services for persons under age 21 (42 U.S.C. 1396d (a)(B)). The Federal administration of this provision has been the subject of much controversy. The Health Care Financing Administration has defined the term "institution for mental disease" (IMD) in guidelines in the State Medicaid Manual.

These IMD guidelines look to such factors as the licensure status of the facility, the way the facility advertises and "holds itself out" to the public, and the facility's level of security. The factor that probably has presented the greatest difficulty for States and providers has been the guideline that considers whether "more than 50 percent of the patients have mental diseases which require inpatient treatment according to the patients' medical records" (ref. 26: Section 4390).

The Federal IMD guidelines have been upheld by the U.S. Supreme Court (7). The clear signal to State agencies and nursing homes from that decision was to carefully monitor the patient mix in order to stay below the 50 percent guideline. Because persons with dementia often have behavioral symptoms, nursing homes have incentives to deny admission to these individuals.

Yet the same Federal guidelines expressly exclude persons with dementia when calculating the 50 percent. The guidelines emphasize that:

. . . in using the ICD-9-CM [International Classification of Diseases, 9th revision, Clinical Modification], it is important to note that, although the senile and presenile organic psychotic conditions listed [including senile dementia, presenile dementia, senile dementia with delusional or depressive features, and arteriosclerotic dementia] . . . are included as mental disorders, these diagnoses represent the behavioral expression of underlying neurological disorders. For this reason, these conditions are not to be considered mental diseases for purposes of IMD identification (ref. 26: Section 4390).

Despite the clear language of that provision, nursing home administrators interviewed during the course of this assessment frequently referred to the IMD exclusion as the reason they are reluctant to admit patients suffering from dementia (4). The incentive to refuse admission therefore persists because administrators prefer not to risk their certification or to jeopardize their substantial Federal funding for intermediate and skilled nursing facility care. Their cautiousness apparently stems from a fear that the IMD guidelines will be applied to include facilities that are not institutions for mental disease (27).

Home- and Community-Based Services

The home- and community-based services waiver, added to the Medicaid statute in 1981 as part of the Omnibus Budget Reconciliation Act, was designed to permit Medicaid funding of services in the community for individuals who would otherwise require placement in a nursing home. Although costs associated with room and board in the community were still excluded, Federal funding became available for the costs of case management, homemaker, home health aide, personal care, adult day health, habilitation, respite care, and other services requested by the State and approved by the Secretary (46 FR 48532). Combining this "services" waiver with the "eligibility" waiver of deeming requirements for persons who would otherwise be at risk of nursing home placement significantly expands the options for families with someone with dementia.

The potential expansion has been largely unrealized, however. The major obstacle appears to be the restrictive interpretation of cost-effectiveness employed by the Health Care Financing Administration and by the Office of Management and Budget in reviewing waiver applications. The Federal statute requires States seeking home- and community-based services waivers to provide satisfactory assurances that "average per capita expenditures . . . with respect to such individuals" will not exceed "the average per capita expenditure . . . for such individuals if the waiver had not been granted" (42 U.S.C. 1396n(c)(2)(D)). The emphasis in that congressional language on "such" individuals indicates that a waiver application should be granted if a State can show that the waiver will be cost-effective for individuals served under the waiver.

By contrast, the regulatory formula for evaluating cost-effectiveness does not simply consider the costs associated with individuals who would be served under the waiver (42 CFR 441.303). Instead, it also considers costs attributable to other recipients under the State plan. The effect has been to limit the scope of the waiver process. If, for example, a State proposed to add home- and community-based services to its plan, some persons could be moved from a nursing home and served in the community. Unless the beds occupied by those persons remained vacant, however, average per capita costs under the regulatory formula might actually increase due to the community costs associated with the recipients now in the community and the nursing home expenditures associated with "substituted" recipients.

Some of these "substituted" recipients are current Medicaid enrollees who could not gain access to nursing home beds and therefore could not generate expenditures. Other "substituted" recipients are not current enrollees because they could not gain access to nursing homes and thereby generate sufficient expenses to meet medically needy spend-down requirements. Costs associated with both classes of "substituted" recipients make it difficult for a State to meet regulatory cost-effectiveness criteria.

The Federal regulatory approach to measuring cost-effectiveness appears to run contrary to the express language of the statute and its legislative history. It effectively "caps" the number of nursing home beds in the State and thereby limits the entitlement aspect of the Medicaid program. It remains, however, the standard applied in evaluating waiver applications. The net effect has been to permit only limited use of the waiver authority, largely in cases when an institution is being closed and therefore no "substitution" can occur.

Community Services

One persistent criticism of the Medicaid program is that it is oriented too much toward institutional care and services. Part of this "bias" is an inevitable result of the low eligibility levels used under the program. Few nonwelfare applicants will be eligible without having incurred substantial medical expenses, which are most likely to be incurred in an institutional setting.

In addition, many State plans do not include the range of community services needed to avoid or delay nursing home placement. Medical day care and personal care services, for example, can qualify for Federal reimbursement without a waiver when provided through a medical model. Few States include such services in their plans and even fewer have been able to attract enough providers to permit recipients broad access to services.

The orientation toward institutional care and services is not illegal under the Medicaid statute. The effect, however, has been to make it more likely that a recipient with dementia will be served in an institutional setting, if at all, since that is often the only service site for which reimbursement will be available.

Intermediate Care Facilities

Unlike the Medicare program, the Federal Medicaid statute authorizes reimbursement for intermediate care facility services (42 U.S.C. 1396d(a)(15)). That provision is an important funding source for long-term nursing home care of dementia patients. Federal regulations define intermediate care to mean services in a facility that:

(1) Fully meets the requirements for a State license to provide, on a regular basis, health-related services to individuals who do not require hospital or skilled nursing facility care, but whose mental or physical condition requires services that—
(i) Are above the level of room and board; and
(ii) Can be made available only through institutional facilities (42 CFR 440.150(a)(1)).

Although this definition is less stringent than that of skilled nursing care under either Medicare or Medicaid (42 CFR 440.40), it may still restrict access for persons with dementia.

The restrictions usually stem from implementation of the words "can be made available only through institutional facilities." Although most individuals with dementia will require more than room and board (such as skilled observation and behavior management) due to their mental condition, few require nursing home placement for this level of care. In fact, many families can and do manage home care of spouses and relatives suffering from dementia through services both in and outside the home (such as respite care, personal care, attendant care, and adult day care).

Despite the potential problems that the intermediate care requirement poses, most States interpret the standard in a lenient manner. Instead of considering the theoretical availability of noninstitutional care, many utilization reviewers look to the practical availability of that care. Nevertheless, different interpretations of this criterion for coverage have spawned large variations from State to State and even within States.

REIMBURSEMENT PRACTICES

Reimbursement practices are often thought of as a matter between the bill-paying agency and the provider of services that does not really affect program beneficiaries. But these practices directly influence provider participation and, therefore, access to services. Moreover, the level of reimbursement will influence the amounts that program beneficiaries have to pay for covered services.

Medicare

Diagnosis-Related Groups

The adequacy of Medicare reimbursement for hospital services has received considerable public scrutiny recently. The introduction of reimbursement for hospital services based on diagnosis-related groups (42 U.S.C. 1395ww) resulted in complaints of dumping of "heavy-care" patients —those likely to generate costs during a stay above the average for that class of diagnosis. Such dumping has special implications for patients with dementia.

Medicare reimbursement for inpatient hospital services related to a diagnosis of Alzheimer's disease or another form of dementia tends to be adequate to cover services needed. However, adequacy of reimbursement does not guarantee access to care.

Once a person has been diagnosed as suffering from dementia, he or she must ultimately be discharged to an appropriate family, community, or institutional care setting. To the extent that these service settings are not available, patients may become "backed-up" in hospitals, which can push costs above the available reimbursement. Such difficulties in placement may then dissuade hospitals from admitting persons likely to be difficult to discharge—including those with dementia (although there is no quantitative evidence of this).

A related problem arises when a person with dementia is admitted for a condition unrelated to the underlying illness. Patients with dementia are commonly perceived as being more difficult to manage. More intensive staff services for supervision and patient management may be required. Hospitals may therefore have a financial incentive to discourage admission of such patients.

Hospitals are also prevented from simply shifting costs to a patient:

> A hospital may not charge a beneficiary for any services for which payment is made by Medicare [under the prospective payment system], even if the hospital's costs of furnishing services to that beneficiary are greater than the amount the hospital is paid under the prospective payment system (42 CFR 412.42).

Physician Reimbursement

Medicare reimbursement for physician services has also been the subject of congressional action. Most Medicare beneficiaries have difficulty finding physicians willing to accept Medicare assignment for the costs of care. Under Part B of the Medicare program, a physician is not generally required to accept Medicare reimbursement as reimbursement in full. Instead, reimbursement is limited to 80 percent of a fee established for that provider. When a physician accepts assignment, the Medicare program makes reimbursement directly to the physician, and the Medicare beneficiary is responsible for paying the remaining 20 percent. In nonassignment cases, the Medicare program still pays only 80 percent of the established fee. However, the beneficiary is liable for paying the difference between the Medicare-established fee and the actual fee. Since actual fees generally exceed the Medicare-established fees significantly, the beneficiary is usually liable for far more than the 20 percent of the established nonassignment cases.

Congress attempted to remedy this situation in the Deficit Reduction Act of 1984 by establishing a voluntary participation system for physicians and suppliers willing to accept assignment for all services provided to Medicare patients during a fiscal year (42 U.S.C. 1395u(h)).

The incentive to encourage participation included listings in directories and toll-free telephone lines, electronic transmission of claims, and certificates of participation. Probably the most significant factor, however, was an expected exemption from freezes on fees to Medicare beneficiaries.

Under the Medicare and Medicaid Budget Reconciliation Amendments of 1984 (enacted as part of the Deficit Reduction Act of 1984), beginning July 1984, all customary and prevailing charge levels for physicians' services were "frozen" at the levels in effect from July 1983 to June 1984. That freeze prohibits both participating and nonparticipating physicians from passing on increases in charges during that period. However, participating physicians would receive a retroactive "catchup" in their fee profiles (42 U.S.C. 1395u(b)(4)).

Although this approach held out some promise of increasing the number of physicians willing to accept assignment, the physician fee freeze may have undercut most of the benefits anticipated. That problem, which adversely affects all Medicare beneficiaries, may have special consequences for persons with dementia.

If a physician believes the costs of treating a patient outweigh the financial benefits, access to care may be reduced. Because the fee for providing a specific service is the same for light-care and heavy-care patients, a physician is more likely to see the light-care patient unless too few patients are scheduled to fill the workday.

The management problems frequently associated with patients with dementia, along with the high frequency of related problems and the limited rehabilitation potential, lead many providers to view patients with dementia as needing heavy care. Although the Medicare regulations permit an adjustment in fee levels for special factors (42 U.S.C. 1395u(b)(3); 42 CFR 405.506), the cumbersome administrative machinery for invoking this adjustment is generally not worth the effort. The effect, therefore, is to discourage equal access to care for the population of persons with dementia.

Nursing Home Reimbursement

Although hospitals are now reimbursed on the basis of diagnosis-related groups, the Medicare program continues to use a retrospective reasonable-cost reimbursement system (42 U.S.C. 1395f(b); 42 U.S.C. 1395x(v)). The theory behind that system is that a provider's actual and reasonable costs related to patient care will be reimbursed by the program.

The effect of that system on recipients requiring heavy care is to discourage access to nursing homes. Since most homes are for-profit facilities, they have a financial incentive to maximize revenues in relation to costs. This incentive will be advanced most by admitting light-care patients. The nursing home will receive its actual costs related to providing services and will receive the same return on equity capital.

A nursing home that admits a heavy-care patient will still receive only its actual costs of providing care for that individual. As it will receive no increase in profits, and as heavy-care patients are more trouble for the facility, the nursing home has an incentive to admit the "cream"—light-care patients—and to discourage those perceived as needing more care.

Data on whether persons with dementia actually require more care are still preliminary. Some studies indicate that residents with dementia need more care and attention from nursing staff, with one study reporting that nursing staff spent approximately 36 percent more time on patients with "senile dementia" than the minimum time required for nursing care in general (19). However, as indicated in chapter 7, that additional requirement may be largely due to inhospitable physical environments and inappropriate care approaches.

Whatever the ultimate findings, access patterns are now sculpted by the perception that individuals with dementia need extra care. Nursing home administrators interviewed for this assessment reported almost unanimously that it is more difficult for persons with dementia to gain access because of heavy-care requirements (4). So long as these perceptions control admissions practices, access for persons with dementia will continue to be more difficult.

Medicaid

For many years the Federal Medicaid regulations have recognized the direct link between provider participation and fee levels. (Several studies have noted this link but also that fee levels are not the only factor affecting access and they may not even be the most significant factor in some cases (e.g., 9,22).) Thus, Federal regulations require fees to "be sufficient to enlist enough providers so that services under the plan are available to recipients at least to the extent that those services are available to the general population" (42 CFR 447.204).

In practice, that goal has not been realized. Medicaid recipients do not have the same access to services as the general population. Thus not only do persons with dementia in general have difficulty obtaining appropriate care, the problems are compounded if they are dependent on Medicaid.

Nursing home reimbursement under Medicaid must be "reasonable and adequate to meet the costs that must be incurred by efficiently and economically operated providers to provide services in conformity with applicable State and Federal laws, regulations, and quality and safety standards" (42 U.S.C. 1396a(13); 42 CFR 447.253(b)(1)). In practice, most States have established a per diem rate for each facility based on some statewide limits on allowable costs.

Under a per diem system, facilities have a strong financial incentive to deny admission to persons they perceive will need heavy care. Since the facility in such a State receives the same amount regardless of the needs of the individual, a light-care patient will be more profitable for the facility. The present reimbursement model in many States therefore discourages access for persons with dementia.

Other States use weighted systems, following a "case mix" or "patient mix" reimbursement methodology, that reimburse facilities based on the service needs of individual residents. These systems have the potential to eliminate any bias in admissions against patients regarded as needing heavy care, such as those with dementia. They could also improve patient care.

To the extent that the assessment tool used in these systems accurately reflects the functional disability of the individual and the associated service needs, higher reimbursement will be available for persons with greater service needs. Nursing homes would then have no incentive to limit admissions to light-care patients. In addition, to the extent that greater reimbursement is available to fund care for an individual, more services can be provided to meet that person's needs.

These potential benefits may not automatically be realized, however, simply because a State uses a case mix system. Some of these systems focus primarily on the medical needs of the individual and do not give sufficient weight to the person's supervision and behavior management needs (see chs. 6 and 8). Unless these other needs are accounted for, the service needs determined for the patient and the associated reimbursement will not be adequate. The bias against admitting persons with dementia will persist, and promises of appropriate care may not be realized.

ADMINISTRATIVE PROCEDURES

Barriers Under Medicare

The administrative procedures that raise barriers to beneficiaries with dementia are the same as those for others using Medicare. Obtaining information about services from fiscal intermediaries or carriers or about eligibility from Social Security district offices is frequently difficult. It may take years to overturn an initial erroneous denial of eligibility for benefits and, thus, to obtain coverage.

Appeals of denial of eligibility are often delayed, especially at the reconsideration and administrative law judge levels. Appeals about coverage of services are subject to the same limitations applicable generally: Hearings will not be granted under Part A unless the amount in question is $100 or more, and judicial review will only be available if at least $1,000 is in dispute (42 U.S.C. 1395ff(b)(2)). Appeal rights under Part B are more restrictive—a hearing will not be granted unless $100 or more is in question, and no judicial review is available for dissatisfied beneficiaries (42 U.S.C. 1395u(b)(3)(C); see also, 15).

Barriers Under Medicaid

Similar administrative barriers exist in the Medicaid program. Eligibility determinations are often subject to substantial delays, above and beyond those associated with the underlying social security or welfare determinations. But there are some additional barriers unique to Medicaid.

Civil Rights Enforcement

The Medicaid eligibility rolls tend to include more people belonging to racial and ethnic minorities than do the Medicare rolls. The traditional access problems experienced by minority persons may therefore be present to a greater degree under Medicaid. Discrimination in violation of Title VI of the Civil Rights Act of 1964 (42 U.S.C. 2000d) may take many forms.

People in minority groups tend to have poorer health and may need more services. Yet in many States black Medicaid recipients 65 and older use only half the amount of services used by white Medicaid recipients of similar age. (See, e.g., 20.)

Recipients with dementia may also experience discrimination on the basis of national origin. Someone who learned English as a second language may revert to his or her original language after the onset of dementia. That person will face substantial difficulties obtaining services if providers do not communicate in the same language.

Discrimination on the basis of handicap (in violation of Section 504 of the Rehabilitation Act of 1973 (29 U.S.C. 794)) may also be a problem. Bias against individuals perceived by nursing homes as needing heavy care persists despite the issu-

ance of letters of findings by the Office for Civil Rights of the Department of Health and Human Services. For example, the Office for Civil Rights has found a violation where a nursing home excluded persons with colostomies and ileostomies (28). Persons with dementia may experience such discrimination in attempting to gain access to day care and other providers as well.

Without civil rights enforcement by States (which are primarily responsible for limiting participation in the Medicaid program to providers who comply with Title VI and Section 504) and by the Federal Government (which through the Office for Civil Rights of the Department of Health and Human Services is ultimately responsible for enforcing compliance with the civil rights laws under both Medicare and Medicaid), these patterns and practices may persist.

Independent legal challenges by dissatisfied beneficiaries and recipients have been successful in some cases. However, the scope of the potential problem and the magnitude of the resources that may be needed suggest that private civil rights actions cannot substitute for government enforcement.

Fair Hearings

Medicaid recipients have a broad legal right to administrative hearings under the program. This hearing right could be used to check erroneous actions by agencies or providers. Its use, however, is limited.

Although statistics are no longer being collected, quality control data collected by DHHS prior to 1981 show that fewer than 5 percent of all recipients challenged actions taken in violation of Federal law to withhold, terminate, or deny benefits. Thus, at least 95 percent of the recipients subjected to negative case actions allow themselves to be deprived of their entitlements.

The problem is compounded by incentives created by the quality control process. States can have Federal financial participation disallowed only for erroneous State payments (see 42 CFR 431.804 for Federal policy after Jan. 1, 1984). A State can be penalized for overpayments or for inappropriate coverage. Yet, if a State erroneously fails to make a payment or makes too small a payment, no meaningful Federal check exists. States thus have a Federal incentive to reduce payments or services, but not to ensure full payments for all eligible persons.

OTHER FEDERAL PROGRAMS

Before reviewing the issues that should be considered in reforming Medicare or Medicaid to better assist persons with dementia and their families, it is important to recognize that other Federal programs also provide services to this population. Although their funding levels are not as great, these programs often fill important gaps for Medicare and Medicaid beneficiaries and provide significant funding for those ineligible for either program.

Among these other Federal programs are the Legal Services Corporation Act (providing civil legal assistance for indigent persons) (42 U.S.C. 2996 et seq.) and the Food Stamp Act (providing funding for purchases of food by indigent persons) (7 U.S.C. 2011 et seq.). But probably the two most important programs affecting persons with dementia are the Older Americans Act (42 U.S.C. 3001 et seq.) and the Social Services Block Grant (42 U.S.C. 1397 et seq.).

The Older Americans Act is a Federal formula grant program that provides grants to States that submit approved plans for the provision of services to persons 60 years of age or older. Funding is available under the act for such services as legal assistance, meal programs at designated congregate sites, and home-delivered meals. In addition, funding can be provided for supportive services designed to prevent unnecessary institutionalization.

The Social Services Block Grant operates in a similar manner with a target population of low-income children and adults. Again, States must submit an approved State plan. Many use this funding to provide support for adult day care, respite care, home modifications, and similar community services that can improve the quality of life for persons with dementia and their families.

Because these two programs have limited funding, many States try to use these funds only for persons or services that cannot be reimbursed through programs such as Medicare and Medicaid. A State survey conducted in conjunction with this assessment revealed, however, that communication and coordination between the agencies administering these different programs is not always ideal (4). As a result, services are not always maximized.

In some instances, for example, formula grants fund services that could be reimbursed under Medicaid. In others, the failure to provide funding under a formula grant for a service (such as in-home respite care) that cannot be reimbursed under Medicaid without a waiver means that unnecessary placement of a person with dementia in a nursing home may occur as families become exhausted.

CONSIDERATIONS FOR REFORM OF THE MEDICARE AND MEDICAID PROGRAMS

Three different types of options are available if it is decided to expand Federal support for persons with dementia and their families. Within each, decisions would have to be made about eligibility, scope of services, the method of reimbursement, and the nature of the administering agency or agencies.

Under the first option, Congress could decide to overhaul the existing Medicare and Medicaid programs. Apparent inequities and inefficiencies could be eliminated, eligibility requirements could be simplified, and services could be expanded to all groups in need of financial assistance. Various proposed national health insurance and catastrophic health insurance plans fall under this option. As a group that would be affected by any such changes, persons with dementia would be aided as others are.

Under the second option, Congress could decide to make incremental changes to the existing programs in order to improve Federal funding for persons with dementia. These changes could focus on the disease-neutral and other criteria that are inconsistent with public policy.

For example, the Listing of Impairments could be amended to specifically include dementia as a qualifying diagnosis. Similarly, a fairer division of marital income and assets could be mandated to bring many spouses living in the community above the poverty level. Case mix reimbursement systems could be mandated to eliminate any disincentives that may exist for the treatment of persons with dementia. Education of beneficiaries could be improved to foster a clearer understanding of the scope and limitations of the programs and to improve families' planning and decision-making. These incremental approaches and others would substantially improve the quality of life for persons with dementia and for their families.

Under the third option, if Congress concludes that insufficient support exists for significant reform of Medicare and Medicaid, it could still recognize the need for some additional Federal role to lessen the hardship of people with dementia and their families. Reform could consist of a specialized program to assist these groups. To the extent that such an approach is based on a closed appropriation, costs could be controlled while testing various financing and service delivery models. These models could then be expanded when additional funding became available.

Each approach has advantages and disadvantages. Before deciding on the most appropriate model, several questions should be answered.

First, should the approach be categorical? Many of the problems identified for long-term care of persons with dementia are shared by elderly persons and other groups. Should the solution to these problems be limited only to a single category of disabled persons?

Second, should the approach be limited to those most in need? A social insurance program like Medicare provides benefits to the wealthy as well as to the poor. Should a solution be limited to only those who require governmental assistance based on some means test?

Third, should the approach be built around existing medical reimbursement programs? Medicare and Medicaid generally fund medical services. The long-term care services required by persons with dementia include medical, social, and other services. Should these nonmedical services qualify for support?

Fourth, what role should relative responsibility play? How should any changes be made so that they encourage the continued provision of voluntary care by relatives or others and do not simply substitute government-funded services for private care?

These are among the major questions that must be asked and answered before reform is undertaken. Incremental or broad reform can then be initiated to address the critical unmet needs of persons with dementia and their families. Whatever approach is undertaken, because the size of this population is potentially so large and the unmet needs so great, any significant improvement in the current situation will necessitate a significant commitment of governmental financial resources. Thus, the current suffering can be significantly ameliorated, but only at a significant fiscal cost.

CHAPTER 11 REFERENCES

1. *Atkins* v. *Rivera*, 106 Sup.Ct. 2456, 91 L.Ed.2d 131 (1986).
2. *Caldwell* v. *Blum*, 621 F.2d 491 (2nd Cir. 1980).
3. *Charleston Memorial Hospital* v. *Conrad*, 693 F.2d 324 (4th Cir. 1982).
4. Chavkin, D.F., "Interstate Variability in Medicaid Eligibility and Reimbursement for Dementia Patients," contract report prepared for the Office of Technology Assessment, U.S. Congress, 1985.
5. *City of New York* v. *Heckler*, 578 F.Supp. 1109, 1115 (E.D.N.Y. 1984), affirmed *Bowen* v. *City of New York*, 106 Sup.Ct. 2002, 90 L.Ed.2d 462 (1986).
6. Commerce Clearinghouse, *Medicare and Medicaid Guide*, Washington, DC.
7. *Connecticut Dept. of Income Maintenance* v. *Heckler*, 105 Sup.Ct. 2210, 85 L.Ed.2d 577 (1985).
8. *Curtis* v. *Taylor*, 625 F.2d 645 (5th Cir. 1980).
9. Davidson, S.M., "Physician Participation in Medicaid: Background and Issues," *Journal of Health Politics, Policy, and Law* 6:703-717, 1982.
10. Davidson, S.M., Cromwell, J., and Shurman, R., "Medicaid Myths: Trends in Medicaid Expenditures and the Prospects for Reform," *Journal of Health Politics, Policy, and Law* 10:699-728, 1986.
11. *DeJesus* v. *Perales*, 770 F.2d 316 (2nd Cir. 1985).
12. *Fabula* v. *Buck*, 598 F.2d 869 (4th Cir. 1979).
13. *Friedman* v. *Berger*, 547 F.2d 724 (2nd Cir. 1976).
14. *Gilliland* v. *Heckler*, 786 F.2d 178 (3rd Cir. 1986).
15. *Gray Panthers* v. *Schweiker*, 652 F.2d 146 (D.C.Cir. 1981).
16. *Gray Panthers* v. *Secretary*, 335 F.2d 1393 (D.C.Cir. 1979), reversed sub nom. *Secretary* v. *Gray Panthers*, 333 U.S. 911 (1981).
17. *Harris* v. *McRae*, 448 U.S. 297 (1980).
18. *Hogan* v. *Heckler*, 769 F.2d 886 (1st Cir. 1985).
19. Hu, T., Huang, L., and Cartwright, W., "Evaluation of the Costs of Caring for the Senile Demented Elderly: A Pilot Study," *The Gerontologist* 26:158-173, 1986.
20. Maryland Department of Health and Mental Hygiene, Maryland Medical Care Programs, "The Year in Review" (Fiscal Year 1984), Baltimore, MD, 1985.
21. *Mattingly* v. *Heckler*, 784 F.2d 258 (7th Cir. 1986).
22. Mitchell, J.B., and Shurman, R., "Access to Private OB-GYN Services Under Medicaid," *American Journal of Obstetrics and Gynecology* 33:332-341, 1985.
23. *Purser* v. *Rahm*, 104 Wash.2d 159 (Wash.Sup.Ct. 1985).
24. *Rousseau* v. *Bordeleau*, 624 F.Supp. 355 (D.R.I. 1985).
25. *Secretary* v. *Gray Panthers*, 333 U.S. 911 (1981).
26. U.S. Department of Health and Human Services, Health Care Financing Administration, *State Medicaid Manual*.
27. U.S. Department of Health and Human Services, Office for Civil Rights, "In Re: *Gurley* v. *Covington Manor Nursing Home*," Policy Interpretation, Nov. 18, 1980.
28. U.S. Department of Health and Human Services, Office for Civil Rights, "In Re: Crestwood Manor Compliance Review," Policy Clarification, Jan. 14, 1981.
29. Urban Systems Research and Engineering, "Short-Term Evaluation of Medicaid: Selected Issues," Contract report prepared for Health Care Financing Administration, U.S. Department of Health and Human Services, Baltimore, MD, 1984.

Financing Long-Term Care for Persons With Dementia

"[Most people would] prefer to live as short a time as possible, once they have become permanently and seriously demented, but think it important not to suffer pain or indignity so long as they do live. . . . People would purchase only enough insurance coverage to provide minimum conditions of dignity, and to relieve pain; they would not seek to ensure funds, at the greatly increased premium charges that would be required, for life-prolonging medical treatment."

—Ronald Dworkin
"Philosophical Issues in Senile Dementia" contract report for the Office of Technology Assessment,
U.S. Congress, August 1986.

CONTENTS

Financing Long-Term Care for Persons With Dementia*

Individuals with dementia and their families must deal not only with the emotional and physical burdens of this tragic condition but also with its financial consequences. The care needed by someone with dementia is an enormous drain on a family's resources. People do receive help from friends, from private charity, and from government at the local, State, and Federal levels, but for a variety of reasons the help is less effective than it might be. For example, families complain about the need to impoverish themselves to obtain assistance, inflexibility in the forms in which aid is provided, arbitrary variations in availability with place of residence and family structure, and a host of other problems. In an era of fiscal constraint, government administrators worry about meeting Federal and State requirements and balancing the needs of those with dementia against the needs of others. Recent hearings before the

Public/Private Sector Advisory Committee on Catastrophic Illness, sponsored by the U.S. Department of Health and Human Services, have emphasized the spotty and inconsistent coverage of services needed by those with dementia and other chronic diseases.

This chapter considers current private and public sources of financing for the care of persons with dementia, emphasizing long-term care. The focus is not on the problems of financing long-term care in general, but on financing care for individuals with dementia, a large portion of the population using long-term care, especially in formal settings. The best estimates place the prevalence of dementia among nursing home residents at more than 50 percent (12). By sheer numbers, then, the problems of the long-term care system are the problems of persons with dementia. Moreover, these people fall into two subgroups facing stricter limits on financing: individuals requiring personal care and those requiring care because of impaired mental functioning.

_____
*This chapter is a contract report by Mary Ann Baily, George Washington University, Washington, DC.

SIZE OF THE FINANCING PROBLEM

As summarized in chapter 1, estimates of dementia's total cost to society range from $24 billion to $48 billion (4,24). Gauging such costs is unusually difficult and there is a large margin of uncertainty in all cost estimates.

Individuals with dementing disorders need many services. They need acute medical care both to diagnose their disease and monitor its progress, and to treat other conditions that may worsen symptoms of dementia (see ch. 2). And they need long-term care—not only nursing but also counseling, personal care, and social services. Patients can live as long as 25 years after the onset of the disease; the average duration for the most common forms of dementia is 6 to 8 years (3). Over that period, medical care costs may be dwarfed

by those of providing supervision and assistance in activities of daily living. Finally, it can be argued that the cost of care for dementia includes counseling and respite services for family members, who are also, in a sense, victims of the disease (see ch. 4).

Individual needs vary. Exactly which services are appropriate and in what quantities depend on the severity of an individual's symptoms, the personal and financial help that can be expected from family and friends, and the services available in the community. Thus, estimates of aggregate cost require information not only on the prevalence of dementia but also on its distribution along dimensions relevant to the cost of treatment, such as age at onset, severity of symptoms, place of residence, and family situation. Moreover, given the complexity of each situation, exploring the needs and available resources—case management—may be an important part of the cost of care.

Measuring the cost of any specific treatment plan is not straightforward. The true cost of required medical services included is difficult to determine, since cost accounting in health care is underdeveloped and charges to the individual or to a third-party payer often bear little relation to true economic cost. Nonmedical services may be even more difficult to value. Where should the line be drawn between ordinary living costs and costs attributable to the disease, and how should services provided by family and friends be valued?

The answer depends on the use to be made of the numbers. If the object is to minimize Federal outlay, only the charge to the Federal Government matters. If the object is to consider what the Federal share should be, then the full economic cost of care must be determined. The time and energy invested by family and friends in caring for the person have a social value, although they do not represent cash outlays. If true costs, including those borne by family and friends, are not measured, cost comparisons will give misleading results. For example, nursing home costs usually include room and board, whereas estimates of the cost of home care do not; that inflates the cost of nursing home care relative to home care.

Estimates of the cost of care that exist are based on small samples and methods constrained by practical reality. Moreover, current cost figures are based on current patterns of care. If—as previous chapters have suggested—many individuals are receiving inadequate care, it could cost more to bring care to an acceptable level. On the other hand, not enough is known about the most effective ways to manage the care of someone with dementia. Research might make it possible to achieve the same or higher levels of quality at lower cost.

PROPER DISTRIBUTION OF RESPONSIBILITY
FOR FINANCING CARE

Who should bear the financial burden? Lack of agreement on the answer is a major obstacle to policy formation. In the absence of an answer, programs for persons with dementia have been shaped by historical accident, rather than by considered principles.

The problem does not exist in isolation. It is part of the Nation's larger unsolved problem of financing and delivering all forms of health care. It is widely accepted today that Americans should be able to obtain important health care regardless of whether they can afford it. But there is no consensus on what care is important, how much a person should be able to obtain, what share of the cost that person should pay, and who should pay the rest. Currently, the level of access to care and the distribution of its cost are determined in an ad hoc manner.

Perhaps this is not surprising, since questions of how much and who should pay are hard to answer. Ensuring access to all beneficial care would be prohibitively expensive. Rather, implicit in American health policy is the assumption that only a basic level of care must be available to everyone—a "decent minimum" or "adequate level" (34). Deciding what this "adequate level" comprises, however, requires assessing relative benefits and costs and comparing relative need among patients. These judgments are so difficult that no one wants to make them—yet if they are not made, it is difficult to decide who should pay.

Taking on the responsibility to help others is unappealing when the responsibility is open-ended. When individuals bear the full cost themselves, at least they have the incentive to consider the cost as well as the benefit of care; with less direct financial responsibility, they may use more services. Existing public programs to ease the burden of health care costs show the tension between the desire to help people in need and the concern that public subsidies will get out of control. The tension is often resolved by writing generous programs and then restricting the availability of services in indirect and arbitrary ways.

The problem is particularly severe in long-term care. For a patient with appendicitis, there may be relatively few choices in formulating a treatment plan; for a person with a chronic illness, there is likely to be a wider range of choices at different levels of quality and cost. In these circumstances, the definition of need is particularly elastic, and no clear line exists between health needs and the need for housing and general income support. Moreover, since families can supply many of these services, the benefits and costs depend not only on the person's health but also on the availability of informal support. Finally, the costs of caring for a severely debilitated person can be enormous, and the benefits of the care may be more controversial, particularly for those who are very old or cognitively impaired. For all these reasons, it is particularly difficult to reach a consensus on what is a decent minimum of long-term care.

Two types of care have been especially problematic: personal services (i.e., assistance with activities of daily living such as eating, bathing, and dressing); and mental health services. The consensus is less clear about the extent to which these kinds of care should be part of a decent minimum. Moreover, use of these services is thought to be more responsive to price. Thus, the existing long-term care system places more restrictions on funding for these services than for medical and skilled nursing services.

In deciding who should pay for care, the key issue is the extent to which individuals and their families should be responsible for the cost of their own health care. This country has a strong tradition of individual responsibility; Americans are expected to provide for their own needs. Yet it is recognized that this may not always be possible, given the potentially catastrophic cost of health care and natural limits on the ability to provide for the future. Moreover, the need for care is quite uneven and largely outside an individual's control.

In the case of long-term care, the issue of family responsibility takes on special importance. Families have always been the major providers of care for elderly and disabled relatives. Their personal involvement with the care of individuals is irreplaceable. Yet society is undecided about how much they should be expected to bear, especially when the burden falls so unevenly. Children whose parents die suddenly at age 65 are in a much different position from those whose parents live until 90 and require years of costly custodial care. Elderly people who have several children with the resources to help them are in a different position from the childless. Is there a societal obligation to even out the burdens on these different groups? Even if there is no obligation, would we make a collective decision to do so as a matter of prudent policy—since we do not know to which group we are likely to belong?

If the responsibility for care is to be shared, the challenge is to develop a system for sharing it that is both efficient and equitable. It must deliver a level of care that balances individual need and societal resources, and it must distribute the cost so that all pay their fair share. The amount of care received and the cost paid should not vary arbitrarily; those with similar needs and similar personal and financial resources should receive similar amounts of help. The existing system does not always meet this ideal.

PRIVATE FINANCING

Direct Financing by Individuals and Families

Most long-term care is financed directly by the recipient and the family at the time of need (see chs. 1 and 4). The majority of care is informal, consisting of goods and services provided by family and friends. For example, the 1982 Long-Term Care Survey showed that 77 percent of elderly persons needing assistance with activities of daily living received no formal long-term care services (45). Much of the cost of formal care is paid out of pocket: Half of nursing home expenditures, which average $22,500 annually per person, are made directly by residents or their families. Since outside assistance is more limited for personal service care, home-based care, and mental-health services than for medical and skilled nursing care, families of individuals with dementia probably bear an even higher share of costs over the course of an illness than do families of other long-term care recipients.

The provision of informal support is often a serious drain on family resources. Moreover, trends in family composition and working patterns may be making it more difficult for families to provide support. Smaller family size, greater instability of marriages, geographical mobility, and greater involvement in work outside the home are all likely to increase the number of people with dementia who are isolated and without family members available to help (6,9) (see ch. 4).

When formal care is required, the heavy burden of costs is a major threat to financial well-being. Five to ten percent of individuals who develop dementia do so before age 65 (12). They are particularly vulnerable since the disease interferes early with their ability to work. Loss of employment not only means loss of income; it may also mean loss of employer-provided group health insurance, and higher out-of-pocket costs for acute care. (The loss of employment-based health insurance will be delayed for many by the passage of Public Law 99-272, which extends the options of group health insurance for 18 months to 3 years after termination from a job in most cases.) The person is not eligible for Medicare until totally and permanently disabled, and even after disability has been established, the waiting period is about 2½ years (see ch. 11).

Those stricken after retirement may also find themselves in serious difficulty, although the financial position of the elderly as a group has improved considerably in recent years, thanks to improved private pension systems and social security. Poverty rates for those age 65 or older dropped from 35.2 percent in 1959 to 12.4 percent in 1984 (16). One study found that the elderly have about 90 percent of the income of the nonelderly after adjustments for tax rates, asset income, and living arrangements (45). Medicare

now provides important protection against the cost of hospital and ambulatory care. Nevertheless, two studies of Massachusetts residents revealed that two-thirds of individuals and one-third of couples aged 65 and older would spend themselves into poverty within 13 weeks if they developed a chronic illness requiring nursing home care (39). Elderly women and members of minority groups are particularly likely to lack the financial resources to meet extraordinary medical and personal care expenses (26,31).

For many older people, the problem is not a lack of financial resources, but the fact that most of their wealth is tied up in home equity. In 1980, almost three-quarters of people aged 65 or older owned their own homes, and nearly 80 percent of these had no outstanding mortgages. In 1982, the average net equity of older people with homes approached $60,000 (22). To use this wealth for current living expenses, such as home care services, they would have to sell the house and uproot themselves.

One solution to this problem is *home equity conversion*. There are two basic approaches: reverse mortgages and sale leasebacks. In the first, the homeowner retains possession of the house during his or her lifetime but receives monthly payments from the mortgage holder; when the occupant dies, the mortgage holder receives title to the house. Under the second, the house is sold and title transferred but the seller has the right to rent the home for his or her lifetime (2,28). These financing mechanisms could allow some people in the early stages of dementia to afford in-home care in familiar surroundings.

Only a handful of home equity conversions have been done to date. Current Medicaid eligibility rules discourage the use of home equity to finance long-term care by making a home a protected asset (see ch. 11). Moreover, the concept is unfamiliar, and the transaction entails significant risk on both sides. The risk could be reduced, although not eliminated, by developing the institutional structure and resolving legal and tax uncertainties. However, the value of home equity conversion as a source of financing long-term care depends on the extent to which the group that needs care overlaps with the group that has substantial equity, now and in the future (2). That in turn depends on the housing market; future generations may not make such large capital gains from equity conversion, and thus the potential of this device may fade.

Another factor can reduce the incentive to convert home equity to pay for long-term care. As noted homes are generally exempt from consideration as assets in determining financial eligibility for Medicaid. Converting home equity into liquid assets removes this special protection and is thus unfavorable from the individual's point of view (see ch. 11).

To summarize, direct financing by individuals and their families is an important source of funds for long-term care. However, the large amount of resources required for the long-term care of those with dementia makes such financing difficult. Even middle-class families face impoverishment; at the very least, they find their assets eroded and the possibility of legacies to heirs diminished.

Financing Through Private Risk-Pooling

A natural response to the risk of a financial catastrophe is to seek insurance against it. Insurance would allow people to bear the costs of long-term care as a group, assuring access to care while protecting the living standard of family members and conserving assets for heirs. Although long-term care insurance seems like a desirable product, little has been sold. In 1982, only $200 million of the estimated $30 billion spent on long-term care came from private insurance policies (36).

The situation reflects both demand and supply factors. Until recently, consumers showed little interest in insurance against costs of long-term care. Relatively few people lived into their retirement years and even fewer went into nursing homes. Many retirees were poor and had trouble meeting basic living expenses. Those who felt the need to insure against heavy health care expenses saw health insurance for acute care to be more pressing.

The introduction of Medicare (and private supplemental "Medigap" insurance) met the need for acute care coverage and provided a little cover-

age for skilled nursing home and home health care. Medicaid paid for nursing home care for the eligible poor. Neither program provided good protection against the cost of long-term care, given strict limits on eligibility, scope of services, and reimbursement levels (see ch. 11). But consumers have been poorly informed about both the size of the risk and the extent of their protection. A study by the American Association of Retired Persons, for example, revealed that 79 percent of the elderly people surveyed thought that Medicare would pay for an extended stay in a nursing home (1).

Insurance companies have also been reluctant to market comprehensive long-term care policies. Companies considered the risk difficult to insure profitably, given the problems of estimating future liability. There may be a long period between initial issuance of the policy and payout. Company expenditures depend on trends subject to unpredictable change—trends in mortality and the incidence of long-term disability, costs of services, the availability of informal social support, and the personal preferences of policyholders.

Perhaps most important, by lowering financial barriers, the insurance itself may increase the use of services, a phenomenon known as "moral hazard." In deciding whether a service is worth having, an insured individual tends to look only at the out-of-pocket cost, not the total cost. Policyholders may realize that collectively they bear the cost in the form of higher premiums, but the cost of each decision is spread over the whole group, so no one has an incentive to economize. (The classic example of moral hazard is a group restaurant check: When people dine out and agree in advance to split the check, each person has an incentive to order more expensively than he or she would if paying separately. Yet in the end each person bears the cost of the collective "overordering" that results.)

Companies offering long-term care policies have tried to structure them to minimize such insurance-induced demand. Usually this has meant an emphasis on coverage for nursing home care and an indemnity payment structure (in which the company pays a fixed amount independent of the actual cost of the services used). The company limits the types of services covered and pays a fixed amount per unit of service (the indemnity), leaving the individual or the family to select services. The fact that most people view nursing homes as a last resort, while coverage for home-based care is limited or absent, serves as a check on the use of services. To control utilization, policies may also impose deductibles and coinsurance rates, require a hospital stay prior to nursing home admission, exclude mental health problems, require a physician to recommend or review care, or require a firm diagnosis of organic disease (32). Clearly, many of these provisions lessen the value of the policies as protection against the cost of a dementing illness.

Companies must also allow for the possibility of a phenomenon called adverse selection. A company may accurately predict the average use of long-term care for the population and then discover that its policyholders use care at a higher rate—because people at higher risk are more likely to purchase insurance. That phenomenon occurs when risk factors for ill health and the use of care are not evenly distributed and consumers have a better idea of their risk than the insurance company. The importance of attitudes toward nursing home placement and the availability of informal support in the decision to use formal care makes adverse selection especially likely in long-term care insurance, particularly if people are free to opt in and out of the insurance from year to year.

To minimize adverse selection, companies do their best to identify risk factors and structure their coverage accordingly. They vary premiums with age, screen applicants for health status, and exclude preexisting conditions. Some exclude selected illnesses from coverage. Most insurers give themselves an escape clause in the renewable provision of the policy. All individually marketed policies reserve the right to raise premiums (32).

Marketing policies on a group basis is another way to lessen the impact of adverse selection. For example, the fact that insurance for acute care expenses is sold through the workplace—and workers have few choices of policies—decreases the importance of adverse selection in that market. Little long-term care insurance is provided through the workplace, however (25). Younger workers prefer other benefits over long-term care coverage, given their low risk. Employer-sponsored health insurance for retirees (held by about 16 percent of the population 65 or older in 1983) is a more natural place for long-term care coverage, but these policies also have few or no long-term care benefits (43).

The prospects for expanding coverage of such costs as a retirement benefit are slim, since employers are backing away from postretirement health benefits rather than planning to add to them. When these benefits were introduced, most employers assumed they could modify the benefit at the firm's discretion, or by negotiation with a union (controlled by the current labor force). Recent court decisions have generally found to the contrary; firms cannot unilaterally alter or terminate benefits. Given the uncertainties surrounding the cost and utilization of health care and the longevity and age distribution of a firm's retirees, employers are likely to be reluctant to provide the existing benefits to new retirees, let alone add an even more unpredictable long-term care benefit (43).

The problems in developing long-term care insurance are formidable. Nevertheless, interest seems to be increasing among both consumers and insurers. Improvement in the financial status of the elderly population and growing awareness of the risk of heavy long-term care expenses are generating demand, and supply is beginning to increase. At least 25 companies already write individual policies, typically offering indemnity benefits ranging from $10 to $70 per day in skilled nursing facilities for 3 to 4 years (23). Some policies also cover custodial, intermediate, and home health care. Premiums vary with age, choice of indemnity level, and waiting period, generally ranging from $20 to $110 or more per month (8, 16,25,30,32). Other insurers are preparing to enter the market, although the signs are mixed. For example, Prudential has been test marketing a long-term care policy under an arrangement with the 22-million-member American Association of Retired Persons. On the other hand, United Equitable, with more than 10 years experience, still considers the product experimental and is cutting back its marketing efforts because of unexpectedly adverse claims experience.

How large a role private insurance plays in long-term care financing depends on its affordability for those who need it most—the elderly. A study done for the Department of Health and Human Services estimated what fraction of the population at least 65 could afford a long-term care policy under various assumptions about benefits, premiums, and the availability of discretionary income. For example, a $450 Firemen's Fund policy premium would be less than 5 percent of cash income for 47 percent of the population aged 65 to 69, and less than 10 percent of cash income for 81 percent of this age group (25). Whether that is an appropriate standard of affordability, and whether elderly Americans will actually be willing to spend that much for long-term care insurance, are unresolved questions, given the substantial out-of-pocket expenses they already incur for Medicare and Medigap insurance premiums, copayments and deductibles, and uninsured medical care.

Long-term care insurance deals only with financing; the insured person must still find the services. Moreover, premiums are not adjusted for the availability of informal support, despite its importance in the decision to purchase care. People require less formal care if they live in an environment that minimizes the demand for it. Thus the concept of combining insurance and service delivery in the same package is attractive.

One example of such packaging is the *life care community*. These provide housing tailored to the needs of an aging population and medical services as needed, including nursing home care, usually in the same complex. Each resident pays a substantial deposit, which may not be refundable if the person leaves the community, and a monthly fee (25,33). With easy access to important services and a supportive community, a person may be able to live independently for a longer time after the onset of disability. If nursing home care is eventually required, the person has automatic access to a familiar facility that he or she has chosen. These communities are expensive, however; one study estimates that only about 20 percent of the population 65 or older could af-

ford to enter one (25). Some communities levy substantial additional charges when a resident enters the nursing home. There is a risk that the facility will not be well managed—that the quality of services may not be maintained or the facility may become financially insolvent. Several life care communities have become financially unstable in recent years, and now see government-backed reinsurance as a means of reducing their actuarial risks. And depending on the exact financial arrangements, a resident may lose flexibility in later decisions about housing and health care.

Life care communities, like long-term care insurers, must consider adverse selection. A small discrepancy between the forecast number and the actual number of persons requiring heavy care can make a big difference in the organization's financial status. As a result, life care communities require people to be healthy at entry into the community, and some exclude dementia from coverage. Such approaches limit their value for individuals with dementing disorders, especially those already exhibiting symptoms.

Another example of the packaging of insurance and service delivery is the *social health maintenance organization* (S/HMO), a new system operating on an experimental basis in some locations. Like a health maintenance organization (HMO) an S/HMO is paid a flat amount per enrollee for a fixed period. In exchange, it provides the enrollee with all needed medical care and social support services for acute and chronic conditions that period. Ideally, the S/HMO puts together a bundle of medical and nonmedical services tailored to the individual in a framework that includes incentives to weigh costs against benefits. The same objective can also be attained by financial arrangements between HMOs and nursing homes in joint ventures.

The obvious advantages of the S/HMO are the elimination of arbitrary boundaries between types of care and the incorporation of the case management function. The disadvantages are also obvious. The S/HMO has an incentive to minimize the quantity and quality of services provided; it is difficult to specify the nature of the contract between the S/HMO and the person, given the wide array of options for handling each case, making quality review difficult. Moreover, managing an ordinary HMO is a formidable task; adding these additional responsibilities makes the task still more difficult.

S/HMOs must also consider adverse selection. As in the case of life care communities, inaccurately forecasting the number of heavy users could bankrupt the S/HMO. Generally, S/HMOs have an incentive to manipulate the mix of enrollees to keep out heavy users. To minimize this problem, fees can be scaled by age or by other factors associated with greater use of services. Quotas can be established on individuals at high risk of needing expensive care. Reinsurance mechanisms (government or private insurance that limits the maximum amount a company will have to pay) can provide financial backing to S/HMOs that experience unexpectedly adverse enrollee mixes for a short time (17).

Adverse selection and the methods insurers use to handle it raise broader questions. The private insurance market groups people according to their level of risk and sets their premiums accordingly. Premiums rise with age, for instance. Society may wish to redistribute the cost of long-term care to a greater extent and along different dimensions than reliance on the market yields—for example, to include the young and the old or those with favorable and unfavorable genetic endowments in the same risk pool.

Someone already showing symptoms or with a family history of dementia would be likely to want long-term care insurance (or his or her family would want it). Given the potentially catastrophic level of costs associated with dementing diseases, the private insurance market would charge such a person a higher premium, or perhaps refuse to insure the individual at all. Requiring insurance companies to treat such people as if they were of average risk would raise premiums for all—or it might encourage companies to seek more subtle screening devices or to avoid the long-term care insurance market altogether. Including these people in a broader risk pool may require direct government intervention.

Private risk-pooling, through long-term care insurance or other means, is an attractive option

for allowing people to meet their own needs. However, the characteristics of dementia and the needs it generates make it a more difficult risk to insure privately than other conditions generating a need for long-term care. Individuals with dementia need the kinds of services that may be more susceptible to moral hazard—mental health services, personal care, chore services, and respite care. The duration of illness may be long; the person may end up in a nursing home, staying beyond the maximum 3 or 4 years covered by private policies. The slow onset of the disease may make it difficult to administer a preexisting condition clause in a manner that allows insurance companies reasonable protection against adverse selection while maintaining the value of the policy as protection against the costs of dementia.

Private Charity

Private charity is any assistance given by people outside a person's family but not paid for by government. It may take the form of services given informally by friends or unpaid volunteers or, more formally, by professionals paid out of charitable contributions. Such assistance is important in long-term care. Neighbors help care for homebound individuals so that family caregivers can get out. Organized groups provide services in the home such as meals on wheels and friendly visitors. Churches and philanthropists subsidize not-for-profit nursing homes and life care communities. Individuals with dementia and their families benefit from the activities of support groups such as the Alzheimer's Disease and Related Disorders Association (ADRDA). A recent innovation, the consumer health cooperative, promotes the sharing of information on sources of public and private financing and the development of a network of providers offering members discounts on long-term care services.

Volunteerism and private charity provide a dimension to long-term care that cannot easily be made available in any other way. Private individuals and groups can often be more flexible than government agencies. Charitable efforts add to people's sense of community. But, private charity is inherently unsystematic. People tend to respond to visible suffering and to victims with whom they can identify. Charitable efforts often depend on the organizational efforts of particular individuals.

Thus, private charity is limited in its ability to help meet a need as large as that of everyone with dementia.

PUBLIC FINANCING

Subsidies to Private Charity

Government provides some aid to volunteer efforts. The Administration on Aging (AOA), for example, has begun a project to support and train senior volunteers to provide in-home supervision of persons with dementia. AOA, the National Institute on Aging, and the National Institute of Mental Health have also provided training materials, seed money, and evaluation of family support groups such as ADRDA. The Department of Health and Human Services has provided a start-up grant to the United Seniors Consumer Cooperative in Washington, D.C.

Subsidies Through the Tax System

The government indirectly provides two kinds of assistance to those with dementia and their families through the tax system. One is tied to expenditures on patient care and lowers the effective cost of such care. The other is tied to other expenditures or to saving and raises the general level of family resources available for care or insurance premiums.

Examples of subsidies tied to expenditures on care are the medical expense deduction and the dependent care credit. Currently, the Federal tax code allows medical expenses above 5 percent of adjusted gross income to be deducted (this will change to 7.5 percent for 1987 and later years), provided the taxpayer itemizes deductions; it allows a tax credit for dependent care expenses when the care is required to allow the taxpayer to work. State income tax codes generally include these provisions as well.

Such tax breaks are subsidies because in forgiving a tax debt that someone would otherwise have to pay, the government loses and the taxpayer gains, just as if the government had sent the taxpayer a check. The value of the subsidy depends on the person's tax position, however, and on the amount spent and the goods purchased.

To benefit from a special *deduction*, the taxpayer must have enough deductible expenses to warrant itemizing. Middle- and upper-income people are more likely than low-income people to be in this position, especially if they are paying interest on home mortgages. The value of the subsidy is the individual's tax rate; the higher the tax bracket, the greater the subsidy.

A tax *credit* is subtracted from the individual's final tax liability, and thus does not vary with the marginal tax rate; some credits are scaled with income so that they are larger for low-income persons. But if a person is too poor to owe any tax, the tax credit is of no benefit, unless it is "refundable" (i.e., the person receives in cash the amount of the credit that exceeds his or her tax liability).

Thus, subsidies provided through the income tax system tend to vary inversely with financial need. This limits their usefulness as a method of evening out the distribution of the cost of long-term care.

In their current form, these tax provisions are of limited benefit to the families of individuals with dementia. The medical expense deduction has a medical orientation and thus does not apply to many of the expenditures caused by dementia. In the case of in-home care, only services performed for medical aid or treatment are deductible; if a nurse performs other services, the wages must be apportioned and nonmedical care cannot be deducted. Board and lodging in a nursing home are deductible only if the resident is confined for medical treatment; in judging whether to allow a deduction, the Internal Revenue Service looks to see whether the resident entered on direction of a doctor and whether the confinement had direct therapeutic effect on the individual's medical condition.

The dependent care provision does allow the credit for expenditures on personal care, but only if required to allow the taxpayer to work. The credit varies from 20 to 30 percent of expenditures up to $2,400, depending on income; it is not refundable. Thus, to cite a hypothetical but not uncommon situation, a retired couple living on a low to moderate fixed income, one of whom has Alzheimer's disease and requires in-home custodial care, would get little help from these tax provisions.

Several tax code provisions potentially increase the resources available to pay for care. Elderly and disabled taxpayers receive a higher personal exemption. (This extra exemption has been eliminated in 1987, and has been replaced by a special deduction of lower dollar amount.) Medicare benefits are nontaxable and social security benefits are taxed at a lower rate than other income. The government subsidizes saving for retirement by allowing taxpayers to delay tax on income received during their working years by putting income into employer pension plans or special savings instruments known as individual retirement accounts (IRAs) or self-employment (Keogh) plans until retirement. This effectively means lower taxes, since the income earns interest over the years and will usually be taxed at a lower rate after the person has left the labor force. (This tax deferrel feature of IRAs is retained in the new tax law, although new contributions to IRAs are no longer tax exempt.)

Tax subsidies for saving have similar drawbacks to those for expenditures on care. The value of the subsidy depends on the tax rate—the higher the tax bracket, the greater the subsidy. Moreover, the subsidy goes only to those who can afford to put money aside for retirement; for many, current needs are so pressing that they cannot spare money to provide for the future. For example, only 23 percent of taxpayers eligible to contribute to IRAs have taken advantage of the opportunity.

IRAs and other tax-deferred savings mechanisms are most likely to be used by middle income groups. In tax year 1983, for example, 59 percent of IRA deductions were taken by those with incomes from $20,000 to $50,000; 74 percent by those with incomes from $20,000 to $75,000 (27). Tax incentives might reduce pressures on publicly subsidized health and welfare programs by providing an alternative funding source for those

with middle and high incomes, but would not assist those most likely to become financially dependent.

On the other hand, tax subsidies, even if restricted to a minority of those needing to pay for long-term care, can nevertheless increase an individual's control over savings and spending. This may thus reduce demand for public programs that finance care, such as Medicaid.

Government Provision of Care

State mental institutions used to be a major source of care for elderly persons with dementia. The movement toward deinstitutionalization drastically reduced the population of mental hospitals and, in particular, ended the role they played as a source of care for that group. Direct government provision of care, as opposed to subsidization of care provided in private institutions, is now the exception rather than the rule.

The principal example of direct provision of care is the Veterans Administration (VA), the largest single provider of long-term care services in the country (see ch. 6). VA's role in long-term care illustrates a classic example of the ad hoc nature of the U.S. health care system. The VA system was originally developed to treat veterans with service-connected medical conditions, but gradually care for non-service-connected medical conditions (including long-term care) was made available to veterans on a space-available basis. The clientele served tended to be low-income veterans who lacked access to health insurance and non-VA health care. In 1986, VA began to apply means tests to certain services for veterans with non-service-connected disabilities (see ch. 6).

Long-term care has had low priority in the VA health care system. As the cohort of World War II veterans reaches retirement age, however, pressure on the long-term care segment of the VA is expected to increase (see ch. 1). The cost and scarcity of nursing home care may lead veterans who would not otherwise use the VA system to press for access to it.

During the most recent Congress, however, the trend was away from extending the number and type of benefits available to veterans at no charge. Public Law 99-272, which became law on April 7, 1986, established nine categories of veterans and criteria for how much veterans will pay for VA services. Services needed because of service-connected disability, and those delivered to veterans eligible for Medicaid or receiving VA income support, will continue to be available at no charge to the veteran. Most veterans seeking VA services because of dementia will not fit into these categories, however, and will pay a fraction of the costs of hospital, nursing home, or domiciliary care on 90-day cycles, with the maximum payment set by the prevailing Medicare deductible.

Finally, direct provision of care includes a variety of social and personal care services and mental health services provided by States, often funded partially or completely by Federal funds. Long-term care services are provided under Social Services Block Grants and Title III of the Older Americans Act, for example (see ch. 6). These efforts, like those of private charity, aid persons with dementia in an unsystematic way, with the availability of services varying arbitrarily from one locality to another, depending on factors such as local political priorities.

Subsidies for the Purchase of Care

Most public assistance to individuals with dementia comes through the Medicare and Medicaid programs. Medicare was initiated in 1965 to provide standard health insurance for people over 65; disabled and end-stage renal disease patients were added 7 years later. These groups had difficulty obtaining insurance because the private health insurance system was based on employment, leaving those outside the labor force at a serious disadvantage. The program's coverage structure was based on private policies, which emphasized medical care for acute conditions and did not cover long-term care.

Medicaid provides medical assistance to indigent people, another group largely left out of the private health insurance system. It was not introduced as a new national program designed to meet the needs of all the poor, however, but rather as an afterthought to the Medicare bill—a consolidation of existing Federal-State programs to pay

for medical care for people in certain federally assisted welfare programs. Thus, unlike Medicare, a uniform national program, Medicaid's structure varies considerably among the States.

Like Medicare, however, Medicaid emphasizes medical care for acute conditions and was not originally designed to meet long-term care needs. As there was no other source of funding for the growing population in need of long-term care, Medicaid took on the role. The program has become a backup financing source for nursing home care for middle-class people, not just for poor individuals. The high cost of residential care, the limited availability of affordable alternatives, and the relative absence of a private way to insure against this financial risk have created a group of people who are poor because expenditures on nursing home care have exhausted their resources. It has been estimated that 30 to 40 percent of nursing home residents supported by Medicaid "spent down" until they reached eligibility standards (36).

In discussing Medicare and Medicaid as financing sources for dementia patients, four aspects are important: eligibility, scope of services, reimbursement, and administration. Chapter 11 describes these in detail. This chapter reviews more briefly the features most relevant to policy options.

Eligibility

Eligibility standards for Medicare are national and independent of financial status. For people at least 65 who receive social security (the overwhelming majority), eligibility is automatic. People under 65 must qualify on the basis of permanent disability. To do so, they must have worked in social security-covered employment for 5 of the 10 calendar years before becoming disabled, and prove they meet the program's definition of permanent disability. The definition and the regulations and administrative processes that interpret it impose a heavier burden of proof on the mentally impaired than on the physically impaired. Many patients in the early stages of dementia have difficulty establishing their eligibility. Moreover, after establishing it, they must wait nearly 2½ years before benefits begin. The House and Senate Appropriations Committees have asked the Social Security Administration to review these policies in consultation with the National Institutes of Health.

Medicaid eligibility is more complicated. Enrollees must meet two kinds of requirements, categorical and financial, that vary by State. The categorical requirements are based on the eligibility requirements for certain federally assisted welfare programs. To meet them, the applicant must belong to one of several categories of persons considered in need of help, defined by age (at least 65), disability (either blindness, or total and permanent disability), or family status (member of a family containing dependent children deprived of the support of one parent for a reason such as absence, disability, unemployment, or death). Most individuals with dementia establish eligibility on the basis of age or disability. Proving disability under Medicaid raises the same problems for these people as it does under Medicare.

The financial eligibility requirements set the maximum net income and assets (after certain exclusions) a person can have and still be eligible for Medicaid. The upper limits vary across categories and by State but are always low (generally $1,500 or less in gross assets); to qualify, families must have incomes below the poverty line. Moreover, the rules on exclusions cause the impact of these financial requirements to be quite uneven among beneficiaries. Individuals with the same level of wealth receive different treatment depending on their State of residence, marital status, and the form in which they hold their assets or receive their income.

Some States have fixed income tests, others have flexible income tests. Under the first, the limit is applied without regard to medical expenses; under the second, the upper limit applies to the level of income after the cost of medical care has been deducted (in other words, the individual may "spend down" to a net income that makes him or her Medicaid-eligible). In either case, when someone enters a nursing home, the person's income above a small personal allowance, including any financial resources received as gifts, must generally be applied to the cost.

States can consider the financial assets of some family members determining whether the applicant meets financial eligibility requirements. If the spouse of an applicant, or the parent of an applicant under 21, has income and assets, these may be "deemed" to be available to the applicant (whether they actually are accessible or not) and thus included in the applicant's income. On the other hand, if the applicant's resources are deemed to be required to support a spouse or children, some portion may be excluded from consideration in applying the tests. Specific rules vary from State to State, but they are generally quite restrictive, and require that family members live at an impoverished level. Since deeming from family member to applicant usually ends with nursing home placement or divorce, it has the perverse effect of encouraging these events.

The financial assets of other family members, such as adult children, are generally not taken into account. According to the Health Care Financing Administration, States have the option of requiring relatives to contribute toward nursing home costs and a few have considered experimenting with "relative responsibility" laws (7). However, that interpretation of the Medicaid statute is disputed. Moreover, if the option does exist, the laws must be carefully drawn to be consistent with other provisions of the statute, such as the requirement that any provision in the State program must be "of general applicability."

Idaho, the only State to put a relative responsibility program into effect, found the results disappointing. The amount collected was low, it proved impossible to collect from out-of-State relatives, and the law was politically unpopular. The experiment ended after only 7 months when the Idaho Attorney General ruled that the law did not conform to the general applicability requirement (7).

The long duration of a dementing illness and the high probability that nursing home care will eventually be required makes Medicaid eligibility extremely important to persons with dementia and their families. These factors also mean that these people may be more likely than other long-term care recipients to be able to plan ahead for Medicaid eligibility and to use legal methods to arrange financial affairs appropriately. However, such planning takes a measure of financial awareness and possibly money for legal advice. Paradoxically, given Medicaid's welfare orientation, it may be the better-off families who gain the maximum advantage from the program, because they are sophisticated enough to appreciate the need for advance planning and can afford good legal advice. That adds a further inequity to the substantial ones inherent in the program's structure.

Scope of Services

Medicare covers only some of the services needed by individuals with dementia, and then only to a limited extent. A major problem is its orientation toward curative, narrowly defined medical services, reducing the coverage of care related to mental functioning or to nonmedical personal needs. Outpatient coverage for counseling and psychotherapy is limited to $250 per year. Coverage for personal care is restricted to skilled nursing care: services ordered by a physician, requiring the skills of technical or professional personnel such as registered nurses or physical therapists, and furnished by or under the supervision of such personnel. The coverage is designed to allow someone who has had an acute illness to convalesce briefly in a nursing home or at home rather than in a hospital to save on hospital expenditures—not to provide long-term care to someone chronically impaired.

If nursing care is provided in a nursing home, the facility must be certified as a skilled nursing facility (SNF). Coverage comes into effect only after a hospital stay of at least 3 days, and cannot exceed 100 days. Each case is reviewed retrospectively to determine whether the person actually needs that level of care; if not, reimbursement is denied. The actual average length of stay is only 30 days. As a result of these provisions, Medicare pays for less than 2 percent of nursing home care (15). If care is provided at home, no limit is imposed on the number of visits, but the definition of skilled care and the supervision requirements effectively restrict coverage to persons recovering from acute illness.

It is more difficult to summarize the scope of services under Medicaid, since coverage varies by State. Like Medicare, Medicaid is medically oriented. Federal requirements mandate coverage of certain basic services such as inpatient hospital services, physician services, laboratory and X-ray services, and they allow States to select others from a list of additional medical services; nonmedical services are generally not eligible for Federal cost-sharing. States may limit the amounts of services as long as the limits are applicable generally. This has been interpreted to mean unrelated to health condition or place of residence within the State; payment is usually restricted to a fixed number of hospital days per year or physician visits per month.

The major difference between Medicare and Medicaid is in the coverage of nursing home care. Medicaid reimburses for care at an intermediate level as well as at the skilled nursing level. Purely custodial care is nominally excluded from coverage, but the definition of intermediate care is sometimes interpreted to cover it. Unlike Medicare, Medicaid does not impose fixed time limits on the amount of nursing home care that will be reimbursed. As a result, Medicaid is a major source of financing for nursing home care, paying nearly 43 percent of total national expenditures (7).

Medicaid funding for home- and community-based services is more limited. Also, under both Medicaid and Medicare, if a person is cared for in the community, room and board costs remain the responsibility of the individual; if the person is placed in a nursing home, not only is the necessary medical care covered, but also room and board. Although Medicaid recipients must surrender income, except for a small personal allowance, any family contributions, in money or in kind, can cease. It has been argued that this creates a bias toward nursing home placement. Studies suggest that the physical and emotional burdens of care are more important than the financial incentive in the decision to move someone to a home (6,11). Nevertheless, that feature clearly leads to inequity in the distribution of the cost of care. Families that accept the burden in time and emotional strain of providing personal care to a dependent relative also bear a greater share of the financial cost than families of nursing home residents on Medicaid.

For those with dementia, a major weakness in both Medicare and Medicaid is that they direct services entirely toward program enrollees and thus do not cover services needed by the families, such as counseling. This orientation also leads to undervaluing of the benefits of services to individuals that at the same time provide respite for family caregivers. Adult day care, a few hours a day or week of personal services, or a week or two a year of institutional care can lighten the burden of caregiving to family members and perhaps enable them to remain effective in that role for a longer time (see ch. 4).

Concern over the high cost of nursing home care, and awareness of Medicaid's bias toward nursing home placement, led to a modification in the Medicaid statute that allows States to experiment with covering of home- and community-based services as a cost-containment measure. The "2176 waiver" program, introduced in 1981, allowed States to request waivers of standard Medicaid requirements in order to introduce new programs on a trial basis. For example, they could fund special programs for groups defined by health condition or place of residence and broaden the scope of services to include nonmedical ones (e.g., case management, homemaker and home health aide services, or adult care). Several States have used the 2176 waiver program to set up special programs for persons with Alzheimer's disease (20,44).

The value of the 2176 program has been limited by its emphasis on preventing nursing home placement, rather than on improving the care available to all patients in need. States had to demonstrate that the program would not cost any more, nor serve any more people than would have been served without the waiver. In other words, the program had to be narrowly targeted at those who would otherwise have entered a nursing home. It is difficult to predict who will enter a nursing home solely on the basis of physical and mental condition. Moreover, targeting those who would have entered a nursing home for special services raises questions of fairness. On the other hand, if subsidized home- and community-based care are simply made more available, expenditures are likely to rise, since many people in the community now receive inadequate care because of insufficient funds or unavailability of appropriate services (20,38,44).

Reimbursement

Eligibility for Medicare or Medicaid gives a person the financing for services, but imposes no requirement on anyone to provide them. Reimbursement largely determines whether individuals are able to obtain care, how much care they receive, what services they can use, and the quality of what they obtain. Although generous reimbursement does not guarantee good quality—particularly for those with dementia, who are poorly equipped to monitor provider performance—low reimbursement levels ensure that even the most dedicated and competent providers cannot deliver acceptable quality.

Reimbursement methods also affect the level and distribution of cost. Payment incentives influence a provider's attention to efficiency. When reimbursement covers less than full cost, the rest must be paid by the provider, the recipient, the person's family, or other people receiving the service.

Reimbursement policy under Medicare and Medicaid shows the conflict among access, quality, and cost objectives. Historically, Medicare and Medicaid have reimbursed facilities on a cost basis and individual providers on a fee-for-service basis. That system minimizes problems in access or quality if the full cost of care is covered and if physician fees match fees in the private sector. Hospitals and nursing homes may be able to charge higher prices to private individuals in the short run, but unless there are barriers to entry into the industry, new beds will be added until all who want care are placed. But such a system exerts no restraint on expenditure.

Fear of excessive impact on Federal and State budgets has caused restrictions on reimbursement, especially in State Medicaid programs. Cost formulas restrict allowable costs. Government payments for service are maintained at below market levels, especially under Medicaid, and limits are placed on the type and amount of services covered.

In the case of *hospital care*, rising expenditures have led Medicare to introduce a prospective payment system for hospitals based on case mix. Patients are classified by medical condition and other easily measured variables into 468 groups expected to require roughly the same resources. These are known as diagnosis-related groups, or DRGs. Hospitals are paid a fixed price for each patient's care based on the patient's DRG (except for a small number of "outlier" patients with unusually high resource use for their DRG). When the system is fully implemented in October 1987, the DRG price will be a national price based on average cost in a base period, adjusted for the hospital's urban or rural location and the area wage rate. Special payments are made for the direct and indirect costs of medical education, and the cost of capital is reimbursed separately, although efforts are now under way in Congress to find a way to include the latter in the new system (40).

Most State Medicaid programs still reimburse hospitals on a cost basis, although the cost formulas and restrictions on the amount of reimbursable services make the effective reimbursement rate lower for Medicaid patients than for others. A few States have adopted the Medicare payment system, however, and others are expected to do so in the future.

Reimbursement for *nursing home care* has been a particular target for budget-cutters. Medicare interprets the skilled nursing care benefit narrowly, reviewing cases retrospectively and often denying payment (18). (This policy was more important than the actual reimbursement level in limiting Medicare expenditures for nursing home care.)

Five State Medicaid programs pay nursing homes a flat per diem rate for all patients, whatever their condition, based on statewide limits on allowable costs. Equally important, many States restrain increases in nursing home capacity, creating a shortage of beds and therefore a queue for placement (38). The majority of Medicaid programs pay for nursing home services on a facility-specific cost basis but limit the degree to which costs are assessed.

Reimbursement restrictions often mean reimbursement at less than full cost, especially for individuals using more than an average level of resources. The national average rate for intermediate care under Medicaid was $38 per day in 1983. Providers have the choice of operating at a loss, lowering quality, manipulating resident mix by accepting only those who would have low costs, or avoiding Medicare or Medicaid recipients altogether. Also, because of low reimbursement levels, many private practice physicians choose not to participate in Medicaid; as a result, Medicaid patients have difficulty getting outpatient care in physicians' offices, and often end up in more costly settings such as hospital emergency rooms.

Nursing homes are reported to take private pay residents ahead of Medicaid and Medicare recipients (18,38). Nursing homes that are reimbursed on a flat-rate basis have an incentive to choose the lowest cost individuals from the queue, sometimes those who do not need to be in a nursing home at all. To ensure that Medicaid nursing home placement is appropriate, some State Medicaid programs have introduced preadmission screening. People often circumvent this screening process by "jumping the queue"—entering a nursing home on a private pay basis, then applying for Medicaid after spending down their assets; at that point, continued nursing home placement is likely to be the only realistic alternative (38).

To eliminate the bias against heavy-care nursing home residents and provide more equitable compensation to homes that accept them, seven State Medicaid programs have adjusted reimbursement for case mix (the type of residents). Some derive an overall average rate for each facility based on a case-mix index of the facility's population; others set a rate for each individual based on the level of care a person requires. One particularly comprehensive system (RUG-II) is conceptually similar to Medicare's new system for hospital reimbursement. Individuals are classified into 16 groups expected to be predictable in their use of resources; these are called Resource Utilization Groups, or RUGs.

The RUG classification is based on an assessment of need for skilled nursing and rehabilitative care; ability to perform three basic activities of daily living (eating, toileting, and transferring to and from bed or chair); and manifestation of four severe types of problem behavior (regression, aggression, verbal abuse, and hallucinations). Each RUG is assigned a fixed price per unit per day derived from average historical cost, and the nursing home is paid that amount for each resident based on the RUG classification. Residents are reassessed every 6 months and the RUG classification is adjusted, if necessary. The system has just been implemented in New York State (35). Other States are considering adopting their own case-mix-based reimbursement systems.

Current case mix systems were developed before special care units for those with dementia were widespread. They may thus understate the true costs of care tailored to the needs of those with dementia (see ch. 7). Special nursing home units report additional costs of $5 to $15 per day, although the basis for these costs has not been publicly documented. If these higher costs are borne out in further studies, case mix reimbursement may need to take account of eligibility for care on special units, or to revise upward the reimbursement levels for those who have dementia.

The effects of Medicare's new prospective payment system for hospitals are not yet known. However, certain effects are likely, given the financial incentives created. For example, DRGs create incentives for increased admissions but rapid discharge, economizing on the use of services during a person's stay, and for avoiding patients who use more resources than average. Since patients are likely to be sicker at time of discharge from a hospital, the new payment system increases the likelihood that patients will be discharged to nursing homes for short-term nursing care rather than to their homes. That may cause pressure to reduce the availability of beds for longer-stay nursing home residents, such as those with dementia.

In considering the effects of reimbursement on access, quality, and cost, it is important to recognize both the great variability in reimbursement levels and restrictions on supply across the country. Thus the impact of reimbursement on individuals depends very much on where they live, particularly for Medicaid recipients. (See table 10-1 in ch. 10, for a summary of Medicaid nursing home reimbursement rates by State.)

Looking specifically at the effects of reimbursement on individuals with dementia, a key question is whether they are, or are perceived to be, persons who use disproportionate amounts of

staff time or require services for which reimbursement is unusually low in relation to cost. It is dangerous to generalize about the answer to this question (see chs. 6 and 7). Persons with dementia vary greatly in their ability to care for themselves and their tendency to exhibit hostile or disruptive behavior. Systematic data are lacking on the distribution of symptoms across individuals and over time, as well as on the effects of symptoms on the cost of different types of care, under either existing or optimal conditions.

What data there are relate to overall nursing home care. For example, data collected for the RUG-II nursing home reimbursement system showed that persons with dementia were distributed across all groups, but on average used 5 to 6 percent more resources because they were more heavily concentrated in the higher disability groups (19). The designers of the RUG-II system found that the cognitive measures they used did not prove to be significant in designing the resource utilization groups. Assessment of the medical need, activities of daily living, and behavioral variables already mentioned was sufficient to group patients for cost purposes. In other words, once these characteristics were assessed, the additional information that the person has dementia is not a strong predictor of additional resource use for that individual. (If it is shown that residents benefit from services and activities specifically designed for those with dementia, then such services should be assessed in future case-mix studies.)

That result has been controversial. Identification of persons with dementia in the data is based on recorded diagnosis and an index of cognitive and behavioral variables. Some critics have argued that residents with dementia in the sample may not have been correctly identified, because the diagnoses were inaccurate and the measures of cognitive and behavioral variables used are inadequate. In particular, it has been argued that the RUG-II data did not discriminate well between those with dementia and others in the group of residents with the lowest levels of medical need and physical disability (19).

The intensity of the debate about whether persons with dementia require extra care suggests that even if they do not, many providers believe they do. That perception may lead to problems with access. Documenting the extent to which individuals with dementia experience greater than average problems with access to care is not easy, given the problems in identifying them. A study by the General Accounting Office showed that patients with mental and behavioral problems and those with significant dependency in activities of daily living were the ones who were likely to be found in hospital beds awaiting admission to a nursing home (38; see also 17). That finding and the extensive anecdotal evidence collected in an OTA survey of Medicaid programs suggest that access to care is a problem for individuals with dementia (10).

People may obtain access to care but then fail to receive appropriate care. Reimbursement policy must be made jointly with quality assurance policy, especially when providers can receive financial benefits by cutting quality (see ch. 10). Moreover, the policy must allow for change over time. For example, when reimbursement is adjusted for case mix, it is based on existing patterns of resource use. If persons with dementia are receiving suboptimal care now, that pattern may be frozen in place, since providers will not be adequately reimbursed for more appropriate care if it is more costly to provide.

In addition to the effects on access and quality, current reimbursement methods lead to inequitable distribution of the cost of care. The extent of subsidy varies arbitrarily across types of care, geographical areas, and providers, leading to quite different cost burdens for families with similar needs.

Administration

A program's structure on paper tells only part of the story of its impact on beneficiaries. The actual administration of the program is equally important.

Administrative barriers to obtaining Medicare services do exist. It is often difficult to obtain information about eligibility and scope of services from fiscal intermediaries and local social security offices. It may take several years to overturn an initial incorrect denial of eligibility for disability benefits. Administrative hearing rights are limited to situations in which the amount in question is at least $100; judicial review is only available if the amount is at least $1,000.

Medicaid has similar barriers. Its complexity makes the problem of obtaining accurate information about eligibility and coverage even more difficult than for Medicare. Eligibility determinations are often subject to substantial delays over and above those associated with the underlying social security or welfare determinations. Although Medicaid recipients have a broad legal right to administrative hearings in the event of erroneous actions by agencies and providers, quality control information collected by the Department of Health and Human Services suggests that fewer than 5 percent of recipients challenge incorrect negative case actions (i.e., actions to withhold, terminate, or deny benefits in violation of Federal law) (see ch. 11). Moreover, the only penalty a State incurs if it does make an error is disallowance of the Federal fraction of payment. Thus, there is no meaningful Federal check on giving a Medicaid enrollee too few benefits, but a substantial financial penalty for giving too many.

Administrative barriers exist for all individuals but are likely to be a greater problem for uneducated, poor, minority-group, and mentally handicapped persons. Those with dementia are likely to have problems unless they have active, involved family members to ensure that they get the services to which they are legally entitled. Particularly troubling is the indirect evidence that black individuals with dementia may have greater unmet needs (31). In OTA's survey of State Medicaid programs, in nearly every State that had utilization data available by race white Medicaid recipients 65 or older were receiving about twice as many services as black recipients (10).

ISSUES AND OPTIONS

Clearly, there are problems with the existing system of financing long-term care for persons with dementia. In evaluating proposals for change, decisionmakers must consider several basic questions. This section presents several key issues that must be addressed by public policy and then describes various proposed options. Because many of the options touch on several different issues, the discussion of issues and options is different from that in other chapters.

Issues

ISSUE 1: How Much Responsibility Should Government Take For the Care of Persons With Dementia?

One answer is, the government should take no responsibility. The problem of financing care for persons with dementia could be considered a private one, to be solved by individuals and their families, with the help of insurance markets and voluntary private charity. Although the private market and private charity have not solved the problem in the past, the future might be different. People are becoming more aware of the risk of developing a dementing illness and the needs such an illness creates, so there will be more private initiatives. The long-term care insurance market is developing, introducing new policies and marketing strategies. The population most at risk has greater financial resources than in the past. Financing devices such as home equity conversion may help free assets to pay long-term care insurance premiums. As the condition achieves higher visibility, more private charity will become available.

On the other side, however, there is reason to question the ability of the private market and private charity to solve the problem. Long-term care insurance is expensive, and moral hazard and adverse selection limit the degree of risk-spreading that can be achieved privately, especially for persons with dementia. Even if prudent members of the middle and upper classes could provide for themselves through private insurance, the poor and the imprudent would remain. Although the financial status of older Americans as a group has improved considerably, there are still major subgroups that are too poor to provide for long-term care at the time of use or through insurance. And there will always be those who can afford insurance but out of ignorance or poor judgment do not buy it. Given the expense of care, private charitable efforts are unlikely to be sufficient to meet their needs.

A decision that no government assistance is in order would be radical, since government at the Federal, State, and local levels already provides some assistance to persons with dementia. Withdrawal of government aid from these people, or from all who need long-term care, raises serious issues of fairness if other government health programs are left intact. It would be difficult to justify providing extensive assistance through Medicare for those who need hospital care and providing no assistance for long-term care, when long-term care can clearly be a greater burden.

A second position is, the government should encourage private initiatives to finance care but should not finance the care itself. In the case of dementia, government might encourage the development of long-term care insurance, home equity conversion, continuing care communities, social health maintenance organizations and long-term care savings funds. Government might encourage the formation of self-help groups and volunteer networks. Government might also fund research on the disease and educate the public about the need to make provisions for long-term care.

In the long run, these actions might help middle-class individuals with dementia but they will not solve the problems of the poor and the improvident. Therefore it might be argued that the government should subsidize the provision of long-term care. If it is decided that access to adequate long-term care should be guaranteed to all, special provision must be made for the poor and for those who fail to provide for their own needs in advance. Such provisions could be in addition to facilitating the development of private solutions. This position is implicit in existing policy. However, it raises complex questions about the proper structure of the subsidies, and these differ markedly among the various options described below.

ISSUE 2: Should Special Subsidies Be Set Up for Persons With Dementia?

Many proposals have been made for special treatment for those with dementia, such as extra tax deductions and exemptions for families and special services under Medicaid. It would be convenient to be able to help individuals with dementia and their families without having to fix the entire long-term care system, or the entire health care delivery system. It is widely recognized that these systems require fundamental changes, but the changes will not happen overnight; in the meantime, this group is suffering.

On the other hand, the categorical approach raises questions of fairness. Individuals with dementia have characteristics in common with others needing long-term care, who are also suffering. It is the combination of problems that makes the situation so difficult for someone with dementia, not the uniqueness of any one problem. There is also a practical difficulty. As chapter 8 discussed, there is no easy way to identify the members of the category. People with dementia already form a large fraction of the long-term care population; if there were financial incentives to having the diagnosis, instead of disincentives (as now), the number of people so classified would almost certainly increase.

ISSUE 3: Should Subsidies Be Provided on a Social Insurance or a Welfare Basis (i.e., be made available to all or only to the poor)?

Restricting subsidies to the poor and relying on private, market-oriented approaches to solve the problems of the other income groups would require a smaller government outlay. It would also be more in accord with American traditions of personal responsibility and limited government involvement in the health care system. Private enterprise may be more efficient and more responsive to consumer preferences than government bureaucracy.

On the other hand, history suggests that it can be difficult to maintain subsidies at a level suffi-

cient to guarantee adequate care, when the subsidies are provided only to a group with little political power. Government outlays may be lower under a welfare approach, but total social outlays may be greater in a mixed public-private system without the control over utilization and adverse selection that would be possible in a broad-based, compulsory social insurance system. A universal, compulsory system would also eliminate the inequity that results when prudent middle-class taxpayers must provide not only for themselves and the poor, but also for the imprudent.

ISSUE 4: How Should the Cost of the Subsidies Be Distributed?

If subsidies take the form of social insurance, should there be redistribution across generations, or should each generation bear the full cost of its own long-term care? Should there be redistribution across income classes? If subsidies are provided as welfare, what should be the income limits? Should close relatives be held responsible for the cost of care, and to what extent? Whatever the solution pursued, financing mechanisms should strive to avoid the abrupt discontinuities in program eligibility by income and in types of covered services that plague the current system.

ISSUE 5: What Is the Proper Relationship Between the Long-Term Care Subsidy Program and the Rest of the Health Care System?

Whether government subsidization is designed as welfare or social insurance, policymakers must consider the fit between public and private sectors, between long-term care and acute care delivery, between third-party payment for acute and long-term care, and between subsidies for health needs and subsidies for other needs, such as housing and nutrition. Because Medicare and Medicaid are such a large part of the health care market, they exert a profound effect on the entire delivery system. Coverage and reimbursement policies lead providers toward provision of services that are covered and reimbursed and away from others. Innovation and integration of services must take place within a structure that creates financial incentives for them. This assessment has described the inefficiencies and inequities that result from lack of coordination in the existing system. Moreover, government programs sometimes fail to solve a problem, yet by their very existence weaken the incentive to solve the problem privately. For example, some argue that Medicaid has been an obstacle to the development of private long-term care insurance, even though it hardly provides satisfactory protection against the long-term care risk, because the public does not realize how strict Medicaid income and asset restrictions are.

ISSUE 6: To What Extent Should the Availability of Assistance Vary With Place of Residence?

It would be impossible to provide exactly the same level of services everywhere in the United States, in remote rural areas and in large cities. On the other hand, in the existing system, the assistance available to those with dementia varies dramatically and arbitrarily with place of residence.

ISSUE 7: What Is the Role of Each Level of Government—Federal, State, and Local—in Subsidizing Care?

Providing assistance at the State and local levels puts it closer to the populations being served. On the other hand, it increases the likelihood of inequitable variations in access to services and distribution of cost.

POLICY OPTIONS*

The Federal Government could **encourage private initiatives to attack the financing problems of dementia patients**. Some efforts could be directed specifically at persons with dementia; equally important, Government could ensure that the special characteristics of that population are kept in mind when considering solutions to the long-term care financing problem in general. Some activities could be carried out without additional Government expenditure, e.g., by refocusing the activities of existing agencies or by serving as a catalyst for efforts funded by private entities. Other activities would require some funding but would not involve continuing subsidies to individuals. These include the following:

Develop the Knowledge Base About the Disease. —Information about dementia's epidemiology, progression, and optimal management would obviously be desirable for medical reasons. It is also of vital importance for developing private financing mechanisms, such as long-term care insurance.

Educate the Public About the Size of the Risk and the Need To Protect Against It.—It is tempting to allow Medicare recipients and their families to continue to believe that they are better protected against the costs of long-term care than they are. Only an unfortunate minority will discover the truth; the rest have peace of mind without the budgetary expense required to make the illusion of protection real. But an equitable and efficient solution to the long-term care problem requires a more accurate public perception of its nature and importance.

Promote an Appropriate Regulatory Framework. —Government regulation sets the framework within which private initiatives can occur. In the case of private long-term care initiatives, the objective of regulation is consumer protection. That objective is pursued through standards for product design and disclosure of information, and rules for the promotion of orderly competition and adherence to contracts among suppliers. Home equity conversion, private long-term care insurance, and life care communities are examples of issues subject to government regulation. The potential for exploitation and abuse—particularly of individuals with dementia—is clearly substantial. On the other hand, if not carefully structured, regulation can stifle innovation and deprive consumers of the benefit of new ways to meet their needs.

---

*Substantial parts of this section are based on "Financing Care for Patients with Alzheimer's Disease and Related Disorders," a paper commissioned by OTA from Karen Davis and Patricia Neuman (13).

Table 12-1.—Federal Policy Options (for explanation of options, see text)

Encourage private initiative to finance long-term care:
Develop knowledge base about dementia.
Educate public about risk and need for protection.
Promote appropriate regulatory framework.
Sponsor reverse mortgage insurance demonstration.
Provide reinsurance for private long-term care (LTC) insurance.
Promote efforts of private organizations to aid persons with dementia.

Subsidize individual efforts to meet LTC needs privately:
Subsidize savings for LTC through tax system.
Modify IRAs to allow tax-free withdrawal for LTC expenses after age 59 and allow tax-free accumulation to continue until age 75.
Authorize tax-deferred contributions solely for health and long-term care expenditures through IMAs (Individual Medical Accounts).
Subsidize family contributions to care through tax system.
Allow an additional exemption for dependents with dementia.
Allow itemized deduction or exemption for contributions toward care of a parent, whether or not parent is a dependent or child contributed more than 50 percent of parental support.

Increase direct Federal provision of services:
Expand VA LTC system with special emphasis on dementia-related services.

Modify Medicare and Medicaid:
Modify eligibility:
   Make dementia a presumptive cause of disability for Medicare.
   Combine above with elimination of two-year waiting period.
   Develop a uniform national treatment of income and assets for Medicaid eligibility.
   Allow people to avoid Medicaid spend-down by purchasing private LTC insurance.
Modify scope of services:
   Expand Medicaid and/or Medicare benefit package to include some or all of: case management, adult day care, personal care, chore services, attendant care.
   Increase coverage for mental health services; include counseling for caregivers.
   Include respite care services.
Modify reimbursement:
   Adopt case-mix reimbursement for nursing homes, with provision for any dementia-related extra costs.
   Give a major role to S/HMOs.

Modify administration:
   Provide better information about programs to those seeking services.
   Develop effective Federal sanctions for incorrect denial of benefits.

Support comprehensive reform of long-term care financing:
(for all who need LTC or dementia patients only)
Davis-Rowland proposal: Add a new *voluntary* LTC benefit to Medicare, financed by income-related premiums and general revenues. Benefits include nursing home, expanded home health, and community services. Benefits are subject to copayment with ceiling on total out-of-pocket expenditures per year.
Harvard proposal: Add *mandatory* LTC coverage to Medicare financed by beneficiary payments, payroll tax, and general revenues. Benefits include expanded nursing home, home health, and mental health services with copayment; geriatric assessment teams for case management. Nursing homes are reimbursed on prospective basis subject to a national or regional cap.
Kane and Kane Canadian model: Provide mandatory, universal LTC insurance coverage to all regardless of age or income, financed by block grants to states. Benefits are based on degree of impairment as assessed by gatekeepers; they include nursing home care, home nursing services, and homemaking services. Home care is free but subject to cap.
LTC Block Grants to States: Provide general Federal block grants to States for LTC; specify eligible population, covered benefits, payment and control mechanisms, or leave these entirely to States.
Bowen proposals: Support a major public education program; allow tax-free withdrawals from IRAs for long-term care expenses; create Individual Medical Accounts to encourage tax-free savings accumulation and limited risk-pooling; encourage long-term care insurance through a tax credit for premiums, expanding income-accumulation, and removing employer disincentives to cover long-term care as an employee benefit; add long-term care as an optional benefit for Federal employees.

SOURCE: Office of Technology Assessment, based on K. Davis and P. Neuman, "Financing Care for Patients With Alzheimer's Disease and Related Disorders," paper prepared for the Office of Technology Assessment workshop on Financing Care for Patients With Alzheimer's Disease and Related Disorders, May 19, 1986.

Most of the regulatory activity occurs at the State level. The Federal Government could, however, encourage States to consider appropriate regulation that accounts for the particular characteristics of those with dementia, and could encourage cooperation among States to ensure more uniformity in market conditions.

Sponsor Reverse Mortgage Insurance on a Demonstration Basis.—Freeing up home equity could

provide funds for the direct purchase of long-term care services or private long-term care insurance. This might save money in the Medicaid program by enabling people to provide for their long-term care needs out of their own assets, without forcing them to leave their homes. Development of home equity conversion instruments is hampered by the absence of mortgage insurance. A Federal demonstration program could stimulate the market and encourage private insurers to move in;

it could also be used to provide a model of disclosure and consumer counseling—important given the significance of the consumer's decision and its unfamiliarity.

Provide Reinsurance for Private Long-Term Care Insurance.—Government could set standards on private long-term care insurance and make qualified plans eligible for Federal Government reinsurance against adverse risk selection or high expenses. Reinsurance protection could include a stop-loss provision that would protect private plans against losses above a given level, or could assume coverage once some threshold was passed (e.g., 3 years of nursing home care or $100,000 per beneficiary).

An obstacle to developing long-term care policies is the profound uncertainty companies have about their future liability, given the unknowns of adverse selection; moral hazard; and trends in mortality, morbidity, and cost of long-term care. The availability of reinsurance might make companies more willing to experiment with long-term care policies. The reinsurance might more than pay for itself if the availability of private risk-pooling decreased the number of people who spent down to Medicaid eligibility. And even if it did not pay for itself, there might still be a substantial social benefit if many people were able to avoid the painful and demeaning spend-down process and government funds were targeted to the most needy. Such an approach would be of special value to those with dementia, since they are particularly likely to experience catastrophic expenses and thus to be considered unattractive risks by insurance companies.

On the other hand, if insurance companies are not effective in controlling insurance-induced demand and if the availability of third-party payment causes long-term care costs to rise significantly, reinsurance could be costly, and could drain funds from more needy groups to subsidize those able to afford long-term care insurance.

Promote Private Voluntary Efforts to Aid Persons With Dementia.—The Federal Government could encourage the activities of specialized organizations such as ADRDA in developing support groups, consumer cooperatives for the purchase or exchange of long-term care services, and in-

formation networks and referral services for individuals and families. It could encourage private organizations with a general health and welfare mission to pay attention to the special needs of those with dementia. Government encouragement could include coordinating, providing information, providing seed money for demonstration projects, or ongoing subsidies. This would encourage private innovation and initiative, while stretching scarce government funds to help more people. Its effectiveness would, of course, be limited by the availability of that private initiative.

The Federal Government could **increase its direct provision of services**. This approach would be more costly.

Expand the VA Long-Term Care System, with Special Attention to Services for Persons With Dementia.—VA already has experience in providing long-term care. Direct provision of services provides the opportunity for direct control of cost and quality. The population the VA has traditionally served is aging, will require a large volume of services in the years to come, and may expect to receive it from VA. By accepting responsibility for this group, VA would decrease the pressure on the rest of the system.

On the other hand, it may not be easy to control cost and quality in a large, geographically dispersed public system serving the chronically ill. Singling out veterans for better access to care for a non-service-connected disability raises questions of fairness. Fairness suggests that if the Federal Government is to provide long-term care services directly, it should be in a context of more general availability.

The Federal Government could **directly subsidize the efforts of private individuals to provide for their long-term care needs**. This approach would also be more costly.

Provide tax subsidies to encourage savings for the purchase of long-term care.

Modify Individual Retirement Accounts (IRAs) to Encourage their Use for the Purchase of Long-Term Care.—IRA savings withdrawn and used for health or long-term care after age 59 could be exempted from income taxation. IRA savings withdrawn and used for other purposes would be counted as taxable income, as at present. The current requirement that savings be withdrawn by age 70½ could be extended to age 75 or 80, when individuals are more likely to require long-term care.

Authorize Additional Tax-Deferred Contributions through Individual Medical Accounts (IMAs) with the Proceeds Restricted to Health and Long-Term Care Expenditures.—DHHS Secretary Otis R. Bowen and Thomas R. Burke have outlined a plan with the following features (5). At age 40 or 45, individuals would be given the option of procuring an IMA. Contributions would be sheltered from income and estate taxes, and would be held by the Federal Government in a health bank and invested at money market or high-yield government securities rates. If an individual dies before using the IMA funds, the original contributions, with some share of the investment income, would be returned to his or her estate. There would be no long-term care insurance component; individual's would have access only to those funds they saved. If long-term care expenses exceeded the IMA contributions, however, the balance would be met from the interest income that accumulates in the health bank. Individuals choosing not to contribute to IMAs would be at risk for all chronic care expenses and would have to spend down to Medicaid eligibility should they require long-term chronic care.

These options encourage individuals to save for future long-term care expenditures and give families the flexibility to use savings for services they feel best meet their needs. They also encourage the private sector to develop and market more services.

The value of the subsidy increases with income. Experience with IRAs suggests that they do little to increase total savings but merely shift savings from one form to another. Moreover, as noted, less than a quarter of taxpayers eligible to contribute to IRAs took advantage of the opportunity; these were predominantly higher income individuals (27). Savings incentives, however, could reduce the likelihood of reliance on Medicaid for a fraction of the population. These options do not pool the risk across individuals and provide no assurance that savings will be adequate to meet long-term care needs.

Modify Tax Laws.—Possible changes to tax laws could include the following:

- Provide tax subsidies to families contributing to the care of persons with dementia.
- Allow an additional tax exemption for dependents with dementia.
- Permit adult children of persons with dementia to claim an itemized deduction or exemption from income for financial contributions toward medical equipment, drugs, home health, and personal and nursing home care. This would not necessarily be conditional on demonstrating that the parent was a dependent or that the adult child contributed more than 50 percent toward the care of the parent.

The tax code, even after reforms made in 1986, already contains many subsidies for other purposes. They are intended to encourage people to do socially useful things by lightening the tax burden of those who do them. Taking care of someone with dementia is socially useful, and the families are certainly as much in need of help as those with other kinds of deductible expenses. It would be easier to get congressional approval for assistance in this form, since it does not appear in the budget. The cost might be offset to some extent by savings in the Medicaid program.

On the other hand, like tax subsidies for savings, subsidies for care would benefit higher income individuals more than lower income individuals, and would provide only minimal help to families in greatest need. This is particularly undesirable if there are direct subsidies to the poor and indirect subsidies to the better off; the poor are likely to be subjected to stricter limitations than middle and upper income groups. (The rising cost of Medicaid has attracted much more legislative attention than the rising cost of tax subsidies to health insurance for the employed.) The current trend is toward simplifying the tax code and eliminating rather than adding tax subsidies. Unlike direct expenditure programs, tax subsidies do not provide any opportunity for directly controlling the price or assuring the quality of long-term care services. Tax subsidies targeted specifically at individuals with dementia and their families raise issues of fairness, and would be difficult to administer given the uncertainties in diagnosis. Finally, the lower overall tax rates for 1988 and beyond make tax subsidies less valuable.

The Federal Government could **support incremental modifications in Medicare and Medicaid** to improve their ability to meet the financing needs of persons with dementia. The following possible modifications could be adopted individually or in combination:

Modify Eligibility

- Make it easier for those with dementia to establish eligibility for Medicare on the basis of disability by making dementia a presumptive cause of disability. This could be combined with a specification of an appropriate diagnostic procedure.
- Combine the above option with elimination of the 2-year waiting period.

These options would make acute care coverage available to those not eligible for Medicare on other grounds. However, the second option gives Medicare another diagnosis-specific category of patients in addition to end-stage renal disease.

- Develop a uniform national treatment of income and assets for eligibility for Medicaid.

The differences in treatment by income, assets and their composition, marital status, and place of residence are a major source of inequity in the existing Medicaid program. They also create perverse incentives with respect to purchase of private long-term care insurance, transfer of assets, and contributions to care in money and in kind by family members.

On the other hand, national standards would decrease State autonomy, and it would be difficult to achieve a consensus on a fair plan, given the wide differences in existing eligibility standards and State ability to pay.

- Allow people to avoid Medicaid spend-down by purchasing private long-term care insurance. For example, someone who purchased a specified level of long-term care coverage (e.g., 4 years of nursing home coverage or $100,000 of total long-term care expenses) could become eligible for Medicaid automat-

ically if his or her expenses exceeded the coverage level, without spending down assets. This option might foster the development of private long-term care insurance and thereby decrease Medicaid expenditures on the middle class. On the other hand, it would change the orientation of the program from welfare to social insurance and could conceivably raise expenditures rather than lower them, if utilization increased.

Modify Scope of Services

- Expand the Medicare, Medicaid, or both benefit packages to include some or all of the following: case management, adult day care services, personal care services, chore services, attendant care.
- Increase the limit on covered expenditures for mental health services; include counseling for caregivers.
- Include respite care services. For example, the benefit could be a specified number of days (e.g., 30 days for persons with severe dementia) during the year, which could be used by caregivers to spend time away from the ill person. They could have the option of taking the days in blocks of time (e.g., 2 weeks twice a year) or on an ongoing basis (e.g., half a day every week). The care could take the form of an attendant in the home or placement in a nursing home or hospital. Alternatively, the value of the benefit could be specified in dollar terms.

These options would make it easier to put together a package of services that would meet the needs of a person with dementia. Counseling and respite services for families would reduce stress on caregivers, improving their quality of life and, in some cases, postponing nursing home placement of the person with dementia.

On the other hand, such an expansion of coverage would be costly unless effective methods for restraining the use of services were developed. It might decrease the amount of informal support provided to individuals. Costs could be limited, however, by setting a maximum dollar amount on the extent of subsidy.

Modify Reimbursement

- Adopt case-mix reimbursement for nursing homes, with careful attention to any extra costs associated with dementia.

If properly structured, case-mix reimbursement could help eliminate bias against individuals with dementia in nursing home admission and provide financial incentives to give quality care. Data collection for case-mix reimbursement systems should incorporate accurate and effective assessment measures to identify those with dementia and establish baseline resource use for these residents. Provision should be made for quality review and for changes in reimbursement to reflect changes in the technology of managing people with dementia.

- Modify reimbursement to give a major role to S/HMOs.

Currently Medicare is testing the Social Health Maintenance Organization concept on a demonstration basis. If it proves successful, it could be instituted on a nationwide basis for Medicare or Medicaid, or both.

The advantage of the S/HMO is that it integrates acute care, long-term care, and social services. In providing managed care, it can offer individuals more of the services they want and need to remain in the community and at home, while incor-porating a mechanism for restraining utilization. It may even be able to save money by reducing inappropriate use of hospital, nursing home, and other medical services.

On the other hand, the extent of patient acceptability and the feasibility of cost savings have not been demonstrated. It would not be easy to determine capitation rates and manage the problem of adverse selection.

Modify Administration

- Provide complete and accurate information about the programs to those seeking long-term care services.
- Develop effective Federal sanctions for incorrect denial of benefits.

These changes would probably raise program expenditures, since the evidence, although incomplete, suggests that administrative errors and lack of information are more likely to deprive people of services to which they are entitled rather than the reverse. However, the changes would reduce the burden of obtaining benefits and distribute them more equitably.

The Federal Government could **support comprehensive reform of long-term care financing**. Several major long-term care financing options have surfaced recently. These options could

Table 12-2.—Summary of Comprehensive Reform Options

	Davis-Rowland	Harvard	Kane & Kane	Block Grants
Eligibility:				
Level of impairment	—	—	X	—
Age	X	X	—	—
Benefits:				
Assessment	—	X	X	—
Home- and community-based services	X	X	X	X
Nursing home	X	X	X	X
Respite	X	—	—	—
Case management	—	—	X	X
Counseling; mental health	—	X	—	—
Day care	X	—	—	—
Financial, other support for family	X	X	X	—
Financing:				
Medicare	X	X	—	—
Medicaid	X	—	—	—
General revenues	X	X	X	X
Copayments	X	X	X	—
Surcharge payroll tax	—	X	—	—
Public/private	X	X	X	—

be supported as designed, to apply to all elderly and disabled people, or they could be redesigned to apply only to persons with dementia.

Voluntary Medicare Coverage of Long-Term Care.—This option would add a new voluntary long-term care benefit to Medicare and finance it with an income-related premium administered through the income tax system (14).

The option has several major features. Covered benefits include nursing home care (both in qualified skilled nursing facilities and intermediate care facilities), expanded home health services (without many of the restrictions in the current Medicare program), and day hospital services. Benefits would be subject to a 10-percent coinsurance charge and would have an annual $3,000 ceiling on out-of-pocket costs. All persons age 60 or older would be eligible to enroll, but benefits would not be available until the person had been enrolled for at least 5 years. No one could enroll after age 70. A direct grant program to public and nonprofit community organizations would provide home services such as attendant care, personal care services, and chore services. The long-term care benefit would be financed with an income-related premium set at 4 percent of income for those who enroll at age 60 (with higher premium rates for those delaying enrollment) with a minimum annual premium of $200. Federal general revenues would be used to meet any long-term care expenditures not covered by premium revenues. Categorical Federal grant funds would be used to finance home help service programs. Medicaid long-term care coverage would continue as a residual program for those low-income people not choosing to purchase Medicare coverage. The Federal financial participation for residual Medicaid long-term care coverage would be reduced by one-half the current contribution rate.

Provide Mandatory Medicare Coverage of Long-term Care.—A study group has recently proposed mandatory coverage of long-term care under Medicare (21). The major provisions of the option are the following. The Medicare benefit package would be expanded by removing current restrictions on home health services and mental health services subject to 10 percent copayment. Home- and community-based services such as personal

care, chore services, attendant care, respite care, and adult day care would not be covered. Coverage for nursing home care would be broadened and custodial care added. Nursing home residents would pay a residential copayment to cover the room and board cost of a nursing home. This copayment would be set at 80 percent of social security benefit payments (or, for a couple, at 80 percent of the difference between the individual's and the couple's social security benefit payments). In addition, residents would pay a one-time, one-month nursing home deductible. Geriatric assessment teams would serve as gatekeepers to determine eligibility for benefits. Nursing homes would be paid on a prospective basis, subject to national or regional budget caps. Expanded benefits would be financed through a combination of payments by beneficiaries (25 percent of total cost), payroll (55 percent of cost), and Federal general revenues (20 percent). Beneficiary contributions would include copayments as specified above, premiums, and a 10 percent income tax surcharge.

Canadian Model of Long-Term Care Financing.—Two researchers have studied universal long-term care benefits in three Canadian provinces (Ontario, Manitoba, and British Columbia) and suggested that a similar approach would be feasible and desirable in the United States (29). Universal long-term care insurance in Canada replaced an earlier system of long-term care for the indigent. Although each provincial program is slightly different, the major features of this approach as applied to this country are the following:

Federal block grants would be made to States for universal long-term care insurance to all individuals regardless of age or income. Benefits would be based on degree of functional impairment, and would include nursing home care, home nursing services, and homemaking services. Residents would pay daily copayments of $10 to $15 for nursing home care. Payment to nursing homes would be set by level of care (e.g., personal care, intermediate care, psychogeriatric care, extended care for bedridden residents) and type of facility. Facilities would be paid on a negotiated per diem rate or a negotiated budget basis. Access to services would be determined on the basis of assessment by specified gatekeepers such as physicians, care managers, or home care coordinators. Homemaking services would be limited to a fixed number of hours per month or to a maximum cost not to exceed nursing home care. Home care would be free to the individual. Home nursing and homemaking services would either be provided by salaried public employees or purchased from for-profit or nonprofit agencies.

Long-Term Care Block Grants to States.—Another approach suggested in the United States is a more **general long-term care block grant from the Federal Government to the States. The grant could either specify the eligible population, covered benefits, payment, and control mechanisms required in a State program as a condition of Federal financial support, or it could leave these features solely to State discretion.**

The major financial burden for individuals with dementia is nursing home care. Although enabling as many people as possible to continue to function in their homes is a desirable objective, it is an unrealistic goal for many, particularly those in advanced stages of the disease. Therefore, some reform of long-term care financing will be required to provide adequate financial protection to families of those with dementia.

Otis Bowen, Secretary of the Department of Health and Human Services, recently released a report dealing with coverage of catastrophic illness. Coverage of long-term care was a major theme in the discussion, and recommendations included several options discussed in other sections of this chapter. The primary recommendations for long-term care coverage included:

- major education program involving the Federal Government and the private sector to acquaint the public with the risks, costs, and financing options for long-term care;
- tax-free withdrawal of IRA savings for long-term care payments, and establishment of Individual Medical Accounts to permit tax-free savings and permit limited risk-pooling;
- encouragement of private long-term care insurance by establishing a tax credit for long-term care premiums, permitting tax-free accumulation of savings analogous to life insurance, and removing provisions in current Federal law that discourage employers from

including long-term care insurance as an employee benefit; and
- establishment of long-term care coverage as an optional health benefit for Federal employees (41).

These recommendations are based in part on a report submitted to Secretary Bowen by the Private/Public Sector Advisory Committee on Catastrophic Illness, which held hearings and meetings throughout the country in 1986 (42). The final recommendations have been submitted to President Reagan for consideration.

All the comprehensive reform options discussed above would address coverage of nursing home care. The first three would provide financing for a broad range of long-term care services, including nursing home care. Coverage would not be conditional on an income eligibility test. Each would require some individual contributions toward nursing home care.

These options have the advantage of lightening the financial burdens now borne by those with dementia and their families. They are undoubtedly costly and would require substantial public budgetary outlays. Sources of revenue would need to be identified to meet these outlays. In addition, all the options would require mechanisms for assessing individual functional impairment in order to define eligibility and match services to needs. Each option is likely to improve the supply of long-term care services and choices among willing providers. To prevent abuses, however, each option would also require carefully designed quality control and payment provisions.

The option of voluntary long-term care benefit under Medicare has added advantages. It is designed to be self-financing and would pool risk across a large group of elderly persons. It would make spend-down less likely, reducing the need for middle-income elderly individuals to depend on Medicaid. It would expand the service options open to older Americans. Its major disadvantages are the possibility of adverse selection and the difficulties of dealing with those who require long-term care but did not enroll in advance.

Mandatory Medicare coverage would provide full coverage for all beneficiaries and pool the risk across all of them. It would not be affected by adverse selection. It avoids any gaps for those who might fail to purchase the voluntary benefit package. Similarly, it would have the greatest impact on reducing dependence on Medicaid. Its major disadvantages are the recommended increases in the payroll tax and drain on Federal general revenues, as well as opposition to new entitlement programs. As designed, it also does not deal with the types of home care services most useful to persons with dementia.

Supporting State programs for long-term care provides opportunities to consolidate and coordinate fragmented delivery systems and target attention and resources on the long-term care population. These approaches would be less likely to tie long-term care services to a medical model. Both run the risk of diverting financial responsibility for long-term care to the States, possibly leading to differences in adequacy of coverage, as well as political opposition from the States. Federal block grant allocations would be politically vulnerable since they are part of the annual appropriations and budget debate. Creation of a new program for long-term care could generate additional problems if it failed to coordinate with Medicare and Medicaid. Standards would need to be built into requirements for State programs to prevent the wide variations that now characterize the Medicaid program.

CHAPTER 12 REFERENCES

1. American Association of Retired Persons, "Long Term Care Research Study," survey conducted by the Gallup Organization, Jan. 30, 1984.
2. Bagby, N.S., "Home Equity Conversion," American Enterprise Institute, Washington, DC, 1986.
3. Barclay, L.L., Zemcov, A., Blass, J.P., et al., "Survival in Alzheimer's Disease and Vascular Dementias," *Neurology* 35:834-840, 1985.
4. Battelle Memorial Institute, "The Economics of Dementia," contract report prepared for the Office of Technology Assessment, U.S. Congress, 1984.
5. Bowen, O.R., and Burke, T.R., "Cost-Neutral Catastrophic Care Proposed for Medicare Recipients," *FAH Review*, 42-45, November/December 1985.
6. Brody, E., "Parent Care as a Normative Family Stress," *The Gerontologist* 25:19-29, 1985.
7. Burwell, B., "Shared Obligations: Family and Government Contributions to Long-Term Care," Medicaid Program Evaluation Working Paper 2.1, U.S. Department of Health and Human Services, Health Care Financing Administration, Office of Research and Demonstrations, February 1986.
8. Cahan, V., and Pave, I., "The Big Boys of Insurance Move Into Nursing Home Care," *Business Week*, Aug. 12, 1985.
9. Cantor, M.H., "The Family: A Basic Source of Long-Term Care for the Elderly," *Long-Term Care Financing and Delivery Systems: Exploring Some Alternatives*, P.H. Feinstein, M. Gornick, and J.N. Greenberg (eds.), Conference Proceedings, Jan. 24, 1984, HCFA Pub. No. 03174 (Bethesda, MD: U.S. Department of Health and Human Services, 1984).
10. Chavkin, D., "Interstate Variability in Medicaid Eligibility and Reimbursement for Dementia Patients," contract reported prepared for the Office of Technology Assessment, U.S. Congress, 1986.
11. Colerick, E.J., and George, L.K., "Predictors of Institutionalization Among Caregivers of Patients With Alzheimer's Disease," *Journal of the American Geriatrics Society* 34:493-498, 1986.
12. Cross, P.S., and Gurland, B.J., "The Epidemiology of Dementing Disorders," contract report prepared for the Office of Technology Assessment, U.S. Congress, 1986.
13. Davis, K., and Neuman, P., "Financing Care for Patients With Alzheimer's Disease and Related Disorders," paper prepared for the Office of Technology Assessment workshop on Financing Care for Patients With Alzheimer's Disease and Related Disorders, May 19, 1986.
14. Davis, K., and Rowland, D., *Medicare Policy: New Directions for Health and Long-Term Care* (Baltimore, MD: The Johns Hopkins University Press, 1986).
15. Doty, P., Liu, K., and Wiener, J., "Special Report: An Overview of Long-Term Care," *Health Care Financing Review* 6:69-78, 1985.
16. Employee Benefit Research Institute, "Financing Long-Term Care," *EBRI Issue Brief* No. 48, November 1985.
17. Eggert, G.M., "Medicare Coverage of Dementia: Current Opportunities and Future Directions," presented at Financing Dementia Symposium, California Alzheimer's Disease Task Force, Sacramento, CA, Feb. 20, 1986.
18. Feder, J., and Scanlon, W., "The Underused Bene-

fit: Medicare's Coverage of Nursing Home Care," *Milbank Memorial Fund Quarterly/Health and Society* 60:604-632, 1982.

19. Foley, W.J., "Dementia Among Nursing Home Patients: Defining the Condition, Characteristics of the Demented, and Dementia on the RUG-II Classification System," contract report prepared for the Office of Technology Assessment, U.S. Congress, 1986.

20. Greenberg, J.N., Schmitz, M.P., and Lakin, K.C., "An Analysis of Responses to the Medicaid Home- and Community-Based Long-Term Care Waiver Program (Section 2176 of Public Law 97-35)," Center for Residential and Community Services and Center for Health Services Research, University of Minnesota, submitted to the National Governors' Association Center for Policy Research, Washington, DC, June 1983.

21. Harvard Medicare Project, "Medicare: Coming of Age, A Proposal for Reform," Center for Health Policy and Management, John F. Kennedy School of Government, Harvard University, Cambridge, MA, March 1986.

22. Health Policy Forum, "Home Equity Conversion," Jan. 31, 1986.

23. Health Policy Forum, "The Developing Market for Long Term Care Insurance," Feb. 10, 1986.

24. Huang, L.F., Hu, T.W., and Cartwright, W.S., "The Economic Cost of Senile Dementia in the United States, 1983," contract report prepared for the National Institute on Aging, No. 1-AG-3-2123, 1986.

25. ICF Inc., "Private Financing of Long Term Care: Current Methods and Resources: Phase I-II; Final Report," submitted to the Office of the Assistant Secretary for Planning and Evaluation, U.S. Department of Health and Human Services, Bethesda, MD, January 1985.

26. ICF Inc., "The Role of Medicare in Financing the Health Care of Older Women," submitted to the American Association of Retired Persons, Washington, DC, July 1985.

27. Internal Revenue Service, Statistics and Income Division, *Individual Income Tax Returns/1983*, Publication No. 1304 (4-86).

28. Jacobs, B., and Weissert, W., "Home Equity Financing of Long-Term Care for the Elderly," *Long-Term Care Financing and Delivery Systems: Exploring Some Alternatives*, P.H. Feinstein, M. Gornick, and J.N. Greenberg (eds.), Conference Proceedings, Jan. 24. 1984, HCFA Pub. No. 03174 (Bethesda, MD: U.S. Department of Health and Human Services, 1984).

29. Kane, R., and Kane, R., "The Feasibility of Universal Long-Term Care Benefits," *New England Journal of Medicine* 312:1357-1364, 1985.

30. Lane, L., "Insurers' Response Growing to Consumer Demand for Long-Term Care Plans," *Business and Health* 3(3):49, 1986.

31. Lockery, S.A., "Impact of Dementia Within Minority Groups," contract report prepared for the Office of Technology Assessment, U.S. Congress, 1986.

32. Meiners, M.R., and Gollub, J.O., "Long-Term Care Insurance: The Edge of an Emerging Market," *Long-Term Care: Challenges and Opportunities*, Health Care Financial Management Association (ed.) (Oakbrook, IL: 1985).

33. Pies, H.E., "Life Care Communities for the Aged— An Overview," *Long-Term Care Financing and Delivery Systems: Exploring Some Alternatives*, P.H. Feinstein, M. Gornick, and J.N. Greenberg (eds.), Conference Proceedings, Jan. 24, 1984, HCFA Pub. No. 03174 (Bethesda, MD: U.S. Department of Health and Human Services, 1984).

34. President's Commission for the Study of Ethical Problems in Medicine and Biomedical and Behavioral Research, *Securing Access to Health Care, Volume One: Report* (Washington, DC: U.S. Government Printing Office, 1983).

35. Schneider, D.P., Fries, B.E., Foley, W.J., et al., "Development of RUG-II Case Mix Measurement System for Long-Term Care," Proceedings of the Annual Conference of the Health Service Division, IIE, American Hospital Association, Chicago, IL, February 1986.

36. SRI International, *Increasing Private Financing of Long-Term Care: Opportunities for Collaborative Action*, Report of Conference on Private Financing of Long-Term Care (Menlo Park, CA: 1986).

37. U.S. Congress, General Accounting Office, "The Elderly Should Benefit From Expanded Home Health Care, But Increasing These Services Will Not Insure Cost Reductions," GAO Pub. No. IPE-83-1, Washington, DC, Dec. 7, 1982.

38. U.S. Congress, General Accounting Office, "Medicaid and Nursing Home Care: Cost Increases and the Need for Services Are Creating Problems for the States and the Elderly," GAO Pub. No. IPE-84-1, Washington, DC, Oct. 12, 1983.

39. U.S. Congress, House Select Committee on Aging, *America's Elderly at Risk*, Committee Pub. No. 99-508 (Washington, DC: U.S. Government Printing Office, 1985).

40. U.S. Congress, Office of Technology Assessment, *Medicare's Prospective Payment System: Strategies for Evaluating Cost, Quality, and Medical Technology*, OTA-H-262 (Washington, DC: U.S. Government Printing Office, October 1985).

41. U.S. Department of Health and Human Services,

"Catastrophic Illness Expenses," Report to the President, November 1986.

42. U.S. Department of Health and Human Services, Private/Public Sector Advisory Committee on Catastrophic Illness, Report to the Secretary of Health and Human Services, Aug. 19, 1986.

43. U.S. Department of Labor, Office of Policy and Research, Pension and Welfare Benefits Administration, "Employer-Sponsored Retiree Health Insurance," Washington, DC, May 1986.

44. Weissert, W., "Innovative Approaches to Long-Term Care and Their Evaluation," paper presented to the Conference on the Impact of Technology on Aging in America, Feb. 16-18, 1983, Millwood, VA, as revised Sept. 30, 1983.

45. Wiener, J.M., "Financing and Organizational Options for Long-Term Care Reform: Background and Issues," paper presented at the New York Academy of Medicine Annual Health Conference: The Role of Government in Health Care: A Time for Reappraisal, New York, May 3, 1985.

Basic Biomedical Research Policy

"[In a time of budgetary constraint] with NIH being a discretionary program, that does create some difficult decisions."

—Otis R. Bowen, M.D.
Medical World News, Apr. 14, 1986.

"It is in the laboratory that we will solve this problem, but I do not know which laboratory."

—Peter Davies
Alzheimer's Disease Research Hearings,
U.S. House of Representatives, Sept. 20, 1984.

CONTENTS

Tables

Figures

Chapter 13
Basic Biomedical Research Policy

This chapter identifies some promising avenues of biomedical research that might lead to amelioration of disorders causing dementia. It also examines ways in which such research might be encouraged or enhanced by Federal action. An attempt is made to identify the advances needed to deal with the problem, and the degrees of progress that might be anticipated from different strategic approaches.

DEMENTING DISORDERS AND PUBLIC HEALTH

Dementing disorders are among the most costly public health problems the Nation is likely to face in the next 50 years. The personnel and scientific tools needed to begin to confront this problem already exist and have been mobilized. What remains is the need to focus the appropriate resources.

The magnitude of public health problems can be considered in a number of ways. These include ranking deaths attributable to specific causes (see table 13-1), measuring the economic costs associated with particular diseases, or counting the number of afflicted persons. Each of these simple measures is likely to understate the magnitude of the problem posed by disorders causing dementia.

Although significant numbers of people die with a dementing disorder, few deaths are attributed to dementia per se. One leading authority (13) has estimated that if dementia were listed as the cause of death for those suffering from it when they died, it would rank as the third or fourth leading cause (after heart disease, cancer, and stroke, but before accidents).

Table 13-1.—Mortality From Selected Causes, United States, 1981

Rank	Disease	Number	Percent of total	Cost (in billions)[a]
1	Heart	753,884	38.1	$14.5
2	Cancer	422,094	21.3	13.1
3	Stroke	160,504	8.3	5.1
4	Accidents	100,704	5.1	19.2
5	Lung	58,832	3.0	NA
	Total	1,977,981		

[a]Approximate 1980 expenditures on health care associated with these diseases.

SOURCE: Based on U.S. Department of Health and Human Services, National Institutes of Health, National Cancer Institute, *NCI Fact Book* (Bethesda, MD: 1985).

Measures of economic costs are particularly deceptive and difficult to apply to dementing disorders. Because of the insidious onset and extended care burden imposed by the most common cause of dementia (Alzheimer's disease), the economic impacts are more diffuse than with many acute diseases. Furthermore, any strictly quantitative measure, such as those imposed by economic models, obscures one of the major tolls of dementing disorders—that on the quality of life. Quality of life is diminished not only for the patient, but for family members who often must drastically reorder their lives in order to provide the necessary extended care. In spite of these enormous uncertainties, the best economic estimates to date confirm dementing disorders to be an enormous and growing problem (see ch. 1), costing between $24 billion and $48 billion a year in the United States (4).

Potentially the most precise method of estimating the size of the problem is through epidemiology and demographics—measuring the frequency with which dementing disorders are observed in the population, and identifying the extent to which different groups are at risk of developing such diseases. Yet problems and uncertainties with diagnosis make it difficult to determine precisely the size of the affected cohort. A recent report by the U.S. Department of Health and Human Services estimates that Alzheimer's disease appears to show a "ten- to twenty-fold increase in age-specific prevalence between the ages of 60 and 80, exceeding 20 percent by 80 to 85 years," and notes that these numbers "are generally agreed to be underestimates of the true prevalence" (30). Demographic data on the age distribution of the

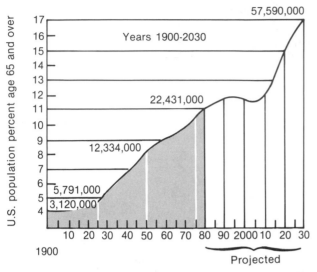

Figure 13-1.—Number and Proportion of U.S. Population 65 or Older, 1900-2030

SOURCE: Adapted from D. Watts and M. McCally, "Demographic Perspectives," *Geriatric Medicine, Vol. II. Fundamentals of Geriatric Care*, C.K. Cassel and J.R. Walsh (eds.) (New York: Springer-Verlag, 1984).

U.S. population show that the population at greatest risk (those age 65 or over) numbered more than 23 million in 1985, and may reach nearly 58 million by the year 2030 (see figure 13-1). Even making the conservative assumption that only 6 percent of this population is likely to be affected by severe dementia, the size of the affected cohort is enormous. Under that assumption, 1.38 million people would be afflicted in 1985, with more than 100,000 dying with Alzheimer's disease each year. By the year 2030, 3.4 million individuals could be affected.

WHY SUPPORT BASIC RESEARCH?

Basic research, the pursuit of knowledge for its own sake, is an enterprise with an irregular history of support by different societies. It is a legitimate question to ask why it should be supported in the United States today.

The first and most fundamental response is that the health of a free society depends absolutely on the widest possible dissemination of accurate information so that a citizenry called on to make vital judgments does so on the basis of information, rather than misinformation or wishful thinking. On a more immediate level, it has been argued that basic research is the fuel that powers the engine of applied research, the effort to take information and turn it in some way to material use or advantage. A host of examples can be drawn from experience with dementing disorders.

One major problem with the principal dementing disorder, Alzheimer's disease, is that no definitive diagnostic test is yet known. Diagnosis is by elimination of other known causes of dementia (e.g., head injury, adverse drug reactions, stroke, or cardiovascular disease). The lack of a specific diagnostic test is a serious clinical problem with

agonizing consequences for patients and their families. In searching for diagnostic tests and therapeutic measures, a number of different avenues can be explored.

Some types of dementia (e.g., Parkinson's disease, in which at least one-third of the 400,000 diagnosed patients suffer from dementia) (22) are known to be associated with a decrease in one of the chemical messengers by which nerve cells communicate with each another. By supplementing either these chemical messengers, or the precursors from which they are formed in the body, it is possible to bring about a partial remission of some of the motor symptoms of patients with Parkinson's disease. Although preliminary work along similar lines with Alzheimer patients has not proved fruitful, it is entirely possible that, over time, a better understanding of the distribution and function of such chemical messengers in the brain may lead not only to diagnostic criteria but also to possible therapies.

It is also known that metabolic activity (especially as monitored by the consumption of energy) varies between different structures in the brain, and at different times is associated with several brain activities. There is some indication that portions of the brain showing structural changes associated with Alzheimer's disease also show altered metabolic activity (9). That finding has been detected by studies using either computerized axial tomography (CAT or CT) scanning, magnetic resonance imaging (MRI), or positron emission tomography (PET) scanning. These are esoteric methods of producing high-resolution images of brain structure or chemical activity. None of these techniques would have been possible were it not for the serendipitous application of advances in a broad variety of unrelated fields—computer analysis, image processing, electronic circuit design, nuclear physics, nuclear medicine, and basic biochemistry. Yet these brain imaging techniques are among the tools holding bright promise for increasing scientists' understanding of the structural and metabolic processes involved in dementing disorders (see ch. 3).

It has been observed that dementia due to Alzheimer's disease is associated with several different structural changes in nerve cells in certain portions of the brain, e.g., neurofibrillary tangles and neuritic plaques (see ch. 3). The causes of these structural abnormalities are not clear. But preliminary reports suggest there may be biochemical changes (specifically, the presence of a specific protein) that accompany these morphological changes and may be unique to the brains of Alzheimer patients (36). Whether that particular finding fulfills its initial promise or not, it is advances of this sort that will lead to diagnostic tests for Alzheimer's disease.

These examples begin to illustrate what is perhaps the single most important feature of the neuroscience that is fundamental to understanding all dementing disorders—its broad, interdisciplinary nature. Its importance can be seen more clearly by reiterating the prominent theories on the causes of Alzheimer's disease, and by examining their implications in terms of the knowledge needed to deal with the disease if one or more of these causes is confirmed.

Postulated Causes of Alzheimer's Disease

At least five major candidates have been identified as possible causes of Alzheimer's disease (see ch. 3):

1. genetic factors,
2. environmental factors,
3. immunologic factors,
4. neurotransmitter deficit or differential nerve cell death, and
5. intrinsic metabolic factors.

These possible causes are not mutually exclusive. It is entirely possible that what is known as Alzheimer's disease is in fact a constellation of disorders of different cause but similar result, or that a dementia is the result of interactions among one or more of several causes. In any case, considerably more information on and understanding of this disease are needed.

If the genetic factors hypothesis is correct, a great deal more will need to be learned about both clinical human genetics and molecular mechanisms of genetic control. It is also true that to whatever extent any of the other theories are shown to be accurate, they will likely involve a significant genetic component. This is true not only because familial forms of dementia are known, but because all the mechanisms of neurochemistry, biochemistry, immunology, and susceptibility to environmental toxins or infectious agents inevitably have a genetic component.

If environmental factors such as metal exposure (e.g., to aluminum), head trauma, or infectious agents are shown to play a major role in the cause of dementing disorders, the prospects for prevention are excellent. But establishing the necessary correlations of cause and effect will require an enormous amount of work in epidemiology and environmental biology.

If immunologic factors are found to play a significant role, it will only be at the cost of a great deal of work in fundamental immunology and genetics. The prospects for treatment in this case may well be significant, though the evidence suggesting the importance of this hypothesis is weaker than for the others described here.

If neurotransmitter deficits or differential nerve cell death are shown to be of general importance in dementing disorders, researchers need to learn a great deal before their understanding will be sufficient to cure the disease. While it is agreed that disrupted nerve cell circuits are responsible for many of the cognitive deficiencies seen in individuals with dementia, those disrupted circuits are themselves symptomatic of underlying change. That more fundamental defect is the ultimate cause of the dementia.

Although significant progress has been made in the past 20 years, scientists' understanding of the fine-scale anatomy of the brain and the way specific populations of cells interact through time is rudimentary. Whereas it was once thought that the important chemical messengers between nerve cells numbered perhaps three or four, present estimates are that there may be 200 or more different neurotransmitters. Each of these is produced by specialized nerve cells whose distribution, function, and action through time and space are largely unknown today. A staggering number of studies of brain biochemistry are likely to be needed to clarify these relationships.

If metabolic factors are shown to play a major role, the extent of researchers' ignorance is similarly humbling. The great number of biochemical pathways involved in the synthesis and transport of the neurotransmitters and concomitant structures important to the genetic hypothesis will need to be elucidated and their manifold interactions understood. The prospect of therapeutic intervention here seems hopeful, but it is far too early to have any firm expectations.

In light of these various possible causes, it is understandable that one prominent neuroscientist has asserted that the level of complexity involved in the neurosciences is "at least four orders of magnitude greater than that involved with either heart disease or cancer" (23). To make this comparison more meaningful, it is illustrative to review the nature of the research effort that brought about the spectacular advances in treatment of heart disease over the past several decades.

Research Effort on Heart Disease

Heart disease is the single largest killer in the United States today, claiming 753,884 lives (38.1 percent of all deaths) in 1981 (33). The third most common cause of death, stroke, is also caused by vascular disease and hypertension. These diseases are the focus of the second largest component of the National Institutes of Health (NIH)—the National Heart, Lung, and Blood Institute (NHLBI). Established in 1948, this institute has seen substantial increases in funding since its inception (see table 13-2).

Appropriations (in real dollars) peaked in 1979 and have declined somewhat since then. The results of the support for research into the causes and treatments of cardiovascular disease have been unambiguous. NHLBI data clearly record a decline in the number of deaths per year from heart disease, especially over the past two decades (33). But the most interesting and instructive lessons of heart disease research have less to do with patterns of funding than with the types of research that are most productive in stimulating advances in clinical treatment. This question has long been interesting to the research and clinical communities and to academia.

In a definitive study published in 1977, two physicians and respiratory physiologists asked a group of 90 physicians and surgeons to select the 10 most important clinical advances in a broad field—cardiovascular and pulmonary medicine—that had made major contributions to saving or prolong-

Table 13-2.—NHLBI Appropriations, 1972-83 (in millions)

Year	Obligation	Amount in 1972 constant dollars
1972	$232.6	$232.6
1973	255.7	244.1
1974	327.3	293.7
1975	327.8	265.8
1976	368.6	278.0
1977	396.5	277.0
1978	447.8	291.2
1979	510.0	306.4
1980	527.1	290.3
1981	549.7	274.5
1982	559.6	260.5
1983	624.1	276.4

SOURCE: U.S. Department of Health and Human Services, National Institutes of Health, *NIH Data Book*, 1985, p. 9.

ing the lives of their patients, preventing disease, or decreasing disability or suffering (5). The study was undertaken because the researchers recognized the need for empirical data relevant to questions about the benefits of different types of research (as impressions of benefits were at that time largely anecdotal). The practitioners selected these 10 developments:

1. open-heart surgery,
2. blood vessel surgery,
3. treatment for hypertension,
4. management of coronary heart disease,
5. prevention of poliomyelitis,
6. chemotherapy of tuberculosis and acute rheumatic fever,
7. cardiac resuscitation and cardiac pacemakers,
8. oral diuretics (for treatment of high blood pressure and congestive heart failure),
9. intensive care units, and
10. new diagnostic tests.

The investigators then conducted a comprehensive literature survey of over 6,000 scientific papers in these fields and selected about 3,400 for closer scrutiny. Of these, 663 "key articles" were identified as having been essential to one or more of the top 10 clinical advances selected. An analysis of the 663 key articles found that 42 percent of them reported research done by scientists "whose goal at that time was *unrelated* to the later clinical advance." This was "untargeted" or "undirected" research that "sought knowledge for the sake of knowledge" and was not primarily concerned with addressing any particular clinical problem. Some 61.5 percent of the 663 articles reported research that was "basic," in that it sought to understand fundamental mechanisms of biological function or activity; 20 percent reported on descriptive clinical investigations that did not involve any experimental work on fundamental mechanisms; 16.5 percent described the development of new apparatus or techniques; and 2 percent involved review and synthesis of previous work (5).

The study also showed that while the majority of the key research was done in colleges, universities, and medical schools and their associated hospitals, important contributions came from other areas, including agriculture, dentistry, pho-

tography, veterinary medicine, and industrial laboratories. Clinical advances were fueled by a wide spectrum of developments in far ranging disciplines, many of them unexpected and unpredictable. A corollary to this observation is found in the nature of public perception of biomedical advances. Although significant advances are nearly always associated in the public eye with particular individuals (e.g., polio vaccine with Salk and Sabin, penicillin with Fleming, or the structure of DNA with Watson and Crick), these breakthroughs are in fact the products of enormous amounts of work by great numbers of contributing scientists. The individuals receiving the majority of public credit for significant advances were often fortunate to have pieced together the final elements in the solution of a problem.

The authors concluded that:

> The real problem in the allocation of federal research dollars is not whether they should be allocated to one *or* the other (clinically-oriented *versus not* clinically-oriented research or to applied *versus* basic research) because all have made essential contributions; the problem is *how much* to one and *how much* to the other. . . . [T]he first priority should be to earmark a generous portion of the nation's biomedical research dollars to identify and then to provide long-term support for creative scientists whose main goal is to learn how living organisms function, without regard to the immediate relation of their research to specific human diseases (5).

Research Effort on Cancer

The second leading cause of death in the United States is cancer. The diseases grouped under this name are the focus of the largest research effort carried out by NIH. Responding to a presidential initiative in 1971, Congress has continually increased funding for the National Cancer Institute until it reached $1 billion per year in 1980, a level around which it has since fluctuated (31).

This example is not nearly so clear-cut, nor hopeful, on first glance as is that provided by heart disease. Mortality statistics for cancer show slight increases from 1950 to 1982 (2) even though survival rates have also increased, and spectacular successes have been achieved against some specific, rare types of cancer (e.g., testicular cancer and childhood leukemia). Some have argued that the "war on cancer" is being lost, and have questioned the massive funding that research has consumed (16). Others have argued that the data illustrate the need for a shift in emphasis from treatment to prevention. Since the largest single cause of deaths due to cancer is essentially self-inflicted—from smoking—a simple change in community behavior would have a major impact on public health and economic burdens (2).

But it is also true that with the spectacular advances in knowledge of genetics and immunology, especially in the understanding of genetic mechanisms of disease exemplified by oncogenes, researchers now have a clear idea of what avenues of investigation will produce the additional information needed to improve clinical prevention and treatment of cancers. The unanticipated results of this massive research effort over the past two decades include the development of recombinant DNA technologies and monoclonal antibodies, and, thus, the biotechnology industry.

Implication for Neuroscience

Although some may dispute that the intellectual problems dementing disorders present to neuroscience are four orders of magnitude more complex than those posed by cardiovascular disease, one sentiment is broadly shared within the neuroscience community. That is that the level of complexity involved in understanding dementing disorders and the need for a broadly based approach are greater than with any previous public health initiative. In addition to clinical progress in dealing with dementing disorders, investment in basic research can be expected to shed much light on the nature of memory and the mechanisms of cognition (10,22,27). The impact that effect will have on the understanding of humanity will be significant.

Fruits of Basic Research

It is difficult to calculate precisely the relationship between the amount of money spent in efforts to solve a public health problem such as Alzheimer's disease and an improvement in public health. There is a variety of confounding factors.

For example, while the successes against smallpox and polio in the United States have led to enormous decreases in infant mortality and a commensurate increase in expected lifespan, the extended lifespan has acted to increase the incidence of cancer, arthritis, and other diseases associated with older ages. On the other hand, no reliable method exists to calculate the increased productivity due to those lives saved from smallpox though the individuals later die of cancer.

Independent of this type of problem, cost/benefit analyses of whatever sort are, at best, potentially misleading aids to guiding public health policy (20,28,35). The objective of biomedical research is public health, not parsimony (29), and it is widely recognized that using economic efficiency as the major criterion in assessing health care would lead quickly to a host of unacceptable practices. Maximum efficiency, for example, would mean that such treatments as dialysis be restricted to younger people, and that cardiovascular surgery and long-term care for the elderly be curtailed.

Although a precise understanding of the relationship between public health and biomedical research cannot be obtained, the general outlines are clear. The increase in average lifespan of the U.S. population is well known (figure 13-2).

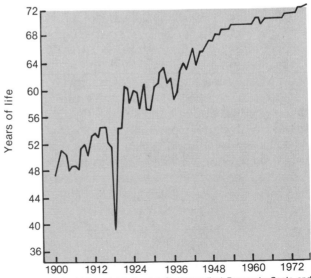

Figure 13-2.—Life Expectancy at Birth, United States, 1900-76

SOURCE: S.J. Mushkin and J.S. Landefeld, *Biomedical Research: Costs and Benefits* (Cambridge, MA: Ballinger Publishing Co., 1979).

The Federal Government has recognized that market economics do not support biomedical research adequately (28,29). A major reason is that federally supported research is related to the production of a public good (i.e., health), the primary nature of which is not measured in economic terms. Congress has therefore appropriated increasing amounts for this research, particularly since World War II. Total U.S. expenditures for basic research are divided among industry, other private sources, and the Federal Government, but a rough gauge of the shift in funding patterns for basic research can be seen in the growth of NIH relative to these other sectors (see figure 13-3).

While Federal support for health research and development channeled through NIH was proportionally the same in 1984 as in 1972 (at 36 percent of the total national effort), when measured in current dollars, inflation resulted in an erosion of nearly 20 percent in purchasing power over the 12 years. Additionally, while the fraction of

total spending by NIH has remained the same, spending by other Federal agencies for health research has declined from 25 percent of the total to 16 percent over the same period. The amount invested by industry has risen from 26 percent in 1972 to 39 percent in 1984, and that by all other sources has declined from 13 to 9 percent (31).

In 1982, for the first time the amounts spent by NIH and industry were roughly equal, at 37 percent each of the total. Since then, NIH spending has been surpassed by that of industry (33). This change is likely to diminish the leadership role Congress has intended NIH to assert in biomedical research; furthermore, it is important to recognize that NIH spending is likely to be qualitatively different from much of the spending by industry. Investment by industry is more likely to be directed at specific applications designed to return a profit. NIH spending is more likely to lead to broad advances over an entire field of understanding.

Figure 13-3.—National Support for Health R&D, by Source, 1972-85 (dollars in millions)

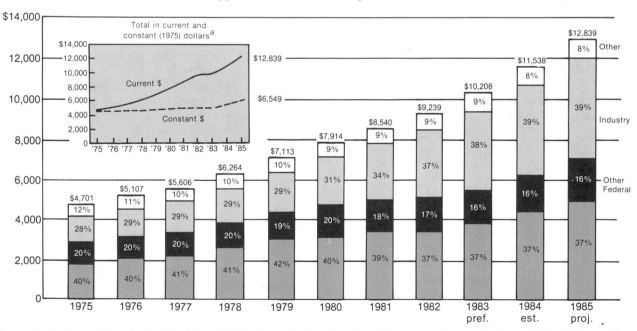

aConstant dollars based on biomedical R&D price index, 1975-1984. Projected to 196.06 for 1985, based on percentage increase in estimated GNP implicit price deflator.
SOURCE: U.S. Department of Health and Human Services, National Institutes of Health, *NIH Databook* (Bethesda, MD: 1985).

EFFORT DIRECTED AT ALZHEIMER'S DISEASE AND RELATED DISORDERS

Epidemiologic studies to date (6,17,26) suggest that the prevalence of severe cognitive impairment in those over 65 is about 6 percent. Some two-thirds of that is judged to be due to Alzheimer's disease (15). Post-mortem analysis confirms the presence of Alzheimer's disease in approximately 80 percent of diagnosed cases (25). One study in Finland found that an additional 4.3 to 15.4 percent of the population studied suffered from milder forms of impairment, for a total prevalence that "may be close to 20 percent" (26). A recent estimate for the United States is that 10 to 15 percent of Americans over 65 suffer from Alzheimer's disease or related forms of organic dementia (3).

That would mean that as many as 3.5 million people could suffer from Alzheimer's disease or other forms of cognitive impairment in the United States today. One estimate is that Alzheimer's disease may rank as the third or fourth leading cause of death in the Nation (13,14). The magnitude and range of these estimates demonstrate the need for better epidemiology studies and more precise measures of affected populations, especially among certain ethnic or minority groups.

The Federal Government's largest funder of research on Alzheimer's disease and related disorders is the National Institute on Aging (NIA) of NIH. Since 1979, this institute has funded the majority of research on these diseases. The other principal vehicle has been NIH's National Institute of Neurological and Communicative Disorders and Stroke (NINCDS), with significant efforts also funded by NIH's National Institute of Allergy and Infectious Diseases and the National Institute of Mental Health (NIMH), which is not part of NIH. Because of NIA's dominant role, its funding levels illustrate the Federal commitment to this problem. These data are given in table 13-3, which also includes the portion of NIA's budget directed toward Alzheimer's disease and related disorders.

Figures for the entire Federal effort in research relevant to Alzheimer's disease and related disorders are given in table 13-4. Although these numbers show nearly a tenfold increase in funding levels since 1976, Alzheimer's disease research is still receiving at least an order of magnitude less

Table 13-3.— NIA Appropriations, 1976-86 (in millions)

Year	Appropriation	Amount devoted to Alzheimer's disease and related disorders
1976	$19.2	$0.857
1977	29.9	1.500
1978	37.1	1.960
1979	56.5	4.140
1980	69.7	4.210
1981	75.6	5.190
1982	81.7	8.050
1983	93.9	11.850
1984	114.9	21.500
1985	144.4	28.800
1986	150.9	32.100
1987	—	32.100

SOURCE: U.S. Department of Health and Human Services, National Institutes of Health, *NIH Data Book* 1985.

funding than heart disease or cancer. Each of these diseases, it can be argued, poses public health problems of roughly equal, or even slightly smaller, magnitude by one or another relevant measure (e.g., estimated economic burden, anticipated rate of growth, or imposed societal burden).

Although analysts have abandoned the linear model that sees a simple progression from basic research to applied research to product development or treatment, the crucial role of basic research in medical advances and in economic growth is recognized (28). Because econometric models are inadequate to the task of measuring returns or monitoring the progress of basic research, researchers have begun to develop a science of bibliometrics, by which they seek to quantify patterns of publication. One of this field's crude but widely used estimates of progress is the number of publications on a specific topic.

Table 13-5 presents the results of a survey of all papers in biomedical journals from 1970 through 1985 that included Alzheimer's disease, dementia, or senility in their titles. If changes in funding research actually have an impact on scientific progress in an area, it would be expected that the number of papers published would follow funding levels with a lag of 3 to 5 years (28). The lag is imposed by the processes of conducting experiments, interpreting data, writing papers, peer review, and publication.

Table 13-4.—Total Federal Obligations for Alzheimer's Disease and Related Disorders, by Agency, 1976-86 (in millions)

Institute	1976	1977	1978	1979	1980	1981	1982	1983	1984	1985	1986[a]
NIA	$0.86	$1.50	$1.96	$4.14	$4.21	$5.19	$8.05	$11.80	$21.50	$28.80	$32.10
NINCDS	2.31	2.33	2.42	2.84	4.96	5.43	6.24	8.68	11.70	12.83	13.20
NIAID	—	—	—	1.38	1.78	1.39	1.26	1.04	1.34	1.21	1.01
DRR	—	—	—	—	—	—	—	0.60	0.70	1.03	1.01
AOA	—	—	—	—	—	—	—	—	0.16	1.13	0.60
NIMH	0.73	0.82	0.79	1.32	2.15	4.70	4.80	5.00	5.65	5.75	6.00
Total	3.90	4.65	5.17	9.68	13.10	16.71	20.35	27.12	41.05	50.75	53.92

[a]NIH estimates.
KEY: NIA=National Institute on Aging; NINCDS=National Institute on Neurological and Communicative Disorders and Stroke; NIAID=National Institute on Allergy and Infectious Diseases; DRR=Division of Research Resources, National Institutes of Health; AOA=Administration on Aging; NIMH=National Institute of Mental Health.
SOURCE: Office of Technology Assessment, from NIH data, 1986.

Table 13-5.—U.S. Research Publications on Alzheimer's Disease, 1970-85[a]

Year	Number of publications
1970	69
1971	58
1972	30
1973	81
1974	72
1975	89
1976	87
1977	130
1978	141
1979	88
1980	159
1981	226
1982	289
1983	317
1984	381
1985	548

[a]Based on a search of the database MedLine for all papers that included the words "Alzheimer's disease," "dementia," or "senility" in their titles.
SOURCE: Office of Technology Assessment, 1986.

The major, precipitous increases in funding research in dementing disorders to date came between 1978 and 1980 (see table 13-4). Table 13-5 shows substantial increases in publication after 1980, suggesting strongly that funding shifts have dramatic impacts on the conduct of research.

In spite of the increases in support of this research, a considerable amount of work judged likely to lead to significant advances in understanding of the disease processes involved is not being done because of a lack of funds. NINCDS was able to fund only 5 of 22 approved grants (22.7 percent) in 1983, and 10 of 43 (23.3 percent) in 1984. One of the most relevant divisions of NIA, the Molecular and Cellular Biology Branch, was able to fund only 6 of 35 (17 percent) proposals received in 1984 (34). The strong consensus among scientists in this field is that good proposals are definitely going unfunded. Some have stressed that valuable opportunities for progress are being missed or delayed.

Following a strategy that has been productive for other research, in fiscal year 1984 Congress appropriated $3.5 million for the establishment of five Alzheimer's Disease Research Centers to be administered by NIA. The announcement of the program resulted in the submission of 22 applications to establish centers. An additional five centers have been funded since. The centers are located at:

- Duke University,
- Harvard Medical School/Massachusetts General Hospital,
- The Johns Hopkins Medical Institutions,
- Mt. Sinai School of Medicine in New York,
- University of California at San Diego,
- University of Kentucky,
- University of Pittsburgh,
- University of Southern California,
- University of Washington, and
- Washington University in St. Louis.

Each center will provide shared resources for established investigators working on basic, clinical, and behavioral studies of Alzheimer's disease and related disorders. They will also fund new research projects and train scientists and health care providers new to Alzheimer's research. The present number—10—is about one-sixth the number of cancer centers that have been funded—

58, and two-thirds the number Congress initially mandated in 1971—15.

Grants to centers like these have been shown to be a more effective mechanism for supporting clinical research than for supporting basic science (11). The most effective mechanism for stimulating progress in basic research is widely agreed to be the investigator-initiated research grant (known to scientists as the R 01). These grants originate with a research proposal being submitted by an individual scientist, or by a small group of scientists working together. Applications are critically examined in a peer review process, which is widely considered to do an excellent job of evaluating the scientific merit of a particular proposal. The process involves rigorous review by 15 to 20 recognized authorities (the "study section") in the same or related disciplines. The applications are then either approved or rejected.

For grant applications approved as worthy of funding, a numerical priority score from 100 (best) to 500 is calculated to act as a guide in the distribution of funds. Most excellent proposals receive scores in the range from 130 to 160. Present funding levels (which vary among institutes and programs) lead to funding cutoffs in the range of 135 to 145, leaving many excellent proposals unfunded (22). Additionally, peer review tends to act against proposals that are perceived to be particularly bold or risky. In such cases, factors other than strict scientific merit can come into play. A major saving grace of the process is that program administrators may act to fund a particular proposal in spite of a priority score otherwise insufficient to assure funding, but they are naturally reluctant to overuse this prerogative.

In spite of the successes of peer review, the impossibility of supporting more than a fraction of excellent proposals approved (at current research funding levels) sometimes inhibits progress from developing as quickly as it might, as several specific examples illustrate. Parkinson's disease is associated with the loss of cells in the substantia nigra found deep within the brain. When a former chemistry student in California manufactured a heroin-like drug in his home several years ago, the chemical process involved a side reaction that introduced a dangerous contaminant into the final product. This contaminant, 1-methyl-4 phenyl-1,2,

3,6-tetrahydropyridine, known as MPTP, caused the selective destruction of the same cells in the substantia nigra whose loss is associated with the symptoms of Parkinson's disease (24) (see ch. 3). This unfortunate "natural experiment" provided an animal model for Parkinson's disease, but extremely stiff competition for scarce research funds meant the researcher who first elucidated this model was unable to exploit it fully for several years. That inability to obtain funding quickly serves to substantiate the widespread perception that valuable progress is being delayed.

Another example of the effects of scarce funding is found in the recent publication of results describing the presence of an unusual structural protein, possibly diagnostic, in the brains of Alzheimer's patients (36). A proposal to NIA to conduct this research was given a peer review priority score of about 230 (the lower the score, the higher the priority; present funding cutoff at NIA is near 140). The program administrators were unsuccessful in arguing that the proposal be funded in spite of the score. Although it does not commonly happen, another source of funds (in this case NIMH) was found by the principal investigator and the work was done, with its exciting, promising result. Although it is entirely possible that this particular finding may not live up to its initial promise, it is clear that work of this type offers great hope.

A logical consequence of combining peer review with limited funding is that "safe" projects will preferentially tend to be approved and funded—projects that the reviewers all agree have a high likelihood of producing results, even though they may not be earthshaking or revolutionary in their implications. This naturally conservative inclination brought about by limited resources often makes it difficult for a researcher to secure funds for imaginative or innovative types of work. It also militates against precisely the sort of interdisciplinary work so urgently needed in research on dementing disorders, wherein a scientist with one type of background and expertise reaches into a new discipline for tools to help in the primary work. As one such researcher has stated:

If I put a grant in to do what I am actually doing in the lab now, it would not get funded because the study section would say, "He has no experience, no training, and no reputation in the area of molecular genetics" (7).

Thus, although centers for research are vitally important, and contribute to valuable progress, the same is true of the investigator-initiated grants. For the best possible results to be derived from limited funding for research, a balance needs to be crafted between the two types of researchers competing for the limited funds available: neither should be overlooked in favor of the other (see table 13-6). As one commentator notes:

> While the need for interdisciplinary research performed by large units centered around sophisticated equipment is there, creativity, originality, and innovation remain, by and large, individual

traits. We must not stifle creativity by allocating insufficient funds to individual investigators or researchers (18).

It may well be that neuroscience stands in relation to Alzheimer's disease and related disorders as molecular biology and immunology do to cancer. The specific results of substantial increases in funding for research in the neurosciences are predictable only in the narrowest sense: more money will lead to more research, and more answers to particular questions. The serendipitous products of such research are—like restriction enzymes, monoclonal antibodies, and the biotechnology industry—wholly unpredictable.

ROLE OF NONGOVERNMENTAL ORGANIZATIONS

There are several areas where nongovernmental organizations, including private industry and philanthropy, have a logical role to play and may supplement or supplant Federal activities.

Private Industry

It is logical to expect private industry to be willing to invest in research that ultimately promises a profitable return. The most obvious of these, for dementing disorders, is the development of therapeutic drugs. Some work of this sort is already taking place (see, e.g., 12) in a way that illustrates the need for coordination among different groups.

The selection of drugs to be tested must be informed by an understanding of the biochemical defects involved in dementing disorders. In most cases these are not yet known, but this knowledge is the sort that will come from studies of fundamental neuroscience. Once candidate drugs have been selected, appropriate mechanisms of delivery must be identified and tested. The standard practices of injection or oral delivery are not likely to be effective with chemical therapies for dementing disorders because many drugs will not cross the blood/brain barrier. Novel technologies such as implantable infusion pumps are therefore being tested (12).

For drug trials to be useful, they must be carried out in a rigorously monitored environment by skilled clinicians. Thus, for pharmaceutical companies to contribute to research in dementing disorders, they must cooperate with clinicians in exploring avenues opened by advances in basic neuroscience.

Philanthropy

Private giving can make valuable contributions to scientific progress. The magnitude of the problems associated with dementing disorders puts effective philanthropy out of reach of all but the wealthiest individuals, and even of many foundations. But in some key areas philanthropy can make a crucial difference. These include funding creative or pilot programs, as well as fellowships for new, young investigators.

The Howard Hughes Medical Institute (HHMI) is potentially the largest source of private funds. It has targeted neuroscience as one of four major program areas for concentration of funding in biomedical research (the others being genetics, immunology, and cell biology and regulation). Twenty-two separate HHMI units are affiliated with universities and hospitals around the country. Neuroscience research is a major focus at seven of them (Yale, Columbia, Massachusetts Gen-

Table 13-6.—Future Research Areas Relevant to Dementing Disorders

Biological question	Techniques	Examples
Role of genes	Recombinant DNA technologies; Southern blots	Localization of Huntington's disease gene demonstration of retrovirus in brain tissue of patients with acquired immune deficiency syndrome (AIDS)
RNA changes	Assays of RNA distribution and activity; Northern blots; in situ hybridization	Reduced RNA in Alzheimer's patients; retrovirus present in brain cells in AIDS patients
Protein changes	Amino acid incorporation studies; SDS gels; immunocytochemistry	Reduced protein synthesis in Alzheimer's patients; phosphorylation of 200-kd neurofilament protein associated with neurofibrillary tangles (NFT) in Alzheimer's disease and with Lewy bodies in Pick's disease (PD)
Character of proteins in abnormal organelles	Purification and analysis of constituents; immunocytochemistry; freeze-fracture and deep-etch	Decoration of paired helical filaments with specific antibody; tubulin in granulovacuolar degeneration; actin in Hirano bodies; amyloid protein in congophilic angiopathy
Axonal transport of proteins	Radiolabeling and gel fluorography	Impaired transport of neurofilament proteins; aluminum poliomyelopathy
Altered transmitters enzymes	Neurochemical assays; radioimmunoassay	In Alzheimer's disease, reduced enzymes cortical cholinesterase acetyl transferase, somatostatin, and corticotropin releasing factor (CRF)
Changes in receptors	Binding assays; in vitro autoradiography	In Alzheimer's disease, reduced somatostatin and M2 cholinergic receptors in cortex; increased cortical CRF receptors
Changes in neuron shape and size	Golgi stains	Abnormal dendritic arborizations in Alzheimer's and Huntington's diseases
Structural abnormalities types of neurons	Immunocytochemistry	NFT in cholinergic and in specific somatostatinergic neurons; nonadrenergic neurites in plaques
Pathologic changes in specific brains	Computer-assisted morphometric methods	Reduced number of neurons in the nucleus basalis, hippocampus, and neocortex in Alzheimer's disease
Roles of specific systems in behavior	Lesion studies; behavioral tests	Memory impairments following bilateral lesions of the nucleus basalis in nonhuman primates
Demonstration of abnormalities in specific regions	Computerized tomography; PET and NMR imaging	Cerebral atrophy in Alzheimer's disease; hypometabolism in striatum in Alzheimer's disease infarcts in multi-infarct dementia
Role of infectious agents	Inoculation studies culture of virus	Transmission of Creutzfeldt-Jakob disease (CJD) to nonhuman primates; isolation of virus in AIDS
Nature of infectious agents	Methods of molecular virology	Characterization of AIDS retrovirus; description of unconventional nature of CJD virus
Treatment strategies	Drug trials; tissue grafts	L-dopa in PD; neural grafts improve functions of animals with lesions in the substantia nigra pars compacta

SOURCE: Based on D.L. Price, "Basic Neuroscience and Disorders Causing Dementia," contract report prepared for the Office of Technology Assessment, U.S. Congress, February 1986.

eral Hospital, Johns Hopkins, University of Texas at Dallas, and the University of California at San Diego and at San Francisco). Total outlays for research in all HHMI units and programs are on the order of $190 million to $200 million per year. Although neuroscience is the most recently declared of the four major program areas and precise figures are not available, a significant portion of this total is directed toward nondisease-related basic research in the neurosciences.

Another nongovernmental organization funding basic research in neuroscience is the Alzheimer's Disease and Related Disorders Association (ADRDA), with headquarters in Chicago. A little more than one-quarter of ADRDA's total annual expenditures goes toward supporting biomedical research (with the other two-thirds to public education, family and patient support, and advocacy efforts). A history of the funding the association has provided for research (most of it basic) is given in table 13-7. Total commitments in 1986 were $2.34 million, distributed among pilot grants, faculty scholar awards, and investigator-initiated grants. The Medical and Scientific Advisory Board of ADRDA finds that half of the proposals they receive are worthy of funding, yet ADRDA is able to support only about 16 percent of the applications received.

The growth rate in its receipt of good proposals is such that the award rate will continue to decline (8).

One of the few foundations making a focused effort in the dementing disorders is the John Douglas French Foundation for Alzheimer's Disease, in Los Angeles, founded in 1983. The major scientific thrust of the French Foundation has been to establish a fellowship program to provide primary salary support for investigators who have shown promise in research (see table 13-8). The foundation also has "a small grants program designed to supply seed money for creative research projects with a maximum funding of $30,000 per year" (19). In addition, twice a year the foundation sponsors workshops to foster exchange between basic and clinical scientists.

Other groups that may play a significant role include the American Federation for Aging Research and other private charities. But given the magnitude of the scientific problems that must be addressed, these organizations are unlikely ever to play more than an ancillary role in finding effective prevention or treatment for dementing disorders.

Table 13-7.—Research Supported by the Alzheimer's Disease and Related Disorders Association, Inc., 1982-86 and to Date

Year	Program	Proposals received	Proposals funded[a]	Amount
1982	Pilot Research Grants	67	7 (10)	$ 78,000
1983	Pilot Research Grants	75	11 (15)	132,000
1984	Pilot Research Grants	95	20 (21)	240,000
	Faculty Scholar Awards	17	3 (18)	342,000
	Total	112	23 (21)	582,000
1985	Pilot Research Grants	94	21 (22)	252,000
	Faculty Scholar Awards	34	6 (18)	684,000
	Parsons/ADRDA Grants	60	4 (7)	395,000
	Total	188	31 (16)	1,331,000
1986	Pilot Research Grants	210	35 (17)	691,000
	Faculty Scholar Awards	17	3 (18)	360,000
	Investigator-Initiated Research Grants	102	12 (12)	1,288,000
	Total	329	50 (15)	2,339,000
To date:	Pilot Research Grants	541	94 (17)	1,393,000
	Faculty Scholar Awards	68	12 (18)	1,386,000
	Parsons/ADRDA Grants	60	4 (7)	395,000
	Investigator-Initiated Research Grants	102	12 (12)	1,288,000
	Total	771	122 (16)	$4,462,000

[a]Number in parentheses gives percent of proposals received that were funded.

SOURCE: Alzheimer's Disease and Related Disorders Association, Inc.

Table 13-8.—Research Supported by the John Douglas French Foundation for Alzheimer's Disease, 1984-85

Year	Grants		Fellowships			Total value
	New	Renewals	Applications	Approved	Funded[a]	
1984	9	0	—[b]	12	4 (33)	$390,000
1985	3	3	150	38	12 (32)	$540,000

[a]Number in parentheses gives percent of approved grants that were funded.
[b]Program not established.

SOURCE: B. Miller, Scientific Coordinator, John Douglas French Foundation for Alzheimer's Disease, Los Angeles, CA, personal communication, 1986.

ISSUES AND OPTIONS

There is widespread agreement that major progress in the understanding, diagnosis, treatment, or prevention of dementing disorders will be based on the foundation of a strong, multidisciplinary research effort. How the Federal Government might best influence this progress is the primary issue with respect to research.

A strong program in basic research is clearly needed. Basic research must be balanced with a complementary program of clinical research. Both of these must be linked with research in health care services (discussed in ch. 1). The Federal Government historically has led such efforts by adjusting patterns of funding to meet perceived needs. The government has also acted to partition responsibilities among relevant agencies, and to effect coordination among them. The primary vehicle for administering funding in biomedical research has been NIH, with large efforts also at NIMH and the Veterans Administration.

With dementing disorders, the importance of NIMH is clear. For example, NIMH funding precipitated the explosion of work on neurotransmitters that brought a Nobel Prize to one researcher, made valuable contributions to the development of positron-emission tomography, and is playing a major role in the development of appropriate drug delivery technologies. With their expertise in epidemiology and demographics, the Centers for Disease Control also must be considered. Other agencies have mounted smaller efforts.

ISSUE: Should Congress act to balance and coordinate the research effort on dementing disorders?

Option 1: Designate a single entity as the lead agency for research relevant to dementing disorders.

Option 2: Empower a single advisory body to make recommendations on the coordination of research activities.

In any field of biomedical science relevant to human health, the best balance of basic and clinical research is difficult to determine. It will vary with the characters of the health problems addressed, the nature of the science involved in the relevant research programs, and the way these change and influence one another over time. As the authors of the definitive study on the connection between advances in basic research and advances in cardiovascular medicine pointed out, there is little reason to suspect that the problems in achieving the optimum balance could not best be handled by permitting the natural forces that govern the relationship between clinical and basic research to operate. At the same time, it is most important:

> . . . to earmark a generous portion of the nation's biomedical research dollars to identify and then provide long-term support for creative scientists whose main goal is to learn how living organisms function, without regard to the immediate relation of their research to specific human diseases (5).

Recent surveys show that essentially all major disciplines that can have a bearing on dementing disorders currently are being funded at some level, by one agency or another (22,30). That finding raises the issue of coordination.

In the past, Congress has met the challenges of coordinating a wide-ranging program of scientific research in several different ways. In some cases, a single agency or institute has been designated as the lead agency to administer and coordinate. In other cases a special task force has been given the authority to resolve conflicts of overlapping responsibility and to make recommendations. Reflecting the complexity and far-reaching nature of the scientific problems common to dementing disorders, elements of both these strategies can be discerned in the approach Congress has taken to date. Funding levels for research certainly reflect the importance of the efforts sponsored by the National Institute on Aging, which receives more money than all other relevant agencies combined. On the other hand, the Department of Health and Human Services has established a special Task Force on Alzheimer's Disease to oversee efforts within that agency.

Option 1 would have a number of advantages, many of them administrative. Research programs could be monitored with precision, expenditures adjusted easily, coordination maximized, and overlap minimized. The disadvantages would be scientific. Especially in times of limited funding, a single administrative source of funds would increase the likelihood that a promising grant or program might fail to be awarded due to vagaries of the peer review process or oversights in administration. A sole source of funding would be likely to decrease the variety and vitality of the research efforts within the scientific community.

If there is a major gap in the coordination of Federal efforts directed toward dementing disorders, it seems to be in coordinating health care services research with efforts in clinical research, and, ultimately, basic biomedical science. An authoritative advisory body (option 2) with the power to make specific recommendations to the President, the Secretary of Health and Human Services, or Congress could help effect such coordination. Such a body need not be nested within any designated lead agency. Indeed, it might be more valuable as an independent entity. The existing Secretary's Task Force theoretically has this power, but it has no legislative authority and is not an independent body.

ISSUE: Should Congress change the current level of funding for research on dementing disorders?

Option 1: Decrease research funding from current levels.

Option 2: Continue research funding at current levels.

Option 3: Increase funding modestly.

Option 4: Increase funding significantly.

The advantage of option 1 would be to make immediate, short-term, small contributions to deficit reduction efforts. Such an advantage must be weighed against the impact on a wide range of scientific disciplines. The total of current Federal spending in this field (approximately $54 million in fiscal year 1986) is small by comparison with many other Federal programs. If this spending were eliminated entirely, the Nation's operating deficit for fiscal year 1986 could be reduced by one-half of 1 percent. The long-term effects of reducing or eliminating funding cannot be quantitatively predicted. The most likely outcome would be to reduce the probability of finding causes, treatments, and means of prevention for dementing disorders.

The advantage of continuing funding at current levels (option 2) would be to avoid exacerbating budgetary problems while permitting some of the high-quality research that is possible within the existing infrastructure.

A modest funding increase, under option 3, is here taken to mean on the order of 20 to 60 percent ($10 million to $30 million per year). ADRDA has recommended "that federal support for research on Alzheimer's disease be assigned a high priority" at the National Institute on Aging, the National Institute of Neurological and Communicative Disorders and Stroke, the National Institute of Allergy and Infectious Diseases, and the National Institute of Mental Health, and that "funding for research . . . be increased to at least $75 million in fiscal year 1987" (1). The National Committee to Preserve Social Security and Medicare has recommended that Congress "double federal research spending to $100 million to find a cure for Alzheimer's disease" (21).

The largest contribution an increase of this magnitude could make to the Nation's deficit in the fiscal year 1986 operating budget would be approximately one-quarter of 1 percent. Funding increases on this order of magnitude would increase the amount of high-quality research possible within the existing infrastructure from between 10 and 20 percent to between 20 and 40 percent of projects now approved by peer review.

Although the social burden of dementing disorders is difficult to compare with that presented by other types of illness, it is of generally the same magnitude as cancer and heart disease. Yet research spending per patient is an order of magnitude lower. Such funding increases would also make it possible to begin preparing a skeletal framework within which to accommodate the increasing amount of medical care and biomedical research that will be needed to deal with the inevitable consequences of an aging population.

If option 4 were followed, and funding were dramatically increased (for example, to $1 billion per year), an immediate, short-term negative impact would be felt in deficit control efforts. (That additional spending would exacerbate current deficit figures by as much as 2 percent per year.) Such an increase would, however, make it possible to accommodate most, if not all, of the high-quality research now known to be possible by scientists in the relevant disciplines. It would also make spending per affected individual for research comparable to that for individuals affected by cancer or heart disease. Rapid, large increases in funding for research in this field also would likely lead to the funding of proposals that would be relatively weak by comparison with research now unfunded in other scientific disciplines.

Gradual increases in funding to a much higher level would surely improve researchers' understanding of principles and problems in mental health, psychiatry, learning disorders and disabilities, speech and memory defects, neurophysiological conditions, artificial intelligence, and many other fields. It would also enable the construction of the medical care infrastructure that will be needed to cope with the public health problems of an aging population. And in the event that this research leads, as all hope, to treatments or cures for dementing disorders, an investment in research could more than pay for itself by offsetting the tremendous and increasing economic and emotional burdens now borne by society.

CHAPTER 13 REFERENCES

1. Alzheimer's Disease and Related Disorders Association, Inc., *National Program To Conquer Alzheimer's Disease* (Chicago, IL: 1986).
2. Bailar, J., and Smith, E.M., "Progress Against Cancer?" *New England Journal of Medicine* 314(19): 1226-1232, 1986.
3. Barclay, L.L., Zemcov, A., Blass, J.P., et al., "Survival in Alzheimer's Disease and Vascular Dementias," *Neurology* 35:834-840, 1985.
4. Battelle Memorial Institute, "The Economies of Dementia," contract report prepared for the Office of Technology Assessment, U.S. Congress, 1984.
5. Comroe, J.H., and Dripps, R.D., *The Top Ten Clinical Advances in Cardiovascular-Pulmonary Medicine and Surgery Between 1945 and 1975: How They Came About* (Bethesda, MD: National Heart, Lung, and Blood Institute, National Institutes of Health, 1977).
6. Cross, P. S., and Gurland, B.J., "The Epidemiology of Dementing Disorders," contract report prepared for the Office of Technology Assessment, U.S. Congress, 1986.
7. Davies, P., U.S. Congress, House Committee on Science and Technology, Subcommittee on Investiga-tions and Oversight, *Alzheimer's Disease Research*, Hearings, Aug. 30 and Sept. 19-20, 1984, Committee Print 98-135 (Washington, DC: 1985).
8. Drachman, D., Chairman, Medical and Scientific Advisory Board, Alzheimer's Disease and Related Disorders Association, Chicago, IL, personal communication, July 28, 1986.
9. Duara, R., Grady, C., Haxby, J., et al., "Positron Emission Tomography in Alzheimer's Disease," *Neurology* 36:879-887, 1986.
10. Finch, C.E., "Alzheimer's Disease: A Biologist's Perspective," *Science* 230:1109, 1985.
11. Gee, H.H., "Resources for Research Policy Development at the National Institutes of Health," paper presented at the Health Policy Research Working Group, Harvard University, Mar. 20, 1985.
12. Harbaugh, R.E., Roberts, D.W., Coombs, D.W., et al., "Preliminary Report: Intracranial Cholinergic Drug Infusion in Patients With Alzheimer's Disease," *Neurosurgery* 15:514-518, 1984.
13. Katzman, R., "The Prevalence and Malignancy of Alzheimer Disease," *Archives of Neurology* 33:217-218, 1976.
14. Katzman, R., and Karasu, T.B., "Differential Diag-

nosis of Dementia," *Neurological and Sensory Disorders in the Elderly*, W. Fields (ed.) (New York: Stratton Intercontinental Medical Book Co., 1975).

15. Katzman, R., Laster, B., and Bernstein, N., " Accuracy of Diagnosis and Consequences of Misdiagnosis of Disorders Causing Dementia," contract report prepared for the Office of Technology Assessment, U.S. Congress, 1986.

16. Kolata, G., "Is the War on Cancer Being Won?" *Science* 229:543-544, 1985.

17. Kramer, M., German, P.S., Anthony, J.S., et al., "Patterns of Mental Disorders Among Elderly Residents of Eastern Baltimore," *Journal of American Geriatrics Society* 33:236-245, 1985.

18. Massey, W.E., "A National Research Strategy," *Issues in Science and Technology* 2:124-125, 1986.

19. Miller, B.L., Scientific Coordinator, John Douglas French Foundation for Alzheimer's Disease, Los Angeles, CA, personal communication, 1986.

20. Mushkin, S.J., and Landefeld, J.S., *Biomedical Research: Costs and Benefits* (Cambridge, MA: Ballinger Publishing Co., 1979).

21. National Committee To Preserve Social Security and Medicare, "Legislative Plan for Alzheimer's Disease," Washington, DC, 1986.

22. Price, D.L., "Basic Neuroscience and Disorders Causing Dementia," contract report prepared for the Office of Technology Assessment, U.S. Congress, Washington, DC, February 1986.

23. Purpura, D., Dean, Albert Einstein College of Medicine, Bronx, NY, personal communication, Dec. 11, 1985.

24. Stein, Y., and Langston, J.W., "Intellectual Changes in Patients With MPTP-Induced Parkinsonism," *Neurology* 35:1506-1509, 1985.

25. Sulkava, R., "Accuracy of Clinical Diagnosis in Primary Degenerative Dementia: Correlation With Neuropathological Findings," *Journal of Neurology, Neurosurgery, and Psychiatry* 56:9-13, 1983.

26. Sulkava, R., *et al.*, "Prevalence of Severe Dementia in Finland," *Neurology* 35:1025-1029, 1985.

27. Thompson, R.F., "The Neurobiology of Learning and Memory," *Science* 233(4767):941-947, 1986.

28. U.S. Congress, Office of Technology Assessment, *Research Funding as an Investment: Can We Measure the Returns?* OTA-TM-SET-36 (Washington, DC: U.S. Government Printing Office, April 1986).

29. U.S. Congress, Office of Technology Assessment, *Technology and Aging in America*, OTA-BA-264 (Washington, DC: U.S. Government Printing Office, June 1985).

30. U.S. Department of Health and Human Services, *Alzheimer's Disease: Report of the Secretary's Task Force on Alzheimer's Disease*, DHHS Pub. No. ADM84-1323 (Washington, DC: U.S. Government Printing Office, 1984).

31. U.S. Department of Health and Human Services, National Institutes of Health, *NIH Data Book* (Bethesda, MD: 1985).

32. U.S. Department of Health and Human Services, National Institutes of Health, National Cancer Institute, *NCI Fact Book* (Bethesda, MD: 1984).

33. U.S. Department of Health and Human Services, National Institutes of Health, National Heart, Lung, and Blood Institute, *Fiscal Year 1984 Fact Book* (Bethesda, MD: 1985).

34. Warner, H., Acting Chief, Molecular and Cellular Biology Branch, National Institute on Aging, National Institutes of Health, personal communication, July 2, 1985.

35. Weisbrod, B.A., *Economics and Medical Research* (Washington, DC: American Enterprise Institute, 1983).

36. Wolozin, B.L., Pruchnicki, A., Dickson, D.W., et al., "A Neuronal Antigen in the Brains of Alzheimer Patients," *Science* 232:648-650, 1986.

Appendixes

The Characteristics of Nursing Home Residents With Dementia

At the start of this assessment, OTA looked for a large database on nursing home residents that might be used to determine what proportion have dementia, how nursing home residents with dementia differ from other residents, and whether residents with dementia require more staff time or cost more to care for than other residents. In 1984, the New York State Case Mix Reimbursement Project collected detailed information on 3,427 residents in 52 New York State nursing homes as a basis for a new Medicaid reimbursement system, RUG-II. OTA contracted with Rensselaer Polytechnic Institute for retrospective analysis of that data.

The nursing homes included in the study had been selected to be representative of nursing homes in New York State in terms of location, size, type of ownership, levels of care, and staffing. A 10-page questionnaire, the Patient Assessment Instrument (PAI), was used to collect information on resident characteristics. Relative resource use by different residents was determined on the basis of a time and motion study that measured the amount of time spent by staff with each resident during a 24-hour period.

The PAI recorded residents' diagnoses using ICD-9 codes—i.e., numbers assigned to specific diagnoses in an international coding system. There is no ICD-9 code for dementia. Rather, the dementia syndrome is associated with many different ICD-9 codes (see ch. 1). Analysis of the database using the ICD-9 codes most likely to indicate dementia showed that 41 percent of all nursing home residents had one or more diagnoses associated with dementia (including primary, secondary, and tertiary diagnoses).

In general, residents with one or more diagnoses associated with dementia had greater impairment in activities of daily living (ADLs) (eating, dressing, bathing, toileting, bladder control, bowel control, and personal hygiene) and behavior (wandering, verbal abuse, physical aggression, and regressive or inappropriate behavior) than residents with no such diagnoses. However, residents with diagnoses associated with dementia varied greatly in ADLs and the behavioral characteristics measured by the PAI. Some had no self-care deficits, for example.

OTA and Rensselaer assumed that part of the reason for this variation was differences in severity of dementia; that is, residents with mild dementia were assumed to have different characteristics from those with severe dementia. Since the PAI does not include any measure of cognitive ability, severity of dementia cannot be ascertained directly from the data. However, a rough index of severity was constructed retrospectively by Rensselaer, in consultation with OTA. The five PAI items used to develop the index of severity are listed in table A-1, along with the resident descriptors and score values for each descriptor. A score value of 0 indicates that these descriptors are generally not characteristic of or specific to dementia. Higher score values are assumed to indicate increasing severity of dementia.

Residents were given a total score between 0 and 15 based on their scores on each of the five PAI items. Overall, 6 percent of residents with one or more diagnoses associated with dementia had a severity score of 0 (defined as "none"); 34 percent had scores between 1 and 5 (defined as "low"); 32 percent had scores between 6 and 10 (defined as "middle"); and 29 percent had scores between 11 and 15 (defined as "high").

Tables A-2 through A-11 show the proportion of residents with impairment in each of seven ADLs and four behavioral problem categories, according to whether they had any diagnoses associated with dementia and, if so, the severity of dementia. (Percentages have been rounded and may not total 100 percent.) The data demonstrate that as the severity of dementia increases (as measured by the index of severity), impairment in ADLs and behavioral problems also increase.

The New York State RUG-II system groups nursing home residents into 16 categories that differ in terms of clinical characteristics and use of resources. In general, residents with diagnoses associated with dementia were found in categories with higher disability more often than other residents. Further, residents with diagnoses associated with dementia had 5.6 percent greater resource use overall than other residents.

It should be noted, however, that these figures represent actual, not ideal resource use. In particular, residents with diagnoses associated with dementia were cared for in nursing homes that treat all kinds of patients, not special care facilities for persons with dementia. It is not known whether resource use is greater or less for dementia patients in special care facilities.

The index of severity used in this analysis is far from ideal for several reasons. First, it was developed retrospectively. Second, the five PAI items used to develop it require a subjective judgment by the interviewer; no standard tests were used to derive the response given. Finally, many of the descriptors used to develop the index of severity could apply to some persons who do not have dementia.

These problems point to the need, emphasized throughout this report, to include measures of cognitive ability in surveys of elderly and long-term care populations. While the reliability and validity of such measures are far from perfect, they do address the central features in dementia and are therefore more likely to accurately reflect severity of dementia than measures of other patient characteristics.

Both Texas and Massachusetts are or will soon be collecting data on nursing home residents to develop State Medicaid reimbursement systems. In Texas, the Mini-Mental State Exam (MMSE) (see ch. 8) is being used to measure residents' cognitive abilities. It is not known whether a measure of cognitive abilities will be included in the Massachusetts study (1).

Appendix A References

1. Cornelius, E., project officer, Health Care Financing Administration, Baltimore, MD, personal communication, Nov. 10, 1986.

Table A-1.—Resident Descriptors Used To Develop the Index of Severity

Questionnaire item	Score value
Expressive communication:	
1. Speaks and is generally understood	0
2. Speaks, but is understood with difficulty	0
3. Uses only structured sign language, writing, or yes or no responses	0
4. Uses only gestures, grunts, or primitive symbols to communicate. This includes a special cueing system developed with the patients (e.g., aphasiac)	1
5. Cannot convey needs (e.g., comatose)	2
6. Cannot determine	0
Receptive communication/comprehension:	
1. Generally understands oral communication	0
2. Has limited comprehension or oral communication; needs repetition or simplified explanations	1
3. Depends on lip reading, written material, or structured sign language	0
4. Understands only primitive gestures, facial expressions, simple pictograms, and/or recognizes environmental cues	2
5. Unable to understand or no indication by patient (e.g., comatose)	3
6. Cannot determine	0
Learning ability:	
1. Listens, retains, and comprehends directions or teaching instructions. Knows what to do and when	0
2. Difficulties retaining or comprehending instructions. Needs clues or continuous reminding	1
3. Cannot comprehend and retain instructions. Must be shown every time	2
4. Cannot comprehend and retain instructions. No instructions given	3
5. Cannot determine	0
Motivation:	
1. High—initiates activity, keeps appointments, willing to tolerate discomfort/pain to achieve goals	0
2. Moderate—will work toward goals but needs to external support and urging	0
3. Minimal—passive, participates in activities when told to when it is required. Activities may be performed in a slow, mediocre or inaccurate fashion	1
4. Poor—resists activity, feels someone else should do everything	2
5. None—due to organic causes	3
6. Cannot determine	0
Refusal to care for oneself:	
1. Performs routine activities (e.g., ADLs) to the extent physically capable	0
2. Performs routine activities (e.g., ADLs) but not to the extent physically capable. Activities are performed incompletely or are of mediocre quality	0
3. Resists assistance by others in performing routine activities (e.g, ADLS), though needs assistance from others	0
4. Refuses to perform routine activities (e.g., ADLs), of which physically capable. Staff must perform the activities	0
5. Unable mentally to perform routine activities (e.g, ADLs) regardless of willingness	4

SOURCE: W.J., Foley, ''Dementia Among Nursing Home Patients: Defining the Condition, Characteristics of the Demented, and Dementia on the RUG-II Classification System,'' contract report prepared for the Office of Technology Assessment, U.S. Congress, Washington, DC, 1986.

Table A-2.—Eating: Proportion of Nursing Home Residents by Eating Ability

Level of impairment	No dementia diagnosis	One or more dementia diagnoses				
		All levels of severity	None	Low	Middle	High
1. Independent—generally feeds self without supervision or physical assistance. May use adaptive equipment.	29%	13%	61%	26	3	1
2. Minimal supervision and/or physical assistance—requires intermittent verbal encouragement or guidance and/or physical assistance with minor parts of feeding, such as cutting food, buttering bread and opening milk carton, setting up equipment.	45	37	35	56	38	14
3. Continous supervision—requires constant one-on-one guidance, teaching and encouragement. May occasionally need help with eating.	11	20	2	12	33	17
4. Hand-fed—totally fed by hand. This includes syringe feeding.	13	27	1	6	22	61
5. Tube or parenteral feeding.	3	3	—	—	3	7

NOTE: Because of rounding, figures may not add to 100%.

SOURCE: W.J., Foley, "Dementia Among Nursing Home Patients: Defining the Condition, Characteristics of the Demented, and Dementia on the RUG-II Classification System," contract report prepared for the Office of Technology Assessment, U.S. Congress, Washington, DC, 1986.

Table A-3.—Dressing: Proportion of Nursing Home Residents by Dressing Ability

Level of impairment	No dementia diagnosis	One or more dementia diagnoses				
		All levels of severity	None	Low	Middle	High
1. Independent—uses no supervision or physical assistance. This includes obtaining clothes and managing buttons, socks and shoes.	18%	6%	38%	10%	1%	—
2. Minimal supervision and/or physical assistance—a person does not have to be constantly present to insure the patient dresses self. May need verbal directing and motivating for the proper arrangement and retrieval of clothing or speed in dressing, and/or putting on artificial limb.	21	11	35	24	1	—
3. Continuous supervision—requires a person to be present to guide, teach, and motivate patient during the entire task, (e.g., needs physical assistance with difficult parts of dressing, such as fasteners).	7	6	11	14	4	—
4. Continuous physical assistance—patient participates in task, but needs constant help with major parts of dressing (e.g., putting blouse/shirt over shoulders).	15	12	10	22	10	2
5. Total assistance—has to be completely dressed by another person; resident does not participate.	35	61	6	30	81	87
6. Patient generally wears a bed gown (60% or more of the time).	4	4	—	1	4	11

NOTE: Because of rounding, figures may not add to 100%.

SOURCE: W.J., Foley, "Dementia Among Nursing Home Patients: Defining the Condition, Characteristics of the Demented, and Dementia on the RUG-II Classification System," contract report prepared for the Office of Technology Assessment, U.S. Congress, Washington, DC, 1986.

Table A-4.—Bathing: Proportion of Nursing Home Residents by Bathing Ability

Level of impairment	No dementia diagnosis	One or more dementia diagnoses				
		All levels of severity	None	Low	Middle	High
1. Independent—requires no supervision or support. May use special equipment and water may be drawn for the patient.	3%	1%	7%	1%	—	—
2. Minimal supervision and/or physical assistance—requires intermittent checking and observing. May require physical assistance for minor parts of the task, transferring in and out of bath and bathing back.	23	9	45	18	1	—
3. Continuous supervision—requires constant one-on-one observation, motivation and guidance.	9	6	16	12	3	—
4. Continuous physical assistance—patient participates but requires constant help with most parts of bathing.	21	14	20	29	9	1
5. Total assistance—patient does not participate. Patient is bathed in bath, shower, or bed by another person.	44	70	12	41	87	99

NOTE: Because of rounding, figures may not add to 100%.

SOURCE: W.J., Foley, "Dementia Among Nursing Home Patients: Defining the Condition, Characteristics of the Demented, and Dementia on the RUG-II Classification System," contract report prepared for the Office of Technology Assessment, U.S. Congress, Washington, DC, 1986.

Table A-5.—Toileting: Proportion of Nursing Home Residents by Toileting Ability

Level of impairment	No dementia diagnosis	One or more dementia diagnoses				
		All levels of severity	None	Low	Middle	High
1. Independent—can toilet self without supervision or physical assistance. May require special equipment, such as a raised toilet or grab bars.	34%	18%	73%	36%	5%	—
2. Minimal supervision and/or physical assistance—requires intermittent observing and guidance for safety or encouragement reasons. May require physical assistance for minor parts of task, such as clothes adjustment and washing hands.	13	8	15	16	5	1
3. Continuous supervision—requires constant one-to-one guidance and teaching.	2	2	1	3	2	—
4. Continuous physical assistance—patient participates but requires constant help with major parts of the task or task will not be completed (e.g., maintaining balance, transferring, wiping and cleaning.	13	10	6	15	13	1
5. Total assistance—patient does not participate at all; another person assists with all aspects of toileting procedures.	10	12	2	7	18	12
6. Incontinent—taken to toilet on a regular scheduled basis.	16	26	2	16	34	35
7. Incontinent—does not use the toilet	13	25	—	8	23	52

NOTE: Because of rounding, figures may not add to 100%.

SOURCE: W.J., Foley, "Dementia Among Nursing Home Patients: Defining the Condition, Characteristics of the Demented, and Dementia on the RUG-II Classification System," contract report prepared for the Office of Technology Assessment, U.S. Congress, Washington, DC, 1986.

Table A-6.—Bladder Control: Proportion of Nursing Home Residents by Bladder Control Ability

Level of impairment	No dementia diagnosis	One or more dementia diagnoses				
		All levels of severity	None	Low	Middle	High
1. Continent—full control or rarely incontinent (i.e., less than once per week).	50%	24%	83%	47%	10%	1%
2. Occasionally incontinent—lacks bladder control at night and/or 1-3 times per week during the daytime.	11	10	12	17	10	3
3. Frequently or totally incontinent—4 or more times per week during the daytime.	29	58	5	32	74	81
4. Indwelling catheter—self care, no assistance needed.	—	—	—	—	—	1
5. Indwelling catheter—not self care, needs assistance.	7	7	—	3	6	14
6. External (or intermittent) catheter.	2	1	—	2	1	1

NOTE: Because of rounding, figures may not add to 100%.

SOURCE: W.J., Foley, "Dementia Among Nursing Home Patients: Defining the Condition, Characteristics of the Demented, and Dementia on the RUG-II Classification System," contract report prepared for the Office of Technology Assessment, U.S. Congress, Washington, DC, 1986.

Table A-7.—Bowel Control: Proportion of Nursing Home Residents by Bowel Control Ability

Level of impairment	No dementia diagnosis	One or more dementia diagnoses				
		All levels of severity	None	Low	Middle	High
1. Continent—full control or rarely incontinent (i.e., less than once per week).	59%	30%	90%	58%	14%	2
2. Occasionally incontinent—one time or less per week loses control. Is generally aware of the urge to move bowels and maintain control	11	12	4	13	18	5
3. Frequently or totally incontinent—two or more times per week loses. Is generally unaware of urge to move bowels.	29	57	2	28	67	92
4. Ostomy—self care, no assistance needed.	—	—	1	—	—	—
5. Ostomy—not self care, assistance needed.	1	1	2	1	1	1

NOTE: Because of rounding, figures may not add to 100%.

SOURCE: W.J., Foley, "Dementia Among Nursing Home Patients: Defining the Condition, Characteristics of the Demented, and Dementia on the RUG-II Classification System," contract report prepared for the Office of Technology Assessment, U.S. Congress, Washington, DC, 1986.

Table A-8.—Personal Hygiene: Proportion of Nursing Home Residents by Personal Hygiene Skills

Level of impairment	No dementia diagnosis	One or more dementia diagnoses				
		All levels of severity	None	Low	Middle	High
1. Independent—generally responsible for and receives no supervision or assistance with personal grooming.	18%	4%	28%	6%	—	—
2. Minimal supervision and/or physical assistance—requires intermittent verbal cueing or observation; and/or requires assistance with difficult parts of grooming.	24	12	54	26	1	—
3. Requires constant one-on-one observation, guidance and encouragement with all or most of personal grooming.	7	7	6	16	4	—
4. Continuous assistance—participates in personal grooming but needs constant physical assistance to complete grooming adequately or at all.	16	12	9	24	11	1
5. Total assistance—does not participate; another person performs all or most aspects of personal hygiene.	35	65	4	29	83	100

NOTE: Because of rounding, figures may not add to 100%.

SOURCE: W.J., Foley, "Dementia Among Nursing Home Patients: Defining the Condition, Characteristics of the Demented, and Dementia on the RUG-II Classification System," contract report prepared for the Office of Technology Assessment, U.S. Congress, Washington, DC, 1986.

Table A-9.—Wandering: Proportion of Nursing Home Residents Who Wander

Extent of wandering behavior	No dementia diagnosis	One or more dementia diagnoses				
		All levels of severity	None	Low	Middle	High
1. Does not wander.	95%	84%	95%	83%	77%	89%
2. Wanders with no clear direction in usual environment. May wander into another resident's room.	3	11	4	11	15	8
3. Unless supervised or restrained, wanders throughout the facility. Can find way back.	1	2	—	2	2	1
4. Takes every opportunity to wander away from unit. Cannot find way back.	1	3	—	2	5	2
5. Unless supervised or restrained, wanders outside the facility with no clear direction.	0	1	1	1	1	1

NOTE: Because of rounding, figures may not add to 100%.

SOURCE: W.J., Foley, "Dementia Among Nursing Home Patients: Defining the Condition, Characteristics of the Demented, and Dementia on the RUG-II Classification System," contract report prepared for the Office of Technology Assessment, U.S. Congress, Washington, DC, 1986.

Table A-10.—Verbal Abuse: Proportion of Nursing Home Residents Who Are Verbally Abusive

Extent of verbal abuse	No dementia diagnosis	One or more dementia diagnoses				
		All levels of severity	None	Low	Middle	High
1. No verbal abuse or disruption.	73%	57%	76%	53%	50%	66%
2. Occasional verbal abuse or disruption (i.e., three times or less per month).	11	11	12	15	11	6
3. Predictable verbal disruption during specific care routines only (e.g., bathing). Four or more times per month.	7	13	6	14	14	11
4. Short-lived verbal disruption during the day and/or night for no appropriate reason (e.g., not just during care routines). Four or more times per month.	3	5	—	6	6	3
5. Recurring verbal disruption during the day and/or night for no appropriate reason. At least four times per month, but not daily.	3	6	4	5	7	6
6. Daily recurring verbal disruption during the day and/or night for no appropriate reason.	3	9	2	7	12	9

NOTE: Because of rounding, figures may not add to 100%.

SOURCE: W.J., Foley, "Dementia Among Nursing Home Patients: Defining the Condition, Characteristics of the Demented, and Dementia on the RUG-II Classification System," contract report prepared for the Office of Technology Assessment, U.S. Congress, Washington, DC, 1986.

Table A-11.—Physical Aggression: Proportion of Nursing Home Residents Who Exhibit Physical Aggression

	No dementia diagnosis	One or more dementia diagnoses				
Extent of physical aggression		All levels of severity	None	Low	Middle	High
1. No physical aggression.	87%	68%	96%	72%	61%	65%
2. Occasional minor physical aggression (i.e., three times or less per month). Minor aggression refers to physical acts that cannot cause potential physical injury to self or others, but are disruptive).	5	9	2	10	10	9
3. Predictable physical aggression during specific care routines only (e.g., bathing) or as a reaction to normal stimuli (e.g., bumped into). May strike or fight.	5	15	1	11	19	19
4. Occasional extreme physical aggression (i.e., three times or less per month) to the point of potential physical injury to self or others (e.g., throws or pokes with sharp objects).	1	2	—	3	2	1
5. Recurring aggression for no rational reason (e.g., not just during specific care routines). At least four times per month, but not daily.	1	4	—	4	5	4
6. Daily recurring aggression for no rational reason (e.g., not just during specific care routines or reaction to normal stimuli).	1	3	—	2	3	3

NOTE: Because of rounding, figures may not add to 100%.

SOURCE: W.J., Foley, "Dementia Among Nursing Home Patients: Defining the Condition, Characteristics of the Demented, and Dementia on the RUG-II Classification System," contract report prepared for the Office of Technology Assessment, U.S. Congress, Washington, DC, 1986.

Table A-12.—Regressive or Inappropriate Behavior: Proportion of Nursing Home Residents Who Exhibit Regressive or Inappropriate Behavior

	No dementia diagnosis	One or more dementia diagnoses				
Extent of regressive or inappropriate behavior		All levels of severity	None	Low	Middle	High
1. Does not exhibit regressive or inappropriate behavior.	76%	51%	92%	60%	42%	41%
2. Exhibits nondisruptive regressive behavior, such as rocking.	14	23	5	18	28	28
3. Occasionally (i.e., three times or less per month) exhibits inappropriate behavior (e.g., smears feces, throws food, makes sexual advances).	5	7	—	7	9	8
4. Frequently (i.e., four times or more per month, not daily) exhibits disruptive and inappropriate behavior, such as frequently dressing and undressing self, smearing feces, throwing food, stealing, sexually displaying oneself to others.	3	9	2	9	10	9
5. Daily exhibits disruptive and inappropriate behavior.	3	10	1	7	12	15

NOTE: Because of rounding, figures may not add to 100%.

SOURCE: W.J., Foley, "Dementia Among Nursing Home Patients: Defining the Condition, Characteristics of the Demented, and Dementia on the RUG-II Classification System," contract report prepared for the Office of Technology Assessment, U.S. Congress, Washington, DC, 1986.

Contractors and Workshop Participants

Contractors

Linda Starke (Editor, through August 1986)
Washington, DC
Richard Ronca (Editor, September to December 1986)
Washington, DC

George J. Annas and Leonard Glantz
Boston University School of Law

Battelle Memorial Institute,
Columbus Laboratories, Columbus, Ohio

Thomas Beauchamp
Georgetown University

Dan W. Brock
Brown University

Allen Buchanan
University of Arizona

Elias S. Cohen
Community Services Institute
Narberth, Pennsylvania

Dorothy H. Coons
Institute of Gerontology
University of Michigan

Peter Cross and Barry Gurland
Center for Geriatrics and Long-Term Care
Gerontology
Columbia University

Karen Davis and Patricia Neuman
Johns Hopkins University

Randy Desonia
Intergovernmental Health Policy Project
George Washington University

Louise Dunn
Senior Respite Care Program
Portland, Oregon

Ronald Dworkin
University College
Oxford University

William J. Foley
Rensselaer Polytechnic Institute

Carolyn French
Atlanta Area Alzheimer's Disease and
Related Disorders Association

Michael Gilfix
Palo Alto, California

Allen Hammond
Editorial consultant, and
Editor, *Issues in Science and Technology*

Richard Jensen
American Public Welfare Association

Marshall Kapp
Wright State University

Robert Katzman, Bruce Lasker, and Nancy
Bernstein
University of California at San Diego

Korbin Liu
Urban Institute
Washington, DC

Bernard Lo
University of California at San Francisco

Shirley A. Lockery
Center on Aging
San Diego State University

John E. Luehrs
National Governors' Association

Lin Noyes and Richard Wittenborn
Dementia Resource Center and Family
Respite Center
Virginia

Nancy R. Peppard and Associates
Rockville, MD

Diana Petty
Family Survival Project
San Francisco

Donald Price
Johns Hopkins University

Daniel Sands and Judy Belman
Harbor Area Adult Day Care Center
Costa Mesa, California

Sallie Tisdale
Writer
Portland, Oregon

Elizabeth Vierck
Gerontological Consultant
Washington, DC

Audrey Weiner
Hebrew Home for the Aged at Riverdale
Bronx, New York

Thelma Wells
University of Michigan

Yankelovich, Skelly & White, Inc.
New York

Project Workshops

Congressional Agency Workshop on Long-Term Care Research, Apr. 5, 1985

Focus Group on Special Care for Patients With Dementia, June 2, 1985

State Approaches to Financing Long-Term Care of Patients With Dementia, Aug. 15, 1985

Making Medical Decisions for Mentally Impaired Adults, Sept. 23, 1985

Health Services Research on Long-Term Care of Patients With Dementia, Feb. 24 1986

Financing Long-Term Care for Patients With Dementia, May 19, 1986

Alzheimer's Disease and Dementia: How To Cope and Who Will Pay? Sept. 18, 1986

Participants of Workshops

Congressional Agency Workshop on Long-Term Care Research
Apr. 5, 1985

Dorothy Amey
Congressional Budget Office
U.S. Congress

Dorothy Guilford
National Academy of Sciences

Bruce Layton
General Accounting Office
U.S. Congress

James Linz
General Accounting Office
U.S. Congress

Korbin Liu
National Center for Health
  Services Research

Carol O'Shaunessy
Congressional Research Service
Library of Congress

Richard Price
Congressional Research Service
Library of Congress

Roger Straw
General Accounting Office
U.S. Congress

Cleonice Tavani
Office of Social Services Policy
Assistant Secretary for Planning
  and Evaluation,
Department of Health and
  Human Services

Susan Van Gelder
General Accounting Office
U.S. Congress

Focus Group on Special Care for Patients With Dementia
Long Beach, CA
June 21, 1985

Jeff Allen
Clearview Sanatorium
Gardena, CA

Judy Belman
Autumn Cottage
Costa Mesa, CA

Jodie Brandenberger
Alzheimer Service Program
Casa Colina Hospital
Pomona, CA

Hazel Castillo
Alzheimer Program
St. John of God
Los Angeles, CA

Dan Sands, M.Div
Harbor Day Care Center
Costa Mesa, CA

Randa L. Smith
Casa Colina Hospital
Pomona, CA

State Approaches to Financing Long-Term Care for Patients With Dementia
Aug. 15, 1985

Robert Burke
Committee on Nursing Home
  Regulation
Institute of Medicine
National Academy of Sciences

David F. Chavkin, Esq.
Maryland Advocacy Unit for the
  Developmentally Disabled, Inc.

Randy Desonia
Intergovernmental Health Policy
  Program
George Washington University

John E. Luehrs
National Governor's Association

Susan Van Gelder
General Accounting Office
U.S. Congress

Gail Wilenski
Project HOPE

Steve Zuckerman
The Urban Institute

Making Medical Decisions for Mentally Impaired Adults
Sept., 23 1985

Thomas L. Beauchamp
Kennedy Institute of Ethics
Georgetown University

Richard W. Besdine
Hebrew Rehabilitation Center for
  the Aging
Roslyndale, MA

Elias S. Cohen
Community Services Institute, Inc.
Narbeth, PA

Dorothy H. Coons
Institute of Gerontology
University of Michigan

Ronald E. Cranford
Department of Neurology
Hennepin County Medical Center
Minneapolis, MN

Anne J. Davis
Department of Mental Health and
  Community Nursing
University of California, San
  Francisco

Daniel C. Dennett
Department of Philosophy
Tufts University

Nancy Neveloff Dubler
Division of Legal and Ethical
  Issues in Health Care
Montefiore Medical Center
Bronx, NY

Bernard Lo
Division of General Internal
  Medicine
Institute for Health Policy Studies
University of California, San
  Francisco

DaCosta R. Mason, Esq.
Legal Counsel for the Elderly
District of Columbia Corporation
  Counsel

Alan Meisel
School of Law
University of Pittsburgh

Vijaya L. Melnick
Center for Applied Research and
  Urban Policy
University of the District of
  Columbia

Paul Nathanson
University of New Mexico
Institute of Public Law

Cynthia E. Northrop, Esq.
Attorney
New York, NY

John J. Regan
School of Law
Hofstra University
Hempstead, NY

Marion Roach
Journalist
New York, NY

Randa Lee Smith
Alzheimer Program
Casa Colina Hospital
Pomona, CA

David C. Thomasma
Loyola Stritch School of Medicine
Loyola University Medical Center
Maywood, IL

Daniel Wikler
Department of History of
    Medicine
Program in Ethics
University of Wisconsin

Health Services Research on Long-Term Care of Patients With Dementia*
Feb. 24, 1986

Monsignor Charles J. Fahey, *Chairman*
Third Age Center, Fordham University

Carolyn Asbury
Robert Wood Johnson
    Foundation
Princeton, NJ

Jacob A. Brody
School of Public Health
University of Illinois at Chicago

Kathleen C. Buckwalter
University of Iowa
College of Nursing

Gene D. Cohen
Program on Aging
National Institute of Mental
    Health

Betty Cornelius
Health Care Financing
    Administration

Morris H. Craig
Chronic Disease Bureau
Texas Department of Health

Peter Cross
Center for Geriatrics and
    Gerontology
Columbia University

Deborah Curtis
Bureau of Maine's Elders
Department of Human Services

Neil Henderson
Suncoast Gerontology Center
University of South Florida

Rosalie Kane
University of Minnesota School
    of Public Health
Center for Health Services
    Research

Mary Grace Kovar
National Center for Health
    Statistics

David A. Lindeman
Institute for Health and Aging
University of California, San
    Francisco

Korbin Liu
The Urban Institute

Lin Noyes
Family Respite Center
Falls Church, VA

Edwin J. Olsen
Development and Management
    Service
VA Office of Geriatrics and
    Extended Care

Robyn Stone
National Center for Health
    Services Research

T. Franklin Williams
National Institute on Aging

James Zimmer
University of Rochester School of
    Medicine

*Workshop cosponsored by Subcommittee on Aging, Senate Committee on Labor and Human Resources; Subcommittee on Human Services, House Select Committee on Aging; and Alzheimer's Disease and Related Disorders Association

Financing Long-Term Care for Patients With Dementia,* May 19, 1986**

T. Franklin Williams, *Chairman*
National Institute on Aging

David F. Chavkin
Maryland Disability Law Center

Miriam Davis
Office of the Assistant Secretary
for Planning and Evaluation
U.S. Department of Health and
Human Services

Pam Doty
Office of Legislation and Policy
Health Care Financing
Administration

Gerald Eggert
Executive Director, ACCESS
Rochester, NY

Judith Feder
Center for Health Policy Studies
Georgetown University

James Firman
United Seniors Consumer
Cooperative

Robert Friedland
Employee Benefits Research
Institute

Howard Goldman
Mental Health Policy Studies
University of Maryland

Robert L. Kane
School of Public Health
University of Minnesota

Laurence F. Lane
American Health Care
Association

Purlaine Lieberman
Equitable Life Assurance Society
of the United States

David A. Lindeman
Institute for Health and Aging
University of California, San
Francisco

Korbin Liu
The Urban Institute

Mark Meiners
Long-Term Care Section
National Center for Health
Services Research

Brian Rasmussen
Blue Cross/Blue Shield
Association

John Rother
Legislation, Research, and Public
Policy
American Association of Retired
Persons

Randy Teach
Office of the Secretary
U.S. Department of Health and
Human Services

Lewis Weinstein
Attorney
Foley, Hoag, & Elliot

Josh Wiener
The Brookings Institution

Judy Williams
Medicaid Eligibility
Maine Department of Human
Services

---

*Workshop cosponsored by Subcommittee on Aging, Senate Committee on Labor and Human Resources; Subcommittee on Human Services, House Select Committee on Aging; and Alzheimer's Disease and Related Disorders Association.

**Discussion paper by Karen Davis, and Patricia Neuman, Johns Hopkins University.

Alzheimer's Disease and Dementia: How To Cope and Who Will Pay? Sept. 18, 1986*

Linda Hope
Producer
"There Were Times Dear . . .
Living With Alzheimer's Disease

David Drachman
University of Massachusetts, and
Chairman, Medical and Scientific
Advisory Board
Alzheimer's Disease and Related
Disorders Association

Peter J. Whitehouse
Director, Alzheimer's Neuroscience
Center
Department of Neurology
Case Western Reserve School of
Medicine, and
Division of Behavioral Neurology
University Hospitals of Cleveland

The Honorable Olympia Snowe
U.S. House of Representatives

The Honorable Ron Wyden
U.S. House of Representatives

Senator Claude Pepper
U.S. Senate

Senator Charles E. Grassley
U.S. Senate

---

*Luncheon cosponsored with the Congressional Clearinghouse on the Future.

Alphabetical listing by author:

Author	Title	Where available (see listing below)
George Annas and Leonard Glantz	Withholding and Withdrawing of Life-Sustaining Treatment for Elderly Incompetent Patients: A Review of Court Decisions and Legislative Approaches	"Decisions in Decline" *Milbank Memorial Fund Quarterly*, Volume #64, Supplement #2, 1986
Battelle Columbus Laboratories	The Economics of Dementia	Through NTIS, volume 2
Allen Buchanan, with Michael Gilfix and Dan W. Brock	Surrogate Decisionmaking for Elderly Individuals Who are Incompetent or of Questionable Competence	"Decisions in Decline" *Milbank Memorial Fund Quarterly*, Volume #64, Supplement #2, 1986
David Chavkin	Interstate Variability in Medicaid Policies Regarding Long-Term Care of Individuals With Dementia	Through NTIS, volume 4
Dorothy H. Coons	Designing a Residential Care Unit for Persons With Dementia	Through NTIS, volume 3
Peter Cross and Barry J. Gurland	The Epidemiology of Dementing Disorders	Through NTIS, volume 1
Karen Davis and	Financing Care for Patients With Dementia	Through NTIS, volume 2, and the Committee on Labor and Human Resources, U.S. Senate
Louise Dunn	The Senior Respite Care Program (Portland, OR)	Through NTIS, volume 3
Ronald Dworkin	Philosophical Issues In Senile Dementia	Excerpts in "Decisions in Decline" *Milbank Memorial Fund Quarterly*, Volume #64, Supplement #2, 1986
William J. Foley	Dementia Among Nursing Home Patients: Defining the Condition, Characteristics of the Demented, and Dementia on the RUG-II Classification System, With Appendix	Through NTIS, volume 2
Carolyn J. French	Experiences of the Atlanta Area ADRDA in the Development and Management of the Community Services Program	Through NTIS, volume 3
Marshall B. Kapp and Bernard Lo	Legal Perceptions and Medical Decisionmaking	"Decisions in Decline" *Milbank Memorial Fund Quarterly*, Volume #64, Supplement #2, 1986
Robert Katzman, Bruce Lasker, and Nancy Bernstein	Accuracy of Diagnosis and Consequences of Misdiagnosis of Disorders Causing Dementia	Through NTIS, volume 1, and the Committee on Labor and Human Resources, U.S. Senate

Alphabetical listing by author:

Author	Title	Where available (see listing below)
Korbin Liu	Analysis of Data Bases for Health Services Research on Dementia	Through NTIS, volume 2, and the Committee on Labor and Human Resources, U.S. Senate
Shirley A. Lockery	Impact of Dementia Within Minority Groups	Through NTIS, volume 2
Lin Noyes and Richard Wittenborn	The Family Respite Center: Day Care for the Demented	Through NTIS, volume 3
Diana Petty	The Family Survival Project	Through NTIS, volume 3
Donald L. Price	Basic Neuroscience and Disorders Causing Dementia	Through NTIS, volume 1
Dan Sands and Judy Belman	Evolution of a 24 Hour Care System for Persons With Alzheimer's and Related Disorders	Through NTIS, volume 3
Elizabeth Vierck	Health Services Research Related To Dementia	To be printed by the Committee on Labor and Human Resources, U.S. Senate
Audrey S. Weiner	Institutional Approaches to the Care of Individuals With Dementia: Report of a National Facility Survey and the Hebrew Home for the Aged at Riverdale as a Case Example	Through NTIS, volume 3
Thelma J. Wells	Urinary Incontinence in Alzheimer's Disease	Through NTIS, volume 3 Through NTIS, volume 2
Yankelovich, Skelly, and White	Caregivers of Patients With Dementia	

Listing by publication:

"Decisions in Decline" *Milbank Memorial Fund Quarterly*, Volume #64, Supplement #2, 1986, Dan. W. Wikler, (ed.) in press

George Annas and Leonard Glantz	Withholding and Withdrawing of Life-Sustaining Treatment for Elderly Incompetent Patients: A Review of Court Decisions and Legislative Approaches
Allan Buchanan, with Michael Gilfix and Dan W. Brock	Surrogate Decisionmaking for Elderly Individuals Who are Incompetent or of Questionable Competence
Marshall B. Kapp and Bernard Lo	Legal Perceptions and Medical Decisionmaking
Ronald Dworkin	Excerpts of "Philosophical Issues In Senile Dementia"

Dementia Working Papers, Volume 1, Epidemiology, Diagnosis, and Basic Science, National Technical Information Service

Peter Cross and Barry J. Gurland	The Epidemiology of Dementing Disorders
Robert Katzman, Bruce Lasker, and Nancy Bernstein	Accuracy of Diagnosis and Consequences of Misdiagnosis of Disorders Causing Dementia
Donald L. Price	Basic Neuroscience and Disorders Causing Dementia

Listing by publication:

Dementia Working Papers, Volume 2, Economics, Social Science and Health Services Research, National Technical Information Service

Battelle Columbus Laboratories	The Economics of Dementia
Karen Davis and	Financing Care for Patients With Dementia
William J. Foley	Dementia Among Nursing Home Patients: Defining the Condition, Characteristics of the Demented, and Dementia on the RUG-II Classification System, With Appendix
Korbin Liu	Analysis of Data Bases for Health Services Research on Dementia
Shirley A. Lockery	Impact of Dementia Within Minority Groups
Yankelovich, Skelly, and White	Caregivers of Patients With Dementia

Dementia Working Papers, Volume 3, Special Care Programs and Facilities, National Technical Information Service

Dorothy H. Coons	Designing a Residential Care Unit for Persons With Dementia
Louise Dunn	The Senior Respite Care Program (Portland, OR)
Carolyn J. French	Experiences of the Atlanta Area ADRDA in the Development and Management of the Community Services Program
Lin Noyes and Richard Wittenborn	The Family Respite Center: Day Care for the Demented
Diana Petty	The Family Survival Project
Dan Sands and Judy Belman	Evolution of a 24 Hour Care System for Persons With Alzheimer's and Related Disorders
Audrey S. Weiner	Institutional Approaches to the Care of Individuals With Dementia: Report of a National Facility Survey and the Hebrew Home for the Aged at Riverdale as a Case Example
Thelma J. Wells	Urinary Incontinence in Alzheimer's Disease

Dementia Working Papers, Volume 4: Interstate Variability in Medicaid Policies for Long-Term Care of Individuals with Dementia, National Technical Information Service, U.S. Department of Commerce

David Chavkin	Interstate Variability in Medicaid Policies Regarding Long-Term Care of Individuals With Dementia

Reports of the Committee on Labor and Human Resources, U.S. Senate, also available through the Subcommittee on Human Services, Select Committee on Aging, U.S. House of Representatives

Karen Davis and	Financing Care for Patients With Dementia
Korbin Liu	Analysis of Data Bases for Health Services Research on Dementia
Elizabeth Vierck	Health Services Research Related to Dementia

Aging and the Brain, Robert Terry (ed.) (New York: Raven Press), based on a symposium in Brussels, Belgium Oct. 27-28, 1986, in press

Robert Katzman, Bruce Lasker, and Nancy Bernstein	Accuracy of Diagnosis and Consequences of Misdiagnosis of Disorders Causing Dementia

Glossary of Acronyms and Terms

Acronyms

AABD —Aid to the Aged, Blind, and Disabled

AAHA —American Association of Homes for the Aged

AARP —American Association of Retired Persons

ACGME —Accreditation Council for Graduate Medical Education

AD —Alzheimer's disease

ADL —activities of daily living

ADRDA —Alzheimer's Disease and Related Disorders Association

AFAR —American Federation for Aging Research

AFDC —Aid to Families With Dependent Children

AGS —American Geriatrics Society

AHEC —Area Health Education Center

AHPC —Aging and Health Policy Center

AIDS —acquired immune deficiency syndrome

AMA —American Medical Association

ANA —American Nurses Association

ANT —Alzheimer neurofibrillary tangle

APA —American Psychological Association

AOA —Administration on Aging, DHHS

BHPr —Bureau of Health Professionals, HRSA

BPRS —Brief Psychiatric Rating Scale

CARE —Comprehensive Assessment and Referral Evaluation

CDR —Clinical Dementia Rating Scale

CMHC —community mental health center

COBRA —Consolidated Omnibus Budget Reconciliation Act of 1985 (Public Law 99-272)

COPS —Comprehensive Service on Aging Institute for Alzheimer's Disease and Related Disorders, NJ

COTA —certified occupational therapy assistant

CS —Cushing's syndrome

CSF —cerebrospinal fluid

CSWE —Council on Social Work Education

CT —computerized axial tomography (also known as CAT)

DCF —domiciliary care facility (also known as board and care facilities)

DHEW —Department of Health, Education, and Welfare (became DHHS in May 1980)

DHHS —Department of Health and Human Services (formerly DHEW)

DNA —deoxyribonucleic acid

DNS —director of nursing services

DON —director of nursing

DPA —durable power of attorney

DPAHC —durable power of attorney for health care

DRG —diagnosis-related group

DRR —Division of Research Resources, NIH

DRS —Dementia Rating Scale

DSM-III —Diagnostic and Statistical Manual of the America Psychiatric Association, 3rd edition

ECA —epidemiologic catchment area

FAI —Functional Assessment Inventory

FDA —Food and Drug Administration, DHHS

FHT —face-hand test

GAC —geriatric assessment center

GAO —General Accounting Office, U.S. Congress

GDS —Global Deterioration Scale

GEC —Geriatric Education Center, HRSA

GEU —geriatric evaluation unit

GNP —geriatric nurse practitioner

GRECC —Geriatric Research, Education, and Clinical Center, VA

GS —geriatric specialist

GSA —Gerontological Society of America

HDL —high density lipoprotein

HHMI —Howard Hughes Medical Institute

HMO —health maintenance organization

HRSA —Health Resources and Services Administration, DHHS

HTLV —human T-cell lymphotrophic virus (now called HIV: human immunodeficiency virus)

IADL —instrumental activities of daily living

ICD-9 —International Classification of Diseases, 9th revision

ICD-9-CM—International Classification of Diseases, 9th revision, Clinical Modification

ICF —intermediate care facility

IEC —institutional ethics committee

IMA —Individual Medical Account

IMD —institution for mental disease

IQ —intelligence quotient

IRA —Individual Retirement Account

IRB —institutional review board

JCAH —Joint Commission on Accreditation of Hospitals

LPN —licensed practical nurse

LTC —long-term care

LVN —licensed vocational nurse

MAD —Multidimensional Assessment for Dementia scale

MID —multi-infarct dementia

MMSE —Mini-Mental State Examination

MPTP —1-methyl-4-phenyl-1,2,3,6-tetrahydropyridine

MRI —magnetic resonance imaging

MS —medical specialist

MSQ —Mental Status Questionnaire

NCHS	—National Center for Health Statistics, DHHS
NCOA	—National Council on the Aging
NFT	—neurofibrillary tangles
NGF	—nerve growth factor
NHLBI	—National Heart, Lung, and Blood Institute, NIH
NIA	—National Institute on Aging, NIH
NIAD	—National Institute on Adult Daycare
NIH	—National Institutes of Health, Public Health Service, DHHS
NIMH	—National Institute of Mental Health, DHHS
NINCDS	—National Institute of Neurological and Communicative Diseases and Stroke, NIH
NLN	—National League of Nursing
NMFI	—National Master Facility Inventory
NMR	—nuclear magnetic resonance
NOSIE	—Nurses' Observation Scale for Inpatient Evaluation
NP	—nurse practitioner
NPH	—normal pressure hydrocephalus
OAA	—Older Americans Act
OARS	—Older American's Research and Service Center instrument
OASDI	—Old Age and Survivors' Disability Insurance
OME	—Object Memory Evaluation
OT	—occupational therapist
OTA	—Office of Technology Assessment, U.S. Congress
PaCS	—Patient Care and Services (quality assurance instrument, DHHS)
PAMIE	—Physical and Mental Impairment of Function Evaluation
PET	—positron emission tomography
PGDRS	—Psychogeriatric Dependency Rating Scale
PPS	—Prospective Payment System, Medicaid
PSP	—progressive supranuclear palsy
RISA	—radioimmunosorbent assay
RN	—registered nurse
RNA	—ribonucleic acid
RRC	—residency review committee
RUG	—resource utilization group
RUG-II	—resource utilization group system used by New York State case mix evaluation
SCAG	—Sandoz Clinical Assessment Geriatric Scale
SDAT	—senile dementia of the Alzheimer type
S/HMO	—social/health maintenance organization
SNF	—skilled nursing facility
SPECT	—single photon emission computed tomography
SPMSQ	—Short Portable Mental Status Questionnaire
SSDI	—Social Security Disability Insurance
SSI	—Supplemental Security Income
WAIS	—Weschler Adult Intelligence Scale
WMS	—Weschler Memory Scale

Terms

Activities of daily living (ADL): Self-care abilities related to personal care, such as bathing, dressing, eating, and continence.

Acute care: Short-term medical care provided by physicians, clinics, hospitals, mental health centers, and rehabilitation services in response to a medical crisis.

Acute illness: A sharp, severe sickness, having a sudden onset, a rapid rise, and a short course.

Adult day care centers: Centers that provide a range of mental health and social services for physically, cognitively, or emotionally impaired and socially isolated people. Services vary according to the clients they serve. Centers dealing with people with dementia emphasize personal care, supervision, socialization, and activities. Adult day care centers have developed largely without Federal regulation, and thus vary greatly in quality and services. Medicaid and participant fees are their main sources of revenue.

Adverse selection: Situation faced by insurance companies when potential clients know of special risks and therefore wish to buy insurance. This raises financial risk to the insuror and discourages risk-pooling.

Ageism: Discrimination on the basis of age. Often results in the denial of rights and services to the elderly; analogous to racism or sexism.

Agnosia: Failure to recognize things or people; the loss of the ability to comprehend the meaning or recognize the importance of various types of sensory stimulation.

Aid to Families with Dependent Children (AFDC): A State-administered program that provides financial support for children under the age of 18 who have been deprived of parental support or care because of death, continued absence from the home, unemployment of a parent, or physical or mental illness. The family of an individual with dementia may be eligible if he or she has children under the age of 18, although establishing eligibility may be difficult.

Acquired Immune Deficiency Syndrome (AIDS): A disease caused by the retrovirus HIV (human immunodeficiency virus; also known as HTLV-III: human T-cell lymphotropic virus, type III) characterized by a deficiency of the immune system. The depression of the immune system often leads to infections unusual in individuals with normal immunity. A substantial portion of persons with AIDS also develop dementia.

AIDS dementia: A form of dementia that results from brain infections encouraged by the immune dysfunction of AIDS, or caused directly by the AIDS virus. AIDS dementia is now the most common dementia caused by infection, and a large number of AIDS patients develop dementia.

Alzheimer's disease: A chronic progressive disorder that is the major cause of degenerative dementia in the U.S. (affecting 2 to 4 million people). The disease may be a group of diseases grouped under one name because scientific knowledge is incomplete. Possible causes include genetic, environmental, immunologic, or metabolic factors. The disease manifests itself with clinical symptoms of dementia and characteristic microscopic changes in the brain. Definitive diagnosis can be obtained only from examination of brain tissue. There is no fully effective method of prevention, treatment, or cure.

Alzheimer's Disease and Related Disorders Association (ADRDA): A non-governmental organization founded in June 1979 by several family support groups. ADRDA is based in Chicago, but has chapters nationwide. It is now the largest organization focusing on dementia and the needs of caregivers. ADRDA funds basic research in neurosciences, and is involved in public education, family support, and patient advocacy efforts.

Alzheimer's Disease Research Centers: Ten federally funded centers created to conduct basic, clinical, and behavioral research into Alzheimer's disease and related disorders. The centers are at various medical centers and universities around the country. The program is administered by the National Institute on Aging, part of the National Institutes of Health (NIH), U.S. Department of Health and Human Services.

Aphasia: Loss or impairment of the power to use words. Expressive aphasia is impairment in the ability to use language, to speak or write; receptive aphasia is the inability to understand language. In some persons aphasia is the first symptom of dementia.

Apraxia: Impairment of the ability to perform complex coordinated movements, such as buttoning buttons, walking, dressing, eating a meal, or maintaining a sitting position. Unlike the person who is paralyzed or injured, someone with apraxia is unable to perform these functions due to brain damage, although physically capable of doing them. Apraxia is another symptom of dementia.

Assessment: The process by which a physician or health care professional evaluates an individual, generally based on conversation with the person, the family, and other caregivers; and on informal observations of the person's behavior. Assessment is related to, but distinct from diagnosis. Assessment of cognitive abilities is a prerequisite for diagnosis of dementia, and can also provide information about the severity of a dementing condition once it has been diagnosed.

Assessment instruments: Specific tests and scales used to measure and evaluate cognitive and self-care abilities, behavioral problems and other patient characteristics. Few tests were specifically designed to evaluate dementia, and they do not always focus on the full range of problems associated with it; thus there are questions of validity and reliability concerning many of them.

Basic research: The pursuit of knowledge for its own sake, without regard for specific practical or commercial results.

Behavioral problems: Persons afflicted with dementia can exhibit various behaviors, which are often the most burdensome aspects of dementia for caregivers. These behaviors include wandering and getting lost, agitation, pacing, emotional outbursts, suspiciousness and angry accusations, physical aggression, combativeness, cursing, and socially unacceptable sexual behavior. They also include chronic screaming and noisiness; repetition of meaningless words, phrases, or actions; withdrawal and apathy; and sleep disruption. Some of these problems are treatable.

Binswanger's disease: A form of vascular dementia caused by loss of blood supply to the white matter of the brain (rather than the cerebral cortex). Also known as Binswanger's dementia and subcortical arteriosclerotic encephalopathy.

Biomedical research: Research into biological, medical, and physical science. Such research could lead to enhanced knowledge of the brain and yield great benefits, especially in the field of neuroscience. NIH and non-governmental agencies such as ADRDA are providing support for biomedical research into dementia.

Brain imaging: The use of various techniques to directly assess the anatomy of the brain; an essential component in the diagnosis of dementia. The most powerful new technologies use computers to create images of the brain. The techniques include computerized axial tomography, nuclear magnetic resonance, positron emission tomography, and single photon emission computed tomography (cf.).

Bureau of Health Professionals (BHPr): Part of the Health Resources and Services Administration, U.S. Department of Health and Human Services (DHHS). BHPr coordinates, evaluates, and supports development of health personnel. It also disseminates and assesses information on the training and education of health personnel, demonstrates new approaches to education, and provides financial support for educational programs. An example of this last function is BHPr's support of geriatric education centers (GECs).

Catastrophic reaction: Inappropriate behavior episodes often displayed by persons with dementia in reaction to some outside stimulus. These can be minor (shouting or stubbornness) or major (violent and threatening behavior such as hitting or swinging a weapon).

Cerebral infarction: An area of dead tissue in the cerebrum caused by an interruption of blood circulation because of functional constriction or actual obstruction of a blood vessel resulting from a stroke, hemorrhage, or lack of oxygen. Dementia can be a symptom of cerebral infarction.

Cerebrospinal fluid (CSF): The liquid that bathes the brain and the spinal column. Measurement of chemicals and cells in the CSF (obtained by lumbar puncture) can be part of the diagnostic process. Because the test is relatively expensive, causes some discomfort, and picks up relatively few diseases, however, there is some debate over its use in diagnosing dementia.

Cerebrum: The main portion of the brain, occupying the upper part of the cranial cavity.

Chronic illness: Disease (usually incurable) characterized by long duration and frequent recurrence. People suffering from chronic degenerative diseases, such as those that cause dementia, have different medical and social needs from those suffering from short-term acute illness.

Clinical research: The application of basic knowledge to the search for preventive measures, treatments, and methods of diagnosing disease. Clinical research is often conducted in a medical setting and is based on direct observation of the patient.

Clinical Research Centers on Psychopathology of the Elderly: Three clinical research centers established by the National Institute of Mental Health (NIMH), two of which focus on research into Alzheimer's disease.

Cognitive abilities: The functions of memory, intelligence, learning ability, calculation, problem solving, judgment, comprehension, recognition, orientation, and attention. Impairment of these functions is a central feature of dementia, and the primary cause of the self-care and behavioral problems associated with it.

Cognitive assessment: The use of specific test instruments to identify and describe cognitive impairments and to measure the cognitive abilities of persons with dementia. Some of these tests are derived from standard tests, while others have been specifically designed for evaluating individuals with dementia. Such assessments are particularly valuable for research and clinical applications, but they may be less successful in determining an individual's needs for for long-term care or in establishing eligibility for services. Tests include the Dementia Rating Scale, the face-hand test, the Mini-Mental State Examination, the Mental Status Questionnaire, and the Sandoz Clinical Assessment Geriatric Scale. (cf.)

Community Mental Health Centers (CMHCS): Agencies that provide a range of mental health services, primarily on an outpatient basis. The number of persons served by CMHCs is not known, but some CMHCs do have special services for elderly people including some with dementia. CMHCs are jointly funded by Federal and State governments.

Competence: For the purpose of this assessment, competence is defined as the ability to make a decision using communication, understanding, reasoning, deliberation, and a relatively stable set of values. The process whereby the decision is reached is more important than the decision itself in determining competence. Competence may be determined by functional assessment. Legally, an individual is assumed to be competent until a court declares otherwise and appoints a guardian, although informal competency determinations between families, physicians, and psychiatrists are common.

Computerized axial tomography (CAT or CT): A diagnostic device that combines X-ray equipment with a computer and a cathode ray tube to produce images of cross-sections of the body. CT is a useful diagnostic tool in detecting some causes of dementia, such as tumors, and it has also been used to study Alzheimer's disease.

Conservatorships and guardianships: The designation of a surrogate decisionmaker on behalf of an incompetent individual, determined and supervised by a court after evidence of an individual's incompetence has been presented. There are two types of authority: conservatorship or guardianship of estate (covering finances) and possessions and conservatorship or guardianship of person (covering residency, certain kinds of health care and service decisions, and personal matters).

Creutzfeldt-Jakob disease (CJD): An infectious, usually fatal neurological illness believed to be transmitted by an atypical infectious agent, sometimes referred to as a "slow virus." Victims of CJD exhibit symptoms of dementia, involuntary jerks, and, frequently, abnormal gait.

Decubitus: Bedsores.

Deeming: The process by which income and resources that is considered to be available to an applicant for Supplementary Security Income (SSI), and other government programs. An example is pension income received by one spouse being considered available to the other spouse applying for Medicaid. In determining eligibility the "deemed" income will be added to the applicant's own income even if the non-applicant spouse fails to make it available to the applicant.

Degenerative disorders: Diseases whose progression cannot be arrested. These disorders cause progressive deterioration of mental and neurological function often over years. Alzheimer's disease is the most prevalent degenerative dementia. The ultimate cause of such disorders is unknown.

Delirium: A decline in intellectual function with clouded consciousness. It differs from dementia in that it implies a temporary loss of ability. However, persons with dementia frequently develop delirium caused by other illnesses or drug reactions and delirium can be confused with dementia particularly in older individuals.

Delusion: A false, fixed idea. Persons with dementia often suffer from delusions and may maintain them for a long time.

Dementia: Impairment in mental function and global cognitive abilities of long duration (months to years) in an alert individual. Symptoms include memory loss, loss of language function, inability to think abstractly, inability to care for oneself, personality change, emotional instability, a loss of sense of time and place, and behavior problems. Dementia can be caused by over 70 disorders, but the leading cause in the United States is Alzheimer's disease. No cure is currently available for the vast majority of dementing conditions and may last for years to decades. Current criteria for dementia are generally based on the Diagnostic and Statistical Manual (DSM) (cf.). Contrast with delirium.

Dementia pugilistica: Brain damage resulting from repeated head trauma. Also known as boxer's or fighter's dementia.

Dementia rating scales: Multidimensional assessment instruments that define a person's level of mental functioning from least to most impaired, describe an individual's condition over time, and predict the course of the illness. The reliability and validity of these scales are controversial.

Dementing disorders: There are more than 70 dementing disorders, the major one in the United States being Alzheimer's disease. Disease of blood vessels is the second most common cause of dementia. Some of the diseases that cause dementia are AIDS, Down's Syndrome, Creutzfeldt-Jakob disease, Huntington's disease, Binswanger's disease, and normal pressure hydrocephalus (NPH).

Dependent care tax credit: A credit subtracted from an individual's final tax liability. In its current form this provision is not generally useful to people with dementia, as credit for expenditures on personal care is only allowed if they enable the taxpayer to work.

Diagnosis Related Groups (DRGs): Medicare's classification of hospital patients by medical condition and other easily measured variables into 468 groups. Hospitals are paid a fixed price for care based on each patient's DRG. This system will be fully implemented in October 1987.

Diagnostic algorithm: Step-by-step diagnosis procedures that medical personnel learn during their professional training and progressively refine during their practice.

Diagnostic and Statistical Manual (DSM): A set of guidelines for diagnosing mental disorders published by the American Psychiatric Association. The third edition, DSM III, is the most widely used system for classifying the symptoms of dementia. APA plans to revise DSM III (published in 1980) and issue DSM IV sometime in 1989.

Disorders that simulate dementia: These are disorders that may have some of the same symptoms as dementia, but which are more likely to respond rapidly to treatment (e.g., depression in older people). Disorders that that simulate dementia may overlap dementing disorders.

Disorientation: The lack of correct knowledge of person, place, or time; i.e., where a person is, who the people around him or her are, and what time of day, day of the week, or month it is.

Domiciliary board and care facilities: Non-medical residences, usually certified by a State, that provide room, board, and 24-hour supervision for residents. Some also provide personal care and other services. These facilities differ from nursing homes in that they do not provide nursing care. They vary in size from board or foster homes that provide care for one or two individuals, to group homes that may serve as many as 10. The term also embraces retirement homes, homes for the aged, and large domiciliary care facilities, including those operated by the Veterans Administration. The services provided and the number and type of these facilities vary greatly from State to State. State and Federal programs pay a significant portion of board and care charges and costs, primarily through Social Security and pensions. The number of persons with dementia who live in such facilities is unknown.

Down's syndrome: A genetic disorder characterized by mental retardation. The syndrome may also include congenital heart defects, immune system abnormalities, various morphological abnormalities, and a reduced life expectancy. People with Down's Syndrome who survive into middle age frequently develop dementia. There are several unexplained relationships between Down's Syndrome and Alzheimer's disease.

Durable Power of Attorney (DPA): A modification of the standard power of attorney that permits a competent individual to transfer specified powers to another person. When the individual becomes incompetent the power of attorney remains valid, thereby providing a surrogate decisionmaker designation that survives the incompetence of the individual. DPA is authorized by State statute throughout the United States except in the District of Columbia.

Excess disability: Impairments in function that are worse than necessary, considering the underlying biological deficits. Such disabilities are considered "excess" in persons with dementia because they can often be corrected (e.g., with a new hearing aid or treatment of a condition that exacerbates the dementia).

Face-Hand Test (FHT): A neurological test used to differentiate between cognitively normal individuals and those with organic dementia. In this test an individual is touched simultaneously on the face and hand, first with the eyes open and then with the eyes closed. Persons with organic dementia frequently report only one of the two stimuli.

Family care: The care provided by family members to a person with dementia. The majority of people suffering from dementia are looked after by families at home during part or all of the disease. The kind of care provided changes as the disease progresses. Initially, families make decisions for the affected individual and take over financial, legal, and domestic responsibilities. Later the family assumes responsibility for activities of daily living, and also often provide round-the-clock supervision, while at the same time dealing with the difficult behavior problems associated with dementia. Family care often continues even after the ill person enters a nursing home, as families continue to visit the ill person and often assume some of the expense involved. The task of providing such care may last for 10 years or more, and the costs of home care are generally not covered by health insurance, Medicare, or Medicaid.

Family Survival Project: An independent program in San Francisco that provides information, advice and referral, case coordination, legal counseling, and support services to brain-damaged individuals and their caregivers. The program has been successful in serving caregivers and in generating government support for its programs.

Functional assessment: A means of determining competence by evaluating an individual's behavior and assessing his or her ability to function independently on a daily basis. Various assessment methods can be used, most of these involve the evaluation of activities of daily living (ADLs) and instrumental activities of daily living (IADLs) (cf.) using specific assessment instruments.

Geriatric Assessment Centers (GACs): Hospital-based centers designed to provide multidisciplinary assessment (based on functional status and medical, social, and financial needs), short-term treatment, and assistance with long-term planning for elderly patients. GACs are common in England, but are relatively new in the United States, and until recently there were few of them.

Geriatric Education Centers (GECs): Centers sponsored by BHPr that disseminate interdisciplinary and discipline-specific information and offer training models in geriatric care. Four centers were set up in 1983 and 16 more were established under the 1985 appropriations for BHPr.

Geriatrics: A branch of medicine devoted to the diseases and problems of older people. Dementia is primarily, though not exclusively, a geriatric problem.

Global cognitive impairment: Impairment of many areas of mental function.

Hallucinations: Sensory experiences unique to the individual who sees, hears, smells, tastes, or feels something not experienced by other people. Some people with dementia are subject to hallucinations.

Health services research: For the purposes of this report, the multidisciplinary study of those with dementia and the people who serve them (including the community and family). Effective health services research will determine the future basis of public and private activities in financing, quality assurance, training, and service delivery to persons with dementia. Federal health services research is sponsored by agencies of the DHHS and the VA.

Home care services: The provision of medical, social, and supportive services in the home by outside organizations. Services can range from sophisticated (e.g., administering intravenous drugs) to relatively simple (providing home-delivered meals). Other services include skilled nursing care, physical or occupational therapy, personal care, home health aide, homemaker, paid companion, and housekeeping services. Although they can be important to families caring for individuals with dementia, not all are covered by Federal or State programs and their delivery system and regulations governing their use are often fragmentary and complex.

Home health aide: A person, not a physician or nurse, who provides home care services, which may include assistance with medication and exercise; personal care, such as bathing, dressing, and feeding; and homemaker services.

Huntington's disease: A rare genetic disease characterized by chronic progressive disorders of movement and mental deterioration culminating in dementia. Symptoms do not usually appear until late middle age, and death usually results within 15 years. Children of affected parents have a 50 percent chance of developing the disease.

Illusions: The misunderstanding of abstract information, leading to an incorrect or distorted perception of reality.

Intravenous: Situated within a vein, or entering by way of a vein. Often refers to injections.

Instrumental Activities of Daily Living (IADL): Activities that facilitate independence, such as the ability to handle finances, use the telephone, use public transportation, take medication, prepare meals, go shopping, and do housework. (Also see Activities of Daily Living, above.)

International Classification of Diseases (ICD-9): A system used to code medical diagnoses. The usefulness of ICD-9 in refining epidemiological studies of dementia is limited, because many of the diagnostic categories (for example Parkinson's disease) do not separate those individuals who have dementia from those who do not. Revision of ICD-9, to be called ICD-10, is scheduled for 1989.

Idiopathic dementia: Disorders in which the clinical symptoms of dementia are present without abnormal findings in the brain. This kind of dementia is found in approximately 5 percent of cases. It is called idiopathic because its cause and mechanism are unknown.

Licensed Practical Nurse (LPN): A technical nurse licensed by a State board of nursing. LPNs (sometimes known as LVNs, or licensed vocational nurses) provide much of the hands-on care in nursing homes. Most LPNs train in vocational, community, or technical colleges.

Life care community: A facility that provides housing tailored to the needs of aging individuals and that provides medical services as needed, including nursing-home care, usually in the same complex. Such communities are expensive; only about 20 percent of the population aged 65 or older could afford to enter one, estimates say.

Living will: A declaration by a competent individual outlining his or her wishes, especially the intent to refuse life-sustaining procedures, once he or she is incompetent and death is imminent. Because these documents are frequently ambiguous, their legality may be unclear. They are not recognized in all States, and requirements and conditions vary from State to State.

Long-term care: The provision of a continuum of care in a formal (institutional) or informal (home) setting to individuals with demonstrated need. Such services can be provided in nursing homes, board and care facilities, and mental health facilities and are often delivered indefinitely. Services may be continuous or intermittent. They include medical care and a variety of other services. Individuals with dementia are likely to need more long-term supervisory and personal care than medical attention. After informal home care, nursing homes are the most frequently used setting for persons with dementia. Although the United States has no national long-term care policy, the Federal government is extensively involved in providing funding for and regulation of a wide range of long-term care services. Long-term care is among the fastest-growing segments of the health services industry.

Magnetic resonance imaging (MRI): A technique that produces images of the body by measuring the reaction of nucleii in magnetic fields to radio frequency waves. This technique provides sensitive detection of strokes and tumors and good images of the white and gray areas of the brain. The machines are expensive and a CT scan can be used for many of the same purposes.

Medicaid: A joint Federal/State medical welfare program with strict means tests, intended to provide medical and health-related services to low-income individuals. Medicaid regulations are established by each State within Federal guidelines. Eligibility requirements and the long-term care services covered vary significantly from State to State, and are often complicated, especially those that concern individuals with dementia. Medicaid generally pays for nursing home and home health care for eligible individuals. Forty-eight percent of Medicaid spending was for long-term care in 1982. Medicaid pays 43 percent of national nursing home costs, and covers more than 70 percent of nursing home residents (fully or in part). In some States, Medicaid covers adult day care and in-home services. Because services such as respite and custodial care are not generally covered, however, Medicaid is of limited use for home care to individuals with dementia and their families.

Medical expense tax deduction: The deduction of medical expenses above a certain percentage of adjusted gross income. This deduction may be of little help to people with dementia as many of their expenditures are not primarily medical ones.

Medical model of care: Provision of care and diagnostic and treatment services that emphasizes the role of the physician over that of other health and social service professionals.

Medicare: The Federal insurance program, initiated in 1965, designed to provide medical care for elderly people. Generally, only those 65 or older are eligible, although disabled people under 65 and those with kidney diseases may also be eligible. Individuals with dementia who are under 65 may find it difficult to establish eligibility. Medicare provides reimbursement for hospital and physician services and limited benefits for skilled nursing home care, home health care, and hospice care. Medicare does not cover protracted long-term care, and by law it does not cover custodial care. The medical orientation of medicare services and benefits means that its usefulness for individuals with dementia is limited to diagnosis and treatment.

Memory: The power or process of reproducing or recalling what has been learned or retained. There are several different forms of memory: immediate (remembering for a few seconds), short-term (remembering for a few months), and long-term (remembering material learned from year to year). Memory loss is a symptom of dementia, particularly short-term memory.

Mental retardation: Lower than normal intellectual competence, usually characterized by an IQ of less than 70. Although it is not always easy to distinguish from mental retardation, dementia indicates the loss of previous mental ability.

Mental status tests: Short screening tests used by mental health professionals to estimate changes in intellectual performance. Useful mainly for preliminary identification of symptoms.

MPTP: 1-methyl-4 phenyl-1,2,3,6, tetrahydropyridine, a contaminant of a heroin-like drug (originally produced illicitly), which causes symptoms similar to those of Parkinson's disease.

Multidimensional assessment instruments: Tests that focus on various categories of assessment, such as diagnosis, physical condition, cognitive status, self-care abilities, emotional and behavioral characteristics, family and social supports, financial status, and health and social service use patterns.

Multidisciplinary team model of health care: An approach that stresses the use of a wide range of health and social services personnel appropriate to certain care situations. Many consider this the most appropriate approach for dealing with the complexity of a dementing illness.

Multi-infarct dementia (MID): Dementia caused by brain damage resulting from multiple cerebral infarcts (cf).

Nurse's aides: Paraprofessionals who provide most of the direct care in long-term care facilities. Aides have the lowest education and training requirements and the highest rate of turnover among nursing home personnel. The Nurse Training Act of 1975 supports efforts to provide improved training for nurses' aides and other paraprofessionals.

Nursing homes: Facilities that provide 24-hour supervision, skilled nursing services, and personal care. An estimated 40 to 75 percent of nursing home residents are persons with dementia. Nursing homes fall into two categories, skilled nursing facilities (SNFs) and intermediate care facilities (ICFs). State Medicaid regulations that define these types of facility vary, as does the number of nursing homes in each category and the supply of beds. Medicaid pays a significant portion of nursing home costs, but nationally half the cost of nursing home care is borne by residents and their families.

Nursing model of health care: Nursing care of the chronically ill, emphasizing rehabilitative and personal services; the objective is to restore maximum function and independence in the patient.

Nurse Practitioner (NP): A nurse specialist (usually an RN), who has completed an academic program to obtain added medical skills and who can perform many tasks otherwise performed by a physician. Some NPs specialize in geriatrics.

Nurse Specialist: A nurse (usually an RN) who has completed graduate education or fulfilled certification requirements in a particular field (e.g., geriatrics).

Nurse Training Act (PL 94-63): Passed in 1975, this Act and its amendments emphasizes, among other things, the problems of providing health care for the elderly and the need for teaching and training programs specializing in geriatrics and long-term care.

Older Americans Act: This Act, passed in 1965, established the Administration on Aging (AOA) within the Department of Health, Education and Welfare (now DHHS). AOA coordinates grants and contracts to the States for development of new and improved programs for older persons. The Act also deals with the need for improved training and more personnel in the field of geriatrics. A 1984 amendment recognize the increasing need for personnel knowledgeable about the treatment and care of persons with Alzheimer's disease.

Older Americans Act Title III: Part of the Older Americans Act of 1965, Title III provides Federal funding to the States for social services for people over 60. States determine specific services, but Title III funds are often used for home health, homemaker, and chore services; telephone reassurance; adult day care; respite care; case management; and congregate and home-delivered meals. Income tests are not generally used to determine eligibility, but these services are targeted to elderly people with social or economic need.

Parkinson's disease: A disease affecting movement and leading to dementia in approximately one-third of those affected. The disease is associated with destruction of cells in the substantia nigra in the brainstem. The cause is unknown. There are several varieties of Parkinson's disease.

Perseveration: The repetition of meaningless words or actions, a behavioral problem sometimes exhibited by persons with dementia.

Pick's disease: A rare dementing disorder, clinically similar to Alzheimer's disease.

Positron-emission tomography (PET): A scanning technique that measures the body's uptake of radioactively labeled substances. PET provides a dynamic image of the brain's metabolic activity and has been useful in detecting Huntington's disease and Alzheimer's disease. Its use is relatively limited, largely because it requires expensive facilities.

Primary family caregiver: The individual within a family who assumes most of the tasks involved in caring for an individual with dementia. Usually a member of the family related by blood or marriage to the ill person, often a middle-aged woman.

Private charity: Assistance provided by people outside a person's family, but not paid for by Federal or State funds. It may take the form of informal help from friends or unpaid volunteers, or more formal help provided by professionals paid out of charitable contributions.

Progressive supranuclear palsy (PSP): A disorder similar to Parkinson's disease. It differs from Parkinson's disease in that those affected lose the ability to gaze up or down and do not necessarily have a tremor. Half to two-thirds of people with PSP become demented.

Psychological testing: Tests used by physicians to screen for mental condition, including the presence of dementia. These tests are used primarily to confirm diagnoses. They are important in distinguishing between dementia and the normal effects of aging. They are also useful in the tracking the stages of illness.

Psychotropic drugs: Drugs that act on the mind. They are often used to control disruptive behavior in persons with dementia.

Regulatory standards: Nursing homes and home health agencies that participate in Medicaid and Medicare programs are obliged to conform with Federal and State regulations. There are no Federal regulations for board and care facilities but most States do have licensing standards for such facilities, though these vary widely from State to State. Thirty-three States and the District of Columbia also have licensing laws pertaining to home care services. Inspection and enforcement of these standards to ensure quality care is often unsatisfactory.

Registered Nurse (RN): A professional nurse licensed by a State board of nursing. By virtue of their training, RNs are certified to assume responsibilities and duties that other less-qualified personnel are not. Recent surveys show that there is little interest in work in long-term care facilities among RNs.

Representative payee: The guardian of an incapacitated individual's social security or other government benefits. Conservatorship and power of attorney are not recognized by many government agencies. A representative payee is usually appointed at the discretion of the head of the appropriate agency.

Resource Utilization Groups (RUGs): The classification by Medicaid of individuals in nursing homes into 16 groups, based on functional impairment. Each RUG category is assigned a fixed price per unit per day, and the nursing home is paid that amount for each resident based on his or her RUG classification. New York State has just implemented a RUG-based system, and similar systems are under consideration in other States.

Respite care: The intermittent provision of services to provide temporary relief for a family caring for an incapacitated individual. Respite programs include in-home companion care, in-home personal care, adult day care, or short-term stays in a nursing home, hospital, or boarding home. Such services are not always publicly or privately funded and are often difficult for caregivers to find.

Single photon emission computed tomography (SPECT): The use of radiation detection machines (available in hospitals with nuclear medicine facilities) to indirectly measure physiological activity. This technique may eventually be able to perform many of the diagnostic functions now only available through a PET scan though with less precision and resolution. It is currently useful in the detection of strokes, hemmorhage, and poor blood circulation in the brain.

Social Health Maintenance Organization (S/HMO): A new type of health maintenance organization (HMO) that is operating on an experimental basis in a few locations. An S/HMO is paid a flat amount per enrollee for a fixed period. During that period it provides all needed medical care and social support services for acute or chronic conditions suffered by the enrollee.

Social Services Block Grant: Provides Federal funding to the States for social services for the elderly and the disabled. Federal standards do not require provision of specific services, but many States use their grants for board and care, adult day care, home health, and similar community services that can improve the quality of life for individuals with dementia and their families.

Staging: The definition of a series of discrete and reliable steps describing the progress of a disease. The effort to develop accurate measures of the stages of Alzheimer's disease has just begun, and no ideal staging scale or tool is available at present.

Supplemental Security Income (SSI): A Federal income support program that provides monthly payments to aged, disabled, and blind people with incomes below a minimum level.

Surrogate decisionmakers: Persons responsible for making decisions concerning an individual's health care, life-style, and estate once the individual is incapable of making these decisions. A surrogate decisionmaker can be a court-appointed conservator or guardian, or someone legally designated by the individual before he or she became incompetent. De facto surrogates—often spouses or other family members—assume these powers for an incapacitated individual without being formally or legally charged to do so. The limits on and the types of decisions that can be made by surrogate decisionmakers vary from State to State.

Toxic dementia: Dementia caused by exposure to toxic substances, such as alcohol (associated with over a dozen forms of brain disease), or chronic exposure to heavy metals.

Transmissible dementia: Dementia associated with diseases caused by unusual infectious agents. Examples are Creutzfeldt-Jakob disease, Gerstmann-Strassler syndrome, and kuru.

"2176 waiver": A modification of the Medicaid program, introduced in 1981, that allows the waiver of standard Medicaid requirements to introduce new programs on a trial basis. Several States have used this waiver to establish programs for people with Alzheimer's disease.

Vascular dementia: Dementia resulting from brain damage caused by cerebral infarction, or other diseases of disorder due to the blood vessels. Vascular dementia is the second largest cause of dementia in the United States (after Alzheimer's disease).

Veterans Administration (VA): For purposes of this report, the largest single provider of long-term care services in the United States. In 1983, the VA operated 99 nursing homes and 16 large board and care facilities. It also paid for nursing home care, board and care in private homes; 3 provided day care at 5 VA medical centers. These services are provided on a priority basis to veterans with service-connected disabilities. Thus, veterans with dementia are accorded a lower priority. The VA also supports research and education in geriatrics.

Index

Index

Abt Associates, Inc., 355, 356
ACCESS, 160
Accreditation Council for Graduate Medical Education
    (ACGME), 348, 349
ACTION, 29
Activities of daily living (ADLs), 70-72, *71*, 211, 227, 292-
    294, 301, 378-379, 499
  reliability and validity of instruments, 294-299, 317
Acute brain syndrome. *See* Delirium
Adjudication, competence, 172-173
Administration on Aging (AOA), 42, 262, 350
  education and training by, 357-359
  Long-Term Care Gerontology Centers of, 25
  research funding by, 47, 50
  subsidies to private charities by, 455
Adult day care, 228-230, 248-252
Advance Directive Principle, 183
Adverse selection, 452, 453, 454
Ageism
  diagnostic error and, 88
  physicians and, 345
Aging and Health Policy Center (AHPC), 375, 388
Agnosia, 69-70
Aid to Families with Dependent Children (AFDC), maxi-
    mum benefit and need standards of, 422
Aid to the Aged, Blind, and Disabled (AABD), 422
AIDS dementia, 16, 33, 116
Alzheimer, Alois, 97, 98
Alzheimer's disease
  characteristics of, 97-100
  clearinghouse for, 50-51
  diagnosis of, 91-93, 94, 95-96
  diagnostic tests for, 480, 481
  Down's syndrome relationship with, 117-118
  duration of, 14
  familial, 101-102, 103, 116
  funding delay for, 488
  heterogeneity of, 100
  informed consent and, 186-188
  MAD scale and, 308
  Pick's disease relationship with, 117, 118
  possible causes of, 100-106
  postulated causes of, 481-482
  prevalence of, 7, 9, 11, 16, 61, 62-63, 80
  public awareness of, 3
  registry for, 8
  special entitlements for, 38
  specialized care for, 243
  specialized program for, 254
  stages of, 63-67
  symptoms of, 10-11, 61-62
  treatment issues of, 106-111
  See also Disorders, dementing
Alzheimer's Disease and Related Disorders Association
    (ADRDA), 3, 7, 48, 148, 491, 493

adult day care centers and, 229
alternative services used by, 247, 248, 253
Atlanta area chapter of, 249, 250
behavioral problems and, 72
caregiver survey of, 17-18, 20, 23-25, 32, 70-71, 72,
    135-136, 137, 139-143, 145-149, 151, 159, 210, 218,
    222, 232, 245, 245, 247, 247, 248, 251, 252, 255
caregiver training and, 41, 42, 253
"diagnostic approach" conference by, 96
diagnostic criteria of, 39, 60
family support by, 30, 32
Medicaid biases and, 145
multidisciplinary training by, 331
referrals to long-term care services by, 233
research funding by, 4, 47, 50, 490, 491
service coordination by, 22
specialized care cost estimate by, 251
support groups of, 454
Alzheimer's and Related Diseases Task Force, Kansas,
    227
Alzheimer's Disease and Associated Disorders, 4
Alzheimer's Disease and Related Dementias Services Re-
    search Act, 50
Alzheimer's Disease Assessment Scale, 302
Alzheimer's Disease Research Centers, 8, 487
Alzheimer's Family Center, Inc. (California), 251
Alzheimer's Resource Center of New York City, 42
American Association of Homes for the Aged (AAHA),
    45, 256
American Association of Retired Persons (AARP), 28, 154
  long-term care insurance by, 452
  Medicare survey by, 451
  respite care programs of, 154
American Board of Family Practice, 348-349
American Board of Internal Medicine, 349
American Board of Urologic Allied Health Professionals,
    340
American College of Health Care Administrators
    (ACHCA), 353
American Express, 251
American Federation for Aging Research (AFAR), 4, 47,
    491
American Geriatrics Society (AGS), 349
American Health Care Association, 41, 45, 46
  multidisciplinary training by, 331
  peer review by, 394
American Journal of Alzheimer's Care, 4
American Medical Association (AMA)
  certification by, 334
  diagnostic review by, 96
  surrogate decision respect and, 185
American Nurses Association (ANA)
  nurse specialist certification by, 339-340
  professional reviews by, 395
American Psychiatric Association, 7, 12, 39, 60

NOTE: Page numbers appearing in italics are referring to information mentioned in the tables or figures.